Are You Eating Right?

Compare Your Diet to the
to the Official Recommendations
Using the Nutrient Content of 5,000+ Foods

Judi Sakimoto Morrill   David L. Stone   Suzanne Pierce Murphy

Cover by George Willett
Photos by Tuan Pham: San Jose State Univ. students (left to right, from top) Guida Tan, Paul Riccobono, Marlene Anderson, Sidney Mitchell, Lindsay Hyde, Nicholas Hau, Isaac Weintraub, Lara Sumera, Pato Man, Rebecca Fong, Robert Boykin, Tuan Pham, Gina Cozzolino, Joannie Sevilla, Nguyen Vu, Jennifer Lam, Johnross Reyes, Julia Peysakhovich, Yvonne Caprini, Adam Fraser, Benson Ka, Shana Simmons, Nicole Meeks, Jesus Herrera, Rick Reade, Mahshid Barghisavar, Brittain Scott, Jackie Lee, Elisa Coney, Joseph Nakamura, Cynthia Lopez, Katrice Hernandez, Yat Cheung, Debbie Neal, Robert Hart, Alex Casadonte, Theresa Salazar, Marcelo Martinez, Lindsay Leutz, Ngo Chi, Mark Del Rosario, Sterling Scott, Stevie Caceres, Michelle Aurand, Frank De Luna, Christina Dionisio, Darrick Hong, Veronica Navarro, Sabrina Ortega, Nancy Trac, Timmy Leong, Chris Shenkle, Michael Wong, Uy Luong, Lisa Yee, Lester Del Rosario, Bryant Reyes, Marissa DeClercq, Rich Jury, Mariam Etemadi, Joe Anderson, William Lu, Kelly McRitchie, William Chang.
Back cover: Veronica Navarro (top corner), Mariam Etemadi, Robert Hart, Tim Ochinang, Philip Martinez, Heather Molesworth, Thomas Nguyen, Lara Sumera

Copyright © 1992, 1997, 2003 Orange Grove Publishing
ISBN 0-9657951-7-9

Orange Grove Publishing
1239 Bellair Way
Menlo Park, CA 94025-6612
www.orangegrovepub.com

Printed by Entire Printing, Santa Clara, CA

Table of Contents

Additional Information (continued)

Food Composition Table (Nutrient Content of Foods)

Index of Foods in the Food Composition Table

Introduction

Chances are, news articles—or your mother—have made you insecure about your diet. For starters, you may wonder if your diet is deficient in nutrients or excessive in fat. This book will help you evaluate your daily diet by using it to compare what's recommended with what's in the food you eat.

With the constant introduction of new foods and the huge variety—all kinds of spaghetti sauces and salad dressings, chips with less salt, shelves of variously fortified breakfast cereals—you'll use food labels first for nutrition information. We assume they're more current than nutrient databases. You'll use the food composition table for unlabeled food and when the labels don't provide all nutrition information you need.

Such a detailed analysis of your diet may not be necessary. But by doing such an analysis, you can assure yourself that you are, in fact, eating right. Or if you find that your diet can be improved, you'll know where to make the changes.

This book is divided into sections:

- **Dietary Recommendations**: Guidelines put forth by expert committees

- **Assessing Your Diet**: Step-by-step directions

- **Additional Information**: Calculating nutrient content from recipes, etc.

- **Food Composition Table**: Nutrient content of more than 5,000 foods

- **Food Index**: Quickly find a particular food

We hope that after assessing your diet, you'll eat with less worry and more pleasure.

Dietary Recommendations

One goal of a healthy diet is to eat enough; another is to avoid eating too much.

The first goal—to get the nutrients you need—is the simpler one. Scientists know quite a lot about what nutrients we need, their functions, and how much we need. There are, of course, many unanswered questions, but not as many as ads for dietary supplements would have you believe.

The other goal—to avoid unhealthful excesses—is more complex. The main concern is that many of our diets are excessive in calories because we get too little exercise and/or eat too much. We can also get excessive amounts of some vitamins and minerals with all the dietary supplements and fortified foods available today.

What we eat also plays a role in diseases such as heart disease, cancer, and diabetes—diseases which are far more complex than those caused by the lack of a single nutrient. Diets high in animal fat and low in fruits and vegetables, for example, are linked with a higher risk of heart disease and some cancers.

Though it isn't always certain that this is a cause-and-effect link, most of us have much to gain from following the advice to eat less animal fat and more fruits and vegetables. Such advice is the basis of the prudent diet—there are good reasons to believe that following the advice is healthful, and there are few, if any, reasons to believe it's harmful.

Meeting Nutrient Needs

Recommended Dietary Allowances (RDAs)

Dietary Reference Intakes (DRIs) are levels of nutrients used to plan and assess diets. For our purpose here, the most useful DRI is the Recommended Dietary Allowance (RDA) —the amount that should meet our needs, yet not be so much as to risk toxicity. We'll also use the DRI called the Tolerable Upper Intake Level (UL)—the highest daily amount at which adverse effects are unlikely.

The Food and Nutrition Board of the Institute of Medicine sets the DRIs. The National Academy Press publishes them as reports that include the scientific basis of the DRIs. These reports can be read—or purchased—online (www.nap.edu).

- **RDAs are for daily averages**, since diets vary from day to day. You aren't expected to get the recommended amounts every single day. Practically speaking, your average nutrient intake, over several days, should meet the RDA.

- **RDAs are generous**. They allow for such things as individual variations in need, amounts lost in food preparation, and how efficiently the nutrients are absorbed into the body. RDAs also provide for reserves in the body.

- **RDAs are for healthy people**. If you have a long-term illness, they may not apply to you.

- **There are many sets of the RDAs,** differing by age, sex, and whether a woman is pregnant or nursing.

Daily Values

In 1973, the Food and Drug Administration created standards for the nutrient labeling of foods. These standards are called Daily Values on food labels.

Why Daily Values are needed:

- Nutrients are measured in metric units (grams, milligrams, micrograms), which are unfamiliar to most U.S. consumers.

- If told how much of the nutrient is in a food, e.g., 1 milligram of zinc, we can't tell if it's a trivial amount or a lot, unless we know the recommended amount.

- It isn't practical to put the many sets of RDAs on a label.

Daily Values as a solution:

- **One Daily Value set was made from several sets of RDAs** by taking the highest RDA from the 1968 edition (the most current at the time) for each nutrient for people 4 years old or older, excluding pregnant or nursing women. This is the set used for most labels.

    There are 3 other sets of Daily Values: for infants up to 12 months old, children under 4 years, and pregnant women. These are for products intended specifically for these groups, e.g., the set for infants is used for labeling baby food.

- **Nutrient content is given as a percentage of the Daily Value**, e.g., the Daily Value for niacin is 20 mg, so a food having 10 mg of niacin is said to have 50% of the Daily Value. This makes the nutrient content easier to understand.

Most of us don't want to—and shouldn't have to—add up % Daily Values to be assured of getting enough of each nutrient. A **Guide to Daily Food Choices** (see opposite page) was set up by the U.S. Department of Agriculture to help us select a good diet.

- **We're advised to eat a certain number of servings per day from 5 food groups**, shown graphically as the **Food Guide Pyramid** (see below), with the most servings coming from the Grain Group, and the least from foods high in fat and/or sugar, shown as the small section at the tip of the pyramid.

- **Each food group is particularly rich in certain nutrients,** e.g., foods in the Milk Group are generally good sources of calcium, riboflavin, and high-quality protein.

- The idea is that if you include the advised number of servings from each food group and eat a variety of foods, it's likely that you're meeting your nutrient needs.

- **Serving sizes are made to be equivalent in terms of certain nutrients,** e.g., 1 serving in the Milk Group is an amount that has about 300 mg of calcium: 1 cup of milk or 1½ oz of cheddar cheese or 2 cups of cottage cheese.

Servings are called *portions* in the Guide on the opposite page, because the amounts aren't always realistic servings, e.g., most of us don't think of 2 cups of cottage cheese as one serving.

- **Try to average— over several days —the advised portions per day**.

- **The key is to eat a lot of plant foods, and get your nutrients from a variety of healthful foods.**

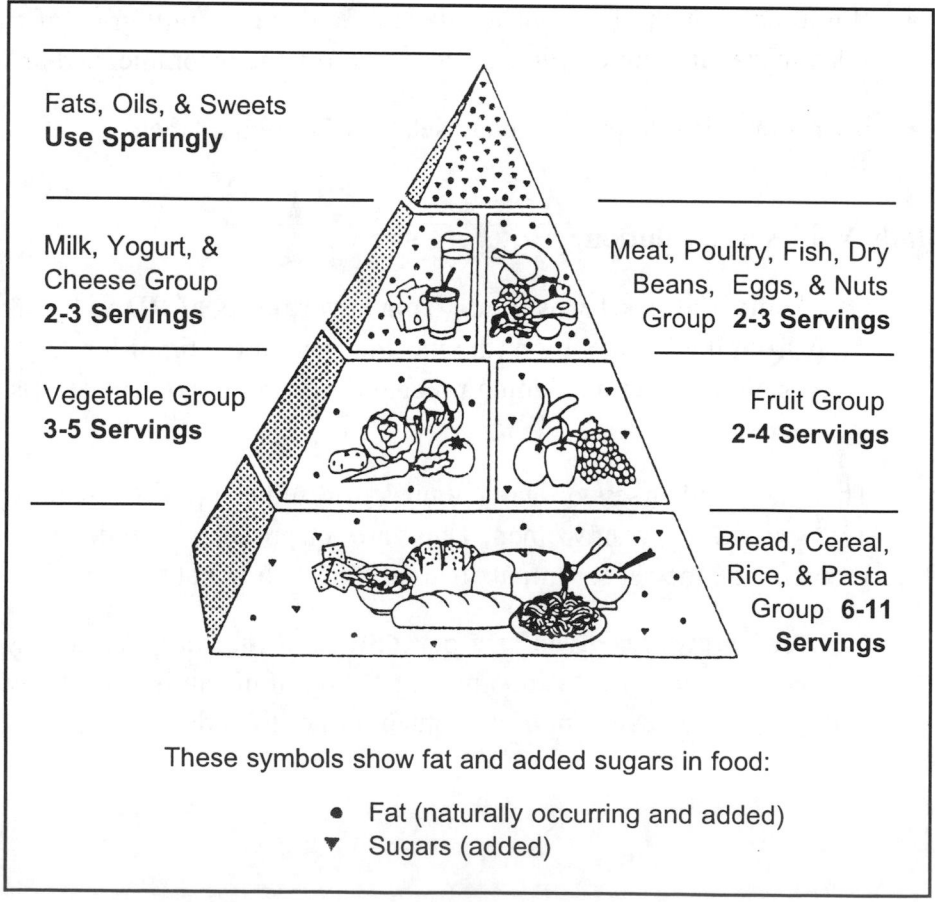

Fats, Oils, & Sweets
Use Sparingly

Milk, Yogurt, & Cheese Group
2-3 Servings

Meat, Poultry, Fish, Dry Beans, Eggs, & Nuts Group **2-3 Servings**

Vegetable Group
3-5 Servings

Fruit Group
2-4 Servings

Bread, Cereal, Rice, & Pasta Group **6-11 Servings**

These symbols show fat and added sugars in food:

- Fat (naturally occurring and added)
▼ Sugars (added)

Guide to Daily Food Choices

- **Grain Group: 6 or more portions for adolescents and adults**; 6 or more smaller portions for children; 7 or more portions for pregnant or nursing women. Emphasize whole grains.

  1 portion = 1 small pancake, slice of bread, tortilla; half a hamburger or hot dog bun; half a bagel or English muffin; 5 saltine crackers; 4 graham crackers; 1 oz dry cereal (= 1 C* cornflakes, $\frac{2}{3}$ C shredded wheat; $\frac{1}{4}$ C Grape Nuts); $\frac{1}{2}$ C cooked rice, pasta, cereal, grits.

- **Vegetable Group: 3 or more portions for adolescents and adults**; 3 or more smaller portions for children; 4 or more portions for pregnant or nursing women (see below for portion sizes).

- **Fruit Group: 2 or more portions for adolescents and adults**: 2 or more smaller portions for children; 3 or more portions for pregnant or nursing women.

  1 portion = 1 medium fruit or vegetable (apple, carrot, banana, potato, etc.); 1 C raw, leafy green vegetable (e.g., lettuce); $\frac{1}{2}$ C fruit or other vegetable (broccoli, canned peaches, cooked spinach, etc.); $\frac{3}{4}$ C (6 fl oz)* fruit or vegetable juice (for fruit drinks, use amount of fruit juice in the drink, as stated on label, e.g., 10% fruit juice). ($\frac{1}{2}$ C beans or peas counts as 1 portion in the vegetable group or $\frac{1}{2}$ portion in the meat group.)

  Include 1 portion of a fruit or vegetable rich in vitamin C (orange, grapefruit, strawberries, green pepper, broccoli, etc.) and 1 portion of a carotene-rich (dark green or orange-colored) fruit or vegetable (carrot, spinach, pumpkin, broccoli, apricot, cantaloupe, etc.; the orange in orange juice isn't carotene).

- **Milk Group: 2 portions for adults age 19-50** and children ages 1 to 10; **3 portions for ages 11-18 and over 50** and women who are pregnant or nursing.

  1 portion = 1 C milk, yogurt, pudding, custard; $1\frac{1}{2}$ C ice cream, ice milk, frozen yogurt; 2 C cottage cheese; $\frac{1}{4}$ C parmesan cheese; $1\frac{1}{2}$ oz (1 oz = 1″ cube) regular cheese (cheddar, swiss, etc.); 2 oz processed cheese (e.g., Velveeta). Cream cheese doesn't count here; it's more like butter.

- **Meat or Meat-substitute Group: 2 portions for adolescents and adults**; 2 smaller portions for children; 3 portions for pregnant or nursing women.

  1 portion = 2 to 3 oz† cooked poultry, fish, meat; 2 frankfurters; 2 eggs; 1 C peas, beans, lentils, soybean curd (tofu); $\frac{1}{2}$ C nuts, sunflower seeds; $\frac{1}{4}$ C (4 Tbs)* peanut butter.

---

* 1 C (cup) = 16 Tbs (tablespoons); fl oz = fluid ounce; a **12 fl oz can of soda, beer = $1\frac{1}{2}$ C.**

† 3 oz lean, cooked poultry, fish, meat is about the size of a deck of cards; a "regular slice" of pre-sliced luncheon meats like bologna = 0.8 oz.

Maintaining Good Health

There's a lot of scientific evidence that one's diet can affect the risk of such diseases as heart disease, chronic liver disease, and cancer of the stomach, colon, breast, lung, and esophagus. The American Heart Association, American Cancer Society, and various government committees evaluating the scientific evidence all give similar dietary advice.

We're bombarded with advice from many sources, such as advertisements, diet and health books, websites, and sports and fitness magazines, not all of which are based on scientific evidence. Often, the advice is tied in with products to sell. This—together with a steady stream of news reports of studies that sometimes seem in conflict—can leave us bewildered. What dietary advice can science give us so far?

The Dietary Guidelines Advisory Committee (made up of our top experts), established by the U.S. Department of Agriculture and U.S. Department of Health and Human Services, recommends a set of *Dietary Guidelines for Americans* (www.health.gov/dietaryguidelines) for ages 2 years and up. First published in 1980, it's revised every 5 years to reflect new scientific knowledge. On the opposite page, the guidelines are in bold print, followed by a brief explanation.

Dietary Guidelines for Americans

Aim for Fitness...

- **Aim for a healthy weight.** If you're at a healthy weight, aim to avoid weight gain. If overweight, first aim to prevent gaining more, and then lose weight to improve your health.

- **Be physically active each day.** Get at least 30 minutes (adults) or 60 minutes (children) of moderate physical activity most, preferably all, days of the week.

Build a Healthy Base...

- **Let the Pyramid guide your food choices.** See pages 4-5.

- **Choose a variety of grains daily, especially whole grains.** Whole grains (e.g., whole wheat, brown rice, oats, and whole grain corn) differ from refined grains in the amount of fiber and nutrients they provide.

- **Choose a variety of fruits and vegetables daily.** These are rich in vitamins, minerals, fiber, and a variety of substances that lower the risk of heart disease and some cancers. They also tend to be low in fat.

- **Keep food safe to eat.** Keep and prepare foods safely in the home; be alert when eating out.

Choose Sensibly...

- **Choose a diet that is low in saturated fat and cholesterol and moderate in total fat.** Aim for less than 10% of total calories from saturated fat, no more than 30% from total fat, and an average of less than 300 mg cholesterol per day.

- **Choose beverages and foods to moderate your intake of sugars.** Sugars provide a concentrated source of calories without otherwise contributing to nutrient intake. Sugars also contribute to tooth decay.

- **Choose and prepare foods with less salt.** Most of us eat more salt (sodium chloride) than we need; excessive amounts may lead to high blood pressure in some of us.

- **If you drink alcoholic beverages, do so in moderation.** Excessive alcohol raises the risk of several diseases such as cirrhosis of the liver. Women who are pregnant or trying to conceive shouldn't drink any alcohol; alcohol can damage the unborn child.

  Moderate drinking = no more than 1 drink/day for women; no more than 2 for men.
  One drink = about ½ oz pure alcohol, e.g., a 12-oz bottle of beer or wine cooler, 5 oz wine,
         1 jigger (1½ oz) vodka, rum, whisky, or gin.

Healthy Weight

To help judge if your weight is "healthy:"

- **Is your weight** (without clothes) **within the range suggested for your height** (without shoes)?*

  A range in weight for a given height allows for different amounts of muscle and bone (e.g., larger or smaller frame). Men have more muscle and bone, so the upper end of a range generally applies to men, and the lower end to women.

  Some of us are overweight without being overfat (e.g., some athletes), but most of us who are overweight are overfat.

  Weighing just under the range may be healthy for some people, but unintentional weight loss can be an early sign of a health problem.

- **Is your waist smaller or no bigger than your hips**? You don't need a measuring tape to do this; a belt, string, or ribbon will do.

  Measure your waist near your navel while standing relaxed (don't pull in your stomach). Measure your hips where they're biggest, over your buttocks.

  A bigger waist than hips suggests excess abdominal fat (*a big belly*), a bigger health risk than excess fat on the hips and thighs. It's linked to high blood pressure, diabetes, early heart disease, and some cancers. Smoking and excessive alcohol tend to put on abdominal fat; vigorous exercise tends to reduce it.

- If your weight is within the suggested range, your waist isn't bigger than your hips, you've gained less than 10 pounds since reaching your adult height, and you don't have a health problem for which your doctor advises weight loss or gain, there's no apparent health advantage to changing your weight.

Height	Weight
4'10"	91-119
4'11"	94-124
5'0"	97-128
5'1"	101-132
5'2"	104-137
5'3"	107-141
5'4"	111-146
5'5"	114-150
5'6"	118-155
5'7"	121-160
5'8"	125-164
5'9"	129-169
5'10"	132-174
5'11"	136-179
6'0"	140-184
6'1"	144-189
6'2"	148-195
6'3"	152-200
6'4"	156-205
6'5"	160-211
6'6"	164-216

---

*Scientists often use Body Mass Index (BMI) to assess body weight. BMI puts weight and height into a single number, but doesn't include a waist-hip ratio and isn't intuitive. BMI is body weight (in kilograms) divided by height (in meters) squared. You can calculate your BMI on page 39.

Other Dietary Advice

Several organizations and government agencies give dietary advice, e.g., the American Heart Association (www.americanheart.org) has a set of recommendations, as does the American Cancer Society (www.cancer.org).

It's reassuring that experts from these various groups come up with remarkably similar advice. There can, however, appear to be discrepancies, primarily because the various organizations update their recommendations at different intervals.

The 2000 update of the Dietary Guidelines for Americans (see page 7), for example, advised that no more than 30% of total calories comes from fat. There was some debate in making this recommendation because of growing scientific evidence that a higher fat diet of "healthier fats" can be healthful.

In 2002, the adult Dietary Reference Intake (see page 2) for fat was recommended to be 20-35% of total calories, with an emphasis on "healthier fats." As the body of scientific evidence evolves, so does expert dietary advice.

Eating for Health and Pleasure

- **Use the Dietary Guidelines for Americans when choosing foods in the Food Guide Pyramid.** For example, if you drink nonfat or low-fat (1-2% fat by weight; 25-35% of calories from fat) milk instead of whole milk (3-4% fat by weight; 45-55% of calories from fat), you're following the guideline to choose a diet lower in saturated fat and cholesterol. Nonfat and low-fat milk also have fewer calories, so this choice can help you lose weight if you're overweight (another guideline).

- **Make changes gradually**. It's hard to switch abruptly from whole milk to low-fat or nonfat milk. Switch gradually by combining whole milk and low-fat milk, gradually increasing the proportion of low-fat milk. Then combine low-fat and nonfat milk. Once you make the switch to nonfat, even low-fat milk may taste like cream. Low-fat milk can then substitute for cream in coffee. Start switching from white to whole wheat bread by making sandwiches with a slice of each.

- **Keep in mind that it's the overall diet, not individual foods, that are "good" or "bad."** Think in terms of being free to eat anything you want—just make a habit of eating foods like candy, hot dogs, and potato chips in smaller amounts or not as often.

- **Eating for health and eating for pleasure can be the same!** Eating is one of life's pleasures, but people often think of healthy food as bland and boring. Many cuisines show us otherwise. What could be less boring, yet so in keeping with dietary guidelines, than a soft taco or burrito topped with a hearty portion of a zesty salsa of red tomatoes, purple onions, bright green cilantro, chili peppers, lime juice, and a dash of olive oil and salt?

Assessing Your Diet

The Plan

- **Record everything you eat and drink for 24 hours** on a typical day. A 3-day record is more accurate, but this can be too tedious for a "first-timer." If needed, make changes afterwards to reflect a more typical day.

- **Categorize the foods you eat by food group, and evaluate your diet using the Guide to Daily Food Choices**. Generally speaking, if you meet the recommendations of this guide, your diet is adequate in nutrients.

- **Do a detailed analysis of your diet** by tabulating the amounts of the various nutrients in your diet, first using label information and then the Food Composition Table.

- **Compare your nutrient intake with the recommended amounts.**

- **See how your diet compares to the Dietary Guidelines.** Determine what changes you can make to improve your diet.

Quick Diet Analysis Using the Food Guide Pyramid

- **On Table 1, record everything you eat and drink for 24 hours**, selecting a "typical day." (If needed, make changes afterwards to make it more typical of what you eat.)

Include everything—coffee, tea, added sugar and cream, diet drinks, oil you cook something in, added salt, mayonnaise in sandwiches, catsup on fries, etc.

Be as accurate as you can in recording amounts in ounces, cups, etc.; we tend to underestimate. For perspective, a can of soda is 12 fluid ounces, which is $1\frac{1}{2}$ cups. See page 35 for conversions and abbreviations, e.g., 1 cup = 16 Tbs; 1 oz = 28 grams.

- **Tabulate the number of portions you had in each food group.** See page 5 for portion sizes. Note that a portion isn't necessarily a typical serving size, e.g., 2 cups of cottage cheese = 1 portion; $\frac{1}{2}$ cup cottage cheese = $\frac{1}{4}$ portion in milk group.

Corn can be in grain group (e.g., corn tortilla) or vegetable group (e.g., corn and peas).

If an item (e.g., candy) isn't in a food group, put a checkmark in the *not in a group* column.

- **For each food group, fill in your recommended number of portions** (see page 5).

- **Answer questions at the bottom.** If you answered yes to these and ate a variety of food (examples of "kinds of grains:" wheat, oats, rice, rye, corn), it's likely you met your nutrient needs.

Table 1: Diet Analysis Using the Food Guide Pyramid

Amount	Food	Grain	Veg	Fruit	Milk	Meat	√ if not in a group
12 fl oz	orange juice			2			
1 cup	Cheerios	1					
½ cup	nonfat milk				½		
16 fl oz	coffee						√
1	McDonald's Big Mac	2			½	1½	
21 fl oz	diet Coke						√
1	banana			1			
2	bean-cheese burritos	2			½	1	
1	carrot		1				
1 cup	iceburg lettuce		1				
2 Tbs	Italian dressing						√
1 cup	nonfat milk				1		
6	Oreo cookies						√
Total number of portions for the day		5	2	3	2½	2½	
Sue's recommended portions		6+	3+	2+	2	2	

Did you eat the recommended number of portions from each of the 5 food groups? yes (no)

Did you eat a vitamin C-rich fruit or vegetable? (yes) no

Did you eat a carotene-rich (dark green of orange colored) fruit or vegetable? (yes) no

Variety: # of kinds of: Grain _2_, Fruit _2_, Vegetable _2_, Meat or Meat Substitute _2_

Table 1: Diet Analysis Using the Food Guide Pyramid

Food or Drink Consumed		Number of Portions					√ if not in a group
Amount	Food	Grain	Veg	Fruit	Milk	Meat	
Total number of portions for the day							
Your recommended portions							

Did you eat the recommended number of portions from each of the 5 food groups?   Yes   No

Did you eat a vitamin C-rich fruit or vegetable?   Yes   No

Did you eat a carotene-rich (dark green or orange-colored) fruit or vegetable?   Yes   No

Variety: # of kinds of : Grain _____, Fruit_____, Vegetable_____, Meat or Meat Substitute_____

You can download this table as an Excel file at www.orangegrovepub.com

Nutrition Facts on Food Labels

Required*	Optional**
Calories per Serving	
Calories from Fat	Calories from Saturated Fat
Total Fat	
Saturated Fat	Polyunsaturated Fat
	Monounsaturated Fat
Cholesterol	
Sodium	Potassium
Total Carbohydrate	
Dietary Fiber	Soluble Fiber
	Insoluble Fiber
Sugars	Sugar Alcohol (e.g., sorbitol)
Protein	
Vitamin A	
Vitamin C	
Calcium	
Iron	Other Vitamins and Minerals

*Except for certain foods, e.g., a soft drink label needn't give values for fat. Trans fat will be required starting 1/1/06 and will be listed directly below saturated fat.

**Required if they've been added, or there are claims, e.g., vitamin E must be listed if it's been added to the food, or the package says *High in Vitamin E*. For more information (e.g., what nutrition/health claims can be made on labels), go to the Center for Food Safety and Applied Nutrition website (www.cfsan.fda.gov/label.html).

For a detailed analysis, it's crucial to use food labels, particularly if you eat a lot of packaged food. If you eat at fast-food or restaurant chains, use nutrition information on their websites www.___.com (burgerking, tacobell, jackinthebox, mcdonalds, dominos, wendys, subway, kentuckyfriedchicken, dairyqueen, dennys, roundtable pizza, jambajuice, etc.).

Besides a huge variety of food, there can be big variations in "simple" foods. One brand of corn tortillas can have ten times the amount of calcium as another, depending mostly on whether the corn was processed traditionally with lime (calcium carbonate). Even canned tuna of the same description (e.g., canned in water) can vary a lot, depending on when and where the tuna was caught and how it was processed.

Fortified foods (foods with specific nutrients added) are easily varied. If you regularly eat the same breakfast cereal, you may be surprised to find that the vitamins and minerals added to your cereal have changed—without a change in taste or appearance—since you bought your first box. Sometimes, even, a product's website with nutrition information will say to look on the product's label for more current information.

Changes in labeling regulations can result in changes in food products. January 1, 2006 is the required-on-the-label deadline for trans fat. Foods high in trans fats (e.g., fried foods, crackers, packaged desserts) are being changed. When trans fat is listed, add it to the amount of saturated fat (both have similar health effects) in doing your diet analysis.

If you want to restrict your diet analysis to those nutrients required on the label, the abbreviated form to do this is on page 47. This abbreviated form works well for a class activity where children bring in labels from favorite foods.

Look carefully at your food labels, particularly the serving size. That 99¢, 3.5-oz bag of chips looks like a bag easily eaten all at once. You glance at the label and see 160 calories, so you buy it and eat it. As you hold the empty bag, you notice that a serving is 1 oz (3.5 servings/bag), so you just ate 560 calories, not 160. Oops!

In using label values for your diet analysis, adjust for the amount you ate if it differs from the 1 serving amount. For that bag of chips, multiply all the nutrients listed by 3.5, e.g., (4%DV iron)(3.5)=14%DV iron. When a label gives an amount only as *less than* or *not a significant source of*, use zero for the amount in doing your diet analysis.

Calculate the % calories from fat: (calories from fat X 100)/total calories = %cal fat. Using the label on the opposite page, (30X100)/90 = 33%cal fat. Whether you eat ½ cup or 9 cups, 33% of the calories in this food comes from fat. The %cal fat stays the same for each food.

Label values are useful in many ways. Say you're trying to decide between bags of Jordan almonds (hard-candy coated almonds). You'd like ones with the thinnest candy coating; they look the same size. Does one brand have smaller almonds with a thicker coating? Serving sizes are the same, but one has more protein and fat—the brand with bigger almonds and thinner coating. Which can of stewed tomatoes has more tomatoes? Which peanut butter has more peanuts? Glean answers from your labels.

Nutrition Facts

Serving Size 1/2 cup (114g)
Servings Per Container 4

Amount Per Serving

Calories 90   Calories from Fat 30

% Daily Value*

Total fat 3g	**5**%
Saturated fat 2g	**10**%
Trans Fat 0g	
Polyunsaturated fat 4g	
Cholesterol 0mg	**0**%
Sodium 300mg	**13**%
Total carbohydrate 13g	**4**%
Dietary Fiber 2g	**8**%
Sugars 4g	
Protein 3g	

Vitamin A 80%   •   Vitamin C 50%

Calcium 4%   •   Iron 4%

*Percent Daily Values are based on a 2000 Calorie diet. Your daily values may be higher or lower depending on your Calorie needs:

		Calories	2,000	2,500
Total Fat	Less than		65g	80g
Sat Fat	Less than		20g	25g
Cholesterol	Less than		300mg	300mg
Sodium	Less than		2400mg	2400mg
Total Carbohydrate			300g	475g
Dietary Fiber			25g	30g

Calories per gram:
Fat 9 • Carbohydrate 4 • Protein 4

% Daily Value (DV) shows how a food fits in your overall diet. Some DVs are upper levels (fat: 65 g *or less*); some are recommended amounts (vitamin C: 60 mg).

50% DV of vitamin C means that 1 serving gives you 50% (30 mg) of what you need to get the recommended amount (60 mg).

The general goal is to choose foods that add up to 100% of the DV for total carbohydrate, fiber, vitamins, & minerals, and add up to less than 100% of the DV for fat, saturated fat, cholesterol, & sodium.

Many women, teenage girls, and less active men use about 2,000 calories/ day.

Many men, teenage boys, and very active women use about 2,500 calories/day.

Detailed Diet Analysis

- **Copy your foods and amounts from Table 1** (page 13) **onto Table 2** (pages 20-21). If you filled in Table 1 as an Excel file, use the copy-paste function to transfer info to Table 2.

- **Use labels and websites to fill in as much as you can** of Table 2, adjusting the values to the amount you ate (if 1 serving is 1 cup, and you had 1½ cups, multiply the values by 1.5). If the amount is given as *less than* or *not a significant source of*, use zero. Be sure all units are consistent, e.g., fat in grams, iron as % of Daily Value.

- **Calculate % calories from fat**: (calories from fat X 100)/total calories = %cal fat. If **trans fat** is given, include it in (i.e., add it to) grams saturated fat. **Circle or shade all the values that came from labels and websites** (see example below).

- For nutrients not listed on the label or website, or for unlabeled food (e.g., apple), get the values from the **food composition table**, again adjusting the values to the amount you ate—is your apple or pizza slice much larger or smaller than what's listed?

- If the food you ate isn't in the food composition table, find the closest match (foods are listed by category and also in the index). If the food is a mixed food, e.g., ham sandwich, it's more accurate to list the parts separately (bread, ham, mustard, etc.) vs. using the values for a "generic" ham sandwich.

- When you use values from the food composition table, put the food number of the food you used in the *food no.* column. Fill in the amount for every nutrient—no blanks.

Table 2: Detailed Diet Analysis

Food No.	Food Amount & Description	wt gm	wt oz	cal	% cal fat	prot gm	carbo gm	fiber gm
125	12 fl oz orange juice, from concentrate	374	13.2	165	1%	3	40	0
3566	1 cup Cheerios	30	1.1	110	14%	3	22	3
557	1½ cup nonfat milk	368	12.9	135	5%	15	20	0
293	16 fl oz cup coffee, black	474	17	10	0%	0	2	0.0
7634	1 McDonald's Big Mac	215	7.6	580	51%	24	47	3
206	21 fl. oz (medium) diet Coke	621	22	0	0%	0	0	0
2031	1 banana	114	4.0	105	5%	1	27	2.7
7723	2 frozen bean-cheese burritos	226	8.0	460	27%	16	70	6
2437	1 carrot	50	1.8	21	4%	1	5	1.5
2537	1 cup iceburg lettuce	55	1.9	7	14%	1	1	0.8
5527	2 Tbs Italian dressing	29.0	1.0	80	88%	0	3	0
1221	6 Oreo reduced-fat cookies	66	2.3	280	23%	4	52	2
	Total from food:			1953		68	289	19
	Total from supplements: Daily Vitamin			0		0	0	0
	Total from food and supplements:			1953		68	289	19
	Recommended amount *(Sue: 120 lb, age 20)*:					43		25

- **List any supplements separately** where indicated on Table 2. Nutrient content is on the label. If you take prenatal supplements, adjust the % Daily Value on the label (see how on page 37); they're based on values specified for pregnant women.

- **Fill in your recommended amounts** as given on page 22 (see below for protein).

- **Calculate and fill in** (on Table 2) **your recommended protein intake.**

  Recommendations are based on age and normal body weight.

  If overweight, use a weight at the high end of the range given for your height on page 8.
  If pregnant or nursing, use your pre-pregnancy weight. During the 2nd half of your pregnancy and while nursing add 25 grams protein to your recommended amount.

Grams protein recommended = body weight X gm/lb (see table just below):

```
┌──────────────┐
│              │  actual or adjusted body weight
└──────────────┘

    ┌──────────────┐
X   │              │  gm/lb
    └──────────────┘
   ─────────────────

    ┌──────────────┐
=   │              │  grams protein recommended
    └──────────────┘
```

Age-years	gm/lb
19 and up	0.36
14-18	0.39
4-13	0.43

Food No.	fat gm	sat fat gm*	choles mg	sodium mg	potas mg	vit A	vit E	vit C	thia	ribo	niac	vit B6	fola	vit B12	calc	phos	mag	iron	zinc
						**% of Daily Value**													
125	0	0	0	22	675	0	1	180	15	4	3	6	22	0	3	6	9	0	2
3566	2	0	0	280	95	10	1	10	25	25	25	25	50	25	10	10	10	45	25
557	0	0	0	210	609	15	0	3	9	30	2	8	4	22	52	38	10	0	10
293	0	0	0	10	256	0	0	0	0	0	6	0	0	0	0	0	6	2	0
7634	33	11	85	1050	420	6	9	4	27	30	38	18	28	45	35	25	11	25	37
206	0	0	0	40	49	0	0	0	2	9	0	0	0	0	0	4	2	0	4
2031	1	0	0	1	451	1	1	17	3	7	3	33	5	0	1	2	8	2	1
7723	14	4	10	920	605	4	6	4	34	27	14	11	56	6	16	51	21	30	21
2437	0	0	0	17	161	140	1	8	3	2	4	2	0	1	2	2	1	1
2537	0	0	0	5	87	2	1	4	2	1	1	1	8	0	1	1	1	2	1
5527	8	1	0	490	4	0	10	2	0	0	0	0	0	1	0	0	0	0	0
1221	7	2	0	400	132	0	3	0	12	9	9	0	9	0	0	12	6	20	3
	65	18	95	3445	3544	178	33	232	132	144	103	106	184	99	119	151	86	127	105
	0	0	0	0	0	100	100	100	100	100	100	100	100	100	0	0	0	0	0
	65	18	95	3445	3544	278	133	332	232	244	203	206	284	199	119	151	86	127	105
			Less than 300	500-2400	3500	70	68	125	73	65	70	65	100	40	100	70	78	100	53

*Include trans fat when on label.

Table 2: Detailed Diet Analysis

Food No.	Food Amount & Description	wt gm	wt oz	calories	% cal fat	prot gm	carbo gm	fiber gm
	Total from food:							
	Total from supplements:							
	Total from food and supplements:							
	Recommended amounts:							

You can download this table as an Excel
file at www.orangegrovepub.com

Food No.	fat gm	sat fat gm*	choles mg	sodium mg	potas mg	vit A	vit E	vit C	thia	ribo	niac	vit B6	fola	vit B12	calc	phos	mag	iron	zinc
			Less than 300																

% of Daily Value

*If trans fat is given on the label, include it
in (add it to) the amount of saturated fat.

-21-

Your Recommended Amounts of Nutrients

As in the food composition table, fiber, sodium, and potassium are given by weight, and the other nutrients that follow are given as % Daily Values. These percentages reflect the recommended amounts for your particular age-and-sex group, as specified by a committee of the National Academy of Sciences. For adults who aren't pregnant or nursing, the committee recommends the range shown for sodium, and an intake of potassium that meets or exceeds the given amount (amounts for children and pregnant or nursing women are extrapolated values).

Example: Sue, age 20, wants to know how the % Daily Value for magnesium applies to her. The table below shows, for females ages 19-30, the number **78** in the magnesium (mag) column. Her recommended amount is 310 mg; the Daily Value is 400 mg. This makes **78** the recommended % Daily Value for magnesium for women ages 19-30 (310 mg is 78% of 400 mg). If Sue gets 78% of the Daily Value for magnesium, she gets the recommended amount.

Age (years)	fiber gm	sodium mg	potassium mg	vit A	vit E	vit C*	thia	ribo	niac	vit B6	fola	vit B12	calc	phos	mag	iron	zinc
									% of Daily Value								
Child 4-8	25	300-1400	2400	40	32	42	40	35	40	30	50	20	80	50	33	56	33
Male																	
9-13	31	400-1900	2800	60	50	75	60	53	60	50	75	30	130	125	60	44	53
14-18	38	500-2400	3500	90	68	125	80	76	80	65	100	40	130	125	103	61	73
19-30	38	500-2400	3500	90	68	150	80	76	80	65	100	40	100	70	100	44	73
31-50	38	500-2400	3500	90	68	150	80	76	80	65	100	40	100	70	105	44	73
51-70	30	500-2400	3500	90	68	150	80	76	80	85	100	40	120	70	105	44	73
71+	30	500-2400	3500	90	68	150	80	76	80	85	100	40	120	70	105	44	73
Female																	
9-13	26	400-1900	2800	70	50	75	60	53	60	50	75	30	130	125	60	44	53
14-18	36	500-2400	3500	70	68	108	67	59	70	60	100	40	130	125	90	83	60
19-30	25	500-2400	3500	70	68	125	73	65	70	65	100	40	100	70	78	100	53
31-50	25	500-2400	3500	70	68	125	73	65	70	65	100	40	100	70	80	100	53
51-70	21	500-2400	3500	70	68	125	73	65	70	75	100	40	120	70	80	44	53
71+	21	500-2400	3500	70	68	125	73	65	70	75	100	40	120	70	80	44	53
Pregnant																	
age <18	28	600-2400	3500	75	68	133	93	82	90	95	150	43	130	125	100	150	87
age 19-30	28	600-2400	3500	77	68	142	93	82	90	95	150	43	100	70	88	150	73
age 31-50	28	600-2400	3500	77	68	142	93	82	90	95	150	43	100	70	90	150	73
Nursing																	
age <18	29	700-2400	3500	120	86	192	93	82	85	100	125	47	130	125	90	56	93
age 19-30	29	700-2400	3500	130	86	200	93	94	85	100	125	47	100	70	78	50	80
age 31-50	29	700-2400	3500	130	86	200	93	82	85	100	125	47	100	70	80	50	80

*If you smoke, add 58 (% Daily Value) to your recommended amount of vitamin C.

Comparing Your Diet to the Recommendations

- **CALORIES:** Your body weight indicates whether the calories you use are in balance with what you eat. Your food intake as recorded on Table 2 is probably less than usual. We tend to underestimate how much we eat and overestimate how active we are. Also, when we record what we eat, we tend to eat less. Calculate your calorie needs on p. 42.

✎ What's your Baseline [calorie] Requirement (excludes physical activity)? ☐
If you don't have more calories than this on Table 2, add more food to Table 2 for a more realistic assessment of your diet.

✎ What's your Daily [calorie] Use (includes physical activity)? ☐

✎ On page 8, is your weight within the range for your height? ☐ Is your waist-to-hip ratio okay? ☐ On page 39, is your BMI at a healthy weight? ☐

✎ If not, what changes in your diet and/or physical activity could you make? Be realistic!

☐

If you need to lose weight, be more active and/or eat less. As you lose weight, you tend to lose muscle as well as fat. By being more active you use more calories, don't have to cut back on food calories as much, and lose less muscle as you lose weight.

Being more active doesn't mean you have to "work out." Use stairs instead of elevators at work or school, meet your friends for a walk instead of coffee. Modest changes are more likely to be long-lasting. Most of the health benefits of physical activity occurs in going from "lightly active" to "moderately active."

Unless under medical supervision, avoid weight-loss diets with calorie counts lower than your baseline requirement (page 42). Losing ½ to 1 pound per week is reasonable. This loss is slow (the same way you gained it), but you're less likely to regain the weight.

- **ALCOHOL:** If you drink alcoholic beverages, do so in moderation. Women who are pregnant or trying to conceive shouldn't drink any alcohol. Alcohol can damage the fetus.

Moderate drinking = no more than 1 drink/day for women; no more than 2 for men.
One drink = about ½ oz pure alcohol, e.g., a 12-oz can or bottle of beer or wine cooler,
5 oz table wine, 1 jigger (1½ oz) vodka, rum, whisky, or gin.

✎ You drink: ☐ not at all ☐ moderately ☐ more than moderately

If you had alcohol on this day, adjust your total calories on Table 2 to exclude calories from alcohol (as shown below). Use this adjusted total calories to calculate the % of calories in your diet that come from protein, carbohydrate, sugar, fat, and saturated fat.

Alcohol content is given in the food composition table as part of the description of the beverage, and is given in grams. There are 7 calories in a gram of alcohol.

✎ Add up the number of grams of alcohol you drank, and multiply the total grams by 7 to get the number of calories that came from alcohol:

Your Calories From Alcohol =

Grams of alcohol you drank ☐ **X 7** cal/gm = ☐

Your Alcohol-adjusted Calorie Intake =

☐ − ☐ = ☐

Total calories   **Calories**   **Alcohol-adjusted**
(from table 2)   from alcohol   **calories**

- **PROTEIN:** Your diet should have the recommended amount (see p. 19), but if you wish to eat more, it's recommended your protein intake not exceed 35% of your total calories.

✏ Do you eat at least the recommended grams of protein? [   ]

✏ Calculate your % of calories from protein, using your *total grams of protein* and *total calories* from Table 2 (or *alcohol-adjusted calories* from page 24):

$$\frac{\boxed{}\ \textbf{X 4}\ \text{calories/gm}}{\boxed{}}\ \textbf{X 100} = \boxed{}\ \textbf{\% of calories from protein}$$

gms protein

total calories

✏ Does less than 35% of your calories come from protein? [   ]

✏ If needed, how can you adjust your diet to bring your protein intake to the recommended level, e.g., what foods would you substitute?

[   ]

Chronically excessive protein intake has been shown to cause kidney damage in some animal studies. It's uncertain whether this is a cause for concern in humans. Some athletes and others take huge doses of amino acid and/or protein supplements over many years. Long-term effects, if any, aren't known.

Protein is absorbed from the intestine as amino acids. When you get more than you need, the extra amino acids aren't stored in the body: the amino part comes off and forms urea, which is excreted in the urine; the calorie-containing part can be converted to carbohydrate or burned for energy. Excretion of urea uses water (we urinate more). It follows that we're thirstier when we consume a lot of protein or amino acid supplements.

- **CARBOHYDRATE:** We're advised to eat a variety of grains (especially whole grains), vegetables, and fruits, with at least 45% of total calories from carbohydrate. Limit <u>added</u> sugar (excludes sugar that's naturally in foods like fruit)—they add empty calories.

🖊 Calculate your % of calories from carbohydrate, using your *total grams of carbohydrate* and *total calories* from Table 2 (or *alcohol-adjusted calories* from page 24):

gms carbohydrate

$$\frac{\boxed{} \textbf{ X 4 } \text{calories/gm}}{\boxed{}} \textbf{ X 100 } = \boxed{} \textbf{ \% of calories from carbohydrate}$$

total calories

🖊 Does at least 45% of your calories come from carbohydrate? $\boxed{}$

🖊 Estimate your grams of added sugar on Table 2; sugared breakfast cereals list gm sugars. Assume all the carbohydrate in soft drinks and candy is sugar. For unfrosted cake and cookies, figure half the carbohydrate is sugar. Make it 2/3 of carbohydrate from sugar in cake and cookies with icing. Calculate your % of calories from added sugar:

gms added sugar

$$\frac{\boxed{} \textbf{ X 4 } \text{calories/gm}}{\boxed{}} \textbf{ X 100 } = \boxed{} \textbf{ \% of calories from added sugar}$$

total calories

🖊 Does less than 10% of your calories come from added sugar? $\boxed{}$

🖊 If needed, what changes might you make in the carbohydrates in your diet?

- **FIBER:** There are many kinds of dietary fiber, and they're found in plants. The typical American diet is low in fiber, and we're advised to choose a diet with plenty of whole grains, vegetables, and fruits. This not only gives us more fiber, but more carbohydrates, vitamins, and minerals.

✎ Did you eat the recommended amount of fiber?

✎ Did the fiber come mainly from a variety of vegetables, fruits, and grain products (rather than from fiber-fortified breakfast cereal, for example)?

✎ If needed, what changes might you make to increase and/or vary your sources of fiber? Look down the column for fiber in the food composition table for ideas.

A low-fiber diet raises the risk of constipation and diverticulosis (outpouchings in the colon wall). But don't go to extremes in consuming fiber-fortified foods or fiber supplements, as this can hamper absorption of minerals. As usual, moderation makes good sense.

- **FAT:** Fat contains essential nutrients but is also a concentrated source of calories. We're advised to get 20-35% of our calories from fat.

✐ Where does most of the fat in your diet come from (see the fat/gm column in Table 2)?

[ ]

✐ Calculate your % of calories from fat, using your *total grams of fat* and *total calories* from Table 2 (or *alcohol-adjusted calories* from page 24):

$$\frac{\boxed{} \text{ gms fat} \quad \textbf{X 9} \text{ calories/gm}}{\boxed{} \text{ total calories}} \quad \textbf{X 100} = \boxed{} \text{ \% of calories from fat}$$

✐ Does 20-35% of your calories come from fat? [ ]

✐ If not, what are practical changes that you can make?

[ ]

Saturated fat (and trans fat) is solid at room temperature; unsaturated fat is liquid. Food fat is a mix of saturated, monounsaturated, and polyunsaturated fats. Whether a fat is solid or liquid depends on which predominates: butter (solid) is mostly saturated, corn oil (liquid) mostly polyunsaturated, olive oil (liquid, but thicker than corn oil) mostly monounsaturated.

- **SATURATED FAT** (and trans fat, found mainly in partially hydrogenated fat) raises blood-cholesterol, thereby raising the risk of heart disease. We're advised to minimize the saturated and trans fat in our diet (grams trans fat, when given, should be added to grams saturated fat on Table 2). Neither is a required nutrient.

✎ Where does most of the saturated fat in your diet come from?

```
┌─────────────────────────────────────────────────────┐
│                                                     │
│                                                     │
│                                                     │
│                                                     │
└─────────────────────────────────────────────────────┘
```

✎ Calculate your % of calories from saturated fat, using your *total grams of saturated fat* and *total calories* from Table 2 (or *alcohol-adjusted calories* from page 24):

gms saturated fat

$$\frac{\boxed{} \textbf{ X 9} \text{ calories/gm}}{\boxed{}} \textbf{ X 100 } = \boxed{} \textbf{ \% of calories from saturated fat}$$

total calories

✎ Does less than 10% of your calories come from saturated fat? ☐

✎ Even if it's less than 10%, what changes might you make to eat less saturated fat?

```
┌─────────────────────────────────────────────────────┐
│                                                     │
│                                                     │
│                                                     │
│                                                     │
│                                                     │
│                                                     │
│                                                     │
│                                                     │
│                                                     │
└─────────────────────────────────────────────────────┘
```

- **CHOLESTEROL** is found only in animal foods (not in plants) and isn't required in our diet. Dietary cholesterol can raise blood-cholesterol, so we're advised to minimize our intake.

✒ Is your cholesterol intake less than 300 mg for this day? ☐

✒ Where does most of the cholesterol in your diet come from?

☐

✒ Would you say that your cholesterol intake averages less than 300 mg per day? ☐

✒ Even if you average less than 300 mg, what changes can you make to eat less cholesterol?

☐

Cholesterol in the diet doesn't raise blood-cholesterol as much as saturated fat does. So it's misleading (and illegal) to label a product *cholesterol-free* when it's high in saturated fat.

The amounts of fat, saturated fat, and cholesterol in food aren't proportional, e.g., salad oil is 100% fat—very high in fat—but low in saturated fat, and has no cholesterol; shrimp is low in fat but rich in cholesterol. Look through the food composition table to see for yourself.

Since most of the cholesterol in a typical American diet comes from egg yolks, we're advised to limit egg yolks to 3 or 4 per week (there's no fat or cholesterol in egg whites).

- **SODIUM** is a required nutrient, but is excessive in the typical American diet. Most of it comes from salt (sodium chloride) in fast food and processed foods such as potato chips, olives, cold cuts, bacon, frankfurters, crackers, and frozen dinners.

  Excessive amounts of salt can raise the risk of high blood pressure in people who are genetically salt-sensitive. But most people eating a high-salt diet don't develop high blood pressure as a result. High blood pressure is more likely when a high-salt diet is low in potassium and calcium. There's no known advantage to a high-salt diet and it's not known beforehand who's salt-sensitive, so we're advised to keep sodium intake to an adequate but not excessive amount.

Which foods in Table 2 are the highest in sodium?

Is your sodium intake within the recommended range?

If not, what changes do you suggest?

- **POTASSIUM** is often low in the typical American diet. Vegetables and fruits are good sources. Those who eat a lot of vegetables and fruits are eating a diet rich in potassium, a diet linked to a lower risk of high blood pressure and stroke. Your diet should have the recommended amount or more.

Does your diet have at least the recommended amount of potassium?

If not, what changes do you suggest?

- **VITAMINS and MINERALS from FOOD** (vitamins and minerals from supplements will be considered separately)

Check it off if your diet has the recommended amount:

❑ Vitamin A	❑ Niacin	❑ Phosphorus
❑ Vitamin E	❑ Vitamin B_6	❑ Magnesium
❑ Vitamin C	❑ Folate	❑ Iron
❑ Thiamin	❑ Vitamin B_{12}	❑ Zinc
❑ Riboflavin	❑ Calcium	

If your **Vitamin A from food** looks extremely high, don't be concerned if most of it came from fruits and vegetables. Vitamin A can be very toxic in big doses, but the vitamin A values given for fruits and vegetables actually represent their carotene content. Vitamin A itself is not found in plants.

Carotene is the most common of about 20 yellow-to-deep-red plant pigments that can be converted to vitamin A in the body. But unlike vitamin A, large amounts aren't toxic. People who drink a lot of carrot juice, for example, get a lot of carotene, an excess that isn't converted to vitamin A. It's stored in body fat, e.g., in the fat layer under the skin, so the skin of those who drink a lot of carrot juice can have a distinct carrot-colored tone.

In the Guide to Daily Food Choices, we're advised to eat a lot of plant foods and to include one portion of a dark green or orange-colored fruit or vegetable each day. (In dark green vegetables, the color of carotene is masked by the dark green color of chlorophyll.) This provides us with carotene as well as other carotene-like substances.

Carotene is also found in some animal foods. Cows and chickens, for example, eat carotene-containing plants, which give a yellow-orange color to butter, egg yolks, and chicken skin. Carotene is added to margarine to give it the color of butter (margarine would otherwise be white).

If your **niacin** is a little low, you needn't be concerned if you meet your RDA for protein. This is because the body can make niacin from tryptophan, an amino acid in protein.

Vitamin B_{12} isn't found in plant foods. Strict vegetarians should get vitamin B_{12} as a supplement or in such foods as fortified cereals. So should people over age 50, since many older people don't absorb B_{12} from food as well.

There are other required nutrients not covered here, mainly because the amounts in many foods haven't been measured. But if you get enough of the nutrients given in Table 2 from a variety of food, you can be quite certain that your diet is nutritionally adequate.

✎ If you didn't meet all the vitamin/mineral recommendations, what foods might **you** eat to raise your intake to the advised level of **each** nutrient you're low in (e.g., if you're low in zinc, look down the zinc column in the food composition table for possibilities)?

- **DIETARY SUPPLEMENTS and/or fortified foods***

✎ Were your supplements/fortified foods* appropriate, i.e., gave you enough of what you were lacking, yet not too much more when you already had enough? ☐

✎ Was your intake below the Tolerable Upper Intake Levels**? ☐

Try to get most of your nutrients from the base of the Food Guide Pyramid—a variety of grains, vegetables and fruit. There are many healthful substances, many yet unidentified, in these foods, e.g., cabbage has indoles that may protect against cancer.

*Even if you don't take supplements, per se, you may be taking them in fortified cereal, fruit drinks, etc. For example, fiber and 100% of the Daily Value of vitamins and minerals are added to many breakfast cereals. In some cases, we're advised to get a nutrient in fortified food or a supplement. Folate deficiency during early pregnancy, for example, can increase the risk of certain birth defects, so women of childbearing age are advised to get 400 mg of folate (folic acid) in a fortified food or supplement. By law, folate is added to refined grains such as white flour, so all foods made from them (bread, cookies, etc.) have added folate.

**See page 38. These are amounts above which there's a potential risk of adverse effects.

SUMMARY: Give an overview and summary of your diet analysis, including discussion of this day's diet as compared to your usual diet.

In an overview, we see that improving the diet in one nutrient also improves the diet in other ways. For instance, you may have suggested eating more vegetables, fruit, and grain in several of the answer boxes that ask for ways to improve your intake of a specific nutrient. By eating more of these plant foods, you get more fiber, vitamins, and minerals, including potassium. Also, these foods tend to be bulky and relatively low in fat and calories—you don't have as much room for extras, making it easier to keep off excess weight.

Even by doing this analysis just once, you may have learned enough so you don't need to do it again. For a while, you can assess your weak spots (e.g., your calcium and fiber intake). After that, your improved nutrition consciousness may be enough to keep you on track.

Once you assure yourself that you're eating right, you're less vulnerable to the steady bombardment of diet-related ads, news reports, etc., that may have caused you anxiety. Also, knowing that your basic diet is good, there's no conflict in eating the likes of an occasional hot fudge sundae. You can eat with less worry and more pleasure.

Additional Information

Conversion Factors and Abbreviations

Weight

1 pound (lb) = 454 grams (gm)

1 pound (lb) = 16 ounces (oz)

1 ounce (oz) = 28 grams (gm)

100 grams (gm) = 3.5 ounces (oz)

1 kilogram (kg) = 2.2 pounds (lb)

1 kilogram (kg) = 1,000 grams (gm)

1 gm = 1,000 milligrams (mg)

1 mg = 1,000 micrograms (μ or mcg)

Volume

1 gallon (gal) = 4 quarts (qt)

1 quart (qt) = 2 pints = 4 cups (C)

1 cup (C) = 8 fluid ounces (fl oz)

1 cup (C) = 16 tablespoons (Tbs)

1 tablespoon (Tbs) = 3 teaspoons (tsp)

1 quart = 0.9464 liters (l)

1 liter (l) = 1.0567 quarts (qt)

1 liter (l) = 1,000 milliliters (ml)

Calories

Fat = 9 calories per gram (cal/gm)

Alcohol = 7 cal/gm

Carbohydrate = 4 cal/gm

Protein = 4 cal/gm

Length

Diameter = dia

Inch(es) = "

Recommended Intakes, Daily Values, Upper Levels

Recommended Intake/Day

	Female (age)			Male (age)			Daily Value[a]	Upper Level[b]
	14-18	19-50	51+	14-18	19-50	51+		
Fat-soluble vitamins:								
Vitamin A (mcg)[c]	700	700	700	900	900	900	1000	3000
Vitamin E (mg)[c]	15	15	15	15	15	15	22	1000
Water-soluble vitamins:								
Vitamin C (mg)[d]	65	75	75	75	90	90	60	2000
Thiamin (mg)	1.0	1.1	1.1	1.2	1.2	1.2	1.5	e
Riboflavin (mg)	1.0	1.1	1.1	1.3	1.3	1.3	1.7	e
Niacin (mg)	14	14	14	16	16	16	20	35
Vitamin B_6 (mg)	1.2	1.3	1.5	1.3	1.3	1.7	2	100
Folate (mcg)	400[f]	400[f]	400	400	400	400	400	1000
Vitamin B_{12} (mcg)	2.4	2.4	2.4[g]	2.4	2.4	2.4[g]	6	e
Minerals:								
Calcium (mg)	1300	1000	1200	1300	1000	1200	1000	2500
Phosphorus (mg)	1250	700	700	1250	700	700	1000	4000/3000[h]
Magnesium (mg)	3600	310/320[i]	320	410	400/420[i]	420	400	350[j]
Iron (mg)	15	18	8	11	8	8	18	45
Zinc (mg)	9	8	8	11	11	11	15	40

[a] Daily Value (see page 3) is used for food labels.

[b] Tolerable Upper Intake Level (maximum intake at which an adverse effect is unlikely) for ages 19 & older.

[c] Vitamins A and E sometimes given in international units (IU) on diet-supplement labels, in which case:
    5 IU vitamin A = 1 mcg vitamin A; 30 IU vitamin E = 22 mg vitamin E.

[d] Recommended amount for smokers is 35 mg more vitamin C

[e] Not determinable due to lack of data; caution advised as to excessive intake.

[f] Women who might get pregnant are advised to get 400 mcg from ortified food or supplements.

[g] 10-30% of elderly may malabsorb B_{12}; age 51+ advised to get B_{12} from fortified food or supplements

[h] Lower value for age 71+

[i] Higher value for age 31-50

[j] Applies to magnesium from pharmaceutical agents only

Adjustment of % of Prenatal Daily Values for Use in Table 2

Some of the *% of [prenatal] Daily Values* on the labels of prenatal supplements must be adjusted for use in Table 2. (The values for vitamins E and C, niacin, iron, and zinc don't need to be changed.) For the nutrients listed below, the percentages given on the prenatal supplement labels should be adjusted as follows:

Vitamin A ☐ % prenatal Daily Value X 1.6 = ☐ Adjusted % Daily Value

Thiamin ☐ % prenatal Daily Value X 1.1 = ☐ Adjusted % Daily Value

Riboflavin ☐ % prenatal Daily Value X 1.2 = ☐ Adjusted % Daily Value

Vitamin B_6 ☐ % prenatal Daily Value X 1.2 = ☐ Adjusted % Daily Value

Folate ☐ % prenatal Daily Value X 2.0 = ☐ Adjusted % Daily Value

Vitamin B_{12} ☐ % prenatal Daily Value X 1.3 = ☐ Adjusted % Daily Value

Calcium ☐ % prenatal Daily Value X 1.3 = ☐ Adjusted % Daily Value

Phosphorus ☐ % prenatal Daily Value X 1.3 = ☐ Adjusted % Daily Value

Magnesium ☐ % prenatal Daily Value X 1.1 = ☐ Adjusted % Daily Value

For example, 800 mcg of folate would be listed on prenatal supplements as 100% of the Daily Value because 800 mcg is the Daily Value for pregnant women. The regular Daily Value (for those 4 years or older who aren't pregnant or nursing) is 400 mcg of folate. Thus, the 100% of prenatal Daily Value for folate is 200% of the regular Daily Value (100% X 2.0 = 200%). This 200% is the adjusted value for folate to use in the row for supplements on Table 2.

Tolerable Upper Intake Level as %DV

A Tolerable Upper Intake Level (UL) is the highest level of daily intake that's unlikely to have an adverse effect. For some nutrients, e.g., thiamin, riboflavin, vitamin B_{12}, there were not enough data to set a UL. For these, we're cautioned to still be careful about exceeding recommended amounts.

Typically, vitamins and minerals in supplements, pharmacologic agents, and fortified food are what push intake to UL levels. The UL for vitamin E, niacin, folate, and magnesium are for amounts from such sources (see footnote). For vitamins A, C, and B_6, and calcium, phosphorus, iron, and zinc, the UL is for total intake from all sources (food, supplements, medications, etc.).

The ULs are given below as % Daily Value (%DV). For example, the UL for vitamin C for a 20-year-old is 2000 mg. Above this amount, vitamin C is increasingly likely to cause diarrhea and other adverse effects. The Daily Value is 60 mg vitamin C for people over age 4, so the UL for vitamin C as %DV is 3333 [(2000mg/60mg) X 100 = 3333% of the DV].

	vit A	vit E*	vit C	niacin*	vit B_6	folate*	calci	phosp	mag*	iron	zinc
Age (years): 4-8	90	1364*	1083	75*	2000	100*	250	300	28*	222	80
9-13	170	2727*	2000	100*	3000	150*	250	400	88*	222	153
14-18	280	3636*	3000	150*	4000	200*	250	400	88*	250	227
19-70	300	4545*	3333	175*	5000	250*	250	400	88*	250	267
71+	300	4545*	3333	175*	5000	250*	250	300	88*	250	267
Pregnant <19	280	3636*	3000	150*	4000	200*	250	350	88*	250	227
Pregnant 19+	300	4545*	3333	175*	5000	250*	250	350	88*	250	267
Nursing <19	280	3636*	3000	150*	4000	200*	250	400	88*	250	227
Nursing 19+	300	4545*	3333	175*	5000	250*	250	400	88*	250	267

*The UL for vitamin E is for supplements of the alpha-tocopherol form of vitamin E. ULs for niacin and folate are for synthetic forms in supplements and fortified food. The UL for magnesium only applies to that taken in pharmacologic agents (e.g., some laxatives are high in magnesium).

Calculate Your Body Mass Index (BMI)

Body Mass Index (BMI) is commonly used to assess body weight. Its main advantage is that it puts height and weight into a single number. It does not, of course, indicate how the weight is distributed (e.g, more on belly than hips) and it presumes (correctly in most cases) that excess weight is mostly excess fat.

BMI = your weight in kilograms divided by the square of your height in meters. You can get the same BMI by multiplying your weight in pounds by 700 and dividing that number by the square of your height in inches:

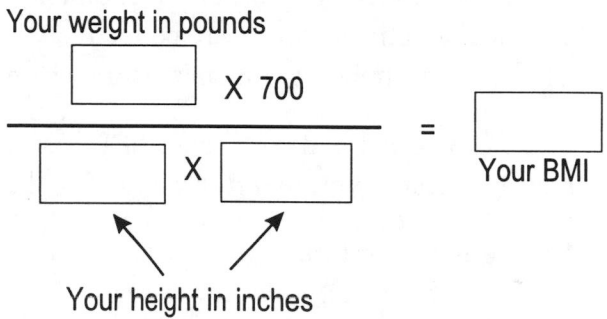

BMI for Adults: less than 18.5 = Underweight
18.5–24.9 = Healthy Weight
25.0–29.9 = Overweight
30.0 and above = Obese

For example, at 170 pounds and 5'7" your BMI = (170 X 700)/(67 X 67) = 26.5 (overweight). Being overweight increases the risk of high blood pressure and such diseases as diabetes, heart disease, and osteoarthritis.

Vitamins and Minerals

There are other vitamins and required minerals besides those in the food composition table, but you can be reasonably certain that your diet is nutritionally adequate if it's adequate in the nutrients assessed in Table 2, and if the nutrients come from a variety of foods rather than from dietary supplements or a few heavily fortified foods.

The table on the opposite page gives for each of the vitamins and minerals assessed:

- **Name of the Nutrient**, with alternate names in parenthesis.

- **Some Functions.** A common function of vitamins and minerals is to take part in a cell's chemical reactions, which are collectively called *metabolism*. For example, vitamin B_6 takes part in amino acid metabolism—chemical reactions involving amino acids.

- **Some Sources**. Foods or groups of foods that are examples of good sources of each nutrient. (Better yet, look for yourself in the food composition table.)

- **Deficiency symptoms**. Some diseases are caused by severe deficiencies of specific nutrients. *Xerophthalmia*, for example, is an inflammation of eye tissue caused by a severe deficiency of vitamin A. In some developing countries, it's a common cause of blindness in children.

  Nutrient deficiencies often cause vague symptoms, an ideal situation for selling supplements. Bleeding gums, for example, can be from a vitamin C deficiency, but a much more common cause is periodontal disease. Similarly, a vitamin deficiency can cause fatigue, but so can depression, lack of sleep, etc. In other words, if you have a symptom of a deficiency, don't automatically conclude you have the deficiency. Besides, you would know from your diet analysis whether you're likely to be deficient.

- **Possible Toxicity from Excessive Amounts**. In general, such excessive amounts come from taking supplements, e.g., birth defects are more common in infants born to women taking high doses of vitamin A. There are exceptions, such as the iron-toxicity disease hemochromatosis, which stems from a genetic defect in which iron is absorbed more efficiently than normal. The result can be severe—even fatal—damage from iron accumulating in various tissues. In genetically susceptible people, the disease occurs more commonly in men, since women regularly "get rid of" iron via menstruation (blood is rich in iron); it follows that there is less disease in regular blood donors.

Nutrient	Functions	Some Sources	Deficiency	Large Excess
Sodium	Water balance	Salty foods, softened water	Weakness, cramps	High blood pressure
Potassium	Nerve function	Citrus fruits, bananas, apricots	Weakness, irregular heartbeat	Irregular heartbeat
Vitamin A	Night vision, maintain various tissues	Yellow-orange and dark-green fruits and vegetables, liver	Night blindness, xerophthalmia	Fatigue, nausea, headache, hair loss
Vitamin E	Antioxidant	Plant oils, whole grains, almonds	Hemolytic anemia	Cramps, diarrhea, dizziness
Vitamin C (ascorbic acid, ascorbate)	Antioxidant, synthesis of connective tissue	Citrus fruits, berries, potatoes, red and green peppers	Scurvy, loose teeth, bleeding gums	Diarrhea, kidney stones
Thiamin (vitamin B_1)	Helps in carbohydrate metabolism	Pork, legumes, whole and enriched grains, liver, nuts	Beriberi, impaired nervous system	Headache, weakness, irritability
Riboflavin (vitamin B_2)	Helps in energy and protein metabolism	Meat, dairy products, enriched grains, eggs, broccoli, liver	Sore, red tongue, inflamed skin, eye disorders	None reported
Niacin (nicotinic acid, niacinamide)	Helps in energy metabolism	Meat, fish, whole and enriched grains, legumes, liver	Pellagra (diarrhea, inflamed skin, dementia)	Flushing of face and hands, liver damage
Vitamin B_6 (pyridoxine)	Helps in amino acid metabolism	Meat, legumes, potatoes, organ meats	Inflamed skin, convulsions in infants	Weak and numb muscles, nerve damage
Folate (folic acid, folacin)	Helps in cell division	Legumes, oranges, green leafy veggies, whole grains, liver	Anemia. risk of neural tube defects in fetus	High folate can delay diagnosis of B_{12} deficiency
Vitamin B_{12}	Helps in cell division	Animal products (meats, eggs, milk)	Anemia, nerve damage	Diarrhea
Calcium	Bone/teeth structure, muscle and nerve function	Milk/milk products, soft fish bones, leafy dark-green veggies	Stunted growth, malformed bones	Kidney stones
Phosphorus	Bone/teeth formation, energy production	Meat, fish, poultry, milk, eggs, legumes, cereals, nuts	Irritability, weakness, muscle ache	Poor bone mineralization if low calcium intake
Magnesium	Helps in metabolism	Whole grains, nuts, legumes, dark-green leafy vegetables	Weakness, muscle pain, cramps, spasms	Loss of reflexes, respiratory failure
Iron	Carries oxygen in blood	Red meat, fortified cereals, liver	Anemia, fatigue	Hemochromatosis
Zinc	Helps in metabolism, development	Oysters, beef, lamb, legumes, whole grains	Retarded growth	Nausea, cramps, diarrhea, fever

Estimate Your Calorie Requirements

Baseline Requirement (calories you need just to breathe, maintain body temperature, blood circulation, muscle tone, etc.) is estimated by multiplying your **body surface area** (see opposite page) by a **basic calorie factor** based on your age and sex (see table below).

Body surface area indicates the amount of surface from which your body can lose heat. The bigger you are and the bigger your surface area, the more baseline calories you need.

Basic calorie factor is affected by whether you're growing and how lean you are. Lean tissue uses more calories than fat tissue. Men are generally leaner than women. Also, as we age, we become less lean. Your basic calorie factor (cal/day/m2) is the estimated calories used each day for basic functions for each square meter of body surface.

$$\boxed{\qquad} \text{m}^2 \quad \text{X} \quad \boxed{\qquad} \text{cal/day/m}^2 \quad = \quad \boxed{\qquad} \text{calories/day}$$

your body surface area   your basic calorie factor   **Your Baseline Requirement**

Daily Use is your baseline use plus what you use for daily activities. If you're very lightly active (a *couch potato*), you use about 30% more than your baseline requirement. At the other extreme, you use about 100% more if you're heavily active (very strenuous activity several hours daily). Estimate your daily use by multiplying your baseline requirement by an activity factor ranging from 1.3 (very lightly active) to 2.0 (heavily active).

$$\boxed{\qquad} \text{cal/day} \quad \text{X} \quad \boxed{\qquad} \quad = \quad \boxed{\qquad} \text{calories/day}$$

your baseline requirement   your activity factor (1.3 to 2.0)   **Your Daily Use**

Basic Calorie Factors (cal/day/m2) by Age and Sex

Age	Male	Female	Age	Male	Female	Age	Male	Female
6	1270	1215	15	1100	960	28-29	955	855
7	1260	1180	16	1095	930	30-34	945	850
8	1245	1130	17	1075	910	35-39	930	845
9	1215	1100	18	1040	880	40-44	910	845
10	1165	1090	19	1015	875	45-49	895	840
11	1130	1085	20-21	995	870	50-54	880	815
12	1120	1065	22-23	980	865	55-59	865	795
13	1110	1030	24-25	965	860	60-64	850	785
14	1105	995	26-27	960	855	65 +	835	775

Your Body Surface Area

Draw a straight line between your height and weight. Read the intersect for your body surface area in square meters (m2), reading to the 2nd decimal point (each segment between numbers is 0.02). The dotted line: a 135-lb, 5'5" person = 1.67 m^2 estimated body surface.

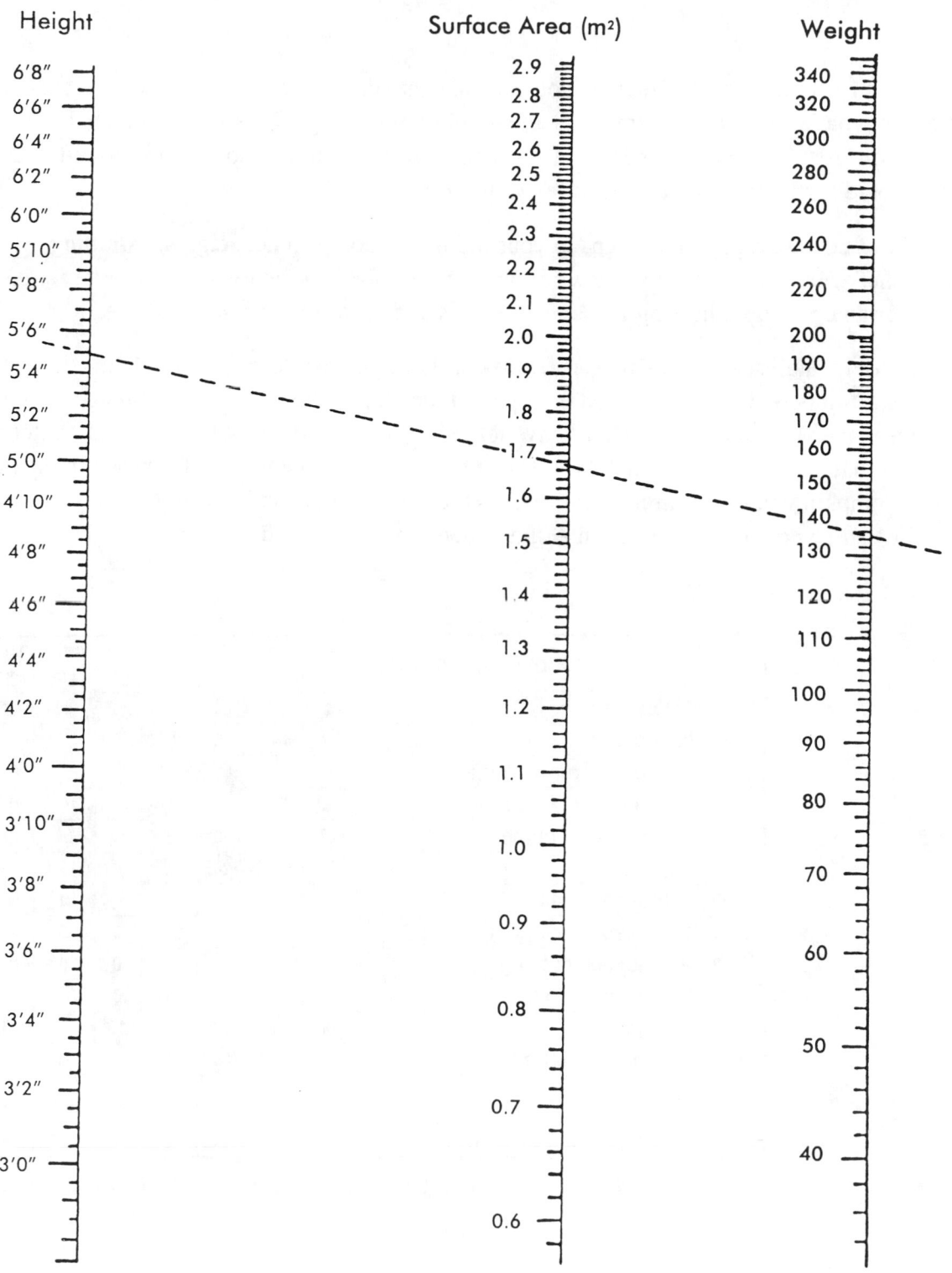

Calculating Nutrient Content from Recipes

As shown for Pumpkin Pie Squares, you can calculate the nutrient content from recipes by adding up what's in it and dividing it by the number of servings. Be sure to use label information first. There are extra lines at the end of sections in the food composition table for you to add what you've calculated for your recipes.

You can, of course, adjust this recipe to your liking and convenience, e.g., substituting whole wheat flour for white flour, low-fat milk for non-fat milk, margarine for butter, 2 egg whites for an egg, and adjusting amounts of spices and sugar to your taste.

In the nutrient analyses of your recipes (and your diet), you can learn a lot by being observant. In this recipe, you see that only plant foods have fiber; only animal foods have cholesterol and B_{12}; and sugar and fat have lots of calories relative to their nutrient content. Note also that you get more than 100% of the Daily Value for vitamin A from one pumpkin square. Pumpkin is a rich source of carotene, which shows as vitamin A in the analysis. Carotene can be converted to vitamin A in the body; plants don't have vitamin A, per se.

Food No.	Food Description & Amount	wt gm	wt oz	cal	% cal fat	prot gm	carbo gm	fiber gm
3128	1 cup flour	120	4.2	400	0%	12	84	0
3479	½ cup oats	39	1.4	140	18%	5	26	4
1782	½ cup dark brown sugar	96	3.4	360	0%	0	96	0.0
5403	½ cup butter (1 cube)	112	4.0	800	100%	0	0	0.0
2708	29 oz canned pumpkin	822	29	270	12%	13	61	33.6
1789	1 cup sugar	192	6.8	720	0%	0	192	0
5743	½ teaspoon salt	3	0.1	0	0%	0	0	0
5711	1½ teaspoon cinnamon	4	0.1	9	11%	0	3	1.8
5728	½ teaspoon nutmeg	1	0	6	62%	0	0	0.2
5712	½ teaspoon cloves	1	0	3	56%	0	1	0.4
939	3 eggs	150	5.3	210	57%	18	3	0
557	1½ cups nonfat milk	368	13.0	135	5%	15	20	0.0
	Total			3053	32%*	63	486	40
	Total/15 = 1 piece (3"x2½")			204	32%	4	32	3

*Calculated value: (107 gm fat X 9 cal/gm)/3053 cal = 0.32 = 32% of calories from fat

Pumpkin Pie Squares

1 cup flour

½ cup oats (dry oatmeal)

½ cup brown sugar

½ cup butter (1 cube)

Mix dry ingredients, and then softened butter (room temperature is about right softness) until crumbly. (If using a food processor, process dry ingredients with cold butter cut into chunks.) Press into 13X9" pan. Bake at 350° until lightly browned (about 15 minutes).

1 large (29 oz) can pumpkin

1 cup sugar

½ teaspoon salt

1½ teaspoon cinnamon

½ teaspoon nutmeg

½ teaspoon ground cloves

3 eggs

1½ cups non-fat or low-fat or whole milk

Mix pumpkin, sugar, salt, and spices (you can use same bowl that you made crust in). Mix in eggs, then milk. Pour over crust. Bake at 350° until knife inserted 1" from side of pan comes out clean (about 45 minutes). For a fancier version, add a layer of whipped cream with lightly toasted chopped walnuts or pecans sprinkled on top. Cut into 15 pieces (3X2½").

Food No.	fat gm	sat fat gm	choles mg	sodium mg	potas mg	vit A	vit E	vit C	thia	ribo	niac	vit B6	fola	vit B12	calc	phos	mag	iron	zinc
												% of Daily Value							
3128	0	0	0	0	160	0	0	0	40	24	32	3	40	0	0	14	7	24	6
3479	2	0	0	0	142	0	1	0	20	4	2	2	3	0	0	10	15	10	8
1782	0	0	0	0	380	0	0	0	0	0	0	0	0	0	8	4	8	12	0
5403	88	56	240	720	32	64	8	0	0	0	0	0	0	0	0	0	0	0	0
2708	3	0	0	34	1688	2021	30	0	13	27	13	23	23	0	13	30	47	27	10
1789	0	0	0	0	0	0	0	0	0	0	0	0	0	0	0	0	0	0	0
5743	0	0	0	1180	0	0	0	0	0	0	0	0	0	0	0	0	0	0	0
5711	0	0	0	1	18	0	0	1	0	0	0	0	0	0	4	0	0	8	0
5728	0	0	0	0	4	0	0	0	0	0	0	0	0	0	0	0	0	0	0
5712	0	0	0	2	34	0	0	1	0	0	0	1	0	0	1	0	1	0	0
939	14	4	645	195	183	18	6	0	6	45	0	9	18	24	6	27	3	12	12
557	0	0	0	210	609	15	0	3	9	30	2	8	4	22	52	38	10	0	10
	107	60	885	2342	3076	2118	45	5	88	130	49	46	88	46	84	123	91	93	46
	7	4	59	156	205	141	3	0	6	9	3	3	6	3	6	8	6	6	3

Pack-Your-Lunch Chart for Children (and Adults?)

It's hard to change eating habits. It's better to have good eating habits from the start. Using this chart, children develop a nutrition consciousness and enjoy making their own lunches.

They can add to the chart, and even convert it to a picture chart made from magazine clippings or from their own drawings. Portion sizes should be proportional to their needs.

Parents: Bite your tongue if their lunch combination is weird—though they might like your calling it weird!

Your Lunch Chart: Go for lots of colors and textures!

Grains (try whole grains!) 2 portions	Fruits, Veggies (different colors) 2 portions	Dairy, Meat (or substitutes) 1 or 2 portions	Extra (optional) (peer pressure!) 1 portion
Bread, Bagel	Fresh Fruit	Milk	Chips
Tortilla	Dried Fruit	Yogurt	Cookie
Cracker	Canned Fruit	Peanut Butter	Sugared Drink
Pancake	Raw Veggie	Meat, Fish	Other Sweets
Noodles, Rice	Cooked Veggie	Cheese	
Cereal	Fruit Juice	Egg	
Granola Bar	Vegetable Juice	Nuts, Beans	

Sample Lunches (weird and not-so-weird):
- Leftover chicken drumstick, leftover pancakes, grapes, tomato juice
- Peanut butter and banana sandwich, carrot, milk, cookie
- Cottage cheese mixed with canned pineapple, raw sugar peas, granola bar, biscuit
- Bean burrito, orange juice, cherry tomatoes, chips
- Celery filled with cheese spread, muffin, cranberry juice, walnuts
- Fruit mixed into yogurt, leftover macaroni and cheese, raisins
- Graham crackers spread with peanut butter, canned peaches, broccoli, cornflakes
- Tuna sandwich with lettuce, chips, apple, dried apricots
- Cheese cubes, melon cubes, waffle, green beans, brownie
- Scrambled egg sandwich with catsup, orange wedges, snap peas, chips

If your child likes the same lunch every day, here's an idea: Roast a chicken for Sunday dinner; don't eat the breast; slice it for sandwiches. Kids can make and freeze sandwiches for the week with the chicken, bread, and mayonnaise (the oil separates out with freezing but tastes fine), mustard, or catsup. Put them in sandwich bags; toss them in the freezer. Fill an equal number of sandwich bags with lettuce; toss them in the fridge. Each morning, fill a lunch bag with a sandwich from the freezer, a bag of lettuce, a fruit, and an "extra."

Table 3: Label Values Only

Food Amount & Description	wt gm	wt oz	calories	protein gm	carbo gm	fiber gm	total fat gm	sat fat gm	choles mg	sodium mg	% of Daily Value			
											vit A	vit C	calcium	iron
Total from food:														
Total from supplements:														
Total from food and supplements:														
Recommended amounts:								less than 300						

You can download this table as an Excel
file at www.orangegrovepub.com

Food Composition Table

Database

The table is adapted from food composition data provided by the Agricultural Research Service, United States Department of Agriculture (USDA) (www.barc.usda.gov/bhnrc/ foodsurvey/Cd98.html). The USDA compiled the data for evaluating the nutritional adequacy of diets in the United States. Many food samples were used for each determination of nutrient content, and the values are averages. There are no missing values in the database; when a chemical analysis of a nutrient in a food was unavailable, they estimated a likely level. Nutrient values are reasonable estimates, not hard-and-fast numbers.

Several foods not in the database (e.g., spices) have been added using another USDA database (www.nal.usda.gov/fnic/foodcomp/Data/SR16/ sr16.html). Nutrient values for some products (e.g., ready-to-eat cereals) have been updated using information from product websites or labels.

Nutrient Values

Nutrient values given for each food are: calories; percent of calories from fat; grams or milligrams of protein, carbohydrate, fiber, fat, saturated fat, cholesterol, sodium, potassium; percent of the Daily Value for 14 nutrients—vitamins A, E, and C, the B-vitamins (thiamin, riboflavin, niacin, B_6, folate, B_{12}), and calcium, phosphorus, magnesium, iron, and zinc.

Values have been rounded, and this can appear to result in discrepancies. For example, if the amount of fat is less than $\frac{1}{2}$ gm, it's rounded to zero, but the trace amount is still used to calculate the % of calories from fat. This can make the % of calories from fat appear abnormally high if the food is extremely low in calories.

There is no express or implied warranty with respect to the information provided in this book. You are advised to read your food labels and refer to USDA databases to update and verify nutrition information.

Portion Size

A description of the portion size for each food is given in brackets after the name of the food. The weight of the portion, given in grams and ounces, applies only to the edible portion (e.g., an orange without the peel, or a rib steak without the bone).

Unless you weigh your food on a scale, it's probably easier to use the description of the portion size, rather than trying to estimate its weight. An ounce is $\frac{1}{16}$ of a pound and, for most foods, isn't the same as a fluid ounce, which is what we measure in a measuring cup (see page 35 for abbreviations and conversions). There are 8 fluid ounces in a cup, but a cup of most foods doesn't weigh exactly 8 ounces (e.g., a cup of milk weighs more than 8 ounces, while a cup of potato chips weighs much less).

Pay close attention to portion sizes. Is your slice of pizza bigger than what's listed in the food composition table? Is that 1 cup or 2 cups of pasta on your plate?

Variation in Foods

Prepared foods can vary a lot. Even batches of spaghetti sauce made by the same person using the same recipe vary. New products are introduced constantly, changes are often made in existing products, and food composition tables can't possibly keep up. This is why **you should first use nutrient values from labels and product websites**, and then look up a similar food in the food composition table to approximate missing nutrient values. For your deli sandwich, it's of course more accurate to list the parts separately, rather than using the values for a generic version.

Foods vary even in their natural state, not only between varieties but within one variety, e.g., the nutrient content of an apple on one side of a tree isn't identical to one on the other. And of course the sizes of apples, carrots, etc., also vary. Other variations (e.g., storage and cooking times) also come into play. As mentioned earlier, nutrient values are reasonable estimates, not hard-and-fast numbers.

There are extra lines at the end of sections in the food composition table for you to add foods. You may want to add brand-name foods that you eat often, but aren't specifically listed in the table. As noted earlier, if there are missing nutrient values on food labels, fast-food websites, etc., you should estimate the values by looking up similar foods in the food composition table. Many food companies have a toll-free number and email address listed on their websites and food labels which you can use to inquire about nutrient content.

You may also want to add foods made from your favorite recipes (see pages 44-45). Some newspapers, magazines, and cookbooks provide nutrient information, including % of Daily Values, for their recipes.

Index of Foods

To help you find a food, the Food Composition Table is organized by categories, and foods are alphabetized within each category. Additionally, the Food Composition Table is followed by an index of the foods.

Beverages, Dairy, Eggs

Beverages, Dairy, Eggs

Food #	Food Description & Amount	wt gm	wt oz	calo-ries	%cal fat	prot gm	carbo gm	fiber gm
	Juices & Juice Drinks (Juice Drinks are not 100% juice; check label for % juice)							
1	Acerola juice [1 cup (8 fl oz)]	249	8.8	57	12%	1	12	0.7
2	Aloe vera juice [1 cup (8 fl oz)]	251	8.9	100	5%	2	23	0.5
3	Ambrosia juice (Include Knudsen's) [1 cup (8 fl oz)]	245	8.6	153	14%	1	32	0.6
4	Apple cider (Include sparkling cider) [1 cup (8 fl oz)]	248	8.7	117	2%	0	29	0.2
5	Apple cider-flavored drink, made from powdered mix, low calorie, with vitamin C added [1 cup (8 fl oz)]	240	8.5	2	0%	0	1	0.0
6	Apple cider-flavored drink, made from powdered mix, with sugar and vitamin C added [1 cup (8 fl oz)]	250	8.8	66	0%	0	17	0.0
7	Apple drink [1 cup (8 fl oz)]	250	8.8	118	0%	0	30	0.0
8	Apple drink with vitamin C added [1 cup (8 fl oz)]	250	8.8	117	0%	0	30	0.0
9	**Apple juice** [1 cup (8 fl oz)]	**248**	**8.7**	**117**	**2%**	**0**	**29**	**0.2**
10	Apple juice drink [1 cup (8 fl oz)]	250	8.8	126	0%	0	32	0.1
11	Apple juice with added vitamin C and calcium [1 cup (8 fl oz)]	248	8.7	116	2%	0	29	0.2
12	Apple juice, with added vitamin C [1 cup (8 fl oz)]	248	8.7	117	2%	0	29	0.2
13	Apple-cherry drink (Include apple-grape, apple-raspberry, apple-pineapple) [1 cup (8 fl oz)]	250	8.8	117	0%	0	30	0.1
14	Apple-cherry juice [1 cup (8 fl oz)]	250	8.8	117	2%	1	29	1.4
15	Apple-cranberry-grape juice drink [1 cup (8 fl oz)]	251	8.9	109	2%	0	28	0.1
16	Apple-grape juice [1 cup (8 fl oz)]	244	8.6	128	2%	1	32	0.2
17	Apple-grape-raspberry juice [1 cup (8 fl oz)]	250	8.8	130	3%	1	32	0.3
18	Apple-orange-pineapple juice drink [1 cup (8 fl oz)]	251	8.9	131	1%	0	34	0.2
19	Apple-pear juice [1 cup (8 fl oz)]	248	8.7	119	2%	0	30	0.2
20	Apple-raspberry juice [1 cup (8 fl oz)]	239	8.4	108	4%	0	26	0.2
21	Apple-white grape juice drink, low calorie, with vitamin C added [1 cup (8 fl oz)]	240	8.5	54	2%	0	13	0.1
22	Apricot nectar [1 cup (8 fl oz)]	251	8.9	141	1%	1	36	1.5
23	Apricot-orange juice [1 cup (8 fl oz)]	250	8.8	123	2%	1	30	1.0
24	Apricot-pineapple juice drink [1 cup (8 fl oz)]	250	8.8	128	1%	0	32	0.4
25	Banana nectar [1 cup (8 fl oz)]	250	8.8	177	2%	1	45	2.1
26	Banana-orange drink [1 cup (8 fl oz)]	250	8.8	126	0%	0	32	0.2
27	Black cherry drink [1 cup (8 fl oz)]	250	8.8	117	0%	0	30	0.4
28	Black cherry drink with vitamin C added [1 cup (8 fl oz)]	250	8.8	117	0%	0	30	0.4
29	Blackberry juice [1 cup (8 fl oz)]	250	8.8	93	15%	1	20	0.3
30	Boka Fruit Juice Cooler [1 cup (8 fl oz)]	250	8.8	121	1%	2	29	0.3
31	Cantaloupe nectar [1 cup (8 fl oz)]	250	8.8	155	2%	1	39	0.8
32	Carbonated noncitrus juice drink (70% juice) [1 can (12 fl oz)]	372	13.1	141	2%	1	35	0.3
33	Carrot juice [1 cup]	236	8.3	94	3%	2	22	1.9
34	Celery juice [1 cup (8 fl oz)]	236	8.3	42	8%	2	9	3.8
35	Cherry drink with vitamin C added [1 cup (8 fl oz)]	250	8.8	117	0%	0	30	0.4
36	Citrus drink with vitamin C added [1 cup (8 fl oz)]	250	8.8	127	0%	0	33	0.0
37	Citrus fruit juice drink (60% fruit juice) (Include 5 Alive Citrus) [1 cup (8 fl oz)]	247	8.7	114	1%	1	28	0.1
38	Citrus juice drink, calcium fortified (Include Citrus Hill Grapefruit Juice Beverage Plus Calcium) [1 cup (8 fl oz)]	240	8.5	112	2%	1	28	0.1
39	Citrus juice drink, low calorie (Include TreeSweet Lite citrus combo) [1 cup (8 fl oz)]	240	8.5	72	0%	1	18	0.2
40	Coconut beverage, Puerto Rican [1 cup (8 fl oz)]	240	8.5	173	41%	2	25	4.3
41	Cranapple-citrus juice drink, low calorie [1 cup (8 fl oz)]	240	8.5	59	0%	0	15	0.2
42	Cranberry cocktail/juice drink with vitamin C added [1 cup (8 fl oz)]	253	8.9	144	2%	0	36	0.3
43	Cranberry cocktail/juice drink, low calorie, with vitamin C added [1 cup (8 fl oz)]	240	8.5	46	0%	0	11	0.0
44	Cranberry juice, unsweetened [1 cup (8 fl oz)]	253	8.9	124	4%	1	32	0.3
45	Cranberry-apple cocktail/juice drink with vitamin C added (Include Crantastic, blueberry-cranberry, raspberry-cranberry, cranberry-apricot, and cranberry-grape juice drink) [1 cup (8 fl oz)]	253	8.9	170	0%	0	43	0.3

| | | | | | | % of Daily Value | | | | | | | | | | | | | |
Food #	fat gm	sat fat gm	choles mg	sodium mg	potass mg	vit A	vit E	vit C	thia-min	ribo-flavin	nia-cin	vit B-6	fol-ate	vit B-12	cal-cium	phos-phorus	magne-sium	iron	zinc
1	1	0	0	7	242	13	0	6640	3	9	5	0	9	0	2	2	7	7	2
2	1	0	0	73	733	1	0	36	15	9	5	28	3	0	6	11	9	6	3
3	2	2	0	11	342	1	0	42	7	4	3	9	8	0	3	3	7	4	2
4	0	0	0	7	295	0	0	4	3	2	1	4	0	0	2	2	2	5	0
5	0	0	0	7	0	0	0	105	0	0	0	0	0	0	3	3	1	0	0
6	0	0	0	8	1	0	0	110	0	0	0	0	0	0	3	3	1	1	1
7	0	0	0	13	48	0	0	0	2	4	0	0	1	0	2	1	1	4	2
8	0	0	0	12	47	0	0	46	2	4	0	0	1	0	2	1	1	4	2
9	0	0	0	7	295	0	0	4	3	2	1	4	0	0	2	2	2	5	0
10	0	0	0	7	75	0	0	138	1	1	0	1	0	0	1	0	1	1	1
11	0	0	0	17	312	0	0	143	0	2	0	4	0	0	28	2	3	4	1
12	0	0	0	7	295	0	0	177	3	2	1	4	0	0	2	2	2	5	0
13	0	0	0	7	31	0	0	1	0	1	0	0	0	0	1	0	1	1	1
14	0	0	0	6	307	1	0	6	4	4	3	4	1	0	2	2	3	5	1
15	0	0	0	6	121	0	0	15	2	2	1	3	1	0	1	1	2	2	1
16	0	0	0	7	303	0	0	2	4	4	2	5	1	0	2	2	4	4	1
17	1	0	0	5	335	1	1	18	5	7	5	6	6	0	3	3	6	5	3
18	0	0	0	7	167	0	0	20	3	2	1	3	3	0	1	1	2	3	1
19	0	0	0	12	347	0	0	5	2	3	3	2	2	0	2	2	4	5	1
20	0	0	0	6	309	1	0	11	3	3	2	4	1	0	2	2	4	6	1
21	0	0	0	12	145	0	0	1	0	1	0	2	0	0	1	1	2	2	1
22	0	0	0	8	286	33	1	3	2	2	3	3	1	0	2	2	3	5	2
23	0	0	0	6	361	19	1	73	6	3	4	7	6	0	2	3	5	6	1
24	0	0	0	5	161	5	0	16	4	2	2	5	5	0	2	1	4	2	1
25	0	0	0	5	347	1	1	13	3	5	2	25	4	0	1	2	7	2	1
26	0	0	0	6	61	0	0	13	1	1	0	2	2	0	1	0	1	0	1
27	0	0	0	7	34	0	0	1	0	1	1	0	0	0	1	1	1	1	1
28	0	0	0	7	34	0	0	136	0	1	1	0	0	0	1	1	1	1	1
29	2	0	0	3	425	4	1	42	3	4	4	5	7	0	3	3	13	13	3
30	0	0	0	21	134	7	0	143	5	3	3	6	7	0	2	1	4	4	1
31	0	0	0	13	277	24	1	49	2	1	3	5	2	0	1	2	3	1	1
32	0	0	0	31	329	0	0	2	4	4	2	6	1	0	3	2	5	4	1
33	0	0	0	68	689	608	0	33	14	8	5	26	2	0	6	10	8	6	3
34	0	0	0	215	670	3	3	24	7	7	4	10	13	0	10	6	7	6	2
35	0	0	0	7	34	0	0	136	0	1	1	0	0	0	1	1	1	1	1
36	0	0	0	7	48	0	0	132	0	1	0	1	0	0	1	0	1	3	1
37	0	0	0	7	275	1	0	111	2	2	2	3	1	0	2	3	4	15	1
38	0	0	0	4	196	0	0	133	4	2	2	3	1	0	32	2	4	1	1
39	0	0	0	7	266	1	0	108	2	3	2	2	1	0	2	2	4	15	1
40	8	7	0	218	589	0	1	9	5	7	1	4	3	0	5	7	15	6	3
41	0	0	0	6	166	0	0	118	1	3	1	2	1	0	2	2	2	8	1
42	0	0	0	5	46	0	0	149	2	1	0	2	0	0	1	1	1	2	1
43	0	0	0	7	53	0	0	129	1	1	0	2	0	0	2	0	1	1	0
44	1	0	0	3	162	1	1	29	3	3	1	8	1	0	2	2	3	3	2
45	0	0	0	5	68	0	0	135	1	3	1	3	0	0	2	1	1	1	1

Beverages, Dairy, Eggs

Food #	Food Description & Amount	wt gm	wt oz	calories	%cal fat	prot gm	carbo gm	fiber gm
46	Cranberry-apple cocktail/juice drink, low calorie, with vitamin C added (Include low calorie or light raspberry-cranberry, cranberry-blueberry, and cranberry-apricot juice drinks) [1 cup (8 fl oz)]	240	8.5	46	0%	0	11	0.2
47	Cranberry-white grape juice mixture, unsweetened (Include Knudsen Cranberry Nectar) [1 cup (8 fl oz)]	253	8.9	142	2%	1	36	0.3
48	Frozen daiquiri mix, from frozen concentrate, reconstituted [1 fl oz]	29	1.0	19	1%	0	5	0.1
49	Frozen daiquiri mix, frozen concentrate, not reconstituted [1 fl oz]	36	1.3	101	1%	0	26	0.5
50	Fruit drink (Include fruit punches and fruit ades, Hawaiian Punch made from canned or frozen) [1 cup (8 fl oz)]	248	8.7	117	0%	0	30	0.2
51	Fruit drink, low calorie [1 cup (8 fl oz)]	240	8.5	43	0%	0	11	0.0
52	Fruit juice blend, 100% juice, all flavors (Include Juicy Juice, Hi-C 100) [1 cup]	250	8.8	132	2%	1	33	0.3
53	Fruit punch, fruit drinks, or fruitades, with vitamin C added (Include Hi-C) [1 cup (8 fl oz)]	247	8.7	116	0%	0	29	0.2
54	Fruit punch, made with fruit juice and soda [1 cup (8 fl oz)]	245	8.6	110	1%	0	28	0.2
55	Fruit punch, made with soda, fruit juice, and sherbet or ice cream [1 cup (8 fl oz)]	256	9.0	164	6%	1	39	0.5
56	Fruit smoothie drink, made with fruit or fruit juice and dairy products [1 commercial smoothie (20 fl oz)]	506	17.8	492	15%	8	104	5.0
57	Fruit smoothie drink, made with fruit or fruit juice only (no dairy products) [1 commercial smoothie (20 fl oz)]	526	18.6	329	3%	2	85	4.9
58	Fruit-flavored beverage, dry concentrate, low calorie, not reconstituted (Include Crystal Light) [1Tbs]	12	0.4	26	0%	1	9	0.0
59	Fruit-flavored concentrate, dry, with vitamin C added (Include Kool-Aid, Hawaiian Punch) [1Tbs]	13	0.4	48	0%	0	12	0.0
60	Fruit-flavored drink, low calorie, calcium fortified (Include Supri drink mix) [1 cup (8 fl oz)]	240	8.5	3	0%	0	1	0.0
61	Fruit-flavored drink, made from powdered mix with high vitamin C added, low calorie (Include Sugar Free Tang) [1 cup (8 fl oz)]	240	8.5	7	1%	0	2	0.0
62	Fruit-flavored drink, made from powdered mix with vitamin C added, no sugar or low calorie sweetener (Include Kool-Aid, Wyler's) [1 cup (8 fl oz)]	240	8.5	90	0%	0	23	0.0
63	Fruit-flavored drink, made from powdered mix, with sugar and vitamin C added (Include Kool-Aid, Wyler's) [1 cup (8 fl oz)]	250	8.8	88	0%	0	22	0.0
64	Fruit-flavored drink, non-carbonated, made from low calorie powdered mix (Include Sugar Free Crystal light) [1 cup (8 fl oz)]	240	8.5	3	0%	0	1	0.0
65	Fruit-flavored drink, non-carbonated, made from powdered mix, with sugar (Include Fla-vor-Aid) [1 can (12 fl oz)]	356	12.6	125	0%	0	32	0.0
66	Fruit-flavored drink, vitamin and mineral fortified (Include Power Burst, Advanced Performance) [1 cup (8 fl oz)]	240	8.5	50	0%	0	14	0.0
67	Fruit-flavored drinks, made from powdered mix, mainly sugar, with high vitamin C added (Include Borden's Instant Breakfast Drink, Keen, Tang Instant Breakfast Juice Drink) [1 cup (8 fl oz)]	240	8.5	119	0%	0	30	0.0
68	Fruit-flavored drinks, punches, ades, low calorie, with vitamin C added (Include low calorie Hi C, Kool-Aid, Wylers) [1 cup (8 fl oz)]	240	8.5	43	0%	0	11	0.0
69	Fruit-flavored thirst quencher beverage, dry concentrate, low sugar, not reconstituted (Include Gatorade) [1Tbs]	13	0.4	46	0%	0	12	0.0
70	Fruit-flavored thirst quencher beverage, low calorie (Include Gatorade Light) [1 cup (8 fl oz)]	240	8.5	26	0%	0	7	0.0
71	Fruit-flavored thirst quencher beverage, low sugar (Include Gatorade, Quick Kick, Powerade, All Sport) [1 cup (8 fl oz)]	240	8.5	60	0%	0	15	0.0
72	Gelatin drink, powder, flavored, with low-calorie sweetener, reconstituted (Include Nutri System Orange Drink) [1 packet dry mix with 1 cup water]	255	9.0	51	0%	13	0	0.0
73	Grape drink with vitamin C added [1 cup (8 fl oz)]	250	8.8	113	0%	0	29	0.0
74	Grape drink, low calorie [1 cup (8 fl oz)]	240	8.5	43	0%	0	11	0.0
75	Grape juice drink [1 cup (8 fl oz)]	250	8.8	125	0%	0	32	0.3
76	Grape juice, unsweetened or low-cal sweetener [1 cup (8 fl oz)]	250	8.8	153	1%	1	37	0.3
77	Grape juice, unsweetened, with added vitamin C [1 cup (8 fl oz)]	250	8.8	152	1%	1	37	0.3
78	Grape juice, with sugar, with added vitamin C [1 cup (8 fl oz)]	250	8.8	128	2%	0	32	0.3
79	Grapeade and grape drink [1 cup (8 fl oz)]	250	8.8	107	0%	0	28	0.0

Food #	fat gm	sat fat gm	choles mg	sodium mg	potass mg	% of Daily Value													
						vit A	vit E	vit C	thia-min	ribo-flavin	nia-cin	vit B-6	fol-ate	vit B-12	cal-cium	phos-phorus	magne-sium	iron	zinc
46	0	0	0	5	65	0	0	128	0	3	1	2	0	0	2	1	1	1	1
47	0	0	0	6	265	0	0	12	4	4	2	8	1	0	2	3	5	3	1
48	0	0	0	23	6	0	0	1	0	0	0	0	0	0	0	0	0	0	0
49	0	0	0	123	34	0	0	5	1	1	0	0	0	0	0	1	0	1	1
50	0	0	0	55	62	0	0	23	3	3	0	0	1	0	2	0	1	3	2
51	0	0	0	50	50	0	0	129	2	3	0	0	1	0	2	0	1	4	2
52	0	0	0	7	328	1	0	100	5	4	3	7	3	0	2	2	5	4	1
53	0	0	0	54	62	0	0	122	4	3	0	0	1	0	2	0	1	3	2
54	0	0	0	10	165	0	0	22	5	2	2	6	7	0	2	1	4	3	1
55	1	1	3	30	272	1	1	60	7	4	2	6	12	1	5	4	5	2	3
56	8	5	28	135	949	9	2	131	12	29	6	36	18	12	27	23	17	7	11
57	1	0	0	14	883	1	2	132	10	12	7	36	15	0	4	6	13	10	2
58	0	0	0	1	447	0	0	99	0	0	0	0	0	0	33	15	0	0	0
59	0	0	0	15	1	0	0	25	0	0	0	0	0	0	2	3	0	0	0
60	0	0	0	11	4	0	0	0	0	0	0	0	0	0	32	1	1	0	0
61	0	0	0	10	71	17	0	112	0	11	11	11	22	0	1	1	2	0	0
62	0	0	0	13	0	0	0	50	0	0	0	0	0	0	1	1	1	0	0
63	0	0	0	34	1	0	0	47	0	0	0	0	0	0	4	5	1	1	1
64	0	0	0	7	45	0	0	10	0	0	0	0	0	0	4	2	1	0	0
65	0	0	0	49	2	0	0	67	0	0	0	0	0	0	5	7	1	1	1
66	0	0	0	26	50	1	24	51	0	0	30	16	31	30	0	0	2	0	0
67	0	0	0	9	59	18	8	123	0	12	12	12	0	0	12	5	1	0	0
68	0	0	0	50	50	0	0	129	2	3	0	0	1	0	2	0	1	4	2
69	0	0	0	84	19	0	0	0	0	0	0	0	0	0	0	2	0	0	0
70	0	0	0	84	24	0	0	25	0	0	0	0	0	0	0	2	1	1	0
71	0	0	0	96	26	0	0	0	1	0	0	0	0	0	0	2	1	1	0
72	0	0	0	37	2	0	0	0	0	2	0	0	1	0	1	1	1	1	1
73	0	0	0	15	13	0	0	142	1	1	0	1	0	0	1	0	1	2	2
74	0	0	0	50	50	0	0	129	2	3	0	0	1	0	2	0	1	4	2
75	0	0	0	3	88	0	0	67	2	1	1	3	1	0	1	1	3	1	1
76	0	0	0	8	330	0	0	0	4	5	3	8	2	0	2	3	6	3	1
77	0	0	0	7	330	0	0	100	4	5	3	8	2	0	2	3	6	3	1
78	0	0	0	5	53	0	0	100	3	4	2	5	1	0	1	1	3	1	1
79	0	0	0	7	33	0	0	0	1	1	0	1	0	0	1	0	1	1	1

Beverages, Dairy, Eggs

Food #	Food Description & Amount	wt gm	wt oz	calo-ries	%cal fat	prot gm	carbo gm	fiber gm
80	Grapefruit juice drink [1 cup (8 fl oz)]	250	8.8	128	1%	0	32	0.1
81	Grapefruit juice drink with vitamin C added [1 cup (8 fl oz)]	250	8.8	128	1%	0	32	0.1
82	Grapefruit juice drink, calcium fortified [1 cup (8 fl oz)]	250	8.8	117	2%	1	29	0.2
83	Grapefruit juice drink, low calorie or light, with vitamin C added [1 cup (8 fl oz)]	231	8.1	32	2%	0	7	0.1
84	Grapefruit juice, canned or bottled, unsweetened or sweetened with low-cal sweetener (Include Ocean Spray) [1 cup (8 fl oz)]	247	8.7	94	2%	1	22	0.2
85	Grapefruit juice, canned, bottled or in a carton, unsweetened [1 cup (8 fl oz)]	247	8.7	94	2%	1	22	0.2
86	Grapefruit juice, canned, with sugar [1 cup (8 fl oz)]	250	8.8	115	2%	1	28	0.3
87	Grapefruit juice, fresh [1 cup (8 fl oz)]	247	8.7	96	2%	1	23	0.2
88	Grapefruit juice, frozen, unsweetened (reconstituted with water) [1 cup (8 fl oz)]	247	8.7	101	3%	1	24	0.3
89	Grapefruit juice, frozen, with sugar (reconstituted with water) [1 cup (8 fl oz)]	248	8.7	118	3%	1	28	0.3
90	Grapefruit-orange juice, canned, unsweetened [1 cup (8 fl oz)]	247	8.7	106	2%	1	25	0.2
91	Grapefruit-orange juice, canned, with sugar [1 cup (8 fl oz)]	249	8.8	127	2%	1	31	0.2
92	Grapefruit-orange juice, fresh [1 cup (8 fl oz)]	247	8.7	104	3%	1	24	0.4
93	Grapefruit-orange juice, frozen, unsweetened (reconstituted with water) [1 cup (8 fl oz)]	247	8.7	106	2%	2	25	0.4
94	Grape-tangerine-lemon juice [1 cup (8 fl oz)]	245	8.6	128	2%	1	32	0.4
95	Guava drink [1 cup (8 fl oz)]	250	8.8	131	1%	0	33	2.0
96	Guava juice drink with vitamin C added (Include Ocean Spray Mauna Lai, Guava Passion Fruit Drink) [1 cup (8 fl oz)]	253	8.9	132	1%	0	34	2.0
97	Guava nectar [1 cup (8 fl oz)]	250	8.8	149	1%	0	38	2.0
98	Lemon juice, canned or bottled [1Tbs (1 fl oz)]	15	0.5	3	12%	0	1	0.1
99	Lemon juice, fresh [1Tbs (1 fl oz)]	15	0.5	4	0%	0	1	0.1
100	Lemon juice, frozen [1Tbs (1 fl oz)]	15	0.5	3	13%	0	1	0.1
101	**Lemonade** [1 cup (8 fl oz)]	**248**	**8.7**	**99**	**1%**	**0**	**26**	**0.2**
102	Lemonade with vitamin C added [1 cup (8 fl oz)]	248	8.7	131	1%	0	34	0.3
103	Lemonade, frozen concentrate, not reconstituted [1 can (6 fl oz)]	219	7.7	396	1%	1	103	0.9
104	Lemonade, low calorie [1 cup (8 fl oz)]	240	8.5	43	0%	0	11	0.2
105	Lemonade-flavored drink, made from low-cal powdered mix, with vitamin C added (Include Sugar Free Country Time) [1 cup (8 fl oz)]	240	8.5	5	1%	0	1	0.0
106	Lemonade-flavored drink, made from sugar and powdered mix, with vitamin C added (Include Country Time) [1 cup (8 fl oz)]	250	8.8	90	0%	0	24	0.0
107	Lemon-limeade [1 cup (8 fl oz)]	248	8.7	133	1%	0	35	0.3
108	Lime juice, canned or bottled [1Tbs (1 fl oz)]	15	0.5	3	10%	0	1	0.1
109	Lime juice, fresh or frozen [1Tbs (1 fl oz)]	15	0.5	4	3%	0	1	0.1
110	Lime juice, frozen [1Tbs (1 fl oz)]	15	0.5	4	3%	0	1	0.1
111	Limeade [1 cup (8 fl oz)]	248	8.7	135	0%	0	36	0.3
112	Mango nectar [1 cup (8 fl oz)]	250	8.8	146	2%	1	38	1.8
113	Nutri System Orange Drink [1 cup (8 fl oz)]	250	8.8	50	0%	13	0	0.0
114	Orange breakfast drink (Include Sunny Delight) [1 cup (8 fl oz)]	250	8.8	110	0%	0	27	0.0
115	Orange breakfast drink, calcium fortified [1 cup (8 fl oz)]	252	8.9	136	0%	0	33	0.3
116	Orange breakfast drink, low calorie (Include Sunny Delight Lite) [1 cup (8 fl oz)]	250	8.8	15	0%	0	4	0.5
117	Orange breakfast drink, made from frozen concentrate (Include Orange Plus, Awake, Bright and Early, Sunny Delight) [1 cup (8 fl oz)]	250	8.8	117	1%	0	29	0.1
118	Orange drink (Include orange ade, Yabba Dabba Dew, Sunny Delight) [1 cup]	249	8.8	115	0%	0	31	0.0
119	Orange drink and orangeade with vitamin C added [1 cup (8 fl oz)]	249	8.8	127	0%	0	32	0.2
120	Orange juice drink, vitamin-fortified [1 cup (8 fl oz)]	249	8.8	132	0%	0	33	0.0
121	Orange juice, canned, unsweetened [1 cup (8 fl oz)]	249	8.8	105	3%	1	25	0.5
122	Orange juice, canned, with calcium added, unsweetened, bottled or in a carton [1 cup (8 fl oz)]	248	8.7	111	1%	2	27	0.5
123	Orange juice, canned, with sugar [1 cup (8 fl oz)]	250	8.8	131	2%	1	31	0.5
124	**Orange juice**, fresh [1 cup (8 fl oz)]	**248**	**8.7**	**112**	**4%**	**2**	**26**	**0.5**
125	Orange juice, frozen, unsweetened (reconstituted with water) (Include reduced acid) [1 cup (8 fl oz)]	249	8.8	113	1%	2	27	0.6

Food #	fat gm	sat fat gm	choles mg	sodium mg	potass mg	% of Daily Value													
						vit A	vit E	vit C	thia-min	ribo-flavin	nia-cin	vit B-6	fol-ate	vit B-12	cal-cium	phos-phorus	magne-sium	iron	zinc
80	0	0	0	5	115	0	0	37	2	1	1	1	2	0	1	1	2	1	1
81	0	0	0	5	115	0	0	132	2	1	1	1	2	0	1	1	2	1	1
82	0	0	0	4	204	0	0	139	4	2	2	3	1	0	33	2	4	1	1
83	0	0	0	5	127	0	0	137	2	1	1	1	2	0	1	1	2	1	1
84	0	0	0	2	378	0	0	120	7	3	3	2	6	0	2	3	6	3	1
85	0	0	0	2	378	0	0	120	7	3	3	2	6	0	2	3	6	3	1
86	0	0	0	5	405	0	0	112	7	3	4	3	7	0	2	3	6	5	1
87	0	0	0	2	400	0	0	156	7	3	2	5	6	0	2	4	7	3	1
88	0	0	0	7	334	0	0	138	7	3	3	5	2	0	2	3	7	2	1
89	0	0	0	7	329	0	0	136	7	3	3	5	2	0	2	3	7	2	1
90	0	0	0	7	390	3	1	120	9	4	3	3	9	0	2	3	6	6	1
91	0	0	0	7	384	3	1	118	9	4	4	3	9	0	2	3	6	6	1
92	0	0	0	2	447	3	1	181	11	4	4	5	13	0	2	4	7	3	1
93	0	0	0	7	405	1	1	150	10	3	3	5	15	0	2	4	7	2	1
94	0	0	0	14	331	2	0	34	6	4	3	7	3	0	3	3	6	3	1
95	0	0	0	7	104	3	1	111	1	1	2	3	1	0	1	1	1	1	1
96	0	0	0	7	105	3	1	142	1	1	2	3	1	0	1	1	1	1	1
97	0	0	0	7	93	2	1	78	1	1	2	2	1	0	1	1	1	1	1
98	0	0	0	3	16	0	0	6	0	0	0	0	0	0	0	0	0	0	0
99	0	0	0	0	19	0	0	12	0	0	0	0	0	0	0	0	0	0	0
100	0	0	0	0	14	0	0	8	1	0	0	0	0	0	0	0	0	0	0
101	0	0	0	8	37	1	0	16	1	3	0	1	1	0	1	0	1	2	1
102	0	0	0	8	48	1	0	21	1	4	0	1	2	0	1	1	1	3	1
103	0	0	0	9	147	2	0	65	4	12	1	3	5	0	2	2	3	9	1
104	0	0	0	7	38	0	0	27	2	1	0	0	2	0	1	0	1	2	0
105	0	0	0	7	0	0	0	10	0	0	0	0	0	0	5	2	1	1	0
106	0	0	0	13	23	0	0	19	0	0	0	0	1	0	5	2	1	1	1
107	0	0	0	7	45	0	0	18	1	2	0	0	1	0	1	1	1	2	1
108	0	0	0	2	12	0	0	2	0	0	0	0	0	0	0	0	0	0	0
109	0	0	0	0	17	0	0	8	0	0	0	0	0	0	0	0	0	0	0
110	0	0	0	0	17	0	0	8	0	0	0	0	0	0	0	0	0	0	0
111	0	0	0	5	43	0	0	14	0	0	0	0	1	0	1	0	1	0	1
112	0	0	0	6	141	29	4	32	3	3	3	6	2	0	1	1	3	1	1
113	0	0	0	36	2	0	0	0	0	2	0	0	1	0	1	1	1	1	1
114	0	0	0	160	103	10	0	54	20	1	1	1	5	0	1	1	2	1	1
115	0	0	0	136	209	10	0	101	20	1	1	3	12	0	25	2	3	1	1
116	0	0	0	138	45	11	0	53	21	0	0	0	1	0	1	0	1	0	1
117	0	0	0	23	323	0	0	258	19	80	2	5	7	0	19	7	4	1	1
118	0	0	0	7	44	0	0	14	1	1	0	1	1	0	1	0	1	1	1
119	0	0	0	40	45	0	0	142	1	0	0	1	1	0	1	0	1	4	1
120	0	0	0	5	105	1	0	62	63	63	62	62	2	62	0	1	2	2	0
121	0	0	0	5	436	4	1	143	10	4	4	11	11	0	2	3	7	6	1
122	0	0	0	2	471	2	2	161	13	3	3	5	27	0	30	4	6	1	1
123	0	0	0	5	425	4	1	139	10	4	4	11	11	0	2	3	7	6	1
124	0	0	0	2	496	5	1	207	15	4	5	5	19	0	3	4	7	3	1
125	0	0	0	7	479	2	1	163	13	3	3	6	28	0	3	4	6	1	1

Beverages, Dairy, Eggs

Food #	Food Description & Amount	wt gm	wt oz	calo-ries	%cal fat	prot gm	carbo gm	fiber gm
126	Orange juice, frozen, unsweetened, not reconstituted [1Tbs]	18	0.6	28	1%	0	7	0.1
127	Orange juice, frozen, unsweetened, with calcium added (reconstituted with water) [1 cup (8 fl oz)]	249	8.8	113	1%	2	27	0.6
128	Orange juice, frozen, with sugar (reconstituted with water) [1 cup (8 fl oz)]	250	8.8	126	1%	2	31	0.6
129	Orange juice, frozen, with sugar, not reconstituted [1Tbs]	18	0.6	32	1%	0	8	0.1
130	Orange-apricot juice drink [1 cup (8 fl oz)]	249	8.8	127	2%	1	32	0.2
131	Orange-banana juice [1 cup (8 fl oz)]	250	8.8	142	3%	2	35	1.9
132	Orange-cranberry juice drink [1 cup (8 fl oz)]	249	8.8	118	1%	0	31	0.1
133	Orange-cranberry juice drink, low calorie, with vitamin C added [1 cup (8 fl oz)]	240	8.5	29	3%	0	7	0.4
134	Orange-grape-banana juice drink [1 cup (8 fl oz)]	234	8.3	100	2%	1	25	0.5
135	Orange-lemon drink [1 cup (8 fl oz)]	249	8.8	125	0%	0	32	0.1
136	Orange-mango juice drink [1 cup (8 fl oz)]	238	8.4	103	1%	0	27	0.1
137	Orange-peach juice drink [1 cup (8 fl oz)]	240	8.5	122	2%	1	30	0.2
138	Orange-raspberry juice drink [1 cup (8 fl oz)]	249	8.8	107	1%	0	28	0.1
139	Orange-white grape-peach juice [1 cup (8 fl oz)]	248	8.7	117	2%	1	28	0.5
140	Papaya juice/drink [1 cup (8 fl oz)]	248	8.7	141	2%	0	36	1.5
141	Papaya juice/nectar [1 cup (8 fl oz)]	249	8.8	134	0%	1	35	1.5
142	Papaya nectar [1 cup (8 fl oz)]	250	8.8	143	2%	0	36	1.5
143	Passion fruit juice (Include Lilikoi) [1 cup (8 fl oz)]	247	8.7	137	2%	1	35	0.5
144	Passion fruit nectar [1 cup (8 fl oz)]	250	8.8	167	0%	0	44	0.2
145	Peach nectar, canned [1 cup (8 fl oz)]	249	8.8	134	0%	1	35	1.5
146	Pear nectar [1 cup (8 fl oz)]	250	8.8	150	0%	0	39	1.5
147	Pear-white grape-passion fruit juice, with added vitamin C [1 cup (8 fl oz)]	246	8.7	149	1%	1	38	0.8
148	Pina Colada mix, nonalcoholic [1Tbs (1 fl oz)]	30	1.1	32	16%	0	7	0.1
149	**Pineapple juice, unsweetened [1 cup (8 fl oz)]**	**250**	**8.8**	**140**	**1%**	**1**	**34**	**0.5**
150	Pineapple juice, with sugar [1 cup (8 fl oz)]	252	8.9	158	1%	1	39	0.5
151	Pineapple juice-non-citrus juice blend, unsweetened, with added vitamin C [1 cup (8 fl oz)]	249	8.8	132	1%	1	33	0.9
152	Pineapple-apple-guava juice, with added vitamin C [1 cup (8 fl oz)]	244	8.6	120	1%	1	30	0.7
153	Pineapple-grapefruit juice drink with vitamin C added [1 cup (8 fl oz)]	250	8.8	118	2%	1	29	0.3
154	Pineapple-grapefruit juice drink, canned [1 cup (8 fl oz)]	250	8.8	118	2%	1	29	0.3
155	Pineapple-grapefruit juice, canned, unsweetened [1 cup (8 fl oz)]	250	8.8	118	2%	1	28	0.4
156	Pineapple-grapefruit juice, canned, with sugar [1 cup (8 fl oz)]	250	8.8	134	1%	1	33	0.4
157	Pineapple-grapefruit juice, frozen (reconstituted with water) [1 cup (8 fl oz)]	250	8.8	116	2%	1	28	0.4
158	Pineapple-orange juice drink [1 cup (8 fl oz)]	250	8.8	45	0%	0	12	0.0
159	Pineapple-orange juice drink with vitamin C added [1 cup (8 fl oz)]	250	8.8	125	0%	3	30	0.3
160	Pineapple-orange juice, canned, unsweetened [1 cup (8 fl oz)]	250	8.8	123	2%	1	30	0.5
161	Pineapple-orange juice, canned, with sugar [1 cup (8 fl oz)]	250	8.8	139	2%	1	34	0.5
162	Pineapple-orange juice, frozen (reconstituted with water) [1 cup (8 fl oz)]	250	8.8	121	1%	1	30	0.5
163	Pineapple-orange-banana juice [1 cup (8 fl oz)]	250	8.8	127	1%	1	31	0.8
164	Pineapple-orange-grapefruit juice drink with vitamin C added (Include Boka Fruit Juice Cooler) [1 cup (8 fl oz)]	251	8.9	122	1%	2	29	0.3
165	Prune juice, unsweetened [1 cup (8 fl oz)]	256	9.0	182	0%	2	45	2.6
166	Prune juice, with sugar [1 cup (8 fl oz)]	258	9.1	199	0%	2	49	2.5
167	Raspberry-flavored drink [1 cup (8 fl oz)]	250	8.8	126	0%	0	32	0.0
168	Soursop (Guanabana) nectar [1 cup (8 fl oz)]	250	8.8	160	1%	0	41	1.2
169	Strawberry juice [1 cup (8 fl oz)]	237	8.4	71	12%	1	17	0.2
170	Strawberry-banana-orange juice [1 cup (8 fl oz)]	234	8.3	126	5%	1	29	2.6
171	Strawberry-flavored drink [1 cup (8 fl oz)]	250	8.8	126	0%	0	32	0.0
172	Strawberry-flavored drink with vitamin C added [1 cup (8 fl oz)]	250	8.8	88	0%	0	22	0.0
173	Tamarind drink, Puerto Rican (Refresco de tamarindo) [1 cup (8 fl oz)]	250	8.8	267	1%	2	69	2.9
174	Tang, dry concentrate [1Tbs]	14	0.5	52	0%	0	13	0.0
175	Tangerine juice, canned, unsweetened [1 cup (8 fl oz)]	247	8.7	106	4%	1	25	0.5

Food #	fat gm	sat fat gm	choles mg	sodium mg	potass mg	% of Daily Value													
						vit A	vit E	vit C	thia-min	ribo-flavin	nia-cin	vit B-6	fol-ate	vit B-12	cal-cium	phos-phorus	magne-sium	iron	zinc
126	0	0	0	1	120	0	0	41	3	1	1	1	7	0	1	1	2	0	0
127	0	0	0	7	478	2	1	163	13	3	3	5	28	0	30	4	6	1	1
128	0	0	0	7	474	2	1	162	13	3	3	6	27	0	3	4	6	1	1
129	0	0	0	1	109	0	0	37	3	1	1	1	6	0	1	1	1	0	0
130	0	0	0	5	199	14	0	83	3	1	2	3	4	0	1	2	2	1	1
131	0	0	0	3	604	2	2	131	12	6	4	22	24	0	2	4	9	2	1
132	0	0	0	6	95	1	0	30	2	1	1	3	2	0	1	1	2	1	1
133	0	0	0	35	110	1	0	115	3	1	1	3	3	0	1	1	2	2	1
134	0	0	0	6	226	1	0	41	4	3	2	8	4	0	1	2	4	3	1
135	0	0	0	8	41	0	0	13	1	1	0	1	1	0	1	0	1	1	1
136	0	0	0	7	74	4	0	19	2	1	1	2	2	0	1	1	2	1	1
137	0	0	0	5	192	14	0	80	3	1	2	3	3	0	1	2	2	1	1
138	0	0	0	6	78	1	0	39	2	2	1	3	2	0	1	1	2	1	1
139	0	0	0	30	409	7	1	14	8	6	3	6	4	0	3	3	6	6	1
140	0	0	0	12	77	3	0	12	1	1	2	1	1	0	2	0	2	5	2
141	0	0	0	17	100	6	0	22	0	2	4	1	1	0	1	1	2	3	1
142	0	0	0	13	78	3	0	13	1	1	2	1	1	0	3	0	2	5	3
143	0	0	0	15	687	39	0	99	0	17	23	7	5	0	1	5	10	4	1
144	0	0	0	10	279	7	0	50	8	7	3	2	1	0	1	5	5	2	1
145	0	0	0	17	100	6	0	22	0	2	4	1	1	0	1	1	2	3	1
146	0	0	0	10	33	0	1	5	0	2	2	2	1	0	1	1	2	4	1
147	0	0	0	9	201	3	0	133	2	4	4	5	1	0	2	2	4	3	1
148	1	0	0	2	21	0	0	2	1	0	0	1	1	0	0	0	1	0	0
149	0	0	0	3	335	0	0	45	9	3	3	12	14	0	4	2	8	4	2
150	0	0	0	3	331	0	0	44	9	3	3	12	14	0	4	2	8	4	2
151	0	0	0	3	361	3	0	147	11	3	3	11	7	0	3	2	6	4	2
152	0	0	0	5	337	3	0	134	7	3	3	7	4	0	2	2	4	4	1
153	0	0	0	35	153	1	0	192	5	2	3	5	7	0	2	2	4	4	1
154	0	0	0	35	153	1	0	192	5	2	3	5	7	0	2	2	4	4	1
155	0	0	0	3	359	0	0	83	8	3	3	7	10	0	3	2	7	3	2
156	0	0	0	3	352	0	0	81	8	3	3	7	10	0	3	2	7	3	2
157	0	0	0	8	339	0	0	95	9	3	3	7	4	0	3	3	7	3	2
158	0	0	0	53	53	0	0	135	2	3	0	0	1	0	2	1	1	4	2
159	0	0	0	8	115	13	0	94	5	3	3	6	7	0	1	1	4	4	1
160	0	0	0	4	386	2	0	94	10	4	4	12	13	0	3	3	8	5	2
161	0	0	0	4	379	2	0	92	9	4	4	11	13	0	3	3	7	5	1
162	0	0	0	8	410	1	0	107	12	3	3	7	17	0	3	3	7	3	2
163	0	0	0	3	433	1	1	100	12	3	3	11	16	0	2	3	7	3	1
164	0	0	0	21	134	7	0	143	5	3	3	6	7	0	2	1	4	4	1
165	0	0	0	10	707	0	0	17	3	11	10	28	0	0	3	6	9	17	4
166	0	0	0	10	698	0	0	17	3	10	10	28	0	0	3	6	9	17	4
167	0	0	0	7	1	0	0	0	0	0	0	0	0	0	0	0	1	0	1
168	0	0	0	11	95	0	1	9	1	1	2	1	1	0	1	1	2	1	1
169	1	0	0	2	393	0	1	112	3	8	2	6	5	0	3	5	6	5	2
170	1	0	0	33	517	0	1	34	19	10	4	20	9	0	3	4	9	7	2
171	0	0	0	7	1	0	0	0	0	0	0	0	0	0	0	0	1	0	1
172	0	0	0	34	1	0	0	47	0	0	0	0	0	0	4	5	1	1	1
173	0	0	0	21	360	0	1	3	16	5	6	2	2	0	5	7	14	9	1
174	0	0	0	1	26	8	4	54	0	5	5	5	0	0	5	2	0	0	0
175	0	0	0	2	440	10	1	121	9	3	3	5	3	0	4	3	5	3	0

Beverages, Dairy, Eggs

Food #	Food Description & Amount	wt gm	wt oz	calo-ries	%cal fat	prot gm	carbo gm	fiber gm
176	Tangerine juice, canned, with sugar [1 cup (8 fl oz)]	249	8.8	125	4%	1	30	0.5
177	Tangerine juice, frozen, unsweetened (reconstituted with water) [1 cup (8 fl oz)]	248	8.7	107	4%	1	25	0.5
178	Tomato and vegetable juice, mostly tomato (Include V-8) [1 cup (8 fl oz)]	242	8.5	46	4%	2	11	1.9
179	Tomato and vegetable juice, mostly tomato, low sodium [1 cup (8 fl oz)]	242	8.5	46	5%	1	11	1.9
180	Tomato juice [1 cup (8 fl oz)]	243	8.6	41	3%	2	10	1.0
181	Tomato juice cocktail [1 cup (8 fl oz)]	243	8.6	46	4%	2	11	1.9
182	Tomato juice with clam or beef juice [1 cup (8 fl oz)]	242	8.5	35	6%	2	8	0.7
183	Tomato juice, low sodium [1 cup (8 fl oz)]	243	8.6	41	3%	2	10	1.9
184	Vegetable and fruit juice drink, with vitamin C added (Include V8 Splash) [1 cup (8 fl oz)]	243	8.6	267	0%	1	68	0.7
185	Vegetable juice, mixed (vegetables other than tomato) [1 cup (8 fl oz)]	246	8.7	70	8%	4	15	4.2
186	Watermelon juice [1 cup (8 fl oz)]	238	8.4	76	12%	1	17	1.2
	Soft Drinks & Miscellaneous Drinks							
200	Ale-type soft drink (Include Ale-8) [1 can (12 fl oz)]	360	12.7	216	2%	1	48	0.0
201	Carbonated water, sweetened (Include tonic, quinine water) [1 can (12 fl oz)]	366	12.9	124	0%	0	32	0.0
202	Carbonated water, unsweetened (Include flavored, club soda, Perrier, seltzer water) [1 can (12 fl oz)]	355	12.5	0	0%	0	0	0.0
203	Chocolate-flavored soda [1 can (12 fl oz)]	369	13.0	155	0%	0	39	0.0
204	Chocolate-flavored soda, sugar-free or sweetened with low-cal sweetener (Include Canfield's Diet Chocolate Fudge Soda) [1 can (12 fl oz)]	355	12.5	4	0%	0	0	0.0
205	**Cola-type soft drink**, plain or flavored, with or without caffeine [1 can (12 fl oz)]	369	13.0	151	0%	0	38	0.0
206	Cola-type soft drink, sugar-free, with or without caffeine [1 can (12 fl oz)]	355	12.5	4	0%	0	0	0.0
207	Corn meal beverage (Atole) [1 cup (8 fl oz)]	249	8.8	210	17%	4	41	0.8
208	Corn meal beverage with chocolate and milk (Champurrado, Atole de Chocolate) [1 cup (8 fl oz)]	254	9.0	277	20%	5	53	1.4
209	Cream soda (Include Almond Smash) [1 can (12 fl oz)]	371	13.1	189	0%	0	49	0.0
210	Cream soda, sugar-free [1 can (12 fl oz)]	355	12.5	0	0%	0	0	0.0
211	Fruit-flavored soft drink (Include orange, lemon, lime, cherry, grape, strawberry, Tom Collins mixer, 7-Up, Sprite, Mellow Yellow, Mountain Dew, Big Red, 7-Up Gold) [1 can (12 fl oz)]	372	13.1	149	0%	0	39	0.0
212	Fruit-flavored soft drink, sugar-free (Include Diet Mountain Dew, Diet 7-Up Gold) [1 can (12 fl oz)]	355	12.5	0	0%	0	0	0.0
213	Ginger ale [1 can (12 fl oz)]	366	12.9	124	0%	0	32	0.0
214	Ginger ale, sugar-free [1 can (12 fl oz)]	355	12.5	0	0%	0	0	0.0
215	Horchata, Puerto Rican (made with almonds, sesame seeds, sugar, water) [1 cup]	240	8.5	246	46%	5	32	2.1
216	Mavi drink [1 can (12 fl oz)]	369	13.0	140	0%	0	38	0.0
217	Oatmeal beverage, Puerto Rican [1 cup (8 fl oz)]	240	8.5	104	2%	1	25	0.5
218	Oatmeal beverage with milk (Atole de avena) [1 cup (8 fl oz)]	255	9.0	209	18%	5	40	0.7
219	Rice beverage, Mexican (Horchata) [1 cup (8 fl oz)]	240	8.5	98	0%	0	25	0.3
220	**Root beer** [1 can (12 fl oz)]	369	13.0	151	0%	0	39	0.0
221	Root beer, sugar-free [1 can (12 fl oz)]	355	12.5	0	0%	0	0	0.0
222	Root beer, made from powdered sugared mix, with vitamin C added, noncarbonated [1 cup (8 fl oz)]	240	8.5	84	0%	0	22	0.0
223	Sugar cane beverage, Puerto Rican [1 cup (8 fl oz)]	247	8.7	169	0%	0	44	0.0
224	Tonic water, sugar-free [1 can (12 fl oz)]	355	12.5	0	0%	0	0	0.0
225	Whiskey sour mix, nonalcoholic (Include Lemix) [1Tbs (1 fl oz)]	31	1.1	26	1%	0	7	0.0
	Coffee & Tea							
280	Bean beverage [1 cup (8 fl oz)]	230	8.1	81	0%	6	14	0.0
281	Cappuccino [1 mug (8 fl oz)]	240	8.5	78	47%	4	6	0.2
282	Cereal beverage (Include Pero, Break Away) [1 mug (8 fl oz)]	237	8.4	10	9%	0	2	0.3
283	Cereal beverage with beet roots, powdered instant, dry (Include Kafix) [1Tbs, dry]	3	0.1	10	9%	0	2	0.3
284	Chicory [1 mug (8 fl oz)]	237	8.4	5	2%	0	1	0.0

Food #	fat gm	sat fat gm	choles mg	sodium mg	potass mg	% of Daily Value													
						vit A	vit E	vit C	thia-min	ribo-flavin	nia-cin	vit B-6	fol-ate	vit B-12	cal-cium	phos-phorus	magne-sium	iron	zinc
176	0	0	0	2	443	10	1	91	10	3	1	4	3	0	4	3	5	3	0
177	0	0	0	2	441	10	1	122	9	3	1	5	2	0	4	3	5	3	0
178	0	0	0	653	467	28	3	112	7	4	9	17	13	0	3	4	7	6	3
179	0	0	0	169	467	28	3	112	6	4	9	17	13	0	3	4	7	6	3
180	0	0	0	877	535	14	7	74	8	4	8	13	12	0	2	5	7	8	2
181	0	0	0	656	469	28	3	112	7	4	9	17	13	0	3	4	7	6	3
182	0	0	0	852	432	10	6	55	6	4	8	10	9	1	2	4	5	6	2
183	0	0	0	24	535	14	7	74	8	4	8	13	12	0	2	5	7	8	2
184	0	0	0	49	437	51	0	101	3	3	1	5	1	0	2	2	2	2	1
185	1	0	0	132	794	199	4	108	11	10	6	15	32	0	14	10	14	20	6
186	1	0	0	5	276	9	1	38	13	3	2	17	1	0	2	2	7	2	1
200	0	0	0	47	29	0	0	3	4	10	20	5	13	1	2	8	6	1	0
201	0	0	0	15	0	0	0	0	0	0	0	0	0	0	0	0	0	0	2
202	0	0	0	75	7	0	0	0	0	0	0	0	0	0	2	0	1	0	2
203	0	0	0	325	185	0	0	0	0	0	0	0	0	0	1	0	1	2	4
204	0	0	0	21	0	0	0	0	1	5	0	0	0	0	1	3	1	1	2
205	0	0	0	15	4	0	0	0	0	0	0	0	0	0	1	4	1	1	0
206	0	0	0	21	0	0	0	0	1	5	0	0	0	0	1	3	1	1	2
207	4	2	15	56	188	3	0	2	9	14	4	3	4	6	14	12	6	4	4
208	6	4	15	60	251	4	1	2	10	15	6	4	4	5	15	14	10	6	5
209	0	0	0	45	4	0	0	0	0	0	0	0	0	0	2	0	1	1	2
210	0	0	0	21	7	0	0	0	0	0	0	0	0	0	1	0	1	1	0
211	0	0	0	41	4	0	0	0	0	0	0	0	0	0	1	0	1	1	1
212	0	0	0	21	7	0	0	0	0	0	0	0	0	0	1	0	1	1	0
213	0	0	0	26	4	0	0	0	0	0	0	0	0	0	1	0	1	4	1
214	0	0	0	21	7	0	0	0	0	0	0	0	0	0	1	0	1	1	0
215	13	1	0	8	158	0	11	0	7	8	5	5	4	0	13	14	20	11	9
216	0	0	0	10	0	0	0	0	0	0	0	0	0	0	1	0	1	0	1
217	0	0	0	7	16	0	0	0	2	1	0	0	0	0	1	2	2	1	1
218	4	2	15	58	189	3	1	2	5	11	1	3	2	6	14	13	6	2	4
219	0	0	0	7	6	0	0	0	1	0	1	0	1	0	1	0	1	2	1
220	0	0	0	48	4	0	0	0	0	0	0	0	0	0	2	0	1	1	2
221	0	0	0	21	7	0	0	0	0	0	0	0	0	0	1	0	1	1	0
222	0	0	0	33	1	0	0	45	0	0	0	0	0	0	4	5	1	1	1
223	0	0	0	43	40	0	0	0	6	2	0	0	0	0	1	1	2	13	1
224	0	0	0	21	7	0	0	0	0	0	0	0	0	0	1	0	1	1	0
225	0	0	0	32	9	0	0	1	0	0	0	0	0	0	0	0	0	0	0
280	0	0	0	5	775	0	0	0	23	14	7	12	35	0	4	21	28	16	6
281	4	3	17	62	250	4	0	2	3	12	2	2	1	6	15	11	6	1	3
282	0	0	0	9	56	0	0	0	1	0	3	1	0	0	1	2	2	1	1
283	0	0	0	2	55	0	0	0	1	0	3	1	0	0	0	2	2	1	0
284	0	0	0	8	80	0	0	0	0	0	3	0	0	0	1	1	2	1	1

Beverages, Dairy, Eggs

Food #	Food Description & Amount	wt gm	wt oz	calo-ries	%cal fat	prot gm	carbo gm	fiber gm
285	Coffee and chicory, dry powder [1Tbs, dry]	3	0.1	7	2%	0	1	0.0
286	Coffee and chicory, made from ground [1 mug (8 fl oz)]	237	8.4	5	0%	0	1	0.0
287	Coffee and chicory, made from powdered instant (Include Luzianne) [1 mug (8 fl oz)]	238	8.4	5	2%	0	1	0.0
288	Coffee and cocoa (mocha) mix, dry powder with whitener and low-cal sweetener (Include Sugar Free Irish Mocha Mint, Suisse Mocha) [1Tbs, dry]	5	0.2	24	60%	0	2	0.1
289	Coffee and cocoa (mocha) mix, dry powder with whitener and sugar (Include Irish Mocha Mint, Suisse Mocha) [1Tbs, dry]	10	0.4	45	33%	0	7	0.1
290	Coffee and cocoa (mocha), made from powdered mix, with whitener and low-cal sweetener (Include Sugar Free Irish Mocha Mint, Suisse Mocha) [1 mug (8 fl oz)]	238	8.4	35	60%	1	4	0.2
291	Coffee and cocoa (mocha), made from powdered mix, with whitener and sugar (Include Irish Mocha Mint, Suisse Mocha) [1 mug (8 fl oz)]	238	8.4	64	33%	1	11	0.2
292	Coffee and cocoa (mocha), made from powdered mix, with whitener and low-cal sweetener [1 mug (8 fl oz)]	238	8.4	92	53%	2	9	0.4
293	**Coffee, made from ground** (Include flavored) [1 mug (8 fl oz)]	**237**	**8.4**	**5**	**0%**	**0**	**1**	**0.0**
294	Coffee, made from liquid concentrate [1 mug (8 fl oz)]	237	8.4	3	2%	0	1	0.0
295	Coffee, made from powdered mix, with whitener and low calorie sweetener, instant (Include Sugar Free Cafe au Lait, French Style Coffee, Orange Cappuccino, Cafe Amaretto, Viennese Coffee mixes) [1 mug (8 fl oz)]	238	8.4	75	60%	1	8	0.4
296	Coffee, made from powdered mix, with whitener and sugar, instant (Include Cafe au Lait, French Style Coffee, Orange Cappuccino, Cafe Amaretto, Viennese coffee mixes) [1 mug (8 fl oz)]	238	8.4	75	43%	1	11	0.0
297	**Coffee, made from powdered** (Include flavored) [1 mug (8 fl oz)]	**238**	**8.4**	**5**	**2%**	**0**	**1**	**0.0**
298	Coffee, Cuban (espresso with brown sugar) [1 espresso cup (2 fl oz)]	61	2.1	17	0%	0	4	0.0
299	Coffee, dry powder (Include Kava) [1Tbs, dry]	3	0.1	6	1%	0	1	0.0
300	Coffee, dry powder, with whitener and low-cal sweetener (Include Sugar Free Cafe au Lait, French Style Coffee, Orange Cappuccino, Cafe Amaretto, Viennese Coffee Mixes) [1Tbs, dry]	5	0.2	22	60%	0	2	0.0
301	Coffee, dry powder, with whitener and sugar (Include Cafe au Lait, French Style Coffee, Orange Cappuccino, Cafe Amaretto, Viennese Coffee Mixes) [1Tbs, dry]	10	0.4	48	43%	0	7	0.0
302	Coffee, **espresso** [1 espresso cup (2 fl oz]	59	2.1	5	18%	0	1	0.0
303	Coffee, **latte** (espresso and whole milk) [1 mug (8 fl oz)]	242	8.5	97	48%	5	8	0.0
304	Coffee, liquid concentrate [1Tbs]	15	0.5	7	2%	0	1	0.0
305	Coffee, Mexican, unsweetened (no milk; not cafe con leche) [1 mug (8 fl oz)]	237	8.4	5	0%	0	1	0.0
306	Coffee, Mexican, with brown sugar (no milk; not cafe con leche) [1 mug (8 fl oz)]	243	8.6	69	0%	0	18	0.0
307	Coffee, **mocha** [1 mug (8 fl oz)]	243	8.6	177	23%	5	32	0.7
308	Coffee, pre-lightened, no sugar, from vending machine [6 fl oz]	177	6.2	26	50%	0	3	0.0
309	Coffee, presweetened with sugar, from vending machine [6 fl oz]	177	6.2	29	0%	0	7	0.0
310	Coffee, presweetened with sugar, pre-lightened, from vending machine) [6 fl oz]	177	6.2	50	26%	0	9	0.0
311	Coffee, Turkish, with sugar [1 Turkish cup (4 fl oz)]	121	4.3	47	0%	0	12	0.0
312	Coffee, with cereal (including barley) [1 mug (8 fl oz)]	237	8.4	5	2%	0	1	0.0
313	Corn beverage [1 mug (8 fl oz)]	242	8.5	70	0%	2	21	0.0
314	Mate, sugared beverage made from dried green leaves (Include Paraguay tea) [1 mug (8 fl oz)]	237	8.4	48	0%	0	13	0.0
315	Postum [1 mug (8 fl oz)]	240	8.5	12	0%	0	2	0.0
316	Postum, dry powder [1Tbs, dry]	7	0.2	23	9%	0	6	0.6
317	Rice beverage/tea, made from brown rice, with oil, salt (Include rice tea, Rice Dream beverage) [1 mug (8 fl oz)]	252	8.9	148	13%	3	29	2.3
318	Tea, chamomile [1 mug (8 fl oz)]	237	8.4	2	0%	0	0	0.0
319	Tea, herb [1 mug (8 fl oz)]	237	8.4	2	0%	0	0	0.0
320	Tea, leaf, presweetened with low-cal sweetener (Include flavored) [1 mug (8 fl oz)]	237	8.4	6	0%	0	2	0.0
321	Tea, leaf, presweetened with sugar (Include flavored) [1 mug (8 fl oz)]	237	8.4	48	0%	0	13	0.0
322	**Tea, leaf** (Include tea bags, green, black, spiced, and flavored teas) [1 mug (8 fl oz)]	**237**	**8.4**	**2**	**0%**	**0**	**1**	**0.0**
323	Tea, made from caraway seeds [1 mug (8 fl oz)]	237	8.4	2	0%	0	0	0.0
324	Tea, made from frozen concentrate (Include flavored) [1 mug (8 fl oz)]	237	8.4	2	0%	0	1	0.0

Food #	fat gm	sat fat gm	choles mg	sodium mg	potass mg	vit A	vit E	vit C	thia-min	ribo-flavin	nia-cin	vit B-6	fol-ate	vit B-12	cal-cium	phos-phorus	magne-sium	iron	zinc
285	0	0	0	1	95	0	0	0	0	0	4	0	0	0	0	1	2	1	0
286	0	0	0	5	128	0	0	0	0	0	3	0	0	0	0	0	3	1	0
287	0	0	0	8	77	0	0	0	0	0	3	0	0	0	1	1	2	1	1
288	2	1	0	16	95	0	0	0	0	3	1	0	0	0	0	2	2	1	1
289	2	1	0	27	105	0	0	0	0	0	1	0	0	0	0	3	2	1	1
290	2	2	0	30	140	0	0	0	0	5	2	0	0	0	1	3	3	2	1
291	2	2	0	45	149	0	0	0	0	0	2	0	0	0	1	4	3	2	1
292	5	5	0	61	322	0	0	0	1	11	4	0	0	0	2	8	6	3	2
293	0	0	0	5	128	0	0	0	0	0	3	0	0	0	0	0	3	1	0
294	0	0	0	8	50	0	0	0	0	0	2	0	0	0	1	0	2	0	1
295	5	4	0	57	297	0	0	0	0	10	3	0	0	0	2	7	5	3	2
296	4	3	0	79	161	0	0	0	1	0	3	0	0	0	1	4	3	1	1
297	0	0	0	8	77	0	0	0	0	0	3	0	0	0	1	1	2	1	1
298	0	0	0	3	45	0	0	0	0	0	1	0	0	0	0	0	1	1	0
299	0	0	0	1	95	0	0	0	0	2	4	0	0	0	0	1	2	1	0
300	1	1	0	42	51	0	0	0	0	0	1	0	0	0	0	1	1	0	0
301	2	2	0	46	103	0	0	0	0	0	2	0	0	0	0	3	1	0	0
302	0	0	0	8	68	0	0	0	0	6	15	0	0	0	0	0	12	0	0
303	5	3	21	78	282	5	1	2	4	15	2	3	2	7	19	15	6	1	4
304	0	0	0	1	106	0	0	0	0	0	4	0	0	0	0	1	2	1	0
305	0	0	0	5	128	0	0	0	0	0	3	0	0	0	0	0	3	1	0
306	0	0	0	11	182	0	0	0	0	0	3	0	0	0	2	1	4	2	1
307	5	3	16	122	379	8	0	2	3	21	18	3	2	7	17	19	24	6	6
308	1	1	0	13	89	0	0	0	0	0	2	0	0	0	1	2	2	1	1
309	0	0	0	6	55	0	0	0	0	0	2	0	0	0	1	0	2	0	0
310	1	1	0	13	86	0	0	0	0	1	2	0	0	0	1	2	2	1	1
311	0	0	0	2	59	0	0	0	0	0	1	0	0	0	0	0	1	0	0
312	0	0	0	8	76	0	0	0	0	0	3	0	0	0	1	1	2	1	1
313	0	0	0	338	203	1	0	15	3	4	6	2	13	0	1	7	6	0	5
314	0	0	0	7	83	0	0	0	0	2	0	0	3	0	0	0	2	0	0
315	0	0	0	10	58	0	0	0	1	0	3	1	0	0	1	2	2	1	0
316	0	0	0	5	127	0	0	0	3	0	6	3	0	0	0	4	4	2	0
317	2	0	0	88	51	0	4	0	6	2	10	9	1	0	2	10	14	3	6
318	0	0	0	2	21	0	1	0	2	1	0	0	0	0	0	0	1	1	1
319	0	0	0	2	21	0	0	0	2	1	0	0	0	0	0	0	1	1	1
320	0	0	0	7	87	0	0	0	0	2	0	0	3	0	0	0	2	0	0
321	0	0	0	7	84	0	0	0	0	2	0	0	3	0	0	0	2	0	0
322	0	0	0	7	88	0	0	0	0	2	0	0	3	0	0	0	2	0	0
323	0	0	0	2	21	0	0	0	2	1	0	0	0	0	0	0	1	1	1
324	0	0	0	7	88	0	0	0	0	2	0	0	3	0	0	0	2	0	0

Beverages, Dairy, Eggs

Food #	Food Description & Amount	wt gm	wt oz	calo-ries	%cal fat	prot gm	carbo gm	fiber gm
325	Tea, made from frozen concentrate, presweetened with low calorie sweetener (Include flavored) [1 mug (8 fl oz)]	237	8.4	6	0%	0	2	0.0
326	Tea, made from powdered instant (Include flavored) [1 mug (8 fl oz)]	237	8.4	4	1%	0	1	0.0
327	Tea, made from powdered instant, presweetened with low-cal sweetener (Include flavored, Lipton Fruit Tea,D402 Crystal Light Fruit Tea) [1 mug (8 fl oz)]	237	8.4	5	2%	0	1	0.0
328	Tea, made from powdered instant, presweetened with sugar (Include flavored) [1 mug (8 fl oz)]	237	8.4	23	0%	0	6	0.0
329	Tea, powdered instant, with sugar, dry [1Tbs, dry]	3	0.1	11	0%	0	3	0.0
330	Tea, powdered instant, unsweetened, dry (Include flavored) [1Tbs, dry]	2	0.1	5	1%	0	1	0.1
331	Tea, Russian (made with sugar, orange drink mix, powdered tea, cloves, cinnamon) [1 mug (8 fl oz)]	237	8.4	138	0%	0	35	0.1
Alcoholic Beverages								
380	Alexander [1 cocktail (2.5 fl oz)] (18 gm alcohol)	74	2.6	176	9%	0	8	0.0
381	Bacardi cocktail [1 cocktail (2 fl oz)] (14 gm alcohol)	63	2.2	117	0%	0	6	0.1
382	Bailey's Irish Cream (Include liqueurs with cream) [1 fl oz] (5 gm alcohol)	31	1.1	101	43%	1	6	0.0
383	Beer (Include ale) [1 can or bottle (12 fl oz)] (13 gm alcohol)	360	12.7	148	0%	1	13	0.7
384	Beer, lite [1 can or bottle (12 fl oz)] (12 gm alcohol)	360	12.7	101	0%	1	5	0.0
385	Beer, nonalcoholic [1 can or bottle (12 fl oz)] (1 gm alcohol)	360	12.7	216	2%	1	48	0.0
386	Black Russian [1 cocktail (3 fl oz)] (26 gm alcohol)	90	3.2	244	0%	0	16	0.0
387	Bloody Mary [1 cocktail (5 fl oz)] (15 gm alcohol)	148	5.2	123	1%	1	5	0.4
388	Bourbon and soda (Include scotch and soda, rum and soda) [1 cocktail (4 fl oz)] (15 gm alcohol)	116	4.1	105	0%	0	0	0.0
389	Brandy (Include applejack, cognac, tequila) [1 fl oz] (9 gm alcohol)	28	1.0	65	0%	0	0	0.0
390	Champagne punch [4 fl oz] (10 gm alcohol)	116	4.1	100	0%	0	7	0.0
391	Coquito, Puerto Rican (coconut, rum) [4 fl oz] (13 gm alcohol)	125	4.4	301	27%	5	20	0.3
392	Daiquiri [1 cocktail (2 fl oz)] (14 gm alcohol)	61	2.2	113	0%	0	4	0.1
393	Eggnog, alcoholic (Include Mexican eggnog, Rompope) [1 cup (8 fl oz)] (17 gm alcohol)	243	8.6	407	29%	9	37	0.0
394	Frozen daiquiri [1 drink (8 fl oz)] (21 gm alcohol)	231	8.1	430	0%	0	16	0.0
395	Fuzzy Navel (peach schnapps and orange juice) [1 cocktail (7 fl oz)] (14 gm alcohol)	213	7.5	254	1%	1	38	0.3
396	Gibson [1 cocktail (2.5 fl oz)] (23 gm alcohol)	71	2.5	158	0%	0	0	0.0
397	Gimlet [1 cocktail (2.4 fl oz)] (19 gm alcohol)	71	2.5	132	0%	0	1	0.1
398	Gin and Tonic [1 cocktail (7.5 fl oz)] (16 gm alcohol)	225	7.9	171	0%	0	16	0.1
399	Gin fizz [1 cocktail (7.5 fl oz)] (17 gm alcohol)	225	7.9	139	0%	0	6	0.1
400	Gin Rickey [1 cocktail (7 fl oz)] (16 gm alcohol)	205	7.2	114	0%	0	1	0.1
401	Gin [1 jigger (1.5 fl oz)] (16 gm alcohol)	42	1.5	110	0%	0	0	0.0
402	Glug (Include glogg, gluhwein) [1 drink (4 fl oz)] (10 gm alcohol)	116	4.1	113	0%	0	11	0.0
403	Gold Cadillac [1 cocktail (4.3 fl oz)] (25 gm alcohol)	125	4.4	377	9%	1	44	0.0
404	Grain alcohol [1 fl oz] (23 gm alcohol)	24	0.8	153	0%	0	0	0.0
405	Grasshopper [1 cocktail (2 fl oz)] (10 gm alcohol)	64	2.3	164	20%	1	15	0.0
406	Highball [1 cocktail (5.5 fl oz)] (15 gm alcohol)	160	5.6	105	0%	0	0	0.0
407	Irish Coffee (Include Coffee Royale) [6 fl oz] (12 gm alcohol)	158	5.6	154	45%	1	4	0.0
408	Liqueur or Cordial (Include amaretto, anisette, benedictine, chartreuse, cointreau, creme de menthe, curacao, drambuie, grenadine, kahlua, kirsch, kummel, sloe gin, tia maria, triple sec) [1 fl oz] (8 gm alcohol)	30	1.1	106	1%	0	13	0.0
409	Long Island iced tea [1 drink (5 fl oz)] (15 gm alcohol)	150	5.3	142	0%	0	11	0.1
410	Mai Tai [1 cocktail (4 fl oz)] (27 gm alcohol)	126	4.4	305	0%	0	29	0.1
411	Manhattan [1 cocktail (2 fl oz)] (17 gm alcohol)	57	2.0	128	0%	0	2	0.0
412	Margarita [1 cocktail (2.5 fl oz)] (18 gm alcohol)	77	2.7	170	0%	0	11	0.1
413	Martini [1 cocktail (2.4 fl oz)] (23 gm alcohol)	71	2.5	158	0%	0	0	0.0
414	Mint julep [1 cocktail (2.3 fl oz)] (20 gm alcohol)	65	2.3	156	0%	0	4	0.0
415	Old fashioned [1 cocktail (2 fl oz)] (20 gm alcohol)	60	2.1	156	0%	0	4	0.0
416	Pina Colada [1 cocktail (4.3 fl oz)] (13 gm alcohol)	133	4.7	231	10%	1	30	0.4
417	Rum and cola [1 cocktail (7 fl oz)] (14 gm alcohol)	211	7.4	159	0%	0	16	0.1

Food #	fat gm	sat fat gm	choles mg	sodium mg	potass mg	vit A	vit E	vit C	thia-min	ribo-flavin	nia-cin	vit B-6	fol-ate	vit B-12	cal-cium	phos-phorus	magne-sium	iron	zinc
												% of Daily Value							
325	0	0	0	7	87	0	0	0	0	2	0	0	3	0	0	0	2	0	0
326	0	0	0	14	48	0	0	0	0	1	0	0	0	0	1	0	1	0	1
327	0	0	0	24	41	0	0	0	0	1	0	0	1	0	1	0	1	1	1
328	0	0	0	8	60	0	0	0	0	0	1	0	0	0	1	0	1	0	1
329	0	0	0	1	29	0	0	0	0	0	0	0	0	0	0	0	0	0	0
330	0	0	0	3	139	0	0	0	0	1	1	1	1	0	0	1	2	0	0
331	0	0	0	8	68	8	4	55	0	6	6	6	0	0	6	3	1	1	1
380	2	1	6	8	23	2	0	0	1	1	0	0	0	1	2	2	0	0	1
381	0	0	0	11	12	0	0	2	1	0	0	0	0	0	0	0	0	0	0
382	5	3	5	29	10	1	0	0	0	1	0	0	0	1	0	2	0	0	0
383	0	0	0	18	90	0	0	0	1	6	8	9	5	1	2	4	5	1	0
384	0	0	0	11	65	0	0	0	2	6	7	6	4	1	2	4	5	1	1
385	0	0	0	47	29	0	0	3	4	10	20	5	13	1	2	8	6	1	0
386	0	0	0	3	12	0	0	0	0	0	0	0	0	0	0	0	0	0	0
387	0	0	0	332	216	5	3	34	3	2	3	5	5	0	1	2	3	3	1
388	0	0	0	16	2	0	0	0	0	0	0	0	0	0	0	0	0	0	1
389	0	0	0	0	1	0	0	0	0	0	0	0	0	0	0	0	0	0	0
390	0	0	0	11	72	0	0	0	0	1	0	1	0	0	1	1	2	2	1
391	9	6	69	68	227	6	1	3	4	13	1	2	3	5	15	16	5	3	5
392	0	0	0	3	13	0	0	2	1	0	0	0	0	0	0	0	0	0	0
393	13	6	367	84	249	20	3	2	6	23	1	7	9	18	21	27	6	6	10
394	0	0	0	12	49	0	0	6	2	0	0	1	1	0	1	1	1	2	1
395	0	0	0	4	313	1	1	107	9	2	2	4	18	0	1	3	4	1	1
396	0	0	0	2	14	0	0	0	0	0	0	0	0	0	0	0	0	0	0
397	0	0	0	3	13	0	0	2	1	0	0	0	0	0	0	0	0	0	0
398	0	0	0	10	12	0	0	2	0	0	0	0	0	0	0	0	0	0	1
399	0	0	0	38	20	0	0	7	0	0	0	0	0	0	1	0	1	0	1
400	0	0	0	32	21	0	0	7	0	0	0	0	0	0	1	0	1	0	1
401	0	0	0	0	1	0	0	0	0	0	0	0	0	0	0	0	0	0	0
402	0	0	0	9	95	0	0	0	0	1	0	1	0	0	1	2	3	2	1
403	4	2	11	18	52	3	0	0	1	3	0	1	0	2	3	3	1	0	1
404	0	0	0	0	0	0	0	0	0	0	0	0	0	0	0	0	0	0	0
405	4	2	11	14	39	3	0	0	1	3	0	1	0	2	3	3	1	0	1
406	0	0	0	25	3	0	0	0	0	0	0	0	0	0	1	0	0	0	1
407	8	5	29	10	73	9	0	0	0	1	1	0	0	1	2	2	2	0	1
408	0	0	0	2	5	0	0	0	0	0	0	0	0	0	0	0	0	0	0
409	0	0	0	7	17	0	0	6	1	0	0	0	0	0	0	0	1	1	0	0
410	0	0	0	11	24	0	0	2	1	0	0	0	0	0	0	1	1	1	0
411	0	0	0	2	14	0	0	0	0	0	0	0	0	0	0	0	0	0	0
412	0	0	0	4	15	0	0	2	1	0	0	0	0	0	0	0	0	0	0
413	0	0	0	2	14	0	0	0	0	0	0	0	0	0	0	0	0	0	0
414	0	0	0	1	1	0	0	0	0	0	0	0	0	0	0	0	0	0	0
415	0	0	0	1	1	0	0	0	0	0	0	0	0	0	0	0	0	0	0
416	3	2	0	8	94	0	0	11	2	1	1	3	4	0	1	1	3	1	1
417	0	0	0	11	25	0	0	3	1	0	0	0	1	0	1	2	1	1	0

Beverages, Dairy, Eggs

Food #	Food Description & Amount	wt gm	wt oz	calo- ries	%cal fat	prot gm	carbo gm	fiber gm
418	Rum [1 jigger (1.5 fl oz)] (14 gm alcohol)	42	1.5	97	0%	0	0	0.0
419	Rum, hot buttered [1 drink (8.7 fl oz)] (28 gm alcohol)	251	8.9	315	34%	0	4	0.2
420	Rum cooler [1 bottle (12.6 fl oz)] (13 gm alcohol)	390	13.8	217	2%	1	33	0.3
421	Sangria [1 drink (8 fl oz)] (11 gm alcohol)	228	8.0	156	0%	0	21	0.1
422	Sangria, Puerto Rican style [1 drink (6.2 fl oz)] (10 gm alcohol)	180	6.3	120	0%	0	16	0.1
423	Screwdriver (Include Harvey Wallbanger, Slo-Screw) [1 cocktail (7 fl oz)] (15 gm alcohol)	213	7.5	182	1%	1	18	0.3
424	Singapore Sling [1 cocktail (7.5 fl oz)] (26 gm alcohol)	225	7.9	229	0%	0	12	0.1
425	Sloe gin fizz [1 cocktail (7.4 fl oz)] (16 gm alcohol)	222	7.8	122	0%	0	3	0.1
426	Stinger [1 cocktail (3 fl oz)] (29 gm alcohol)	92	3.2	283	0%	0	21	0.0
427	Tequila Sunrise [1 cocktail (5.5 fl oz)] (19 gm alcohol)	172	6.1	189	1%	1	15	0.2
428	Tom Collins (Include Vodka Collins) [1 cocktail (7.4 fl oz)] (16 gm alcohol)	222	7.8	122	0%	0	3	0.1
429	Vodka [1 jigger (1.5 fl oz)] (14 gm alcohol)	42	1.5	97	0%	0	0	0.0
430	Whiskey (Include bourbon, scotch, rye) [1 jigger (1.5 fl oz)] (15 gm alcohol)	42	1.5	105	0%	0	0	0.0
431	Whiskey sour (Include scotch sour, vodka sour, soda sour, apricot sour, brandy sour) [1 cocktail (3 fl oz)] (15 gm alcohol)	90	3.2	123	1%	0	5	0.2
432	White Russian [1 cocktail (3.3 fl oz)] (26 gm alcohol)	100	3.5	257	4%	0	17	0.0
433	Wine cooler [1 drink (7 fl oz)] (8 gm alcohol)	210	7.4	105	0%	0	12	0.1
434	Wine spritzer [1 drink (5 fl oz)] (8 gm alcohol)	146	5.1	61	0%	0	1	0.0
435	Wine, Chinese [1 wine glass (3.5 fl oz)] (9 gm alcohol)	100	3.5	70	0%	0	1	0.0
436	Wine, cooking (after cooking) [1 fl oz] (0 gm alcohol)	29	1.0	8	0%	0	0	0.0
437	Wine, dessert, dry [1 wine glass (3.5 fl oz)] (16 gm alcohol)	103	3.6	130	0%	0	4	0.0
438	Wine, dessert, sweet (Include marsala, port, tokay, madeira, muscatel, angelica, sherry, sweet vermouth) [1 wine glass (3.5 fl oz)] (16 gm alcohol)	103	3.6	158	0%	0	12	0.0
439	Wine, red, dry, table [1 wine glass (3.5 fl oz)] (10 gm alcohol)	103	3.6	74	0%	0	2	0.0
440	Wine, rose, dry, table [1 wine glass (3.5 fl oz)] (10 gm alcohol)	103	3.6	73	0%	0	1	0.0
441	Wine, white, dry, table [1 wine glass (3.5 fl oz)] (10 gm alcohol)	103	3.6	70	0%	0	1	0.0
442	Wine, light [1 wine glass (3.5 fl oz)] (7 gm alcohol)	103	3.6	52	0%	1	1	0.0
443	Wine, light, nonalcoholic [1 wine glass (3.5 fl oz)] (0 gm alcohol)	110	3.9	7	0%	1	1	0.0
444	Wine, nonalcoholic [1 wine glass (3.5l oz)] (0 gm alcohol)	102	3.6	6	0%	1	1	0.0
445	Wine, rice (Include sake) [1 fl oz] (5 gm alcohol)	29	1.0	39	0%	0	1	0.0
446	Zombie [1 cocktail (6.5 fl oz)] (46 gm alcohol)	193	6.8	372	0%	0	13	0.1
	Milk, Milk-Based Drinks, Cream							
480	Buttermilk, dry [2Tbs]	15	0.5	58	13%	5	7	0.0
481	Buttermilk, reconstituted from dry [1 cup (8 fl oz)]	245	8.6	93	13%	8	12	0.0
482	Buttermilk (Include Kefir milk) [1 cup (8 fl oz)]	245	8.6	99	20%	8	12	0.0
483	Buttermilk, 2% fat [1 cup (8 fl oz)]	245	8.6	137	32%	10	13	0.0
484	**Chocolate milk** (whole milk with 2Tbs chocolate syrup) [1 cup (8 fl oz)]	250	8.8	206	33%	8	30	0.6
485	Chocolate milk (2%-fat milk with 2Tbs chocolate syrup) [1 cup (8 fl oz)]	250	8.8	163	14%	8	30	0.6
486	Chocolate milk (non-fat milk with 2Tbs chocolate syrup) [1 cup (8 fl oz)]	250	8.8	148	4%	8	30	0.6
487	Chocolate, instant, dry mix, fortified with vitamins/minerals, Puerto Rican style [1Tbs]	8	0.3	29	9%	0	7	0.1
488	Chocolate drink, Spanish/Puerto Rican style (chocolate espanol) (Include chocolate milk beverage made with evaporated milk) [1 cup (8 fl oz)]	240	8.5	277	54%	10	25	1.1
489	Chocolate-flavored drink, whey- and milk-based (Include Yoo-hoo) [1 bottle (9 fl oz)]	274	9.7	145	7%	3	28	1.1
490	Cocoa, hot chocolate, not from dry mix (made with whole milk) [1 cup (8 fl oz)]	250	8.8	193	27%	10	29	2.0
491	Cocoa/chocolate powder with sugar (Include Hershey's Instant, Nestle's Quik) [1Tbs]	8	0.3	29	8%	0	8	0.5
492	Cocoa/chocolate powder with low-cal sweetener [1Tbs]	7	0.2	22	25%	1	4	1.6
493	Cocoa/chocolate powder with nonfat dry milk and sugar (Include Swiss Miss Hot Chocolate; Hershey's Hot Chocolate; Nestle's Hot Chocolate) [1 envelope]	28	1.0	101	10%	3	22	0.3
494	Cocoa/chocolate powder with nonfat dry milk and low-cal sweetener (Include Swiss Miss Sugar-Free Hot Cocoa Mix, Alba Sugar-Free Hot Cocoa Mix) [1 envelope]	17	0.6	54	8%	4	10	0.4
495	Cocoa beverage, Puerto Rican style (whole milk with 5 tsp sugar-cocoa mix fortified with vitamins and minerals) [1 cup (8 fl oz)]	250	8.8	212	35%	9	27	0.2

Food #	fat gm	sat fat gm	choles mg	sodium mg	potass mg	% of Daily Value													
						vit A	vit E	vit C	thia-min	ribo-flavin	nia-cin	vit B-6	fol-ate	vit B-12	cal-cium	phos-phorus	magne-sium	iron	zinc
418	0	0	0	0	1	0	0	0	0	0	0	0	0	0	0	0	0	0	0
419	12	7	31	7	9	11	1	0	1	1	0	0	0	0	1	1	1	1	1
420	1	0	0	14	213	1	1	32	3	4	2	3	4	0	2	2	5	5	2
421	0	0	0	26	156	0	0	19	2	2	1	2	3	0	2	2	4	3	1
422	0	0	0	12	64	0	0	14	1	1	0	1	1	0	1	1	2	1	1
423	0	0	0	2	326	1	1	111	9	2	2	4	19	0	2	3	4	1	1
424	0	0	0	33	19	0	0	6	1	0	0	0	0	0	1	0	1	0	1
425	0	0	0	38	20	0	0	6	1	0	0	0	0	0	1	0	1	0	1
426	0	0	0	3	1	0	0	0	0	0	0	0	0	0	0	0	0	0	0
427	0	0	0	7	179	2	0	55	4	2	2	4	5	0	1	2	3	3	1
428	0	0	0	38	20	0	0	6	1	0	0	0	0	0	1	0	1	0	1
429	0	0	0	0	1	0	0	0	0	0	0	0	0	0	0	0	0	0	0
430	0	0	0	0	1	0	0	0	0	0	0	0	0	0	0	0	0	0	0
431	0	0	0	10	48	0	0	19	1	0	0	1	1	0	1	1	1	0	0
432	1	1	4	7	25	1	0	0	1	1	0	0	0	1	1	1	1	0	1
433	0	0	0	18	95	0	0	6	1	1	0	1	1	0	1	1	3	3	1
434	0	0	0	19	79	0	0	0	0	1	0	1	0	0	1	1	2	2	1
435	0	0	0	8	89	0	0	0	0	1	0	1	0	0	1	1	3	2	0
436	0	0	0	182	26	0	0	0	0	0	0	0	0	0	0	0	1	1	0
437	0	0	0	9	95	0	0	0	1	1	1	0	0	0	1	1	2	1	0
438	0	0	0	9	95	0	0	0	1	1	1	0	0	0	1	1	2	1	0
439	0	0	0	5	115	0	0	0	0	2	0	2	1	0	1	1	3	2	1
440	0	0	0	5	102	0	0	0	0	1	0	1	0	0	1	2	3	2	0
441	0	0	0	5	82	0	0	0	0	0	0	1	0	0	1	1	3	2	0
442	0	0	0	7	91	0	0	0	0	1	1	1	0	0	1	2	3	2	1
443	0	0	0	8	97	0	0	0	0	1	1	1	0	0	1	2	3	2	1
444	0	0	0	7	89	0	0	0	0	1	1	1	0	0	1	2	3	2	1
445	0	0	0	1	7	0	0	0	0	0	0	0	0	0	0	0	0	0	0
446	0	0	0	6	51	0	0	7	2	1	1	1	2	0	1	1	1	1	1
480	1	1	10	78	239	1	0	1	4	14	1	3	2	10	18	14	4	0	4
481	1	1	17	131	382	1	0	2	6	22	1	4	3	15	29	22	7	1	7
482	2	1	9	257	371	2	0	4	6	22	1	4	3	9	29	22	7	1	7
483	5	3	20	211	441	5	0	6	8	30	1	4	4	15	35	20	8	1	4
484	8	5	29	138	403	7	1	4	6	22	1	5	3	13	26	25	13	5	7
485	3	2	9	141	413	13	0	4	6	22	1	5	3	13	27	25	13	5	7
486	1	0	4	144	433	13	0	4	5	19	1	4	3	14	27	26	12	4	7
487	0	0	0	48	95	31	0	20	16	19	20	17	2	0	4	3	2	8	1
488	17	10	39	146	458	7	2	4	4	27	2	3	2	3	35	30	14	5	9
489	1	1	3	206	206	15	0	10	2	10	10	4	1	8	10	10	10	2	4
490	6	4	20	128	500	14	1	4	7	26	2	6	4	15	32	29	18	6	10
491	0	0	0	18	50	0	0	0	0	1	0	0	0	0	0	1	2	1	1
492	1	0	0	17	145	0	0	0	0	2	0	0	0	0	1	3	5	2	2
493	1	1	1	141	199	0	0	1	2	9	1	2	0	6	9	9	6	2	3
494	1	0	1	191	459	0	0	0	3	14	1	3	1	5	10	15	9	5	4
495	8	5	32	230	585	85	1	53	46	70	51	48	7	14	36	29	12	20	7

Beverages, Dairy, Eggs

Food #	Food Description & Amount	wt gm	wt oz	calories	%cal fat	prot gm	carbo gm	fiber gm
496	Cocoa beverage: 2%-fat milk with 2½ tsp sugar-cocoa mix (Include Nestle's Quik, Hershey's Instant) [1 cup (8 fl oz)]	250	8.8	168	16%	8	30	1.2
497	Cocoa beverage: nonfat milk with 2½ tsp sugar-cocoa mix (Include Nestle's Quik, Hershey's Instant) [1 cup (8 fl oz)]	250	8.8	152	6%	9	30	1.2
498	Cocoa beverage: whole milk with 2½ tsp sugar-cocoa mix (Include Nestle's Quik, Hershey's Instant) [1 cup (8 fl oz)]	250	8.8	213	35%	8	29	1.2
499	Cocoa powder, unsweetened, (no dry milk) [1Tbs]	5	0.2	12	54%	1	3	1.8
500	Cocoa beverage: water added to cocoa mix with nonfat dry milk and low cal sweetener (Include Sugar-Free Hot Cocoa Mix, Swiss Miss, Alba) [1 packet plus 6 fl oz water]	197	6.9	49	8%	4	9	0.4
501	Cocoa beverage: water added to high-calcium cocoa mix with nonfat dry milk and low-cal sweetener (Include Alba High Calcium Cocoa) [1 packet plus 6 fl oz water]	197	6.9	62	7%	5	10	0.5
502	Cocoa beverage: water added to cocoa mix with sugar, and dry milk (Include Swiss Miss Hot Chocolate, Hershey's Hot Chocolate, Nestle's Hot Chocolate, Carnation Hot Chocolate) [1 oz packet plus 6 fl oz water]	206	7.3	102	10%	3	22	0.3
503	Cocoa-whey powder with low-cal sweetener, fortified, not reconstituted (Include Ovaltine Sugar-Free Hot Cocoa) [1 envelope]	12	0.4	37	8%	3	7	0.3
504	Cocoa-whey beverage: water added to dry mix with low-cal sweetener, fortified (Include Ovaltine Sugar-Free Hot Cocoa) [1 cup (8 fl oz)]	249	8.8	49	8%	4	9	0.4
505	Cocoa-whey beverage: 2%-fat milk added to dry mix with low-cal sweetener (Include Sugar-free Nestle's Quik, Swiss Miss Sugar-Free Chocolate Milk Maker) [1 cup]	250	8.8	117	26%	9	15	1.4
506	Cocoa-whey powder with low-cal sweetener (Include Sugar-Free Nestle's Quik, Swiss Miss Sugar-Free Chocolate Milk Maker) [1 envelope]	5	0.2	14	52%	1	3	1.3
507	Cream substitute, liquid or frozen (Include Coffee Whitener, Dairy Rich Moca Mix, mocha mix, Coffee Rich, Coffee Tone, Freezer Pak, Poly Perx, Poly Rich) [1Tbs]	15	0.5	20	66%	0	2	0.0
508	Cream substitute, light, liquid [1 cup (8 fl oz)]	242	8.5	167	46%	2	22	0.0
509	Cream substitute, powdered (Include Coffee Mate, Coffee Tone, Cremora, instant coffee creamer, instant creamer, Please, Pream) [1 Tbs]	6	0.2	32	58%	0	3	0.0
510	Cream substitute, light, powdered [1 packet]	3	0.1	13	33%	0	2	0.0
511	Cream, half and half [2Tbs]	30	1.1	39	79%	1	1	0.0
512	Cream, heavy (Include whipping cream, unwhipped) [2Tbs]	30	1.0	103	97%	1	1	0.0
513	Cream, heavy, whipped, sweetened [1 cup]	119	4.2	413	90%	2	10	0.0
514	Cream, heavy, whipped, unsweetened [1 cup]	119	4.2	410	97%	2	3	0.0
515	**Cream, light (Include coffee cream, table cream) [2Tbs]**	**30**	**1.1**	**59**	**89%**	**1**	**1**	**0.0**
516	Cream, light, whipped (unsweetened) (Include coffee cream, table cream) [1 cup]	120	4.2	351	95%	3	4	0.0
517	Cream, whipped, pressurized container (Include Reddiwip, Fashion Whip, Quip) [1 cup]	60	2.1	154	78%	2	7	0.0
518	Eggnog, beads, reconstituted with whole milk [1 cup (8 fl oz)]	254	9.0	218	20%	8	37	0.8
519	Eggnog, made with 2%-fat milk [1 cup (8 fl oz)]	254	9.0	191	38%	12	17	0.0
520	Eggnog, made with whole milk [1 cup (8 fl oz)]	254	9.0	342	50%	10	34	0.0
521	Flavored milk drink, whey- and milk-based, flavors other than chocolate (Include Yoo-hoo) [1 bottle (9 fl oz)]	274	9.7	145	7%	3	28	1.1
522	High calorie milk beverage, powder (Include Nutrament) [2Tbs]	15	0.5	57	4%	4	10	0.0
523	Imitation milk, fluid, non-soy, sweetened, chocolate flavor [1 cup (8 fl oz)]	250	8.8	153	24%	3	29	1.3
524	Instant breakfast, powder, Carnation, include all flavors [1 envelope]	35	1.2	124	4%	5	27	0.1
525	Instant breakfast, powder, sugar-free, Carnation, include all flavors [1 envelope]	20	0.7	72	13%	7	8	0.4
526	Instant breakfast, ready-to-drink, Carnation, include all flavors [1 can (10 fl oz)]	310	10.9	220	12%	12	35	0.0
527	Milk beverage beads, chocolate (Include PDQ) [2Tbs]	14	0.5	49	8%	0	13	0.8
528	Milk beverage beads, not chocolate [2Tbs]	14	0.5	55	2%	0	14	0.4
529	Milk beverage with nonfat dry milk and low-cal sweetener, water added, chocolate (Include Alba) [1 cup (8 fl oz)]	276	9.7	85	8%	7	14	0.5
530	Milk beverage with nonfat dry milk and low-cal sweetener, water added, flavors other than chocolate (Include Alba) [1 cup (8 fl oz)]	276	9.7	104	7%	7	17	0.5
531	Milk beverage powder with sugar, dry milk, and egg white powder, dry mix (Include Banana Frost, Strawberry Frost) [2Tbs]	26	0.9	99	0%	2	23	0.0
532	Milk beverage beads, chocolate, (Include PDQ), whole milk added [1 cup (8 fl oz)]	250	8.8	213	35%	8	29	1.2

Food #	fat gm	sat fat gm	choles mg	sodium mg	potass mg	vit A	vit E	vit C	thia- min	ribo- flavin	nia- cin	vit B-6	fol- ate	vit B-12	cal- cium	phos- phorus	magne- sium	iron	zinc
496	3	2	9	159	480	14	1	4	6	24	2	5	3	14	29	25	13	4	8
497	1	1	4	161	502	14	1	4	6	21	2	5	3	14	29	26	12	4	8
498	8	5	31	156	470	7	1	4	6	24	1	5	3	14	28	24	13	4	8
499	1	0	0	1	82	0	0	0	0	1	1	0	0	0	1	4	7	4	2
500	0	0	1	178	415	0	0	0	3	13	1	2	1	5	9	14	8	4	4
501	0	0	4	165	425	8	0	1	4	17	1	1	0	4	33	24	11	0	5
502	1	1	1	148	202	0	0	1	2	9	1	2	0	6	10	9	6	2	3
503	0	0	1	76	313	4	0	0	2	10	1	2	0	4	17	19	6	3	3
504	0	0	1	107	413	5	0	0	3	13	1	2	1	5	22	25	9	4	4
505	3	2	10	131	512	14	1	4	7	26	2	6	4	15	31	27	14	5	8
506	1	0	0	7	123	0	0	0	1	2	1	0	0	0	1	4	6	4	2
507	1	0	0	12	29	0	1	0	0	0	0	0	0	0	0	1	0	0	0
508	8	2	0	145	428	0	0	0	0	0	0	0	0	0	0	18	0	8	1
509	2	2	0	11	48	0	0	0	0	1	0	0	0	0	0	2	0	0	0
510	0	0	0	7	27	0	0	0	0	0	0	0	0	0	0	0	0	0	0
511	3	2	11	12	39	3	0	0	1	3	0	1	0	2	3	3	1	0	1
512	11	7	41	11	22	13	1	0	0	2	0	0	0	1	2	2	1	0	0
513	41	26	153	42	85	47	2	1	2	7	0	1	1	3	7	7	2	0	2
514	44	27	163	45	90	50	2	1	2	8	0	2	1	4	8	7	2	0	2
515	6	4	20	12	37	5	0	0	1	3	0	0	0	1	3	2	1	0	1
516	37	23	133	41	116	35	2	1	2	9	0	2	1	4	8	7	2	0	2
517	13	8	46	78	88	12	1	0	1	2	0	1	0	3	6	5	2	0	1
518	5	3	25	155	355	11	1	4	6	22	1	5	3	14	28	22	8	2	6
519	8	4	194	155	369	20	2	3	7	32	1	7	8	19	27	27	8	4	8
520	19	11	149	138	420	20	2	6	6	28	1	6	1	19	33	28	12	3	8
521	1	1	3	206	206	15	0	10	2	10	10	4	1	8	10	10	10	2	4
522	0	0	1	34	183	10	0	9	8	3	9	8	9	5	13	11	8	9	8
523	4	3	0	245	78	5	0	0	0	1	1	0	1	0	4	5	4	1	3
524	0	0	4	135	331	35	25	45	20	8	25	20	20	10	25	25	20	25	20
525	1	0	9	80	341	35	25	46	20	8	26	20	20	10	25	25	21	25	21
526	3	1	10	210	470	45	25	50	25	25	25	25	25	25	50	50	25	25	25
527	0	0	0	29	83	0	0	0	0	1	0	0	0	0	1	2	3	2	1
528	0	0	3	22	1	0	0	0	0	0	0	0	0	0	0	0	0	1	0
529	1	1	2	229	637	10	0	1	2	32	2	2	3	11	26	24	16	12	7
530	1	1	4	256	701	9	0	1	2	6	2	2	3	13	29	5	17	14	8
531	0	0	1	38	81	3	0	0	1	6	0	1	1	3	5	4	1	0	1
532	8	5	31	156	470	7	1	4	6	24	1	5	3	14	28	24	13	4	8

Beverages, Dairy, Eggs

Food #	Food Description & Amount	wt gm	wt oz	calo-ries	%cal fat	prot gm	carbo gm	fiber gm
533	Milk beverage, made with whole milk, flavors other than chocolate (Include strawberry Nestle's Quik) [1 cup (8 fl oz)]	250	8.8	221	31%	8	31	0.0
534	Milk beverage powder, dry mix, flavors other than chocolate (Include strawberry Nestle's Quik) [2Tbs]	16	0.6	62	0%	0	16	0.0
535	Milk beverage powder with nonfat dry milk and low-cal sweetener, dry mix, chocolate (Include Alba) [2Tbs]	16	0.6	48	8%	4	8	0.3
536	Milk beverage powder with nonfat dry milk and low-cal sweetener, dry mix, flavors other than chocolate (Include Alba) [2Tbs]	14	0.5	46	7%	3	7	0.2
537	Milk fruit drink made with whole milk, bananas, strawberries, sugar (Include licuado) [1 cup (8 fl oz)]	209	7.4	149	18%	5	27	1.6
538	Milk fruit drink, Puerto Rican style (Champola de frutas) made with evaporated whole milk, mashed papaya, sugar, lime juice [1 cup (8 fl oz)]	240	8.5	207	28%	6	32	0.4
539	Milk shake with malt (Include malted milk with ice cream) [10 fl oz]	283	10.0	404	32%	9	62	0.1
540	Milk shake, fountain type, chocolate [10 fl oz]	283	10.0	367	34%	9	57	1.8
541	Milk shake, fountain type, flavors other than chocolate [10 fl oz]	283	10.0	381	32%	8	60	0.5
542	**Milk shake, thick, fast-food type, chocolate (thick shake mix, milk added) [16 fl oz]**	**401**	**14.1**	**509**	**26%**	**14**	**82**	**3.2**
543	Milk shake, thick, fast-food type, flavors other than chocolate (thick shake mix, milk added) [16 fl oz]	401	14.1	444	24%	14	72	1.7
544	Milk shake, made with nonfat milk, chocolate [1 cup (8 fl oz)]	127	4.5	132	7%	5	28	1.9
545	Milk shake, made with nonfat milk, flavors other than chocolate [1 cup (8 fl oz)]	127	4.5	126	4%	5	27	1.2
546	Milk, chocolate, lowfat milk-based (Include chocolate milk drink) [1 cup (8 fl oz)]	250	8.8	179	25%	8	26	1.3
547	Milk, chocolate, nonfat milk-based [1 cup (8 fl oz)]	250	8.8	144	7%	9	27	1.5
548	Milk, chocolate, whole milk-based [1 cup (8 fl oz)]	250	8.8	208	37%	8	26	2.0
549	Milk, flavors other than chocolate, whole milk-based [1 cup (8 fl oz)]	250	8.8	221	31%	8	31	0.0
550	Milk, condensed, sweetened, undiluted [½ cup undiluted or 1 cup diluted]	306	10.8	982	24%	24	166	0.0
551	**Milk, cow's, whole (Include leche fresca) [1 cup (8 fl oz)]**	**244**	**8.6**	**150**	**49%**	**8**	**11**	**0.0**
552	Milk, cow's, whole, calcium-fortified [1 cup (8 fl oz)]	247	8.7	151	49%	8	11	0.0
553	Milk, cow's, whole, low-sodium [1 cup (8 fl oz)]	244	8.6	149	51%	8	11	0.0
554	**Milk, cow's, 2% fat** (Include acidophilus milk, lactose-reduced milk, Hi-Protein milk, fortified milk) [1 cup (8 fl oz)]	245	8.6	122	35%	8	12	0.0
555	**Milk, cow's, 1% fat (Include acidophilus milk, lactose-reduced milk, Lactaid) [1 cup]**	**245**	**8.6**	**103**	**23%**	**8**	**12**	**0.0**
556	Milk, cow's, 1% fat, calcium-fortified (Include lactose-reduced milk, CalciMilk, CalciMilk with Lactaid) [1 cup (8 fl oz)]	247	8.7	103	23%	8	12	0.0
557	**Milk, cow's, nonfat (Include lactose-reduced) [1 cup (8 fl oz)]**	**245**	**8.6**	**86**	**5%**	**8**	**12**	**0.0**
558	Milk, cow's, nonfat, calcium-fortified (Include lactose-reduced) [1 cup (8 fl oz)]	247	8.7	86	5%	8	12	0.0
559	Milk, cow's, filled with vegetable oil, lowfat [1 cup (8 fl oz)]	245	8.6	105	23%	8	12	0.0
560	Milk, cow's, filled with vegetable oil, whole [1 cup (8 fl oz)]	244	8.6	153	49%	8	12	0.0
561	Milk, dry, whole [2Tbs]	16	0.6	79	48%	4	6	0.0
562	Milk, dry, lowfat [2Tbs]	15	0.5	54	4%	5	8	0.0
563	Milk, dry, nonfat [2Tbs]	8	0.3	30	2%	3	4	0.0
564	Milk, dry, reconstituted, whole [1 cup (8 fl oz)]	244	8.6	157	48%	8	12	0.0
565	Milk, dry, reconstituted, lowfat [1 cup (8 fl oz)]	245	8.6	84	4%	8	12	0.0
566	Milk, dry, reconstituted, nonfat [1 cup (8 fl oz)]	245	8.6	82	2%	8	12	0.0
567	**Milk, evaporated, whole [½ cup undiluted or 1 cup diluted]**	**244**	**8.6**	**169**	**51%**	**9**	**13**	**0.0**
568	Milk, evaporated, 2% fat [½ cup undiluted or 1 cup diluted]	244	8.6	117	19%	9	14	0.0
569	Milk, evaporated, nonfat [½ cup undiluted or 1 cup diluted]	245	8.6	99	2%	10	14	0.0
570	Milk, evaporated, filled with vegetable oil [½ cup undiluted or 1 cup diluted]	244	8.6	167	51%	9	13	0.0
571	Milk, goat's, whole [1 cup (8 fl oz)]	244	8.6	168	54%	9	11	0.0
572	Milk, human [1 cup (8 fl oz)]	246	8.7	171	57%	3	17	0.0
573	Milk, imitation, non-soy, corn-syrup based [1 cup (8 fl oz)]	244	8.6	112	39%	4	13	0.0
574	Milk, imitation, soy based [1 cup (8 fl oz)]	244	8.6	150	50%	4	15	0.0
575	Milk, malted, dry mix, unfortified, not reconstituted, chocolate [2Tbs]	16	0.6	60	9%	1	14	0.1
576	Milk, malted, dry mix, unfortified, flavors other than chocolate [2Tbs]	16	0.6	66	17%	2	12	0.1

Food #	fat gm	sat fat gm	choles mg	sodium mg	potass mg	% of Daily Value													
						vit A	vit E	vit C	thia-min	ribo-flavin	nia-cin	vit B-6	fol-ate	vit B-12	cal-cium	phos-phorus	magne-sium	iron	zinc
533	8	5	31	120	348	7	1	4	6	23	1	5	3	14	27	21	8	1	6
534	0	0	0	6	0	0	0	0	0	1	0	0	0	0	0	0	0	0	0
535	0	0	1	125	358	6	0	0	1	18	1	1	2	6	14	14	8	7	4
536	0	0	2	109	308	4	0	0	1	3	1	1	1	6	12	2	7	6	3
537	3	2	11	67	401	7	1	36	5	16	2	14	5	8	17	14	8	2	4
538	7	4	25	94	388	5	1	49	5	17	2	3	8	2	23	18	7	1	5
539	14	9	55	216	499	14	1	4	12	34	6	8	5	16	32	28	12	2	8
540	14	9	47	182	538	14	1	4	6	25	2	6	5	13	28	29	19	10	9
541	13	8	54	147	422	14	1	26	6	26	2	6	3	14	29	23	8	4	9
542	15	9	52	389	801	9	1	3	15	58	3	10	4	22	45	41	17	7	11
543	12	8	44	329	698	13	1	5	12	43	4	10	3	24	49	41	12	2	10
544	1	1	5	97	302	1	0	2	4	13	1	3	2	9	17	15	7	3	5
545	0	0	4	96	237	1	0	2	4	12	1	2	2	9	17	13	4	1	4
546	5	3	17	151	422	14	0	4	6	24	2	5	3	14	28	25	8	3	7
547	1	1	4	121	486	14	0	4	6	20	1	5	3	15	29	27	11	4	8
548	8	5	31	149	417	7	1	4	6	24	2	5	3	14	28	25	8	3	7
549	8	5	31	120	348	7	1	4	6	23	1	5	3	14	27	21	8	1	6
550	27	17	104	389	1136	25	2	13	18	75	3	8	9	23	87	78	20	3	19
551	8	5	33	120	370	8	1	4	6	23	1	5	3	15	29	23	8	1	6
552	8	5	33	121	373	8	1	4	6	24	1	5	3	15	103	23	8	1	6
553	8	5	33	6	617	8	1	4	3	15	1	4	3	15	25	21	3	1	6
554	5	3	18	122	378	14	1	4	6	24	1	5	3	15	30	23	8	1	6
555	3	2	10	124	382	14	0	4	6	24	1	5	3	15	30	24	8	1	6
556	3	2	10	125	385	15	0	4	6	24	1	5	3	15	55	24	9	1	6
557	0	0	4	126	406	15	0	4	6	20	1	5	3	15	30	25	7	1	7
558	0	0	4	127	409	15	0	4	6	20	1	5	3	16	50	25	7	1	7
559	3	2	5	130	415	0	0	3	6	21	1	4	3	16	30	22	7	1	7
560	8	8	4	138	339	0	0	4	5	18	1	5	3	14	31	24	8	1	6
561	4	3	16	59	213	4	1	2	3	11	1	2	1	9	15	12	3	0	4
562	0	0	3	81	253	11	0	1	4	15	1	3	2	10	18	15	4	0	4
563	0	0	2	47	145	6	0	1	2	9	0	1	1	6	10	8	2	0	2
564	8	5	31	124	421	9	1	5	6	22	1	5	3	17	29	25	7	1	7
565	0	0	5	132	388	16	0	2	6	23	1	4	3	15	28	22	7	1	7
566	0	0	4	132	388	16	0	2	6	23	1	4	3	15	28	22	7	1	7
567	10	6	37	137	381	7	1	4	4	23	1	3	2	3	33	25	8	1	7
568	2	2	10	148	416	17	0	3	4	23	1	3	3	5	37	24	9	2	8
569	0	0	5	150	422	15	0	3	4	23	1	4	3	5	37	25	9	2	8
570	9	8	4	139	414	17	0	1	4	25	1	2	2	5	30	24	8	1	8
571	10	7	28	122	499	14	1	5	8	20	3	6	0	3	33	27	9	1	5
572	11	5	34	42	126	16	7	21	2	5	2	1	3	2	8	3	2	0	3
573	5	1	0	134	366	15	0	0	0	0	1	0	0	0	20	24	1	1	2
574	8	2	0	191	279	0	9	0	2	13	0	0	0	0	8	18	4	5	19
575	1	0	1	40	99	0	0	0	2	2	2	1	1	1	1	3	3	2	1
576	1	1	3	79	121	1	0	1	5	ribo	nia	3	2	2	5	6	4	1	1

Beverages, Dairy, Eggs

Food #	Food Description & Amount	wt gm	wt oz	calories	%cal fat	prot gm	carbo gm	fiber gm
577	Milk, soy, ready-to-drink, not baby's (include reconstituted from canned or dry) [1 cup]	245	8.6	81	52%	7	4	3.2
578	Slim-Fast powder, include all flavors [1 scoop (3Tbs)]	28	1.0	100	5%	5	20	2.0
579	Slim-Fast shake, include all flavors [1 can (11 fl oz)]	340	12.0	220	12%	10	40	5.0
580	**Sour cream [2Tbs]**	**29**	**1.0**	**62**	**88%**	**1**	**1**	**0.0**
581	Sour cream, half and half [2Tbs]	30	1.1	41	80%	1	1	0.0
582	Sour cream, reduced fat [2Tbs]	32	1.1	58	70%	2	2	0.0
583	Sour cream, light [2Tbs]	32	1.1	44	70%	1	2	0.0
584	Sour cream, fat free [2Tbs]	32	1.1	24	0%	1	5	0.0
585	Sour cream, imitation (non-dairy) (Include Imo, Zero) [2Tbs]	29	1.0	60	84%	1	2	0.0
586	Whey, sweet, dry [2Tbs]	18	0.6	64	3%	2	13	0.0
587	Whipped cream substitute, non-dairy, dietetic, made from powdered mix (Include Feather Weight Low Calorie Whipped Topping) [1 cup]	80	2.8	80	54%	1	8	0.0
588	Whipped cream substitute, non-dairy, made from powdered mix (Include Dream Whip, Lucky Whip, Smooth Whip) [1 cup]	80	2.8	151	59%	3	13	0.0
589	Whipped topping, non-dairy, frozen (Include Cool Whip, Handiwhip Whipped Topping, Pet Whip) [1 cup]	75	2.6	239	72%	1	17	0.0
590	Whipped topping, non-dairy, frozen, lowfat [1 cup]	75	2.6	165	54%	2	18	0.0
591	Whipped topping, non-dairy, pressurized can (Include Lucky Whip, Reddiwip) [1 cup]	70	2.5	184	76%	1	11	0.0
	Yogurt							
650	Yogurt, chocolate, nonfat milk (Include Snackwell's chocolate almond yogurt) [1-6 oz container]	170	6.0	190	0%	6	40	2.0
651	Yogurt, chocolate, whole milk [1-6 oz container]	170	6.0	232	21%	6	39	2.0
652	Yogurt, fruit and nuts [1-8 oz container]	227	8.0	268	23%	10	43	0.5
653	Yogurt, fruit variety, lowfat milk (Include custard style) [1-8 oz container]	227	8.0	231	10%	10	43	0.0
654	Yogurt, fruit variety, nonfat milk [1-8 oz container]	227	8.0	213	2%	10	43	0.0
655	Yogurt, fruit variety, nonfat milk, sweetened with low-calorie sweetener [1-6 oz container]	170	6.0	86	3%	7	14	0.9
656	Yogurt, fruit variety, whole milk (Include breakfast yogurt) [1-8 oz container]	227	8.0	270	25%	10	42	0.0
657	Yogurt, plain, lowfat milk [1-8 oz container]	227	8.0	144	22%	12	16	0.0
658	Yogurt, plain, nonfat milk [1-8 oz container]	227	8.0	127	3%	13	17	0.0
659	Yogurt, plain, whole milk [1-8 oz container]	227	8.0	139	48%	8	11	0.0
660	Yogurt, vanilla, lemon, maple, or coffee flavor, lowfat milk (Include liquid yogurt, LeShake, Tuscan) [1-8 oz container]	227	8.0	194	13%	11	31	0.0
661	Yogurt, vanilla, lemon, maple, or coffee flavor, nonfat milk [1-8 oz container]	227	8.0	207	2%	12	40	0.0
662	Yogurt, vanilla, lemon, maple, or coffee flavor, nonfat milk, sweetened with low calorie sweetener [1-8 oz container]	227	8.0	98	4%	9	17	0.0
663	Yogurt, vanilla, lemon, or coffee flavor, whole milk [1-8 oz container]	227	8.0	229	28%	11	31	0.0
	Ice Cream & Frozen Yogurt							
700	Ice cream bar with fruit (Include Carnation Berry Swirl) [1 bar]	41	1.4	65	36%	1	10	0.8
701	Ice cream bar, chocolate or vanilla, chocolate covered [1 bar]	56	2.0	169	66%	2	14	0.2
702	Ice cream bar, chocolate ice cream, chocolate covered [1 big bar]	101	3.6	339	61%	3	36	2.1
703	Ice cream bar, chocolate or caramel covered, with nuts (Include Heavenly Sundae, Vanilla fudge nuts; Heavenly Sundae caramel; Heavenly Sundae) [1 bar]	54	1.9	177	63%	3	16	0.6
704	Ice cream bar, not chocolate or cake covered [1 bar]	56	2.0	113	49%	2	13	0.0
705	Ice cream bar, cake covered [1 bar]	59	2.1	168	38%	3	25	0.7
706	Ice cream bar, rich vanilla ice cream, thick chocolate covering (Include DoveBar) [1 bar]	81	2.9	261	57%	4	27	0.8
707	Ice cream bar, rich vanilla ice cream, chocolate covered, with nuts (Include Haagen Dazs) [1 bar]	113	4.0	369	61%	6	34	1.9
708	Ice cream cone with nuts, chocolate ice cream [1 cone]	78	2.8	212	53%	5	23	1.8
709	Ice cream cone with nuts, flavors other than chocolate [1 cone]	78	2.8	205	57%	5	20	1.2
710	Ice cream cone, chocolate covered or dipped, chocolate ice cream [1 cone]	78	2.8	190	42%	3	27	1.1
711	Ice cream cone, chocolate covered or dipped, flavors other than chocolate [1 cone]	78	2.8	187	46%	3	24	0.6
712	Ice cream cone, chocolate covered, with nuts, chocolate ice cream [1 cone]	78	2.8	224	53%	5	25	2.0

Food #	fat gm	sat fat gm	choles mg	sodium mg	potass mg	% of Daily Value													
						vit A	vit E	vit C	thia-min	ribo-flavin	nia-cin	vit B-6	fol-ate	vit B-12	cal-cium	phos-phorus	magne-sium	iron	zinc
577	5	1	0	29	345	1	0	0	26	10	2	5	1	0	1	12	12	8	4
578	1	0	5	120	230	15	50	30	30	10	35	30	25	20	15	10	25	35	30
579	3	1	5	220	600	35	100	100	35	35	35	35	30	35	40	40	35	15	15
580	6	4	13	15	41	6	1	0	1	3	0	0	1	1	3	2	1	0	1
581	4	2	12	12	39	3	0	0	1	3	0	0	1	2	3	3	1	0	1
582	5	3	11	22	68	4	0	0	1	5	0	0	1	2	5	3	1	0	1
583	3	2	11	23	68	3	0	0	1	2	0	0	1	2	5	2	1	0	1
584	0	0	3	45	41	3	0	0	1	3	0	0	1	2	4	3	1	0	1
585	6	5	0	29	46	0	0	0	0	0	0	0	0	0	0	1	0	1	2
586	0	0	1	196	377	0	0	0	6	24	1	5	1	7	14	17	8	1	2
587	5	3	0	85	21	0	0	0	0	0	0	0	0	0	0	2	0	0	0
588	10	9	8	53	121	4	0	1	1	6	0	1	1	3	7	7	2	0	1
589	19	16	0	19	14	6	0	0	0	0	0	0	0	0	0	1	0	1	0
590	10	8	2	54	76	3	0	0	1	4	0	1	1	3	5	6	1	0	1
591	16	13	0	43	13	3	0	0	0	0	0	0	0	0	0	1	0	0	0
650	0	0	2	230	576	0	0	0	5	22	2	4	5	14	15	28	17	4	13
651	5	3	16	222	558	5	1	0	5	21	2	4	5	14	15	27	16	4	12
652	7	2	9	129	454	3	1	3	9	24	1	5	6	17	34	28	10	2	13
653	2	2	10	133	442	2	0	2	6	24	1	5	5	18	34	27	8	1	11
654	0	0	5	132	440	0	0	3	6	24	1	5	5	18	35	27	9	1	11
655	0	0	2	98	388	0	0	31	5	19	2	4	6	13	26	21	7	2	9
656	7	5	22	130	432	7	1	2	5	23	1	4	5	17	34	27	8	1	11
657	4	2	14	159	531	4	0	3	7	29	1	6	6	21	41	33	10	1	13
658	0	0	4	174	579	0	0	3	7	31	1	6	7	23	45	36	11	1	15
659	7	5	29	105	351	7	1	2	4	19	1	4	4	14	27	22	7	1	9
660	3	2	11	149	498	3	0	3	6	27	1	5	6	20	39	31	9	1	13
661	0	0	4	155	518	0	0	3	7	28	1	5	6	21	40	32	10	1	13
662	0	0	5	134	402	0	0	4	5	22	1	4	5	16	32	25	7	2	10
663	7	5	22	147	488	7	1	3	6	26	1	5	6	20	38	30	9	1	12
700	3	2	10	19	66	3	0	5	1	4	0	1	1	1	3	3	1	1	1
701	13	10	19	36	104	5	0	0	1	6	0	1	1	3	6	5	2	1	2
702	23	14	38	56	260	9	2	0	2	12	2	2	1	4	7	14	16	6	7
703	12	8	17	44	128	5	1	0	3	7	3	2	2	3	6	7	4	1	3
704	6	4	25	45	111	7	0	1	2	8	0	1	1	4	7	6	2	0	3
705	7	2	30	254	139	3	2	0	3	7	2	1	3	2	7	11	4	8	3
706	17	10	40	52	184	12	1	1	3	10	1	2	1	5	11	11	5	2	4
707	25	13	54	65	293	16	6	1	4	15	2	2	3	6	17	18	13	5	8
708	12	4	16	40	218	5	3	1	3	13	3	2	4	4	10	13	12	4	6
709	13	5	28	58	198	8	2	1	3	16	3	2	3	4	11	12	10	3	6
710	9	5	17	43	178	6	1	1	3	8	2	1	2	4	8	8	6	4	3
711	10	6	29	61	161	8	1	1	3	11	2	2	2	4	9	8	5	3	4
712	13	5	15	37	223	5	3	1	3	12	3	2	3	4	10	13	12	5	6

Beverages, Dairy, Eggs

Food #	Food Description & Amount	wt gm	wt oz	calo-ries	%cal fat	prot gm	carbo gm	fiber gm
713	Ice cream cone, chocolate covered, with nuts, flavors other than chocolate (Include Nutty Buddy) [1 cone]	78	2.8	217	57%	4	22	1.4
714	Ice cream cone, no topping, chocolate ice cream [1 cone]	78	2.8	173	39%	3	25	0.7
715	Ice cream cone, no topping, flavors other than chocolate [1 cone]	78	2.8	166	45%	3	21	0.1
716	Ice cream cookie sandwich (Include Chipwich) [1 sandwich]	59	2.1	144	35%	3	22	0.6
717	Ice cream pie (vanilla ice cream with whipped cream topping, no crust) [1/8 of 8"dia]	99	3.5	218	59%	3	21	0.0
718	Ice cream pie, with cookie crust, fudge topping, and whipped cream [1/8 of 8"dia]	230	8.1	698	41%	9	96	2.5
719	Ice cream sandwich (Include Oreo Ice Cream sandwich) [1 sandwich (5"x1¾"x¾")]	59	2.1	144	35%	3	22	0.6
720	Ice cream soda, chocolate [1 soda (10 fl oz)]	240	8.5	222	40%	3	35	1.0
721	Ice cream soda, flavors other than chocolate [1 soda (10 fl oz)]	240	8.5	203	30%	2	35	0.0
722	Ice cream sundae cone (Include Drumstick, all flavors) [1 cone]	107	3.8	284	51%	6	32	1.3
723	Ice cream sundae, chocolate or fudge topping with whipped cream [1 sundae]	165	5.8	437	47%	6	54	1.5
724	Ice cream sundae, fruit topping with whipped cream [1 sundae]	165	5.8	386	42%	4	56	0.5
725	Ice cream sundae, fudge topping, with cake and whipped cream [1 sundae]	175	6.2	490	44%	7	64	1.5
726	Ice cream sundae, caramel or butterscotch topping with whipped cream [1 sundae]	165	5.8	402	51%	5	47	0.4
727	Ice cream sundae, prepackaged type, flavors other than chocolate [1 sundae]	65	2.3	120	29%	3	19	0.0
728	Ice cream with sherbet [1 cup]	163	5.7	267	31%	3	45	0.5
729	**Ice cream, chocolate [1 cup]**	**133**	**4.7**	**273**	**42%**	**5**	**37**	**1.0**
730	Ice cream, flavors other than chocolate [1 cup]	133	4.7	267	49%	5	31	
731	Ice cream, rich, flavors other than chocolate [1 cup]	148	5.2	357	60%	5	33	0.0
732	Ice cream, fried [1 cup]	133	4.7	358	46%	5	46	0.8
733	Ice cream, imitation, chocolate (with vegetable fat) (Include Mellorine) [1 cup]	133	4.7	268	47%	5	33	1.0
734	Ice cream, imitation, flavors other than chocolate (with vegetable fat) (Include Mellorine) [1 cup]	133	4.7	265	46%	5	32	0.0
735	Ice cream, soft serve, chocolate [1 cup]	173	6.1	355	42%	6	48	1.3
736	Ice cream, soft serve, flavors other than chocolate [1 cup]	173	6.1	348	49%	6	41	0.0
737	Ice milk bar or stick, chocolate covered, with nuts (Include Buster bar) [1 bar]	149	5.3	441	65%	9	36	1.8
738	Ice milk bar or stick, with low-calorie sweetener, chocolate-coated (Include Sugar Free Eskimo Pie, Klondike Lite Sugar Free) [1 bar]	53	1.9	113	42%	3	14	1.1
739	Ice milk bar or stick, chocolate-coated [1 bar]	56	2.0	142	61%	2	14	0.2
740	Ice milk cone, chocolate [1 cone]	78	2.8	129	19%	4	23	0.5
741	Ice milk cone, flavors other than chocolate [1 cone]	78	2.8	116	18%	4	20	0.2
742	Ice milk creamsicle or dreamsicle [1 bar]	66	2.3	91	20%	2	18	0.2
743	Ice milk sandwich (Include Dairy Queen) [1 sandwich]	60	2.1	118	20%	3	22	0.6
744	Ice milk sundae, chocolate or fudge topping with whipped cream (Include McDonald's sundaes) [1 sundae]	165	5.8	386	40%	6	53	1.5
745	Ice milk sundae, soft serve, chocolate or fudge topping, no whipped cream [1 cup]	142	5.0	258	21%	7	45	1.0
746	Ice milk sundae, fruit topping with whipped cream (Include McDonald's sundaes) [1 sundae]	165	5.8	335	33%	4	55	0.5
747	Ice milk sundae, soft serve, fruit topping, no whipped cream [1 cup]	142	5.0	173	15%	5	33	0.6
748	Ice milk sundae, caramel or butterscotch topping with whipped cream (Include McDonald's sundaes) [1 sundae]	165	5.8	366	28%	6	64	0.8
749	Ice milk sundae, soft serve, no fruit or chocolate topping, no whipped cream [1 cup]	142	5.0	269	19%	7	50	0.4
750	Ice milk, chocolate [1 cup]	131	4.6	189	20%	6	34	0.6
751	Ice milk, flavors other than chocolate [1 cup]	131	4.6	182	28%	5	30	0.0
752	Ice milk, fudgesicle [1 bar]	73	2.6	104	29%	3	18	0.9
753	Ice milk, premium, chocolate (Include Breyers Light, Hood Light) [1 cup]	136	4.8	245	31%	6	38	0.6
754	Ice milk, premium, flavors other than chocolate (Include Breyers Light, Hood Light) [1 cup]	136	4.8	136	31%	4	21	0.0
755	Ice milk, soft serve, chocolate (Include frozen custard, Tastee Freeze, Dairy Queen, Dairy Queen Blizzard) [1 cup]	175	6.2	243	17%	8	45	0.8
756	Ice milk, soft serve cone, chocolate (Include Dairy Queen) [1 small fast food cone]	186	6.6	278	21%	11	51	3.7

Food #	fat gm	sat fat gm	choles mg	sodium mg	potass mg	% of Daily Value														
						vit A	vit E	vit C	thia-min	ribo-flavin	nia-cin	vit B-6	fol-ate	vit B-12	cal-cium	phos-phorus	magne-sium	iron	zinc
713	14	6	26	55	204	7	2	1	3	15	3	2	3	4	10	12	11	4	6
714	7	4	18	46	168	6	1	1	3	8	2	1	3	4	9	8	4	3	3
715	8	5	32	65	151	9	0	1	3	11	1	2	2	5	10	8	3	1	4
716	6	3	20	36	122	5	0	0	2	7	1	1	1	3	6	6	3	2	3
717	14	9	56	74	182	16	0	1	3	13	1	2	1	6	12	10	3	0	4
718	32	15	53	559	494	23	12	1	8	28	6	5	4	10	20	23	14	10	9
719	6	3	20	36	122	5	0	0	2	7	1	1	1	3	6	6	3	2	3
720	10	6	29	94	213	9	1	1	2	7	1	1	1	4	9	11	9	5	5
721	7	4	27	82	126	7	0	1	2	9	0	1	1	4	9	6	3	0	4
722	16	8	37	78	259	10	3	1	5	14	8	3	5	5	12	15	9	4	9
723	23	13	69	261	387	18	6	1	5	21	1	4	2	8	17	18	10	4	7
724	18	11	68	88	232	18	1	23	3	14	1	3	2	6	14	11	4	3	6
725	24	13	78	318	366	17	7	1	8	22	4	4	4	8	18	18	10	8	7
726	23	15	79	164	285	21	1	2	3	19	1	3	2	7	19	15	5	1	6
727	4	2	8	62	137	2	1	2	2	7	2	2	1	4	8	9	3	1	2
728	9	6	34	98	225	9	0	8	3	13	1	3	2	6	14	11	4	1	6
729	13	8	33	68	295	11	1	1	4	12	1	2	2	8	16	14	7	3	5
730	15	9	59	106	265	16	0	1	4	19	1	3	2	9	17	14	5	1	6
731	24	15	90	83	235	27	0	2	4	14	1	3	2	9	17	14	4	0	4
732	18	9	45	313	246	31	4	22	24	35	22	24	22	7	14	14	6	22	26
733	14	12	0	95	357	0	0	1	4	17	1	4	1	13	18	16	9	3	11
734	14	12	0	97	287	0	0	1	4	17	1	4	1	13	18	14	5	1	9
735	17	10	43	89	384	15	2	2	5	16	1	3	2	11	21	18	9	4	6
736	19	12	76	138	344	20	0	2	5	24	1	4	2	11	22	18	6	1	8
737	32	19	14	89	384	5	5	1	7	18	15	6	8	11	16	22	15	4	12
738	5	3	5	55	162	2	0	0	2	9	0	2	1	3	12	9	4	1	3
739	10	8	6	38	109	2	0	1	2	7	0	1	1	5	6	5	2	1	2
740	3	1	7	53	175	2	1	1	3	9	2	2	3	5	10	9	4	2	3
741	2	1	9	59	166	2	0	1	3	10	2	2	3	6	11	9	3	1	3
742	2	1	6	43	99	2	0	3	2	6	0	2	1	4	6	5	2	0	2
743	3	1	6	39	130	2	0	1	3	8	1	2	1	5	7	7	3	2	2
744	17	10	44	266	397	12	6	2	6	22	1	5	2	12	18	18	10	4	5
745	6	3	14	197	364	3	3	2	5	17	1	4	2	10	20	18	8	3	5
746	12	8	43	91	242	12	1	24	4	16	1	4	2	10	15	11	4	3	5
747	3	2	13	84	264	3	0	10	4	13	1	3	4	9	17	13	4	1	4
748	11	8	26	215	302	7	1	2	4	19	1	4	2	9	19	16	6	1	4
749	6	4	15	161	311	3	1	2	4	16	1	3	2	9	22	17	5	1	5
750	4	3	12	82	310	4	0	2	4	14	1	3	2	10	19	16	6	2	5
751	6	3	18	111	276	6	0	2	5	20	1	4	2	15	18	14	5	1	4
752	3	2	10	60	221	3	0	1	3	12	1	2	1	8	10	10	6	3	3
753	8	5	23	91	343	7	1	2	5	16	1	3	2	11	21	17	7	2	6
754	5	3	19	58	179	4	0	2	3	11	0	2	1	7	14	11	4	0	3
755	5	3	14	109	414	4	0	2	6	19	1	4	3	13	25	21	9	2	7
756	7	4	20	133	658	5	1	2	8	24	5	5	6	14	27	29	20	13	11

Beverages, Dairy, Eggs

Food #	Food Description & Amount	wt gm	wt oz	calo-ries	%cal fat	prot gm	carbo gm	fiber gm
757	Ice milk, soft serve, flavors other than chocolate (Include frozen custard, Tastee Freeze, Dairy Queen, Dairy Queen Blizzard) [1 cup]	175	6.2	221	19%	9	38	0.0
758	**Ice milk, soft serve cone**, flavors other than chocolate (Include Dairy Queen) [1 small fast food cone]	**186**	**6.6**	**267**	**18%**	**9**	**47**	**0.3**
759	Ice milk, with sherbet or ice cream [1 bar]	60	2.1	83	20%	1	16	0.2
760	Milk dessert bar, frozen, lowfat (Include Weight Watcher's Treat Bars) [1 bar]	81	2.9	88	10%	2	19	0.0
761	Milk dessert bar, frozen, lowfat, low-cal sweetener (Include sugar free Fudgsicle Fudge Pops) [1 bar]	41	1.4	24	13%	2	9	4.6
762	Milk dessert bar or stick, frozen, with coconut (Include Frut Stix bar) [1 bar]	129	4.6	198	36%	7	27	2.2
763	Milk dessert sandwich bar, frozen, lowfat (Include Weight Watcher's Sandwich Bars) [1 sandwich bar]	77	2.7	135	9%	4	27	0.7
764	Milk dessert sandwich bar, frozen, lowfat, low-calorie sweetener (Include Sugar Free Eskimo Pie Sandwich) [1 Sandwich]	59	2.1	184	26%	3	31	1.2
765	Milk dessert, frozen, low-calorie sweetener, chocolate [1 cup]	129	4.6	213	43%	6	34	5.6
766	Milk dessert, frozen, low-calorie sweetener, flavors other than chocolate [1 cup]	129	4.6	183	40%	3	26	0.3
767	Milk dessert, frozen, lowfat (Include Weight Watchers) [1 cup]	131	4.6	147	6%	6	29	0.0
768	Milk dessert, frozen, lowfat, chocolate (Include Healthy Choice Premium Low Fat Ice Cream) [1 cup]	144	5.1	226	16%	6	45	1.4
769	Milk dessert, frozen, lowfat, flavors other than chocolate [1 cup]	144	5.1	174	3%	5	37	1.0
770	Milk dessert, frozen, lowfat, low-calorie sweetener, flavors other than chocolate [1 cup]	137	4.8	156	10%	5	33	2.3
771	Milk dessert, frozen, milk-fat free, chocolate [1 cup]	137	4.8	229	5%	6	52	2.7
772	Milk dessert, frozen, milk-fat free, flavors other than chocolate [1 cup]	137	4.8	195	4%	5	43	4.1
773	Milk dessert, frozen, milk-fat free, made with Simplesse, chocolate [1 cup]	179	6.3	279	3%	18	50	1.8
774	Milk dessert, frozen, milk-fat free, made with Simplesse, flavors other than chocolate [1 cup]	179	6.3	240	0%	16	45	1.8
775	Milk dessert, frozen, nonfat, low-calorie sweetener, chocolate [1 cup]	144	5.1	153	16%	6	35	7.7
776	Milk dessert, frozen, nonfat, low-calorie sweetener, flavors other than chocolate [1 cup]	144	5.1	157	3%	4	36	1.2
777	Sherbet, all flavors [1 cup]	193	6.8	266	13%	2	59	1.0
778	Yogurt, frozen, carob-coated [1 bar]	41	1.4	100	42%	2	13	0.3
779	Yogurt, frozen, chocolate, whole milk [1 cup]	174	6.1	221	26%	5	38	4.0
780	Yogurt, frozen, chocolate, lowfat milk [1 cup]	193	6.8	219	15%	10	42	3.0
781	Yogurt, frozen, chocolate, nonfat milk [1 cup]	193	6.8	207	7%	11	43	3.0
782	Yogurt, frozen, chocolate, nonfat milk, with low-calorie sweetener [1 cup]	186	6.6	199	7%	8	37	3.7
783	Yogurt, frozen, chocolate-coated [1 bar]	41	1.4	109	56%	1	12	0.1
784	Yogurt, frozen, flavors other than chocolate, whole milk [1 cup]	174	6.1	221	26%	5	38	0.0
785	Yogurt, frozen, flavors other than chocolate, lowfat milk [1 cup]	193	6.8	203	12%	9	37	0.0
786	Yogurt, frozen, flavors other than chocolate, nonfat milk [1 cup]	193	6.8	191	1%	10	38	0.0
787	Yogurt, frozen, cone, chocolate [1 small cone]	78	2.8	168	39%	4	24	1.1
788	Yogurt, frozen, cone, chocolate, lowfat milk (Include McDonald's) [1 medium cone]	118	4.2	155	15%	6	29	1.9
789	Yogurt, frozen, cone, flavors other than chocolate [1 small cone]	78	2.8	147	26%	3	25	0.2
790	Yogurt, frozen, cone, flavors other than chocolate, lowfat milk (Include McDonald's) [1 medium cone]	118	4.2	99	20%	6	13	0.2
791	Yogurt, frozen, flavors other than chocolate, nonfat milk, with low-calorie sweetener [1 cup]	186	6.6	236	1%	9	52	1.8
792	Yogurt, frozen, sandwich [1 sandwich]	85	3.0	181	22%	4	32	0.4
Cheese								
800	Cheese nuggets or pieces, breaded, baked, or fried (Include Banquet, Beatrice, Firesaver brands) [1 cup]	115	4.1	417	54%	30	17	0.5
801	Cheese spread, cheddar or American cheese base (Include Velveeta, Cheez Whiz, Old English Smokey, Bacon, Yellow in a Jar) [2Tbs]	31	1.1	89	66%	5	3	0.0
802	Cheese spread, cheddar or American cheese base, lowfat, low sodium (Include lowfat, low sodium Velveeta) [2Tbs]	31	1.1	55	35%	8	1	0.0
803	Cheese spread, cream cheese or Neufchatel base [2Tbs]	29	1.0	86	87%	2	1	0.0

Food #	fat gm	sat fat gm	choles mg	sodium mg	potass mg		vit A	vit E	vit C	thia-min	ribo-flavin	nia-cin	vit B-6	fol-ate	vit B-12	cal-cium	phos-phorus	magne-sium	iron	zinc
757	5	3	21	123	387		5	0	3	6	20	1	4	3	15	27	21	6	1	6
758	5	3	21	138	399		5	1	3	8	23	4	4	6	15	28	22	7	3	7
759	2	1	6	39	90		2	0	3	2	6	0	1	1	4	6	4	2	0	2
760	1	0	1	44	107		4	0	1	2	7	0	1	1	4	8	7	2	0	2
761	0	0	1	20	108		2	0	1	1	4	0	1	1	2	5	5	4	2	2
762	8	7	9	165	425		2	1	2	5	16	1	6	3	12	24	19	7	2	7
763	1	1	3	55	183		0	0	1	3	7	1	2	1	7	10	10	4	2	3
764	5	2	2	233	130		0	2	0	6	8	5	1	5	3	5	8	6	8	3
765	10	6	29	42	559		10	1	1	3	12	2	3	2	4	11	20	23	16	9
766	8	5	30	52	157		11	1	2	2	9	0	2	1	6	12	10	3	0	3
767	1	1	7	122	312		1	0	1	3	15	1	3	0	15	22	18	5	1	4
768	4	2	14	101	359		9	0	2	3	16	1	3	2	5	21	18	10	5	6
769	1	0	4	98	344		12	0	0	4	18	1	1	1	4	19	16	5	6	6
770	2	1	8	78	310		2	0	29	4	14	1	4	3	9	18	14	5	1	4
771	1	1	0	133	456		3	0	2	5	21	1	3	2	13	21	17	15	0	4
772	1	1	0	121	255		9	0	0	4	15	1	2	1	7	18	14	5	1	4
773	1	1	20	150	465		3	0	3	6	34	3	4	3	12	22	18	9	4	6
774	0	0	30	131	401		3	0	1	4	31	1	3	3	10	19	14	7	1	6
775	3	1	2	137	570		6	1	2	4	11	4	3	3	7	16	17	13	6	7
776	0	0	2	68	212		7	0	2	3	10	1	2	1	7	14	11	3	0	3
777	4	2	10	89	185		3	0	14	3	8	1	3	2	4	10	8	4	2	6
778	5	4	1	38	125		2	1	1	1	5	1	2	1	3	7	5	2	1	3
779	6	4	23	110	407		5	0	19	5	18	1	3	5	2	17	15	11	4	3
780	4	2	10	113	621		3	0	2	5	23	2	4	5	15	30	30	19	9	14
781	2	1	3	123	655		0	0	2	6	25	2	5	6	16	33	32	19	10	15
782	1	1	7	151	631		0	0	2	5	20	2	4	6	15	30	24	19	0	6
783	7	5	1	28	74		2	0	0	1	4	0	1	1	2	5	4	1	1	1
784	6	4	23	110	271		5	0	2	5	18	1	3	2	2	17	15	4	4	3
785	3	2	10	118	393		3	0	2	5	21	1	4	5	16	31	24	7	1	10
786	0	0	3	129	429		0	0	2	5	23	1	4	5	17	33	26	8	1	11
787	7	4	1	84	197		4	1	1	5	11	3	3	3	3	10	12	8	5	4
788	3	1	6	75	365		1	1	1	4	15	3	5	3	5	17	18	11	7	8
789	4	2	1	90	158		4	0	1	5	11	3	3	3	3	10	10	3	3	2
790	2	1	7	88	267		2	1	1	4	15	2	3	5	10	20	17	5	2	7
791	0	0	3	129	424		0	0	2	6	23	1	4	5	17	32	25	8	1	10
792	4	2	1	57	151		4	0	1	3	9	2	3	2	3	10	10	3	2	2
800	25	13	93	684	150		20	5	0	9	27	6	4	6	10	75	55	9	9	22
801	6	4	17	410	74		6	1	0	1	8	0	2	1	2	17	22	2	1	5
802	2	1	11	2	55		2	1	0	1	7	0	1	1	4	21	25	2	1	7
803	8	5	26	195	32		10	1	0	0	3	1	1	1	2	2	3	0	2	1

Beverages, Dairy, Eggs

Food #	Food Description & Amount	wt gm	wt oz	calo-ries	%cal fat	prot gm	carbo gm	fiber gm
804	Cheese spread, pressurized can [2Tbs]	28	1.0	82	66%	5	2	0.0
805	Cheese spread, Swiss based (Include Swiss Almond cold pack cheese food) [2Tbs]	31	1.1	89	66%	5	3	0.0
806	Cheese with nuts (Include cheese balls) [2Tbs]	30	1.1	123	72%	8	1	0.1
807	Blue or Roquefort (Include Gorgonzola, Stilton) [2Tbs, crumbled]	17	0.6	60	73%	4	0	0.0
808	Brick (Include Beer, Elbinger, Zweiteitige, Wilstermarsch, Bondost, Oka) [1-oz slice]	28	1.0	104	72%	7	1	0.0
809	Brick with salami [1-oz slice]	28	1.0	100	72%	6	1	0.0
810	Brie [1-oz slice]	28	1.0	93	75%	6	0	0.0
811	Camembert [1-oz slice]	28	1.0	84	73%	6	0	0.0
812	**Cheddar or American** type (Include Coon, Longhorn, Wisconsin, New York, Pioneer, Hoop, Tillamook, sharp cheese, Chevres) [1-oz slice]	**28**	**1.0**	**113**	**74%**	**7**	**0**	**0.0**
813	Cheddar or American type, dry, grated [4Tbs]	27	0.9	140	74%	9	0	0.0
814	Cheddar or Colby, low sodium [1-oz slice]	28	1.0	111	74%	7	1	0.0
815	Cheddar or Colby, low sodium, lowfat [1-oz slice]	28	1.0	48	36%	7	1	0.0
816	Cheddar or Colby, lowfat [1-oz slice]	28	1.0	48	36%	7	1	0.0
817	Colby [1-oz slice]	28	1.0	110	73%	7	1	0.0
818	Colby Jack [1-oz slice]	28.4	1.0	109	73%	7	0	0.0
819	Cottage cheese, creamed, large or small curd [1 cup]	210	7.4	217	39%	26	6	0.0
820	Cottage cheese, low sodium [1 cup]	225	7.9	232	39%	28	6	0.0
821	Cottage cheese, dry curd (Include baker's, pressed, dutch, skim, nonfat cottage cheese) [1 cup]	145	5.1	123	4%	25	3	0.0
822	Cottage cheese, lowfat (Include lowfat pot cheese) [1 cup]	226	8.0	164	13%	28	6	0.0
823	Cottage cheese, lowfat, lactose reduced [1 cup]	227	8.0	168	12%	28	7	1.4
824	Cottage cheese, lowfat, low sodium [1 cup]	225	7.9	162	13%	28	6	0.0
825	Cottage cheese, lowfat, with fruit [1 cup]	226	8.0	174	15%	20	17	1.0
826	Cottage cheese, lowfat, with vegetables [1 cup]	226	8.0	151	13%	25	7	0.0
827	Cottage cheese, salted, dry curd [1 cup (not packed)]	145	5.1	121	4%	25	3	0.0
828	Cottage cheese, with gelatin dessert [1 cup]	240	8.5	199	26%	17	19	0.0
829	Cottage cheese, with gelatin dessert and fruit [1 cup]	240	8.5	214	19%	14	31	0.9
830	Cottage cheese, with gelatin dessert and vegetables [1 cup]	240	8.5	205	32%	21	14	0.5
831	Cottage cheese, with fruit (creamed or uncreamed, large or small curd) [1 cup]	226	8.0	279	25%	22	30	0.0
832	Cottage cheese, with vegetables [1 cup]	226	8.0	215	40%	25	7	0.0
833	**Cream cheese [2Tbs]**	**29**	**1.0**	**101**	**90%**	**2**	**1**	**0.0**
834	Cream cheese, lowfat [2Tbs]	29	1.0	68	69%	3	2	0.0
835	Cream cheese, nonfat or fat free [2Tbs]	31	1.1	30	13%	5	2	0.0
836	Farmer's cheese [1 cup]	210	7.4	311	61%	25	5	0.0
837	Feta cheese [1-oz slice]	28	1.0	74	73%	4	1	0.0
838	Fontina [1-oz slice]	28	1.0	109	72%	7	0	0.0
839	Goat cheese [1-oz slice]	28	1.0	101	72%	7	1	0.0
840	Gouda or Edam (Include Caciocavallo, Delft, ball cheese) [1-oz slice]	28	1.0	100	70%	7	0	0.0
841	Gruyere [1-oz slice]	28	1.0	116	70%	8	0	0.0
842	Imitation cheese, American or cheddar type (Include Cheez-ola, Pretend, Country Meadow) [1-oz slice]	28	1.0	67	53%	5	3	0.0
843	Imitation cheese, American or cheddar type, low cholesterol [1-oz slice]	28	1.0	109	74%	7	0	0.0
844	Imitation cheese spread (Include Count Down) [2Tbs]	28	1.0	35	7%	5	3	0.0
845	Imitation cream cheese [2Tbs]	29	1.0	67	83%	1	2	0.0
846	Imitation mozzarella cheese (Include Pizza Mate) [1-oz slice]	28	1.0	69	44%	3	7	0.0
847	Limburger [1-oz slice]	28	1.0	93	75%	6	0	0.0
848	Monterey [1-oz slice]	28	1.0	105	73%	7	0	0.0
849	Monterey, lowfat [1-oz slice]	28	1.0	89	62%	8	0	0.0
850	Mozzarella (Include pizza cheese, string cheese, cheese sticks) [1-oz portion]	28	1.0	78	55%	8	1	0.0
851	Mozzarella, nonfat or fat free [1 cup, shredded]	113	4.0	168	0%	36	4	2.0
852	Mozzarella, low sodium [1-oz slice]	28	1.0	78	55%	8	1	0.0
853	Muenster [1-oz slice]	28	1.0	103	73%	7	0	0.0

Food #	fat gm	sat fat gm	choles mg	sodium mg	potass mg	vit A	vit E	vit C	thia-min	ribo-flavin	nia-cin	vit B-6	fol-ate	vit B-12	cal-cium	phos-phorus	magne-sium	iron	zinc
						% of Daily Value													
804	6	4	16	378	68	5	1	0	1	7	0	2	0	2	16	20	2	1	5
805	6	4	17	410	74	6	1	0	1	8	0	2	1	2	17	22	2	1	5
806	10	5	26	175	43	7	1	0	1	6	0	2	1	5	23	16	3	1	6
807	5	3	13	235	43	4	0	0	0	4	1	1	2	3	9	7	1	0	3
808	8	5	26	157	38	8	0	0	0	6	0	1	1	6	19	13	2	1	5
809	8	5	26	171	40	8	0	0	1	6	1	1	1	7	17	12	2	1	5
810	8	5	28	176	43	5	1	0	1	9	1	3	5	8	5	5	1	1	4
811	7	4	20	236	52	7	1	0	1	8	1	3	4	6	11	10	1	1	4
812	**9**	**6**	**29**	**174**	**28**	**8**	**0**	**0**	**1**	**6**	**0**	**1**	**1**	**4**	**20**	**14**	**2**	**1**	**6**
813	12	7	36	216	34	10	0	0	1	8	0	1	2	5	25	18	2	1	7
814	9	6	28	6	31	8	0	0	0	6	0	1	1	4	20	14	2	1	6
815	2	1	6	6	31	2	0	0	0	0	0	1	1	4	20	14	2	1	6
816	2	1	6	171	18	2	0	0	0	4	0	1	1	2	12	14	1	1	3
817	9	6	27	169	35	8	0	0	0	6	0	1	1	4	19	13	2	1	6
818	9	6	26	162	29	7	0	0	0	6	0	1	1	4	20	13	2	1	6
819	9	6	31	850	177	10	1	0	3	20	1	7	6	22	13	28	3	2	5
820	10	6	34	29	189	11	1	0	3	21	1	8	7	23	14	30	3	2	6
821	1	0	10	19	47	1	1	0	2	12	1	6	5	20	5	15	1	2	5
822	2	1	10	918	193	2	1	0	3	22	1	8	7	24	14	30	3	2	6
823	2	1	9	499	195	2	1	0	3	21	1	8	7	24	12	30	3	2	6
824	2	1	9	29	194	2	1	0	3	21	1	8	7	24	14	30	3	2	6
825	3	2	12	594	218	6	3	3	3	17	3	6	5	17	10	23	3	3	5
826	2	1	7	911	194	9	1	15	2	17	1	6	6	18	13	29	2	1	4
827	1	0	10	580	47	1	1	0	2	12	1	6	5	20	5	15	1	2	5
828	6	4	19	570	110	6	1	0	2	13	1	4	4	13	8	19	2	1	3
829	4	3	15	437	160	6	1	3	2	10	2	6	4	10	7	16	3	2	3
830	7	5	24	673	190	23	1	14	3	16	2	7	6	16	10	23	3	2	4
831	8	5	25	915	151	8	1	0	3	17	1	6	5	19	11	24	2	1	4
832	9	6	32	911	194	17	1	15	2	17	1	6	6	18	13	29	2	1	4
833	**10**	**6**	**32**	**86**	**35**	**11**	**1**	**0**	**0**	**3**	**0**	**1**	**1**	**2**	**2**	**3**	**0**	**2**	**1**
834	5	3	16	87	49	6	0	0	0	5	0	1	1	3	3	4	1	3	1
835	0	0	3	170	51	9	0	0	1	3	0	1	3	3	6	14	1	0	2
836	21	13	61	801	167	21	2	0	3	19	1	7	6	21	12	26	3	2	5
837	6	4	25	313	17	4	0	0	3	14	1	6	2	8	14	9	1	1	5
838	9	5	32	224	18	8	0	0	0	3	0	1	0	8	15	10	1	0	7
839	8	6	21	115	22	11	1	0	2	12	2	2	0	1	12	13	2	3	2
840	8	5	27	258	47	6	1	0	1	6	0	1	1	7	20	15	2	1	7
841	9	5	31	94	23	8	0	0	1	5	0	1	1	7	28	17	3	0	7
842	4	2	10	378	68	4	0	0	1	7	0	2	0	2	16	20	2	1	5
843	9	2	4	188	15	4	1	0	1	6	0	1	1	4	20	15	2	1	6
844	0	0	1	394	82	0	0	0	1	8	0	2	1	2	15	22	2	1	5
845	6	1	0	245	127	0	10	0	0	0	0	0	0	0	0	10	0	1	2
846	3	1	0	192	127	12	2	0	0	7	0	1	1	4	17	16	3	1	4
847	8	5	26	227	36	9	1	0	2	8	0	1	4	5	14	11	1	0	4
848	8	5	25	150	23	7	0	0	0	6	0	1	1	4	21	12	2	1	6
849	6	4	18	160	23	9	1	0	0	6	0	1	1	4	20	13	2	1	6
850	5	3	15	148	27	5	0	0	0	6	0	1	1	4	20	15	2	0	6
851	0	0	20	797	120	23	1	0	2	20	1	5	3	17	100	74	9	2	30
852	5	3	15	4	27	5	0	0	0	6	0	1	1	4	20	15	2	0	6
853	8	5	27	176	38	9	0	0	0	5	0	1	1	7	20	13	2	1	5

Beverages, Dairy, Eggs

Food #	Food Description & Amount	wt gm	wt oz	calo-ries	%cal fat	prot gm	carbo gm	fiber gm
854	Muenster, lowfat [1-oz slice]	28	1.0	77	58%	7	1	0.0
855	Muenster, low sodium [1-oz slice]	28	1.0	103	73%	7	0	0.0
856	Parmesan, dry grated (Include Romano, aged Asiago) [4Tbs]	25	0.9	114	59%	10	1	0.0
857	Parmesan, dry grated, low sodium [4Tbs]	25	0.9	114	59%	10	1	0.0
858	Parmesan, hard (Include Romano, fresh Asiago) [1-oz slice]	28	1.0	110	59%	10	1	0.0
859	Parmesan cheese topping, fat free (Include Kraft and Weight Watchers Fat Free Grated Topping) [4Tbs]	30	1.1	111	12%	12	12	0.0
860	Port du Salut [1-oz slice]	28	1.0	98	72%	7	0	0.0
861	**Processed American** or cheddar-type cheese (Include American Cheese Slices, Cheezes, Cheez Kisses) [¾-oz slice]	21	0.7	70	69%	4	1	0.0
862	Processed American or cheddar type cheese, low sodium [¾-oz slice]	21	0.7	79	75%	5	0	0.0
863	Processed American or cheddar type cheese product, reduced fat (Include Velveeta Light) [¾-oz slice]	21	0.7	50	53%	4	2	0.0
864	Processed American or cheddar type cheese product, reduced fat, reduced sodium (Include Alpine Lace American Flavor Process Cheese Product) [¾-oz slice]	21	0.7	64	63%	4	1	0.3
865	Processed American or cheddar type cheese, lowfat [¾-oz slice)]	21	0.7	38	35%	5	1	0.0
866	Processed American or cheddar type cheese, lowfat, low sodium [¾-oz slice]	21	0.7	38	35%	5	1	0.0
867	Processed American or cheddar type cheese, nonfat (Include Borden Lite, Alpine Lace Fat Free) [¾-oz slice]	21	0.7	31	5%	5	3	0.0
868	Processed American-Swiss cheese [¾-oz slice]	21	0.7	79	75%	5	0	0.0
869	Processed cheese food (Include Handi-Snack) [¾-oz slice]	21	0.7	69	67%	4	2	0.0
870	Processed cheese with vegetables (Include pepper cheese, pimiento) [¾-oz slice]	21	0.7	79	75%	5	0	0.0
871	Processed cheese with wine [¾-oz slice]	21	0.7	69	67%	4	2	0.0
872	Processed Mozzarella cheese, low sodium [¾-oz slice]	21	0.7	59	55%	6	1	0.0
873	Processed Muenster cheese, lowfat, low sodium [¾-oz slice]	21	0.7	35	38%	5	0	0.0
874	Processed Swiss cheese [¾-oz slice]	21	0.7	70	67%	5	0	0.0
875	Processed Swiss cheese, low sodium [¾-oz slice]	21	0.7	70	67%	5	0	0.0
876	Processed Swiss cheese, reduced fat (Include Kraft Light Singles) [¾-oz slice]	21	0.7	44	45%	4	1	0.0
877	Processed Swiss cheese, lowfat [¾-oz slice]	21	0.7	36	27%	5	1	0.0
878	Processed Swiss cheese, lowfat, low sodium (Include Alpine Lace Swiss-Lo Cheese) [¾-oz slice]	21	0.7	43	36%	6	1	0.0
879	Provolone [1-oz slice]	28	1.0	98	68%	7	1	0.0
880	Provolone, reduced fat, reduced sodium [1-oz slice]	28	1.0	77	58%	7	1	0.0
881	Puerto Rican white cheese (queso del pais, blanco) [1-oz slice]	28	1.0	48	67%	3	1	0.0
882	Queso Anejo (aged Mexican cheese) [4Tbs, crumbled]	33	1.2	123	72%	7	2	0.0
883	Queso Asadero (Include Oaxacan-style string cheese) [1-oz slice]	28	1.0	100	71%	6	1	0.0
884	Queso Chihuahua (Include Mennonite cheese) [1-oz slice]	28	1.0	105	71%	6	2	0.0
885	Queso Fresco (Include Hispanic-style farmer cheese) [1-oz slice]	28	1.0	41	52%	3	2	0.0
886	Ricotta [1 cup]	246	8.7	384	60%	28	10	0.0
887	Semi-soft cheese, low sodium [1-oz slice]	28	1.0	110	74%	7	0	0.0
888	**Swiss** (Include Emmentaler, Asiago, Jarlsburg, Samsoe, Danbo, Sweitzer) [1-oz slice]	28	1.0	105	66%	8	1	0.0
889	Swiss, low fat [1-oz slice]	28	1.0	50	26%	8	1	0.0
890	Swiss, low sodium [1-oz slice]	28	1.0	105	66%	8	1	0.0
891	Yogurt cheese [1 cup]	245	8.6	186	2%	19	25	0.0
	Eggs (chicken eggs unless specified otherwise)							
925	Egg casserole with bread, cheese, milk and meat [1 cup]	164	5.8	384	59%	20	18	0.9
926	Egg salad [1 egg]	74	2.6	236	87%	7	1	0.0
927	Egg substitute (from powdered, frozen, or liquid) [1 cup, cooked]	210	7.4	256	51%	28	2	0.0
928	Egg, creamed [1 egg]	145	5.1	218	63%	11	8	0.2
929	Egg, deviled [½ egg]	31	1.1	63	73%	4	0	0.0
930	Egg, duck, cooked [1 egg]	70	2.5	130	67%	9	1	0.0
931	Egg, goose, cooked [1 egg]	144	5.1	267	65%	20	2	0.0
932	Egg, quail, canned [4 eggs]	36	1.3	56	63%	5	0	0.0

Food #	fat gm	sat fat gm	choles mg	sodium mg	potass mg	vit A	vit E	vit C	thia-min	ribo-flavin	nia-cin	vit B-6	fol-ate	vit B-12	cal-cium	phos-phorus	magne-sium	iron	zinc
										% of Daily Value									
854	5	3	18	168	38	5	0	0	0	6	0	1	1	7	15	13	2	1	5
855	8	5	27	5	38	9	0	0	0	5	0	1	1	7	20	13	2	1	5
856	8	5	20	465	27	4	1	0	1	6	0	1	1	6	34	20	3	1	5
857	7	5	20	16	27	4	1	0	1	6	0	1	1	6	34	20	3	1	5
858	7	5	19	448	26	4	1	0	1	5	0	1	0	6	33	19	3	1	5
859	2	1	6	345	180	14	0	0	1	1	0	2	2	6	24	21	3	8	6
860	8	5	34	150	38	10	0	0	0	4	0	1	1	7	18	10	2	1	5
861	5	3	14	257	55	5	0	0	0	5	0	1	0	4	12	10	2	1	4
862	7	4	20	1	34	6	0	0	0	4	0	1	0	2	13	16	1	0	4
863	3	2	11	333	69	5	0	0	1	6	0	1	1	4	11	17	2	0	3
864	4	3	15	148	154	4	0	0	0	4	0	1	0	2	22	16	1	0	4
865	1	1	7	300	38	1	0	0	0	5	0	1	0	3	14	17	1	1	5
866	1	1	7	1	38	1	0	0	0	5	0	1	0	3	14	17	1	1	5
867	0	0	2	321	60	9	0	0	1	6	0	1	1	4	14	20	2	0	5
868	7	4	20	300	34	6	0	0	0	4	0	1	0	2	13	16	1	0	4
869	5	3	13	250	59	5	0	0	0	5	0	1	0	4	12	10	2	1	4
870	7	4	20	300	34	7	0	1	0	4	0	1	0	2	13	16	1	0	4
871	5	3	13	250	59	5	0	0	0	5	0	1	0	4	12	10	2	1	4
872	4	2	11	3	20	4	0	0	0	4	0	1	1	3	15	11	1	0	4
873	1	1	5	1	28	1	0	0	0	4	0	1	1	5	15	10	1	0	4
874	5	3	18	288	45	5	0	0	0	3	0	0	0	4	16	16	2	1	5
875	5	3	18	9	45	5	0	0	0	3	0	0	0	4	16	16	2	1	5
876	2	1	11	259	59	4	0	0	0	4	0	1	0	3	15	7	1	1	5
877	1	1	7	300	38	1	0	0	0	5	0	1	0	3	14	17	1	1	5
878	2	1	6	26	45	3	0	0	0	4	0	0	0	4	19	16	2	1	5
879	7	5	19	245	39	7	0	0	0	5	0	1	1	7	21	14	2	1	6
880	5	3	15	123	39	10	0	0	0	6	0	1	1	7	35	14	2	1	6
881	4	2	14	23	29	4	0	0	0	3	0	1	1	2	6	4	1	1	2
882	10	6	35	373	29	2	0	0	0	4	0	1	0	8	22	15	2	1	6
883	8	5	29	183	24	2	0	0	0	4	0	1	1	5	19	12	2	1	6
884	8	5	29	173	15	2	0	0	0	4	0	1	0	5	18	12	2	1	7
885	2	1	9	37	37	3	0	0	0	3	0	0	1	1	8	5	1	1	3
886	26	16	100	257	282	30	2	0	3	27	1	4	8	13	59	42	8	6	21
887	9	6	25	35	38	6	1	0	2	4	0	1	1	7	25	13	2	1	5
888	8	5	26	73	31	7	0	0	0	6	0	1	0	8	27	17	3	0	7
889	1	1	10	73	31	2	0	0	0	6	0	1	0	8	27	17	3	0	7
890	8	5	26	4	31	7	0	0	0	6	0	1	0	8	27	17	3	0	7
891	0	0	7	186	625	0	0	4	8	33	1	6	7	25	49	38	12	1	16
925	25	11	158	959	323	14	3	2	24	28	14	9	8	15	31	33	8	12	16
926	23	4	235	188	73	11	10	0	2	16	0	9	6	11	3	10	1	4	4
927	15	3	2	489	763	57	7	0	14	39	1	0	6	10	12	28	5	27	20
928	15	4	279	365	207	15	6	1	7	28	2	6	9	16	13	19	4	6	7
929	5	1	122	50	37	5	2	0	1	9	0	2	3	5	1	5	1	2	2
930	10	3	619	102	156	28	2	0	6	16	1	8	11	54	4	15	3	15	7
931	19	5	1227	199	302	55	4	0	12	31	1	16	20	104	9	30	6	29	13
932	4	1	301	190	47	3	1	0	3	17	0	3	6	9	2	8	1	7	3

Beverages, Dairy, Eggs

Food #	Food Description & Amount	wt gm	wt oz	calo-ries	%cal fat	prot gm	carbo gm	fiber gm
933	Egg, white only, cooked, salted [1 white]	33	1.2	17	0%	3	0	0.0
934	Egg, white only, raw (Include cooked unsalted) [1 white]	33	1.2	17	0%	3	0	0.0
935	Egg, whole, baked, salted [1 egg]	45	1.6	75	61%	6	1	0.0
936	**Egg, whole, boiled in shell and salted** or poached without shell in salted water [1 egg]	**50**	**1.8**	**75**	**61%**	**6**	**1**	**0.0**
937	Egg, whole, fried (Include scrambled egg without milk) [1 egg]	46	1.6	91	68%	6	1	0.0
938	Egg, whole, pickled [1 egg]	47	1.7	73	62%	6	1	0.0
939	Egg, whole, raw (include cooked, unsalted) [1 egg]	50	1.8	75	61%	6	1	0.0
940	Egg, yolk only, raw or cooked [1 yolk]	17	0.6	61	78%	3	0	0.0
941	Eggs a la Malaguena, Puerto Rican style (Huevos a la Malaguena) [1 egg]	123	4.3	126	43%	11	8	1.8
942	Eggs Benedict [1 egg]	155	5.5	288	55%	17	15	0.8
943	Huevos rancheros [1 egg]	118	4.2	139	51%	8	10	1.9
944	**Omelet or scrambled egg** (egg, milk, salt), cooked in margarine [1 egg]	**62**	**2.2**	**95**	**65%**	**7**	**1**	**0.0**
945	Omelet or scrambled egg, cooked without fat [1 egg]	60	2.1	79	58%	6	1	0.0
946	Omelet or scrambled egg, with beef and onions [1 egg]	95	3.4	152	63%	11	3	0.1
947	Omelet or scrambled egg, with cheese [1 egg]	67	2.4	127	66%	8	2	0.0
948	Omelet or scrambled egg, with cheese and ham [1 egg]	78	2.8	156	65%	11	2	0.0
949	Omelet or scrambled egg, with chicken [1 egg]	95	3.4	150	53%	15	2	0.0
950	Omelet or scrambled egg, with chorizo [1 egg]	70	2.5	147	69%	9	2	0.0
951	Omelet or scrambled egg, with dark-green vegetables [1 egg]	84	3.0	110	63%	8	2	0.5
952	Omelet or scrambled egg, with fish [1 egg]	88	3.1	136	61%	11	2	0.0
953	Omelet or scrambled egg, with ham or bacon [1 egg]	70	2.5	130	64%	10	1	0.0
954	Omelet or scrambled egg, with mushrooms [1 egg]	69	2.4	88	62%	6	2	0.4
955	Omelet or scrambled egg, with onions, peppers, tomatoes, and mushrooms (Include Spanish omelet) [1 egg]	145	5.1	177	69%	8	6	1.1
956	Omelet or scrambled egg, with peppers, onion, and ham (Include Western omelet) [1 egg]	94	3.3	146	62%	11	3	0.2
957	Omelet or scrambled egg, with potatoes and/or onions (Tortilla Espanola, traditional style Spanish omelet) [1 egg]	156	5.5	199	50%	10	15	1.2
958	Omelet or scrambled egg, with sausage [1 egg]	87	3.1	204	71%	12	2	0.0
959	Omelet or scrambled egg, with sausage and cheese [1 egg]	85	3.0	189	69%	11	2	0.0
960	Omelet or scrambled egg, with sausage and mushrooms [1 egg]	95	3.4	167	67%	11	2	0.1
961	Omelet or scrambled egg, with vegetables other than dark-green vegetables [1 egg]	64	2.3	84	62%	6	2	0.3
962	Omelet or scrambled egg, with chili, cheese, tomatoes, and beans [1 egg]	103	3.6	159	63%	10	4	0.6
963	Omelet with ripe plantain, Puerto Rican style (Tortilla de amarillo) [1 cup]	173	6.1	396	60%	11	32	2.2
964	Scrambled egg, made from cholesterol-free frozen mix (Include Egg Beaters) [1 cup, cooked]	153	5.4	252	65%	16	6	0.0
965	Scrambled egg, made from cholesterol-free frozen mix with cheese (Include Egg Beaters Cheese) [1 cup, cooked]	153	5.4	265	63%	17	7	0.0
966	Scrambled egg, made from cholesterol-free frozen mixture with vegetables [1 cup, cooked]	188	6.6	136	31%	17	5	0.3
967	Scrambled egg, made from dry eggs [1 cup]	214	7.5	461	80%	20	2	0.0
968	Scrambled egg, made from frozen mix (Include Egg Delight) [1 cup, cooked]	140	4.9	174	46%	15	9	0.0
969	Scrambled egg, made from packaged liquid mix (Include Second Nature) [1 cup, cooked]	210	7.4	214	47%	23	4	0.0
970	Scrambled egg, made from powdered mix (Include Eggstra) [1 cup, cooked]	188	6.6	361	66%	21	8	0.0
971	Scrambled eggs with jerked beef, Puerto Rican style (Revoltillo de tasajo) [1 cup]	140	4.9	375	64%	29	4	0.4
972	Shrimp-egg patty (Torta de Cameron seco) (Include dried shrimp patty) [½-cup patty]	43	1.5	184	67%	10	4	0.1
Your Additions								

Food #	fat gm	sat fat gm	choles mg	sodium mg	potass mg	% of Daily Value													
						vit A	vit E	vit C	thia-min	ribo-flavin	nia-cin	vit B-6	fol-ate	vit B-12	cal-cium	phos-phorus	magne-sium	iron	zinc
933	0	0	0	54	47	0	0	0	0	8	0	0	0	1	0	0	1	0	0
934	0	0	0	54	47	0	0	0	0	9	0	0	0	1	0	0	1	0	0
935	5	2	212	63	60	10	2	0	2	14	0	3	4	7	2	9	1	4	4
936	5	2	213	63	61	10	2	0	2	13	0	3	4	7	2	9	1	4	4
937	7	2	212	85	61	11	3	0	2	14	0	3	4	7	3	9	1	4	4
938	5	2	199	58	59	8	2	0	2	14	0	3	5	9	2	8	1	3	3
939	5	2	213	63	61	10	2	0	2	15	0	3	6	8	2	9	1	4	4
940	5	2	218	7	16	10	2	0	2	6	0	3	6	9	2	8	0	3	4
941	6	2	231	513	303	17	4	14	9	19	6	9	9	8	4	15	5	8	7
942	17	6	226	1007	223	15	4	0	24	23	14	15	10	13	9	22	5	10	11
943	8	2	217	249	199	14	5	21	4	16	3	8	10	7	8	15	5	8	6
944	7	2	201	89	87	12	3	0	2	15	0	3	4	8	5	10	2	4	4
945	5	2	201	69	86	10	2	0	2	15	0	3	4	8	5	10	2	4	4
946	11	3	268	123	151	15	3	1	3	21	3	6	6	14	6	15	3	6	8
947	9	4	191	229	110	13	3	0	2	17	0	4	4	9	11	15	3	4	6
948	11	5	198	373	145	13	3	0	7	18	3	6	4	10	11	18	3	5	8
949	9	3	244	114	165	13	3	0	3	18	16	12	5	10	5	18	4	6	6
950	11	4	201	240	132	11	3	0	7	17	3	6	4	11	5	12	2	5	7
951	8	2	223	108	167	22	4	16	3	18	1	5	10	8	7	12	4	7	5
952	9	3	254	186	151	14	4	0	3	20	5	6	6	19	9	17	3	5	6
953	9	3	177	330	133	9	2	0	10	15	5	7	4	9	4	13	3	4	7
954	6	2	177	147	97	10	2	0	3	14	2	4	4	7	4	10	2	4	4
955	14	3	219	170	269	21	7	32	5	21	4	8	7	8	6	14	4	6	5
956	10	3	232	274	161	13	3	9	9	19	4	8	5	10	5	15	3	5	7
957	11	3	282	143	330	18	4	8	7	22	4	13	8	11	8	17	6	7	7
958	16	5	233	443	187	13	3	1	15	20	6	8	5	16	6	16	3	6	9
959	15	5	232	389	168	15	3	1	9	21	3	7	5	14	11	18	3	5	8
960	13	4	267	294	162	15	3	1	9	21	3	7	6	13	6	16	3	6	7
961	6	2	170	98	88	10	2	1	2	13	1	3	4	6	4	9	2	4	4
962	11	4	250	262	200	23	4	6	4	22	1	6	7	11	12	19	4	6	7
963	26	5	346	106	535	24	15	21	6	26	3	18	10	12	4	18	11	10	7
964	18	3	3	320	342	24	11	1	10	31	1	9	4	9	15	13	6	14	9
965	19	4	8	478	348	23	10	1	9	32	1	9	4	8	21	22	6	13	11
966	5	1	1	314	333	9	3	15	2	41	2	3	2	7	7	8	6	1	2
967	41	10	715	502	218	35	18	0	5	37	1	8	13	24	11	35	5	16	15
968	9	2	67	220	208	30	4	1	1	21	1	1	5	5	6	7	4	1	2
969	11	2	3	401	675	47	6	1	12	34	1	1	6	11	17	27	5	21	17
970	27	6	217	561	293	35	13	0	5	38	1	3	9	19	13	19	7	7	5
971	27	6	392	2247	409	16	14	2	7	32	17	17	10	38	5	27	8	23	28
972	14	2	205	347	101	9	8	1	5	12	5	4	5	11	4	11	4	9	6

Many of us don't eat enough fruit. One reason is that many people think it must be fresh fruit, that canned or frozen fruit isn't as good for us. In fact, canned and frozen fruit can be as good for us as fresh fruit. Those trying to cut calories, however, should choose the ones with less added sugar, e.g., fruit canned in juice instead of syrup.

Fresh fruit, of course, doesn't last as long. If it's getting over-ripe, eat it or freeze it before it spoils. (See the Apple Crisp recipe at the end of the next section for how to use apples that have lost their crispness.) Peel the bananas before freezing, and wash fruits like strawberries before freezing. This way, they're ready to make into banana bread, smoothies, etc.

Milk and fruit are a tasty combination, so if you aren't getting enough milk, add milk or yogurt to your fruit smoothies. Below are some milk-fruit (and a milk-pumpkin) recipes for frozen bars.

Mix the ingredients in a blender. Add some sugar if the fruit isn't sweet enough. You can also add chopped nuts. Pour into popsicle molds, and freeze. If possible, use wooden popsicle sticks so that you can transfer the frozen bars to plastic bags and have the molds free to refill (and you don't have to worry about kids not returning the sticks).

Strawberry Milk Bars
1-2 cups fresh or frozen strawberries
2 ripe bananas
½ cup milk

Orange Sherbet Bars
6 oz (1 small can) frozen orange juice concentrate
12 oz milk (use above can to measure 2 canfuls)

Chocolate Bars
1 ripe banana
2 Tbs instant chocolate mix
½ cup milk

Pumpkin Pie Bars
2 cups (1 small can) pumpkin
6 Tbs sugar
1 tsp cinnamon
¼ tsp ginger
¼ tsp cloves
¼ tsp salt
5.3 oz (1 small can) evaporated milk

Desserts and Sweets

Cakes *1000*

Bars *1150*

Cookies *1200*

Pies and Cobblers *1350*

Frozen Desserts *1500*

Puddings *1550*

Pastries *1650*

Jams, Sweeteners, Toppings *1750*

Candy *1850*

Your Additions

End-of-Section Recipes
Meringue Pie with Fruit
Apple Crisp

Desserts & Sweets

Food #	Food Description & Amount	wt gm	wt oz	calories	%cal fat	prot gm	carbo gm	fiber gm
	Cakes							
1000	Cake batter, raw, chocolate [2Tbs]	28	1.0	88	38%	1	13	0.5
1001	Cake batter, raw, not chocolate [2Tbs]	30	1.1	86	26%	1	15	0.2
1002	Cake, angel food, chocolate, no icing [1/12 of 10"dia]	57	2.0	141	2%	4	32	0.5
1003	Cake, angel food, with icing [1/12 of 10"dia]	77	2.7	207	1%	4	49	0.1
1004	Cake, angel food, no icing [1/12 of 10"dia]	57	2.0	143	1%	3	33	0.1
1005	Cake, applesauce with raisins, low calorie, no icing (Include Weight Watcher's Apple Raisin Spice Cake) [1 individual cake]	74	2.6	173	21%	4	32	1.6
1006	Cake, applesauce with raisins, with icing [1/12 of 10"dia]	108	3.8	399	30%	3	69	1.4
1007	Cake, applesauce with raisins, no icing (Include rhubarb, blueberry, apricot, blackberry, apple crunch cake) [1/12 of 10"dia]	87	3.1	313	33%	3	52	1.6
1008	Cake, banana, with icing [1/12 of 10"dia]	108	3.8	327	22%	4	61	1.4
1009	Cake, banana, no icing [1/12 of 10"dia]	87	3.1	262	27%	3	46	1.3
1010	Cake, black forest (chocolate-cherry) [1/12 of 2-layer, 8"dia]	71	2.5	187	43%	2	27	0.9
1011	Cake, Boston cream pie [1/12 of 8"dia]	69	2.4	174	30%	2	30	1.0
1012	Cake, butter, with icing [1/10 of 1-layer, 8"dia]	83	2.9	313	35%	3	50	0.7
1013	Cake, butter, no icing [1/10 of 8"dia]	53	1.9	193	41%	2	27	0.3
1014	Cake, carrot, low calorie (Include Weight Watcher's) [1 individual cake]	85	3.0	179	33%	4	28	1.2
1015	**Cake, carrot, with icing (Include carrot cupcakes with icing) [1/10 of 1-layer, 8"dia]**	**80**	**2.8**	**328**	**46%**	**3**	**43**	**0.9**
1016	Cake, carrot, no icing (Include carrot pudding) [1/10 of 8"dia]	58	2.0	242	50%	2	29	0.8
1017	Cake, chiffon, chocolate, with icing [1/12 of 10"dia]	92	3.2	328	41%	5	47	1.6
1018	Cake, chiffon, chocolate, no icing [1/12 of 10"dia]	66	2.3	227	41%	4	31	1.0
1019	Cake, chiffon, with icing [1/12 of 10"dia]	92	3.2	317	34%	4	49	0.3
1020	Cake, chiffon, no icing [1/12 of 10"dia]	66	2.3	219	36%	4	32	0.3
1021	Cake, chocolate, devil's food, or fudge, pudding-type mix, with icing (Include Pillsbury Plus, Duncan Hines, Betty Crocker Super Moist) [1/12 of 2-layer, 8"dia]	109	3.8	401	38%	4	62	1.9
1022	Cake, chocolate, devil's food, or fudge, pudding-type mix, no icing (Include Pillsbury Plus, Duncan Hines, Betty Crocker Super Moist) [1/10 of 8"dia]	42	1.5	147	48%	2	19	0.8
1023	Cake, chocolate, devil's food, or fudge, pudding-type mix, made by "Lite" recipe (eggs and water added to dry mix; no oil added), with icing [1/12 of 2-layer, 8"dia]	109	3.8	373	29%	4	66	2.1
1024	Cake, chocolate, devil's food or fudge, pudding type mix, made by "no cholesterol" recipe (water, oil, egg whites added to dry mix), with "light" icing [1/10 of 1-layer, 8"dia]	66	2.3	220	29%	2	39	0.8
1025	Cake, chocolate, devil's food, or fudge, pudding type mix, made by "no cholesterol" recipe (water, oil and egg whites added to dry mix), no icing [1/10 of 8"dia]	42	1.5	136	40%	2	20	0.6
1026	Cake, chocolate, devil's food, or fudge, standard-type mix (eggs and water added to dry mix), with icing (Include Jiffy, Washington) [1/12 of 2-layer, 8"dia]	109	3.8	389	30%	4	69	1.7
1027	Cake, chocolate, devil's food, or fudge, standard-type mix (eggs and water added to dry mix), no icing [1/10 of 8"dia]	42	1.5	138	34%	2	22	0.7
1028	**Cake, chocolate, devil's food, or fudge, with icing, made from home recipe or purchased ready-to-eat [1/12 of 2-layer, 8"dia]**	**109**	**3.8**	**410**	**35%**	**4**	**67**	**1.7**
1029	Cake, chocolate, devil's food, or fudge, no icing or filling, made from home recipe or purchased ready-to-eat [1/10 of 8"dia]	42	1.5	152	42%	2	22	0.7
1030	Cake, chocolate, made with mayonnaise or salad dressing, with icing, coating, or filling [1/12 of 2-layer, 8"dia]	139	4.9	487	27%	4	89	2.3
1031	Cake, chocolate, made with mayonnaise or salad dressing, no icing or filling [1/10 of 8"dia]	53	1.9	161	28%	2	28	1.0
1032	Cake, chocolate, with icing, low calorie (Include Weight Watcher's Chocolate Cake) [1 individual cake]	71	2.5	217	25%	5	40	2.8
1033	Cake, coconut, with icing [1/12 of 2-layer, 8"dia]	109	3.8	388	26%	5	69	1.1
1034	Cake, cream (Include Italian rum-cream) [1/10 of 8"dia]	51	1.8	192	35%	3	29	0.3
1035	Cake, Dobos Torte (Include seven-layer cake) [1/12 of 8"dia]	123	4.3	496	50%	8	58	1.4
1036	Cake, frozen yogurt and cake layer, not chocolate, with icing [1/8 of 8"dia]	148	5.2	429	26%	6	75	0.6
1037	Cake, frozen yogurt and cake layer, chocolate, with icing [1/8 of 8"dia]	148	5.2	439	34%	6	71	1.5

Food #	fat gm	sat fat gm	choles mg	sodium mg	potass mg	% of Daily Value													
						vit A	vit E	vit C	thia-min	ribo-flavin	nia-cin	vit B-6	fol-ate	vit B-12	cal-cium	phos-phorus	magne-sium	iron	zinc
1000	4	1	12	95	49	1	1	0	3	3	2	1	3	1	3	4	2	4	1
1001	3	0	14	128	19	1	1	0	3	3	2	1	3	1	3	6	1	2	1
1002	0	0	0	275	91	0	0	0	3	7	1	0	3	0	5	13	3	2	1
1003	0	0	0	284	79	0	0	0	3	7	0	0	3	0	5	13	1	1	0
1004	0	0	0	283	75	0	0	0	3	7	0	0	3	0	5	13	1	1	0
1005	4	1	28	93	195	8	1	2	9	9	5	4	5	2	4	6	3	7	2
1006	13	3	20	163	137	4	6	1	8	7	5	3	5	1	2	4	3	7	2
1007	12	2	22	141	145	1	5	2	9	7	5	3	5	1	2	5	3	8	2
1008	8	2	33	191	178	9	4	5	9	11	6	11	7	1	3	5	4	6	2
1009	8	2	32	181	168	8	4	5	9	10	6	11	7	1	3	5	4	6	2
1010	9	4	39	160	118	3	4	16	1	8	2	3	2	3	3	7	3	4	3
1011	6	2	26	99	27	2	2	0	19	11	1	1	3	2	2	3	1	1	1
1012	12	6	64	313	78	9	3	0	3	6	2	2	4	2	5	11	3	4	2
1013	9	4	56	281	36	6	2	0	3	6	2	2	4	2	4	10	1	3	1
1014	7	2	14	338	109	44	3	5	7	7	4	3	5	2	5	5	2	5	2
1015	17	3	48	82	79	41	10	2	7	8	4	2	5	2	5	5	2	6	2
1016	14	2	39	61	65	35	9	2	6	6	4	2	4	1	4	4	1	5	1
1017	15	5	74	140	152	6	6	0	8	11	5	2	6	3	8	11	8	11	5
1018	10	3	71	111	108	4	5	0	7	10	4	2	5	3	7	9	5	9	3
1019	12	2	71	163	71	6	7	3	8	10	5	1	6	3	7	6	1	8	2
1020	9	1	69	123	62	3	5	0	8	10	5	1	6	3	6	6	1	8	2
1021	17	3	48	407	199	6	9	0	5	8	4	1	5	5	6	15	7	9	4
1022	8	1	29	219	88	1	4	0	3	4	3	1	3	3	3	8	3	4	2
1023	12	3	39	484	187	0	0	0	6	7	5	1	15	5	7	15	5	9	3
1024	7	2	0	273	105	0	2	0	3	4	3	0	2	3	4	8	3	4	2
1025	6	1	0	237	94	0	1	0	3	3	3	0	2	2	3	7	3	4	1
1026	13	3	34	434	221	6	6	0	5	7	4	1	5	1	8	16	8	14	4
1027	5	1	23	257	106	1	2	0	3	4	2	1	3	1	5	9	4	8	2
1028	16	5	31	186	157	6	6	0	8	9	5	1	5	2	10	11	8	11	4
1029	7	2	19	83	61	1	2	0	5	5	3	1	3	1	6	6	4	6	2
1030	14	3	6	459	182	8	6	0	11	9	7	1	7	1	5	9	8	12	4
1031	5	1	4	244	67	1	2	0	7	5	4	1	4	0	2	4	3	6	2
1032	6	2	35	99	293	7	2	0	10	12	6	2	8	4	6	12	11	12	6
1033	11	4	1	310	108	1	0	0	9	12	6	2	6	1	10	8	3	7	2
1034	8	4	57	90	41	9	1	0	8	7	5	1	5	1	6	5	1	8	2
1035	28	9	188	248	133	24	10	0	6	19	4	4	7	6	3	13	8	10	6
1036	13	4	34	456	181	6	3	1	13	16	8	3	8	5	17	15	4	12	4
1037	16	6	35	427	234	7	4	1	10	15	6	3	6	4	17	17	9	12	5

Desserts & Sweets

Food #	Food Description & Amount	wt gm	wt oz	calo-ries	%cal fat	prot gm	carbo gm	fiber gm
1038	Cake, fruit cake, light or dark [1/12 of 7"dia]	113	4.0	366	25%	3	70	4.2
1039	Cake, German chocolate [1/12 of 2-layer, 8"dia]	109	3.8	396	46%	4	54	2.0
1040	Cake, gingerbread [1/10 of 8"dia]	69	2.4	213	30%	3	35	0.8
1041	Cake, graham cracker [1/10 of 9"dia]	45	1.6	159	39%	3	22	0.4
1042	Cake, ice box with fruit and whipped cream [1/10 of cake]	83	2.9	172	21%	4	31	0.4
1043	Cake, ice cream roll (or cake), chocolate [1/10 of roll]	34	1.2	101	44%	1	14	0.4
1044	Cake, ice cream roll (or cake), not chocolate [1/10 of roll]	34	1.2	92	40%	1	13	0.1
1045	Cake, jelly roll [1/10 of roll]	51	1.8	147	14%	3	29	0.2
1046	Cake, Korean Injolmi, made with glutinous rice and dried beans [1 cubic inch]	21	0.7	38	2%	2	8	0.6
1047	Cake, lemon, with icing [1/12 of 2-layer, 8"dia]	109	3.8	385	25%	3	71	0.6
1048	Cake, lemon, no icing [1/10 of 8"dia]	42	1.5	159	43%	2	21	0.2
1049	Cake, lemon, lowfat, no icing [1/10 of 1-layer, 8"dia]	42	1.5	132	23%	2	23	0.2
1050	Cake, lemon, lowfat, with icing [1/10 of 1-layer, 8"dia]	66	2.3	231	24%	2	43	0.2
1051	Cake, marble, with icing [1/12 of 2-layer, 8"dia]	109	3.8	377	31%	5	65	2.1
1052	Cake, marble, no icing [1/10 of 8"dia]	42	1.5	140	30%	2	24	0.7
1053	Cake, nut, with icing (Include butter pecan cake; pistachio cake) [1/12 of 2-layer, 8"dia]	109	3.8	420	42%	3	60	0.8
1054	Cake, nut, no icing (Include butter pecan cake; pistachio cake) [1/10 of 8"dia]	42	1.5	161	50%	2	19	0.5
1055	Cake, oatmeal [1/10 of cake]	78	2.8	282	34%	3	45	1.5
1056	Cake, oatmeal, with icing [1/10 of cake]	110	3.9	409	31%	3	70	1.4
1057	Cake, peanut butter, with icing [1/12 of 2-layer, 8"dia]	109	3.8	410	36%	6	62	1.3
1058	Cake, pineapple, very lowfat, no cholesterol, no icing [1 slice (3¾"x2"x½")]	28	1.0	69	1%	2	15	0.4
1059	Cake, plum pudding (Include date pudding) [1 piece]	42	1.5	131	39%	2	19	0.7
1060	Cake, Poor Man's (spice-type) [1/10 of 8" square]	48	1.7	154	23%	2	28	0.6
1061	Cake, poppy seed, no icing [1/12 of 10"dia]	90	3.2	356	46%	6	43	0.9
1062	Cake, pound, chocolate, with icing [1/10 of loaf]	91	3.2	386	47%	5	49	1.6
1063	Cake, pound, chocolate, very lowfat, no cholesterol [1 slice (3¼"x2¾"x½")]	28	1.0	77	4%	2	17	0.6
1064	Cake, pound, Puerto Rican style (Ponque) [1 slice (3½"x3½"x1")]	90	3.2	411	51%	6	45	0.4
1065	Cake, pound, very low fat, no cholesterol (Include Entenmann's Fat-Free, Cholesterol-Free Golden Loaf Cake) [1 slice (3¼"x2¾"x½")]	28	1.0	79	4%	2	17	0.3
1066	Cake, pound, with icing [1/10 of loaf]	123	4.3	483	35%	7	73	0.5
1067	Cake, pound, no icing (Include toasted cake, yogurt honey pound cake, butter rum cake, whiskey cake, lemon pound cake with glaze) [1/10 of loaf]	91	3.2	354	38%	6	49	0.5
1068	Cake, pound, reduced fat, no cholesterol [1 slice (3½"x 2"x¾")]	28	1.0	86	20%	2	15	0.3
1069	Cake, pumpkin, no icing [1/10 of 8" square]	51	1.8	153	28%	2	26	0.8
1070	Cake, pumpkin, with icing [1/10 of 1-layer, 8"dia]	80	2.8	271	31%	2	46	0.9
1071	Cake, Quezadilla, El Salvadorian style [1/10 of cake]	150	5.3	526	42%	17	60	0.7
1072	Cake, raisin-nut, with icing [1/12 of 2 layer, 8"dia]	133	4.7	486	33%	6	78	1.9
1073	Cake, raisin-nut, no icing (Include prune cake, date-nut cake) [1/10 of 8"dia]	59	2.1	220	35%	3	34	1.0
1074	Cake, Ravani (made with farina) [1/10 of cake]	56	2.0	176	23%	2	34	0.5
1075	Cake, rice flour (Include coconut mochiko, Filipino cake) [1 piece]	45	1.6	148	42%	2	20	1.0
1076	Cake, rum flavored (Sopa Borracha) [1 slice (4"x3"x1¾")]	185	6.5	494	7%	7	105	0.4
1077	Cake, shortcake, biscuit type, with fruit [1 biscuit (2"dia) with fruit]	65	2.3	146	33%	2	23	1.1
1078	Cake, shortcake, biscuit type, with whipped cream and fruit [1 biscuit (2"dia) with fruit and whipped cream]	74	2.6	173	41%	3	24	1.1
1079	Cake, shortcake, sponge type, with fruit [1 cake (3"dia) with fruit]	102	3.6	192	11%	4	40	1.2
1080	Cake, shortcake, sponge type, with whipped cream and fruit (Include strawberry shortcake) [1 cake (3"dia) with fruit and whipped cream]	118	4.2	212	22%	4	40	1.2
1081	Cake, shortcake, with whipped topping and fruit, low calorie (Include Weight Watchers Strawberry Shortcake) [1 individual]	85	3.0	160	22%	3	30	1.2
1082	Cake, soybean [1/10 of 8"dia]	69	2.4	244	36%	6	37	3.2
1083	Cake, spice, with icing (Include walnut cake with whipped cream, Little Debbie Apple Spice, Stir-n-Frost Spice Cake) [1/12 of 2-layer, 8"dia]	109	3.8	368	29%	5	62	1.0

Food #	fat gm	sat fat gm	choles mg	sodium mg	potass mg	% of Daily Value													
						vit A	vit E	vit C	thia-min	ribo-flavin	nia-cin	vit B-6	fol-ate	vit B-12	cal-cium	phos-phorus	magne-sium	iron	zinc
1038	10	1	6	305	173	2	12	1	4	7	4	3	5	1	4	6	5	13	2
1039	20	5	52	363	148	2	8	0	7	8	5	2	4	2	5	17	4	7	3
1040	7	2	24	316	167	1	3	0	9	8	5	1	5	1	5	12	3	13	2
1041	7	1	33	189	50	7	3	0	3	6	3	1	3	2	5	5	2	4	2
1042	4	2	106	33	76	6	1	5	7	10	3	3	5	3	2	6	2	6	2
1043	5	2	15	45	57	2	1	0	3	4	2	1	2	1	4	4	2	3	2
1044	4	2	16	51	46	2	1	0	2	4	1	1	1	1	5	4	1	2	1
1045	2	1	93	30	44	4	1	2	5	9	3	2	4	3	1	5	1	5	2
1046	0	0	0	200	47	0	0	0	2	1	2	1	2	0	1	2	2	1	1
1047	11	2	34	359	53	6	5	2	5	7	4	2	6	2	7	15	1	5	2
1048	8	1	34	221	27	2	6	0	2	4	2	1	3	1	3	11	1	2	1
1049	3	1	24	209	25	1	2	0	5	5	3	1	4	1	4	8	1	3	1
1050	6	1	24	238	30	4	3	0	5	5	3	1	4	1	4	9	1	3	1
1051	13	5	43	248	185	4	6	0	8	11	6	2	7	2	10	21	8	10	4
1052	5	1	23	126	65	1	3	0	4	5	3	1	4	1	4	9	2	4	1
1053	19	3	52	375	73	6	9	0	7	8	3	3	5	2	6	19	3	5	4
1054	9	1	29	190	38	1	4	0	4	4	2	1	3	1	3	11	2	3	2
1055	11	2	20	129	132	1	5	1	9	7	5	3	5	1	2	6	4	8	2
1056	14	3	21	167	142	4	6	1	12	7	6	3	6	1	2	6	4	11	2
1057	16	6	55	500	217	11	6	0	8	9	12	4	8	2	13	11	7	9	4
1058	0	0	0	65	33	0	0	0	4	5	2	1	2	0	2	3	1	2	1
1059	6	3	15	66	199	1	1	1	4	4	3	4	1	1	5	4	6	5	1
1060	4	1	3	125	21	0	0	0	7	5	5	0	5	0	2	3	1	5	1
1061	18	7	81	312	139	10	6	1	16	17	8	3	12	3	11	12	5	9	5
1062	20	6	69	242	123	18	8	0	10	12	6	2	7	3	4	10	7	9	4
1063	0	0	0	82	79	1	0	0	4	5	2	1	2	1	4	5	2	4	1
1064	23	14	173	243	69	24	2	0	13	14	8	2	9	4	2	8	2	13	3
1065	0	0	0	95	31	1	0	0	2	5	1	0	3	0	1	4	1	3	1
1066	19	4	121	280	91	21	9	0	16	17	10	3	11	4	7	10	2	15	4
1067	15	3	112	230	80	17	7	0	15	15	9	2	10	4	6	9	2	14	3
1068	2	0	0	117	41	0	2	0	4	5	2	0	3	0	5	6	1	3	1
1069	5	1	25	89	50	31	2	1	5	5	3	1	4	1	1	3	2	5	1
1070	9	2	26	118	63	39	4	1	6	6	4	1	4	1	2	4	2	5	1
1071	25	11	124	566	133	35	3	0	12	25	7	4	10	7	45	38	6	11	12
1072	18	4	56	316	252	4	9	1	12	14	7	5	9	2	10	27	8	11	4
1073	9	2	29	153	99	1	4	0	6	7	4	3	5	1	4	13	3	5	2
1074	5	1	19	108	30	5	2	2	4	4	3	1	3	1	4	3	1	4	1
1075	7	6	0	45	106	0	1	1	2	0	3	4	1	0	3	5	5	4	2
1076	4	1	148	63	107	7	1	0	7	17	4	7	7	5	3	9	3	8	4
1077	5	1	0	89	74	1	2	24	8	7	5	1	6	0	7	5	2	6	1
1078	8	3	9	101	89	3	3	23	8	7	5	1	6	1	8	6	2	6	2
1079	2	1	96	31	96	4	1	41	6	10	4	3	7	3	2	6	2	7	2
1080	5	2	109	48	114	7	1	45	3	10	2	3	5	4	3	6	2	5	2
1081	4	1	7	16	201	0	3	22	8	7	5	1	6	1	7	11	3	6	2
1082	10	2	1	211	236	10	5	2	7	5	6	5	4	1	4	11	11	7	5
1083	12	3	50	281	136	4	7	0	9	11	6	2	7	2	8	21	3	8	2

Desserts & Sweets

Food #	Food Description & Amount	wt gm	wt oz	calo-ries	%cal fat	prot gm	carbo gm	fiber gm
1084	Cake, spice, no icing [1/10 of 8"dia]	42	1.5	146	30%	2	24	0.5
1085	Cake, sponge, chocolate, with icing [1/12 of 10"dia]	92	3.2	292	22%	7	53	1.7
1086	Cake, sponge, chocolate, no icing [1/12 of 10"dia]	66	2.3	197	18%	5	36	1.0
1087	Cake, sponge, with icing [1/12 of 10"dia]	92	3.2	303	15%	3	62	0.3
1088	Cake, sponge, no icing (Include shortcake-sponge type) [1/12 of 10"dia]	66	2.3	191	8%	4	40	0.4
1089	Cake, sweet potato, with icing [1/10 of 8"dia]	76	2.7	277	40%	4	39	1.1
1090	Cake, torte, raspberry (Include fruit tortes) [1/12 of torte]	76	2.7	223	44%	3	29	0.9
1091	Cake, upside down, pineapple (and/or other fruits) [1/12 of 9"dia]	121	4.3	387	34%	4	61	0.9
1092	Cake, white, pudding-type mix (oil, egg whites, and water added to dry mix), with icing (Include Pillsbury Plus, Duncan Hines, Betty Crocker Super Moist) [1/12 of 2-layer, 8"dia]	109	3.8	400	33%	3	66	0.9
1093	Cake, white, pudding-type mix, no icing (Include Pillsbury Plus, Duncan Hines, Betty Crocker Super Moist) [1/10 of 8"dia]	42	1.5	147	38%	2	22	0.2
1094	Cake, white, standard-type mix (egg whites and water added to mix), with icing (Include Jiffy, Washington) [1/12 of 2-layer, 8"dia]	109	3.8	393	24%	3	74	1.1
1095	Cake, white, standard-type mix (egg whites and water added to mix), no icing (Include Jiffy, Washington) [1/10 of 8"dia]	42	1.5	139	23%	2	25	0.3
1096	Cake, white, with icing, made from home recipe or purchased ready-to-eat (Include wedding cake) [1/12 of 2-layer, 8"dia]	109	3.8	419	31%	3	70	0.3
1097	Cake, white, no icing, made from home recipe or purchased ready-to-eat [1/10 of 8"dia]	42	1.5	155	38%	2	22	0.2
1098	Cake, white, eggless, lowfat [1/10 of 1-layer, 8"dia]	49	1.7	165	20%	2	31	0.4
1099	Cake, whole wheat, with fruit and nuts (Include apple nut loaf, whole wheat banana carob cake) [1/10 of loaf]	63	2.2	244	34%	3	40	2.4
1100	Cake, yellow, pudding-type mix (oil, eggs, and water added to dry mix), with icing (Include Pillsbury Plus, Duncan Hines, Betty Crocker Super Moist) [1/12 of 2-layer, 8"dia]	109	3.8	401	34%	4	64	0.9
1101	Cake, yellow, pudding-type mix (oil, eggs, and water added to dry mix), no icing (Include Pillsbury Plus, Duncan Hines, Betty Crocker Super Moist) [1/10 of 8"dia]	42	1.5	148	41%	2	20	0.2
1102	Cake, yellow, standard-type mix (eggs and water added to dry mix), with icing (Include Jiffy, Washington) [1/12 of 2-layer, 8"dia]	109	3.8	384	25%	3	70	1.1
1103	Cake, yellow, standard-type mix (eggs and water added to dry mix), no icing (Include Jiffy, Washington) [1/10 of 8"dia]	42	1.5	134	26%	2	23	0.3
1104	**Cake, yellow, with icing, made from home recipe or purchased ready-to-eat [1/12 of 2-layer, 8"dia]**	**109**	**3.8**	**402**	**28%**	**4**	**70**	**1.0**
1105	Cake, yellow, no icing, made from home recipe or purchased ready-to-eat [1/10 of 8"dia]	42	1.5	150	31%	2	24	0.2
1106	Cake, zucchini, with icing [1/12 of 2-layer, 8"dia]	133	4.7	552	45%	6	73	1.5
1107	Cake, zucchini, no icing [1/10 of 8"dia]	58	2.0	231	41%	2	32	0.7
1108	**Cheesecake (Include cream cheese pie) [1/12 of 9"dia]**	**128**	**4.5**	**412**	**54%**	**11**	**37**	**0.4**
1109	Cheesecake with cherries (and/or other fruit) [1/12 of 9"dia]	142	5.0	389	45%	9	47	0.7
1110	Cheesecake, chocolate [1/12 of 9"dia]	128	4.5	505	57%	8	49	1.9
1111	Cheesecake, chocolate, reduced fat [1 piece (1/12 of 9"dia)]	128	4.5	334	42%	12	41	2.5
1112	Cheesecake, low calorie (Include Weight Watchers) [1 individual cake (3½ x3½"x1")]	113	4.0	253	37%	6	34	0.9
1113	Cheesecake, low calorie, with fruit glaze (Include Weight Watchers) [1 individual cake (3½"x3½"x1")]	113	4.0	242	36%	6	34	1.2
1114	Cheesecake-type dessert, made with yogurt, with fruit [1/10 of 8"dia]	64	2.3	131	21%	1	26	0.9
1115	Coffee cake, crumb or quick-bread type (Include cinnamon cake) [1/12 of 8"square]	50	1.8	163	28%	3	26	0.6
1116	Coffee cake, crumb or quick-bread type, reduced fat, no cholesterol (Include Dolly Madison Buttercrumb) [1 individual cake]	43	1.5	139	6%	1	32	1.2
1117	Coffee cake, crumb or quick-bread type, cheese-filled [1/12 of 8"square]	47	1.7	144	37%	4	18	0.4
1118	Coffee cake, crumb or quick-bread type, custard filled [1/12 of 8"square]	47	1.7	129	28%	3	21	0.5
1119	Coffee cake, crumb or quick-bread type, with fruit (Include apple pastry cake) [1/12 of 8"square]	47	1.7	158	25%	3	28	0.8
1120	Coffee cake, crumb or quick-bread type, with nuts and icing [1/12 of 8"square]	42	1.5	145	33%	2	23	0.6
1121	Coffee cake, yeast type, with/without nuts (Include coffee bread with icing) [1/8 of 8"dia]	41	1.4	153	40%	3	21	1.0
1122	Coffee cake, yeast type, made from home recipe or purchased at a bakery, with/without nuts (Include coffee bread with icing) [1/8 of 8"dia]	41	1.4	140	24%	3	23	0.8

Food #	fat gm	sat fat gm	choles mg	sodium mg	potass mg	% of Daily Value													
						vit A	vit E	vit C	thia-min	ribo-flavin	nia-cin	vit B-6	fol-ate	vit B-12	cal-cium	phos-phorus	magne-sium	iron	zinc
1084	5	1	24	123	37	1	3	0	4	5	3	1	4	1	3	9	1	3	1
1085	7	3	155	58	150	8	2	2	7	15	4	3	7	5	4	12	8	12	6
1086	4	1	139	42	98	6	1	2	6	13	4	3	6	4	2	9	5	9	4
1087	5	1	62	189	66	6	3	0	10	10	6	2	6	3	5	9	2	9	2
1088	2	1	67	161	65	3	1	0	11	10	6	2	6	3	5	9	2	10	2
1089	12	2	40	204	133	19	6	9	6	7	4	5	5	1	6	12	5	6	3
1090	11	4	65	182	63	12	4	4	5	7	3	1	4	2	3	5	2	5	2
1091	15	4	27	388	140	8	5	3	12	11	7	2	8	2	14	10	4	10	3
1092	14	3	0	352	98	4	8	0	7	7	5	0	5	1	4	14	4	5	2
1093	6	1	0	185	26	0	4	0	4	4	3	0	3	0	2	7	1	2	0
1094	10	2	0	375	129	5	5	0	6	7	3	1	4	1	10	18	4	6	3
1095	4	1	0	221	43	0	2	0	4	4	2	0	3	1	6	11	1	3	1
1096	15	3	1	213	59	6	6	0	8	8	5	1	5	1	9	6	2	8	1
1097	7	1	1	107	36	0	3	0	6	5	4	0	3	0	6	4	1	5	1
1098	4	1	1	74	44	1	2	0	7	6	4	1	5	1	6	5	1	5	1
1099	9	2	22	9	168	1	3	1	6	6	5	4	4	1	2	7	7	6	3
1100	15	3	51	349	95	6	8	0	7	8	5	1	6	2	6	14	4	6	3
1101	7	1	31	182	25	1	4	0	4	5	3	1	4	1	3	8	1	3	1
1102	11	2	34	353	109	6	5	0	5	8	4	2	6	2	7	17	4	6	2
1103	4	1	23	199	30	1	2	0	3	5	2	1	4	1	4	10	1	3	1
1104	13	3	30	141	114	6	5	0	11	10	7	1	7	2	10	16	4	12	3
1105	5	1	19	57	36	1	2	0	7	5	4	1	4	1	6	9	1	6	1
1106	28	5	59	206	130	8	14	4	13	12	7	5	10	2	6	10	6	10	4
1107	11	1	30	90	48	2	7	2	6	6	4	1	5	1	3	4	2	5	1
1108	25	10	86	520	118	25	8	1	3	14	3	3	5	6	7	14	3	6	4
1109	19	8	67	406	124	22	6	2	3	12	3	3	4	4	6	11	3	7	3
1110	32	16	118	239	189	30	7	0	11	17	6	3	8	4	7	14	9	12	6
1111	16	9	112	290	405	22	2	0	3	22	2	4	13	7	14	23	13	15	9
1112	10	5	23	346	115	9	3	0	5	13	7	3	6	4	6	9	3	10	4
1113	10	5	20	304	122	8	2	14	5	11	6	3	7	4	5	8	3	10	4
1114	3	1	0	95	76	0	3	25	2	3	1	1	2	1	2	2	2	2	1
1115	5	1	48	215	43	2	3	0	6	6	4	1	5	2	6	11	2	4	2
1116	1	0	0	147	30	0	0	0	6	4	3	0	3	0	5	8	1	4	1
1117	6	2	42	162	49	4	2	0	4	6	3	1	4	2	8	10	2	3	3
1118	4	1	26	166	57	2	2	0	4	5	3	1	5	1	6	9	2	3	1
1119	4	1	40	182	83	2	3	0	5	5	3	2	4	1	5	10	2	5	2
1120	5	1	18	156	49	2	2	0	5	4	3	1	4	1	5	8	2	3	2
1121	7	1	27	157	46	3	4	1	9	6	5	2	5	1	3	3	2	4	2
1122	4	1	10	9	61	1	1	0	10	9	7	2	9	1	2	5	2	6	2

Desserts & Sweets

Food #	Food Description & Amount	wt gm	wt oz	calo-ries	%cal fat	prot gm	carbo gm	fiber gm
1123	Coffee cake, yeast type, very lowfat, no cholesterol, with fruit (Include Entenmann's Fat-free Cholesterol-free Raspberry or Lemon Twist) [1 piece (5"x1"x1")]	33	1.2	94	2%	3	20	0.6
1124	Cupcake, not chocolate, with fruit and cream filling (Include Fruit & Creme Twinkies) [1 cupcake]	43	1.5	144	28%	2	24	0.4
1125	Cupcake, chocolate, with icing or filling (Include Ho Ho's, Ding Dongs, Tastykake cupcake) [1 cupcake (2¾"dia)]	46	1.6	173	35%	2	28	0.4
1126	Cupcake, chocolate, no icing or filling, with/without nuts (Include chocolate crunch bar) [1 cupcake (2¾"dia)]	33	1.2	102	27%	2	18	0.8
1127	Cupcake, chocolate, with/without icing, fruit filling or cream filling, very lowfat, no cholesterol (Include Nutri System) [1 cupcake]	39	1.4	118	7%	3	25	0.9
1128	Cupcake, chocolate, with/without icing, fruit filling or cream filling, very lowfat, no cholesterol (Include Hostess Lights Cake with Creamy Filling) [1 cupcake]	42	1.5	127	7%	4	27	1.0
1129	Cupcake, chocolate, with/without icing, fruit filling or cream filling, very lowfat, no cholesterol (Include Hostess Lights) [1 cupcake]	49	1.7	148	7%	4	32	1.2
1130	Cupcake, not chocolate, with icing or filling (Include Hostess Twinkies and Snowballs, Crazy Bones, Snackin' Cakes) [1 cupcake (2¾"dia)]	48	1.7	175	28%	1	31	0.2
1131	Cupcake, not chocolate, no icing or filling [1 cupcake (2¾"dia)]	33	1.2	105	26%	2	18	0.3
1132	Cupcake, not chocolate, with icing, reduced fat, no cholesterol (Include Hostess Twinkies Lights) [1 cupcake]	38	1.3	128	15%	3	25	0.6
Bars								
1150	Brownie, butterscotch [1 small brownie]	34	1.2	152	45%	2	20	0.3
1151	Brownie, carob and honey [1 small brownie]	34	1.2	144	57%	2	16	2.0
1152	Brownie, chocolate, no icing, with/without nuts (Include Hostess Brownie Bites) [1 small brownie]	34	1.2	129	32%	2	21	0.7
1153	**Brownie, chocolate,** with icing, with/without nuts (Include Little Debbie Fudge Brownie) [1 small brownie]	**42**	**1.5**	**170**	**36%**	**2**	**27**	**0.9**
1154	Brownie, chocolate, reduced fat, with icing [1 small brownie]	40	1.4	140	18%	2	29	1.5
1155	Brownie, chocolate, fat free, no cholesterol, with icing [1 small brownie]	46	1.6	124	5%	2	30	1.9
1156	Brownie, chocolate, diet, with nuts (Include Weight Watchers Chocolate Brownie) [1small brownie]	34	1.2	131	26%	1	24	1.3
1157	Brownie, chocolate, with cream cheese filling, no icing, with/without nuts [1small brownie]	42	1.5	171	43%	2	23	0.7
1158	Brownie, chocolate, with peanut butter fudge icing [1small brownie]	30	1.1	121	38%	2	18	0.6
1159	Coconut bar [2 small bars]	27	1.0	133	45%	2	17	1.1
1160	Cookie bar, with chocolate, nuts, and graham crackers (Include Magic Cookie Bars) [1 bar]	25	0.9	121	55%	1	13	0.5
1161	Date bar (Include date-nut bar, date macaroon, date pinwheel) [2 bars]	32	1.1	111	19%	1	23	1.5
1162	Fruit-filled bar (Include trail mix cookies, fruitcake cookies, Apple Newton, Blueberry Newton, Cherry Newton, Strawberry Newton) [2 bars]	32	1.1	130	28%	1	22	0.7
1163	Fruit-filled bar, fat free (Include Newton bar, Health Valley Apple Raisin or Apricot bar) [1-2 bars]	38	1.3	124	1%	2	29	0.8
1164	Fig bar (Include Fig Newton, Little Debbie Figaroos) [2 bars]	32	1.1	111	19%	1	23	1.5
1165	Fig bar, fat free (Include Newton) [2 bars]	38	1.3	127	2%	2	30	1.2
1166	**Granola bar,** oats, sugar (including with coconut, raisins, chocolate chips) [1 bar]	**43**	**1.5**	**195**	**35%**	**4**	**29**	**1.3**
1167	Granola bar, oats, fruit and nuts, lowfat [1-oz bar]	28	1.0	106	15%	2	22	1.5
1168	Granola bar, peanuts, oats, sugar, wheat germ [1 bar]	43	1.5	206	40%	5	27	1.8
1169	Granola bar, chocolate-coated [1-oz bar]	28	1.0	130	41%	2	19	1.0
1170	Granola bar with nuts, chocolate-coated [1 bar]	35	1.2	178	55%	3	19	1.3
1171	Granola bar, coated with non-chocolate coating [1-oz bar]	28	1.0	131	44%	2	17	0.8
1172	Granola bar, high fiber, coated with non-chocolate yogurt coating [1-oz bar]	28	1.0	96	27%	3	19	2.2
1173	Granola bar or cluster, with nougat [1 bar or cluster]	34	1.2	138	30%	2	24	1.4
1174	Lemon bar [2 small bars]	33	1.2	143	39%	2	21	0.3
1175	Rice Krispie bar [1-oz bar]	28	1.0	119	36%	2	18	1.0
1176	Toffee bar [2 small bars]	38	1.3	183	42%	2	25	0.9

Food #	fat gm	sat fat gm	choles mg	sodium mg	potass mg	% of Daily Value													
						vit A	vit E	vit C	thia-min	ribo-flavin	nia-cin	vit B-6	fol-ate	vit B-12	cal-cium	phos-phorus	magne-sium	iron	zinc
1123	0	0	0	53	59	1	0	1	6	7	4	1	6	0	2	3	1	4	1
1124	4	1	23	208	33	1	2	1	3	5	2	1	4	2	4	10	1	3	1
1125	7	1	8	196	56	0	3	0	7	8	6	1	3	1	3	4	5	9	2
1126	3	1	18	51	79	1	1	0	5	4	3	1	3	1	3	4	3	6	2
1127	1	0	0	143	130	0	0	0	6	8	4	1	4	1	5	7	4	7	2
1128	1	0	0	154	139	0	0	0	7	9	4	1	4	1	6	8	5	8	2
1129	1	0	1	180	163	0	0	0	8	11	5	1	5	1	6	9	5	9	3
1130	5	1	8	175	43	0	3	0	5	4	3	1	3	1	2	4	1	3	1
1131	3	1	18	156	24	1	2	0	3	4	2	1	4	1	3	8	1	2	1
1132	2	1	0	129	34	0	1	0	5	7	4	0	4	0	2	4	1	4	1
1150	8	1	21	90	72	7	3	0	4	4	3	1	3	1	2	3	2	4	1
1151	9	1	22	90	79	6	3	0	4	4	2	2	1	1	3	5	4	3	4
1152	5	1	12	14	61	0	2	0	5	4	3	1	3	0	1	3	3	6	2
1153	7	2	7	131	63	1	3	0	7	5	4	1	2	1	1	4	3	5	2
1154	3	1	9	103	141	0	2	0	6	6	4	1	4	1	2	5	6	9	3
1155	1	0	0	193	144	0	0	0	2	5	2	1	2	0	9	14	6	6	2
1156	4	2	0	32	107	0	2	0	2	3	2	0	3	0	0	2	1	3	0
1157	8	3	25	43	73	4	2	0	5	5	3	1	4	1	2	4	3	7	2
1158	5	1	8	25	74	0	2	0	4	3	5	1	4	0	1	4	4	5	2
1159	7	3	0	40	62	1	1	0	3	3	2	1	3	1	2	3	4	5	2
1160	7	3	4	56	80	3	2	0	2	3	1	1	1	1	4	4	3	2	2
1161	2	0	0	112	66	0	1	0	3	4	3	1	2	0	2	2	2	5	1
1162	4	1	3	134	36	0	1	0	5	5	4	2	2	0	0	4	1	4	1
1163	0	0	0	207	93	2	0	2	7	6	5	1	4	1	5	7	2	7	1
1164	2	0	0	112	66	0	1	0	3	4	3	1	2	0	2	2	2	5	1
1165	0	0	0	191	101	0	0	0	7	5	4	1	4	1	6	7	2	7	1
1166	8	5	0	120	140	0	1	1	8	3	4	8	9	0	3	12	11	8	5
1167	2	0	0	70	67	5	0	0	9	7	7	11	11	0	1	7	6	8	3
1168	9	1	0	120	131	0	2	0	5	2	3	2	2	0	2	13	12	6	6
1169	6	3	3	50	86	2	2	1	4	4	2	2	2	1	3	6	4	3	2
1170	11	6	4	68	119	1	4	0	2	4	6	2	2	3	4	8	6	3	3
1171	6	1	0	100	88	2	4	1	5	4	4	3	3	1	3	6	4	2	3
1172	3	1	0	6	107	0	2	0	8	3	4	2	2	0	2	11	9	4	4
1173	5	2	0	50	81	0	5	0	6	3	2	2	3	0	2	6	6	3	3
1174	6	1	26	87	22	7	3	2	4	4	2	1	3	1	2	2	1	3	1
1175	5	1	0	138	60	5	2	6	9	7	8	7	7	0	1	5	4	4	3
1176	9	3	0	120	51	0	3	0	6	5	5	1	4	0	1	4	3	6	2

Desserts & Sweets

Food #	Food Description & Amount	wt gm	wt oz	calo- ries	%cal fat	prot gm	carbo gm	fiber gm
	Cookies							
1200	Almond cookie [3 small cookies]	30	1.1	155	55%	3	16	1.0
1201	Applesauce cookie (Include apple snacks, Dutch apple) [2 small cookies]	26	0.9	96	30%	1	16	0.8
1202	Baby cookie (Include Gerber animal-shaped cookie) [5 cookies]	32	1.1	141	27%	4	22	0.1
1203	Biscotti [1 cookie]	32	1.1	146	40%	3	20	1.0
1204	Butter or sugar cookie (Include Pepperidge Farm Sugar, Bordeaux, Chessman, Pirouette) [4 cookies]	36	1.3	171	41%	2	24	0.3
1205	Butter or sugar cookie, with nuts and/or fruit (including coconut) [2 cookies]	32	1.1	128	31%	2	21	0.3
1206	Butterscotch chip cookie [3 small cookies]	30	1.1	150	50%	2	18	0.3
1207	Caramel coated cookie, with nuts [2 small cookies]	28	1.0	140	53%	1	16	0.7
1208	Carob cookie [2 small cookies]	26	0.9	111	42%	3	15	2.7
1209	Chocolate chip cookie, fresh-baked, Toll-House-type recipe (including made with M&M's) [3 small cookies (2"dia)]	30	1.1	147	52%	2	18	0.8
1210	**Chocolate chip cookie**, packaged (Include Congo bar, Chips Ahoy!, Keebler Pecan Chips Deluxe, Pepperidge Farm Chocolate Chunk Pecan) [2 small cookies (2"dia)]	30	1.1	144	42%	2	20	0.8
1211	Chocolate chip cookie, reduced fat (Include Reduced Fat Chips Ahoy!, Snackwells) [3 small cookies]	32	1.1	140	33%	2	23	0.7
1212	Chocolate chip cookie, with raisins (Include date-nut chocolate chip bar) [3 small cookies (2"dia)]	30	1.1	141	41%	2	20	0.8
1213	Chocolate cookie, plain (Include chocolate snaps) [2 small cookies]	24	0.8	104	30%	2	17	0.8
1214	Chocolate fudge cookie (Include chocolate-jelly cookie, Peanut Butter'N Fudge Chocolate Chip Cookie) [2 small cookies]	26	0.9	113	30%	2	19	0.9
1215	Chocolate or chocolate chip cookie, with chocolate filling (Include Keebler Magic Middles, Archway Rocky Road Home Style Cookie) [2 small cookies]	28	1.0	140	55%	1	15	0.8
1216	Chocolate cookie, with chocolate filling or coating, fat free (Include Snackwells) [2 cookies]	32	1.1	110	3%	2	26	0.9
1217	Chocolate cookie, made with rice cereal (Include Little Debbie Star Crunch) [2 cookies]	30	1.1	128	44%	1	20	1.1
1218	Chocolate-covered marshmallow cookie (Include marshmallow puff, pinwheels) [2 cookies]	34	1.2	143	36%	1	23	0.7
1219	Chocolate-covered sugar wafer, creme-filled (Include Little Debbie Fudge Crispy Bar) [2 wafers]	30	1.1	151	46%	1	20	0.5
1220	**Chocolate sandwich-cookie** (Include **Oreos**, Keebler Grasshoppers) [2 double-cookies]	22	0.8	104	39%	1	15	0.7
1221	Chocolate sandwich-cookie, reduced fat (Include Reduced Fat Oreos, Snackwells) [2 double-cookies]	22	0.8	88	14%	1	18	0.6
1222	Chocolate sandwich-cookie, with extra filling (Include Double Stuff Oreo) [2 double-cookies]	28	1.0	140	45%	1	19	0.6
1223	Chocolate sandwich-cookie, chocolate covered (Include Fudge Covered Oreos, Nabisco Mystic Mint) [2 double-cookies]	40	1.4	192	49%	1	26	2.1
1224	Chocolate chip or chocolate and vanilla sandwich-cookie [3 double-cookies]	33	1.2	158	38%	2	23	0.8
1225	Coconut cookie [2 cookies]	32	1.1	141	38%	1	21	0.3
1226	Coconut and nut cookie [2 cookies]	32	1.1	145	42%	1	21	0.4
1227	Cone shell for ice cream, wafer-type [2 cones]	12	0.4	50	15%	1	9	0.4
1228	Cone shell for ice cream, sugar-cone [1 cone]	12	0.4	48	9%	1	10	0.2
1229	Cookie dough, raw, not chocolate [2Tbs]	31	1.1	136	46%	2	17	0.3
1230	Dietetic cookie, apple pastry [1 cookie]	24	0.8	115	55%	1	12	0.2
1231	Dietetic cookie, chocolate chip [3 cookie]	20	0.7	90	34%	1	15	0.3
1232	Dietetic cookie, chocolate flavored [3 cookies]	24	0.8	120	48%	1	15	0.5
1233	Dietetic cookie, coconut [4 thin wafers]	24	0.8	115	55%	1	12	0.9
1234	Dietetic cookie, fruit types [1 cookie]	22	0.8	102	46%	1	13	0.2
1235	Dietetic cookie, oatmeal with raisins [4 cookies]	28	1.0	126	36%	1	20	0.8
1236	Dietetic cookie, sandwich type [2 cookies]	22	0.8	101	43%	1	15	0.9
1237	Dietetic cookie, sugar or plain [4 cookies]	24	0.8	103	27%	1	18	0.2

Food #	fat gm	sat fat gm	choles mg	sodium mg	potass mg	vit A	vit E	vit C	thia-min	ribo-flavin	nia-cin	vit B-6	fol-ate	vit B-12	cal-cium	phos-phorus	magne-sium	iron	zinc
1200	9	2	13	71	66	6	8	0	5	7	4	1	4	1	2	5	6	4	2
1201	3	1	6	56	54	3	2	0	3	2	1	1	1	0	2	3	2	3	1
1202	4	1	0	62	163	0	0	4	32	62	26	96	1	25	3	6	4	8	2
1203	6	1	14	51	56	1	6	0	6	7	4	1	4	0	2	5	5	5	2
1204	8	2	18	150	37	4	3	0	6	5	5	1	4	1	2	4	1	4	1
1205	4	2	13	79	31	2	1	0	5	4	3	1	3	1	2	3	1	3	1
1206	8	2	13	110	45	6	3	0	4	3	2	1	3	1	1	2	2	3	1
1207	8	2	3	47	46	0	4	0	3	2	1	1	1	0	2	4	3	2	2
1208	5	1	19	64	135	1	3	0	3	6	3	3	2	2	8	7	4	3	3
1209	9	2	10	84	67	5	3	0	4	3	2	1	2	0	1	3	4	4	2
1210	7	2	0	95	41	0	3	0	4	5	4	1	3	0	1	3	2	5	1
1211	5	2	0	141	46	0	2	0	6	5	4	0	4	0	2	4	3	5	1
1212	6	2	0	89	53	0	3	0	4	5	4	1	3	0	1	3	2	5	1
1213	3	1	0	139	50	0	2	0	3	4	3	0	3	0	1	3	3	5	2
1214	4	1	1	151	55	0	2	0	4	4	4	0	3	0	1	3	3	6	2
1215	9	2	10	82	54	0	4	0	4	3	2	1	3	0	1	3	3	4	1
1216	0	0	0	62	83	0	0	0	7	4	4	0	4	0	1	4	3	8	2
1217	6	4	0	65	75	3	1	3	4	4	4	4	4	0	1	3	5	4	3
1218	6	2	0	57	62	0	2	1	2	4	1	1	2	1	2	3	3	5	1
1219	8	3	3	36	57	1	2	0	2	4	2	0	2	1	3	4	2	3	1
1220	5	1	0	133	39	0	2	0	1	2	2	0	2	0	1	2	2	5	1
1221	1	0	0	65	44	0	1	0	4	3	3	0	3	0	2	4	2	4	1
1222	7	1	0	138	34	0	4	0	1	2	2	0	3	0	1	3	2	4	1
1223	11	3	0	130	96	0	5	0	3	5	3	1	2	1	1	4	4	7	2
1224	7	1	0	157	44	0	3	0	4	4	4	0	4	0	1	3	2	6	1
1225	6	4	28	66	48	5	1	0	3	3	2	1	2	1	1	2	1	3	1
1226	7	4	28	65	51	5	1	0	4	3	2	1	2	1	1	2	2	3	1
1227	1	0	0	17	13	0	1	0	2	2	3	0	3	0	0	1	1	2	1
1228	0	0	0	38	17	0	0	0	4	3	3	0	2	0	1	1	1	3	1
1229	7	1	15	100	32	7	3	0	6	4	3	1	4	1	2	2	1	3	1
1230	7	2	0	0	22	0	5	0	2	1	2	0	2	0	0	1	2	2	0
1231	3	1	0	2	40	0	2	0	4	2	3	0	2	0	1	2	1	4	1
1232	6	2	0	3	20	0	5	0	3	2	2	1	2	1	1	1	2	2	1
1233	7	3	0	0	22	0	1	0	2	1	2	1	2	1	0	1	3	2	2
1234	5	1	1	0	9	0	2	0	3	1	2	0	2	0	0	1	2	2	0
1235	5	1	0	3	49	0	3	0	6	3	3	1	4	0	1	4	2	5	1
1236	5	1	0	53	65	0	2	0	5	4	3	0	3	0	1	4	4	6	2
1237	3	0	0	1	25	0	2	0	6	3	4	0	3	0	1	2	1	5	1

% of Daily Value

Desserts & Sweets

Food #	Food Description & Amount	wt gm	wt oz	calories	%cal fat	prot gm	carbo gm	fiber gm
1238	**Fortune cookie** [2 cookies]	16	0.6	60	6%	1	13	0.3
1239	Gingersnaps [2 cookies]	24	0.8	100	21%	1	18	0.5
1240	Granola cookie [2 cookies]	26	0.9	119	33%	2	17	1.1
1241	Japanese tea cookie, plain, ginger, or seaweed (Include senbei) [5 cookies]	25	0.9	96	1%	1	23	0.2
1242	Ladyfinger (Include anisette sponge, Stella D'Oro Egg Jumbo, Stella D'Oro Breakfast Treat) [2 ladyfingers]	28	1.0	102	22%	3	17	0.3
1243	Lebkuchen (Include honey nut bar) [2 cookies]	32	1.1	123	14%	2	25	0.9
1244	Lemon wafer, lowfat (Include NuSystem) [0.9-oz package]	26	0.9	105	9%	2	22	0.4
1245	Macaroon [2 cookies]	28	1.0	113	28%	1	20	0.5
1246	Marshmallow pie, chocolate covered (Include moon pies, sweetie pie, mallow pies, scooter pies, whoopie pie) [1 scooter pie]	34	1.2	143	36%	1	23	0.7
1247	Marshmallow cookie, with coconut [2 cookies]	36	1.3	152	36%	1	24	0.7
1248	Marshmallow cookie, with rice cereal (Include Rice Krispies bar cookie) [1 bar (2"square)]	30	1.1	115	24%	1	22	0.1
1249	Meringue cookie (Include angel cup) [5 cookies]	20	0.7	72	0%	1	18	0.0
1250	Molasses cookie (Include hermits, gingerbread man) [2 cookies]	30	1.1	129	27%	2	22	0.3
1251	Multigrain cookie, high fiber (Include Fibbers High Fiber Cookies) [2 cookies]	48	1.7	194	39%	5	31	5.4
1252	Oat bran cookie, sweetened with fruit juice (Include Health Valley Fruit Jumbos, Honey Jumbos, Kathies) [2 cookies]	36	1.3	129	34%	4	22	3.7
1253	Oatmeal sandwich, with creme filling (Include Keebler Chipsies) [2 cookies (1"-1½"dia)]	30	1.1	146	41%	1	20	0.6
1254	**Oatmeal cookie** [2 cookies (2½"dia)]	26	0.9	121	37%	1	18	0.7
1255	Oatmeal cookie, reduced fat, with raisins (Include Snackwells) [2 cookies]	27	1.0	103	13%	2	21	1.0
1256	Cookie, oatmeal, fat free, with raisins (Include Entenmanns, Health Valley) [2 cookies]	22	0.8	72	4%	1	17	1.6
1257	Oatmeal cookie, with chocolate and peanut butter [2 cookies]	68	2.4	281	38%	5	41	2.7
1258	Oatmeal cookie, with chocolate chips or M&Ms or chocolate frosting [2 cookies]	30	1.1	152	56%	2	16	0.8
1259	Oatmeal cookie, with fruit filling [1 cookie (2½"dia)]	27	1.0	115	35%	2	17	0.8
1260	Oatmeal cookie, with raisins or dates, with/without nuts (Include Tastykake Oatmeal Raisin Bars) [2 cookies (2½"dia)]	26	0.9	117	36%	2	18	0.7
1261	**Peanut butter cookie** or peanut cookie (Include chocolate peanut bars, peanut sandwich cookies, peanut butter wafers, Nabisco Nutter Butter, Almost Home Peanut Butter Cream Sandwich) [2 cookies]	32	1.1	153	45%	3	19	0.6
1262	Peanut butter cookie with rice cereal [2 bars (2"square)]	48	1.7	195	32%	3	32	0.5
1263	Peanut butter cookie, with chocolate (Include Pepperidge Farm Nassau) [2 Nassau]	30	1.1	143	46%	3	18	0.7
1264	Peanut butter cookie, with oatmeal [2 cookies]	32	1.1	153	40%	3	21	0.6
1265	Peanut butter filled cookie, chocolate-coated (Include Girl Scout Tagalongs Peanut Butter Patties) [2 cookies]	26	0.9	132	51%	2	15	0.9
1266	Pfeffernusse [2 cookies]	26	0.9	104	22%	2	19	0.4
1267	Pizzelles (Italian style wafer) (Include rosettes) [2 wafers or rosettes]	28	1.0	138	40%	2	18	0.3
1268	Pumpkin cookie (Include carrot bars) [2 cookies]	22	0.8	85	43%	1	12	0.6
1269	Puerto Rican cookie (Mantecaditos polvorones) [2 cookies (2"x2"x¼")]	38	1.3	194	43%	2	25	0.6
1270	Raisin cookie (Include date-nut cookie) [2 cookies]	32	1.1	128	31%	1	22	0.4
1271	Raisin sandwich cookie, cream-filled (Include Little Debbie Raisin Creme Pie) [1 cookie (3½"-4"dia)]	30	1.1	135	41%	1	20	0.2
1272	Rugelach [2 cookies]	28	1.0	119	53%	3	11	0.3
1273	Rum ball (Include bourbon balls) [2 balls]	22	0.8	87	29%	1	14	0.5
1274	S'more, homemade (graham cracker sandwich with chocolate and marshmallow filling) [1 S'more (2-3/8"x2-3/8")]	42	1.5	177	30%	2	30	0.8
1275	**Shortbread cookie** (Include Pecan Sandies, Greek cookies, Pepperidge Farm Shortbread) [2 cookies]	30	1.1	151	43%	2	19	0.5
1276	Shortbread cookie, reduced fat (Include Reduced Fat Pecan Sandies) [2 cookies]	32	1.1	146	35%	1	23	0.4
1277	Shortbread cookie, with chocolate filling (Include Keebler Magic Middles) [2 cookies]	28	1.0	139	46%	2	18	0.7
1278	Sugar wafer [5 wafers]	35	1.2	179	43%	1	25	0.2
1279	Sugar cookie, iced [2 cookies]	32	1.1	134	30%	1	23	0.2
1280	Sugar cookie, with chocolate frosting [2 cookies]	32	1.1	124	26%	1	22	0.3

Food #	fat gm	sat fat gm	choles mg	sodium mg	potass mg	% of Daily Value													
						vit A	vit E	vit C	thia-min	ribo-flavin	nia-cin	vit B-6	fol-ate	vit B-12	cal-cium	phos-phorus	magne-sium	iron	zinc
1238	0	0	2	44	7	0	0	0	2	1	1	0	2	0	0	1	0	1	0
1239	2	1	0	157	83	0	1	0	3	4	4	2	4	0	2	2	3	9	1
1240	4	3	0	86	94	0	0	0	10	4	2	5	5	0	2	9	7	4	3
1241	0	0	0	182	10	0	0	0	4	2	2	0	2	0	0	1	0	2	0
1242	3	1	102	41	32	5	1	2	5	7	3	2	5	4	1	5	1	6	2
1243	2	0	6	11	59	0	3	0	6	5	4	1	4	0	2	3	3	5	1
1244	1	0	0	83	38	0	1	0	9	6	7	1	5	0	1	3	2	6	1
1245	4	3	0	69	44	0	0	0	0	2	0	1	0	0	0	1	1	1	1
1246	6	2	0	57	62	0	2	1	2	4	1	1	2	1	2	3	3	5	1
1247	6	2	0	60	66	0	2	1	2	4	1	1	2	1	2	3	3	5	2
1248	3	1	0	131	13	9	1	7	7	7	7	7	7	0	1	1	1	3	1
1249	0	0	0	14	13	0	0	0	0	2	0	0	0	0	0	0	0	0	0
1250	4	1	0	138	104	0	2	0	7	5	5	4	6	0	2	3	4	11	1
1251	8	1	0	144	182	0	5	0	11	10	14	11	8	0	2	16	17	20	13
1252	5	1	0	221	164	1	4	2	9	3	6	4	2	0	1	12	11	7	5
1253	7	1	3	21	62	0	3	0	5	3	3	1	2	0	2	3	3	5	1
1254	5	1	0	65	26	0	2	0	6	2	3	0	2	0	2	4	2	5	1
1255	1	0	0	118	69	0	1	0	6	4	3	1	3	0	5	10	3	5	1
1256	0	0	0	66	47	0	0	0	2	3	1	1	2	0	1	2	2	3	1
1257	12	2	1	117	168	7	6	0	9	4	7	3	3	1	3	13	12	6	6
1258	10	2	7	80	60	3	3	0	4	3	2	1	2	0	1	3	4	4	2
1259	4	1	2	63	40	0	2	0	6	3	3	1	3	0	2	4	3	4	1
1260	5	1	0	100	37	0	2	0	5	4	3	1	3	0	1	4	2	4	1
1261	8	1	0	133	53	0	4	0	4	3	7	1	5	0	1	3	4	4	1
1262	7	1	0	226	57	14	4	11	12	11	15	13	13	0	1	4	4	5	3
1263	7	2	0	106	59	0	3	0	3	3	6	1	4	0	1	3	4	4	1
1264	7	2	0	118	61	0	3	0	7	5	6	1	4	0	2	6	4	5	2
1265	7	1	0	60	76	0	6	0	5	4	5	1	4	0	1	3	3	4	2
1266	3	1	10	78	105	3	1	0	5	4	4	2	4	0	2	2	4	5	1
1267	6	1	36	126	27	7	3	0	6	6	3	1	4	1	4	4	1	4	1
1268	4	1	9	46	68	18	2	1	4	2	2	1	2	0	3	3	2	4	1
1269	9	4	9	1	24	0	0	0	9	6	6	0	6	0	0	2	1	6	1
1270	4	1	1	108	45	0	2	0	5	4	3	1	4	1	1	3	2	4	1
1271	6	1	0	70	29	0	2	0	3	3	2	1	2	0	1	2	1	3	0
1272	7	1	1	82	31	7	4	0	4	3	3	1	3	1	1	2	1	3	1
1273	3	1	0	57	95	0	1	0	3	2	2	2	1	0	2	2	4	4	2
1274	6	2	0	140	36	0	3	0	7	5	5	1	4	0	1	3	2	5	1
1275	7	2	6	137	30	0	3	0	7	6	5	0	4	0	1	3	1	5	1
1276	6	1	0	110	29	0	2	0	7	3	4	1	4	0	2	4	1	6	2
1277	7	2	4	103	43	0	3	0	5	5	4	0	3	0	1	3	3	4	1
1278	9	1	0	51	21	0	4	0	2	4	4	0	4	0	1	2	1	4	1
1279	4	1	9	63	17	3	2	0	2	3	2	0	2	0	1	2	1	2	0
1280	4	1	8	78	23	1	1	0	4	4	3	0	3	0	3	3	1	3	1

Desserts & Sweets

Food #	Food Description & Amount	wt gm	wt oz	calo- ries	%cal fat	prot gm	carbo gm	fiber gm
1281	Vanilla cookie with caramel, coconut, and chocolate coating (Include Girl Scout Samoas) [2 cookies]	30	1.1	155	56%	1	18	0.7
1282	Vanilla sandwich-cookie, round (Include Pepperidge Farm Brussels Mint) [2 double-cookies]	22	0.8	106	37%	1	16	0.3
1283	Vanilla sandwich-cookie, reduced fat (Include Snackwells) [2 double-cookies]	24	0.9	100	14%	2	20	0.3
1284	Sandwich-cookie, not vanilla or chocolate (Include Keebler Puddin' Cremes) [2 double-cookies]	22	0.8	106	37%	1	16	0.3
1285	Vanilla wafer (Include vanilla cookie) [5 wafers]	20	0.7	88	31%	1	15	0.4
1286	Vanilla wafer, reduced fat [1 cookie]	4	0.1	17	22%	0	3	0.0
1287	Vanilla waffle creme [2 cookies]	18	0.6	92	43%	1	13	0.1
1288	Whole wheat cookie, with dried fruit, nuts [2 cookies]	28	1.0	120	47%	2	16	1.2
	Pies & Cobblers							
1350	Apple cobbler [1 cup]	217	7.7	439	24%	5	81	2.6
1351	Apple pie, one crust (Include apple pie with crumb topping) [1/8 of 9"dia]	150	5.3	371	34%	3	60	2.0
1352	**Apple pie, two-crust (Include apple-peach, apple-berry) [1/8 of 9"dia]**	150	5.3	356	42%	3	51	2.4
1353	Apple pie, individual size or tart [1 tart]	120	4.2	377	45%	4	49	1.7
1354	Apple fried-pie (Include McDonald's) [1 individual pie]	86	3.0	327	53%	3	37	1.2
1355	Apple pie, diet (Include Weight Watchers) [1 individual pie]	85	3.0	193	21%	2	38	1.7
1356	Apple-sour cream pie [1/8 of 9"dia]	159	5.6	339	40%	3	50	2.7
1357	Apricot cobbler [1 cup]	217	7.7	408	21%	6	78	4.5
1358	Apricot pie, two-crust [1/8 of 9"dia]	150	5.3	419	41%	5	59	2.8
1359	Apricot pie, individual size or tart [1 tart]	120	4.2	359	43%	4	48	2.3
1360	Apricot fried-pie [1 individual pie]	86	3.0	316	53%	3	35	1.7
1361	**Banana cream pie [1/8 of 9"dia]**	144	5.1	387	46%	6	47	1.0
1362	Banana cream pie, individual size or tart [1 tart]	117	4.1	279	41%	5	37	1.2
1363	Berry cobbler [1 cup]	217	7.7	507	24%	6	94	4.3
1364	Black bottom pie [1/8 of 9"dia]	99	3.5	273	53%	5	28	0.9
1365	Blackberry pie, two-crust (Include boysenberry) [1/8 of 9"dia]	150	5.3	402	42%	4	56	4.7
1366	Blackberry pie, individual size or tart [1 tart]	120	4.2	348	44%	3	46	3.7
1367	Blueberry pie, two-crust (Include huckleberry) [1/8 of 9"dia]	150	5.3	348	39%	3	52	1.5
1368	Blueberry pie, one crust [1/8 of 9"dia]	137	4.8	293	37%	3	45	2.3
1369	Blueberry pie, individual size or tart [1 tart]	120	4.2	349	44%	3	47	2.3
1370	Blueberry pie filling [1 cup]	262	9.2	272	3%	2	68	3.7
1371	Buttermilk pie [1/8 of 9"dia]	144	5.1	551	43%	6	75	0.6
1372	Cherry cobbler [1 cup]	217	7.7	426	24%	5	78	2.5
1373	**Cherry pie, two-crust [1/8 of 9"dia]**	150	5.3	390	38%	3	60	1.2
1374	Cherry pie, one crust [1/8 of 9"dia]	137	4.8	313	34%	3	50	1.6
1375	Cherry pie, individual size or tart [1 tart]	120	4.2	285	43%	3	39	1.7
1376	Cherry fried-pie (Include McDonald's) [1 individual pie]	86	3.0	287	51%	3	33	1.1
1377	Cherry pie filling [1 cup]	264	9.3	316	6%	2	76	2.3
1378	Cherry pie filling, low calorie [1 cup]	264	9.3	211	9%	2	51	1.6
1379	Cherry pie, made with cream cheese and sour cream [1/8 of 9"dia]	159	5.6	454	42%	5	63	1.0
1380	Chess pie (Include lemon chess pie) [1/8 of 9"dia]	89	3.1	367	44%	5	48	0.9
1381	Chiffon pie, chocolate [1/8 of 9"dia]	99	3.5	318	43%	6	41	1.3
1382	Chiffon pie, not chocolate [1/8 of 9"dia]	99	3.5	291	37%	7	40	0.5
1383	Chiffon pie, with liqueur (Include grasshopper pie) [1/8 of 9"dia]	99	3.5	342	51%	4	33	0.8
1384	**Chocolate cream pie (Include chocolate meringue, chocolate ice box dessert, chocolate pudding pie, Jell-O chocolate mousse pie) [1/8 of 9"dia]**	144	5.1	388	44%	7	50	2.1
1385	Chocolate cream pie, individual size or tart [1 tart]	117	4.1	345	46%	6	42	1.7
1386	Chocolate-marshmallow pie [1/8 of 8"dia]	102	3.6	383	50%	5	47	1.6
1387	Coconut cream pie (Include coconut custard) [1/8 of 9"dia]	144	5.1	429	50%	3	54	1.9
1388	Coconut cream pie, individual size or tart [1 tart]	117	4.1	277	48%	6	30	0.9

Food #	fat gm	sat fat gm	choles mg	sodium mg	potass mg	vit A	vit E	vit C	thia-min	ribo-flavin	nia-cin	vit B-6	fol-ate	vit B-12	cal-cium	phos-phorus	magne-sium	iron	zinc
														% of Daily Value					
1281	10	4	2	46	74	0	3	0	1	2	1	1	1	0	2	3	3	2	2
1282	4	1	0	77	20	0	2	0	4	3	3	0	3	0	1	2	1	3	1
1283	2	0	0	77	38	0	1	0	5	4	3	0	3	1	4	5	1	3	1
1284	4	1	0	77	20	0	2	0	4	3	3	0	3	0	1	2	1	3	1
1285	3	1	12	62	19	0	1	0	4	4	3	1	3	0	1	2	1	3	0
1286	0	0	0	10	4	0	0	0	1	1	1	0	0	0	0	0	0	1	0
1287	4	1	0	26	11	0	2	0	1	2	2	0	2	0	0	1	0	2	0
1288	6	1	15	67	111	4	2	0	3	2	2	3	1	1	2	5	5	4	2
1350	12	3	4	219	197	3	5	5	15	13	9	3	9	2	17	12	4	10	3
1351	14	3	0	15	98	1	6	4	10	7	7	2	6	0	1	3	2	7	1
1352	17	6	0	399	98	5	8	8	3	2	2	3	8	0	2	4	3	4	2
1353	19	4	0	2	77	0	8	2	15	9	9	2	9	0	1	4	2	9	2
1354	19	4	0	5	57	0	9	1	10	7	7	1	6	0	1	3	2	7	1
1355	5	1	0	245	61	0	3	0	7	5	4	1	4	0	1	2	1	5	1
1356	15	5	8	17	218	4	5	6	10	8	6	3	6	0	4	5	4	8	2
1357	10	2	2	177	470	31	8	18	15	13	12	5	9	1	14	11	5	13	5
1358	19	4	0	2	244	17	10	10	16	11	12	3	11	0	2	5	4	12	3
1359	17	3	0	2	185	13	9	8	14	10	10	2	9	0	1	5	3	10	3
1360	18	4	0	3	136	8	9	5	10	7	7	1	6	0	1	3	2	7	2
1361	20	5	73	346	238	10	7	4	13	18	8	10	10	6	11	13	6	8	5
1362	13	3	50	38	199	5	5	4	10	14	6	9	8	3	7	9	5	7	3
1363	13	3	2	260	189	2	9	21	21	17	13	3	12	1	18	13	5	13	4
1364	16	7	90	162	169	16	4	1	3	11	2	3	3	4	8	10	6	7	4
1365	19	4	0	27	166	3	10	22	14	10	10	3	12	0	3	5	5	11	3
1366	17	3	0	20	130	2	9	17	13	9	9	2	11	0	2	4	4	9	2
1367	15	3	0	488	75	5	7	7	1	3	2	3	8	0	1	3	2	3	2
1368	12	2	0	5	67	1	9	2	11	9	7	2	6	0	1	4	2	8	2
1369	17	3	0	23	78	2	9	11	14	9	9	2	8	0	1	4	2	8	2
1370	1	0	0	68	97	2	8	4	5	8	1	4	1	0	1	3	3	5	1
1371	26	6	91	64	103	4	11	0	10	15	6	2	8	4	5	9	3	7	4
1372	12	2	2	223	197	11	5	4	15	14	10	4	10	1	15	11	5	20	3
1373	17	4	0	369	122	8	7	2	2	3	2	3	8	0	2	4	3	4	2
1374	12	2	0	19	106	7	5	3	9	8	6	2	7	0	1	3	3	13	1
1375	14	3	0	16	110	2	6	2	10	8	7	2	7	0	1	4	3	7	1
1376	16	3	0	4	62	2	7	1	9	7	6	1	6	0	1	3	2	9	1
1377	2	0	0	39	201	17	2	7	2	6	2	4	4	0	2	2	3	16	1
1378	2	0	0	24	201	5	2	7	2	5	2	4	3	0	2	2	3	4	1
1379	21	10	78	98	138	19	5	2	7	13	4	3	6	3	6	8	3	10	3
1380	18	8	129	205	53	13	10	0	7	12	4	2	7	4	2	7	2	6	3
1381	15	4	107	53	94	6	5	0	8	12	5	2	7	3	2	9	6	8	4
1382	12	3	139	44	71	6	5	8	8	14	5	3	8	4	2	8	2	7	3
1383	19	8	96	230	88	19	5	0	4	10	3	2	5	4	3	7	4	6	3
1384	19	7	77	44	234	7	6	1	13	17	8	3	9	5	11	17	11	11	7
1385	18	6	57	33	179	5	6	1	13	15	8	3	9	4	9	13	9	10	5
1386	21	10	10	218	202	10	6	1	5	11	4	2	3	4	10	12	7	6	5
1387	24	10	0	367	94	3	8	0	5	7	1	5	3	5	4	12	7	6	6
1388	15	5	74	54	157	6	5	1	10	16	6	3	8	4	9	12	4	7	4

Desserts & Sweets

Food #	Food Description & Amount	wt gm	wt oz	calories	%cal fat	prot gm	carbo gm	fiber gm
1389	Cranberry pie, two-crust (Include juneberry pie, gooseberry pie) [1/8 of 9"dia]	150	5.3	438	43%	4	60	3.6
1390	Cranberry pie, one crust [1/8 of 9"dia]	137	4.8	345	37%	2	54	3.8
1391	Cranberry pie, individual size or tart [1 tart]	120	4.2	377	45%	4	50	2.8
1392	Custard pie (Include custard cream, egg pie) [1/8 of 9"dia]	136	4.8	286	50%	7	28	2.2
1393	Custard pie, individual size or tart (Include custard cream pie) [1 tart]	117	4.1	217	29%	7	31	0.6
1394	Frozen yogurt pie (all flavors) [1/8 of 9"dia]	144	5.1	361	50%	4	42	0.7
1395	Lemon cream pie (Include lemon ice box pie) [1/8 of 9"dia]	144	5.1	399	38%	7	56	0.6
1396	Lemon cream pie, individual size or tart [1 tart]	117	4.1	342	41%	6	46	0.6
1397	Lemon pie (not cream or meringue) [1/8 of 9"dia]	99	3.5	384	36%	5	57	0.9
1398	Lemon pie (not cream or meringue), individual size or tart [1 tart]	120	4.2	478	38%	6	69	1.2
1399	Lemon fried-pie [1 individual pie]	85	3.0	284	51%	4	31	0.6
1400	Lemon meringue pie (Include key lime pie) [1/8 of 9"dia]	137	4.8	367	29%	2	65	1.6
1401	Lemon meringue pie, individual size or tart [1 tart]	117	4.1	301	41%	4	41	0.6
1402	Mince pie, two-crust [1/8 of 9"dia]	150	5.3	434	34%	4	72	3.9
1403	Mince pie, individual size or tart [1 tart]	120	4.2	370	43%	4	51	2.3
1404	Oatmeal pie [1/8 of 9"dia]	114	4.0	447	36%	6	69	1.6
1405	Peach cobbler [1 cup]	217	7.7	425	21%	5	82	3.8
1406	Peach pie, two-crust [1/8 of 9"dia]	150	5.3	335	40%	3	49	1.2
1407	Peach pie, one crust [1/8 of 9"dia]	150	5.3	337	31%	3	57	2.7
1408	Peach pie, individual size or tart [1 tart]	120	4.2	344	43%	4	47	2.0
1409	Peach fried-pie [1 individual pie]	86	3.0	308	54%	3	34	1.5
1410	Peanut butter cream pie [1/8 of 9"dia]	144	5.1	424	45%	12	49	1.8
1411	Pear cobbler [1 cup]	217	7.7	453	21%	5	89	4.3
1412	Pear pie, two-crust [1/8 of 9"dia]	150	5.3	391	41%	4	56	2.6
1413	Pear pie, individual size or tart [1 tart]	120	4.2	342	44%	3	46	2.1
1414	Pecan pie (Include coconut-pecan pie, walnut pie) [1/8 of 9"dia]	114	4.0	456	42%	5	65	4.0
1415	Pecan pie, individual size or tart [1 tart]	85	3.0	363	49%	4	46	1.6
1416	Pie shell, regular [1 pie shell (9"dia)]	172	6.1	884	57%	8	85	1.7
1417	Pie shell, chocolate wafer [1 pie shell (9"dia)]	210	7.4	1063	55%	11	114	3.2
1418	Pie shell, graham cracker [1 pie shell (9"dia)]	210	7.4	1037	45%	9	137	3.2
1419	Pineapple cobbler [1 cup]	217	7.7	416	22%	4	80	1.7
1420	Pineapple pie, two-crust [1/8 of 9"dia]	150	5.3	396	41%	4	56	1.4
1421	Pineapple pie, individual size or tart [1 tart]	120	4.2	342	44%	3	46	1.2
1422	Pineapple cream pie (Include millionaire's pie, Hawaiian pie, sunshine pie) [1/8 of 9"dia]	144	5.1	291	34%	5	43	0.8
1423	Plum cobbler [1 cup]	217	7.7	447	22%	5	86	3.0
1424	Plum pie, two-crust [1/8 of 9"dia]	150	5.3	441	42%	4	61	1.9
1425	Praline mousse pie, with nuts (Include Weight Watchers Praline Pecan Mousse) [1 individual pie]	77	2.7	190	33%	5	27	0.3
1426	Prune pie, one crust [1/8 of 9"dia]	150	5.3	453	29%	6	77	3.5
1427	Pudding pie, chocolate, with chocolate coating, individual size [1 individual pie]	142	5.0	473	50%	5	55	1.7
1428	Pudding pie, flavors other than chocolate, with chocolate coating, individual size [1 individual pie]	142	5.0	492	50%	5	58	1.2
1429	Pudding pie, flavors other than chocolate [1/8 of 9"dia]	144	5.1	322	45%	6	39	0.7
1430	Pudding pie, flavors other than chocolate, individual size or tart [1 tart]	120	4.2	404	53%	4	43	0.7
1431	Pumpkin pie [1/8 of 9"dia]	154	5.4	323	41%	6	42	4.2
1432	Pumpkin pie, individual size or tart [1 tart]	117	4.1	272	53%	6	27	1.8
1433	Raisin pie, two-crust [1/8 of 9"dia]	150	5.3	379	39%	4	56	1.8
1434	Raisin pie, individual size or tart [1 tart]	120	4.2	350	42%	4	49	1.6
1435	Raspberry pie, two-crust [1/8 of 9"dia]	150	5.3	422	43%	4	58	5.4
1436	Raspberry pie, one crust [1/8 of 9"dia]	137	4.8	328	36%	3	52	5.7
1437	Raspberry pie, individual size or tart [1 tart]	120	4.2	377	45%	4	50	2.8
1438	Raspberry cream pie [1/8 of 9"dia]	144	5.1	287	52%	3	33	3.5

Food #	fat gm	sat fat gm	choles mg	sodium mg	potass mg	% of Daily Value													
						vit A	vit E	vit C	thia-min	ribo-flavin	nia-cin	vit B-6	fol-ate	vit B-12	cal-cium	phos-phorus	magne-sium	iron	zinc
1389	21	4	0	30	83	3	9	13	16	10	10	3	10	0	1	5	3	10	2
1390	14	3	0	34	77	3	6	17	10	6	6	3	6	0	1	3	2	6	2
1391	19	4	0	23	68	2	8	10	14	9	9	2	9	0	1	4	2	9	2
1392	16	3	45	326	144	7	5	1	4	17	2	3	7	10	11	15	4	4	5
1393	7	2	78	58	157	7	2	1	11	17	6	3	8	5	10	12	4	7	4
1394	20	10	3	252	166	12	6	10	4	10	2	4	5	5	10	10	4	4	4
1395	17	4	93	115	165	12	7	10	10	17	5	3	7	6	10	12	4	6	4
1396	16	4	68	84	127	9	7	7	9	14	5	3	7	5	7	10	3	6	3
1397	16	3	76	47	67	5	7	10	12	13	7	2	9	2	2	6	2	8	3
1398	20	4	84	52	82	6	9	11	16	16	10	2	12	3	2	8	3	11	3
1399	16	3	49	16	44	2	7	3	10	9	6	1	7	2	1	5	2	7	2
1400	12	2	62	200	122	7	7	7	6	17	4	2	4	3	8	14	5	5	4
1401	14	3	69	23	50	3	6	5	9	10	5	2	7	2	1	5	2	7	2
1402	16	4	0	381	305	0	9	15	15	9	9	5	9	0	3	6	5	12	2
1403	18	4	1	14	203	0	8	2	16	11	10	3	10	0	3	5	5	13	2
1404	18	4	87	154	85	10	8	0	13	12	5	3	7	3	2	11	6	9	5
1405	10	2	2	190	325	7	7	11	14	14	15	2	9	1	14	11	5	10	3
1406	15	2	0	405	188	3	9	3	6	3	2	2	9	0	1	4	2	4	1
1407	12	2	0	1	210	5	7	9	10	8	11	1	6	0	1	4	3	7	2
1408	16	3	0	1	139	3	8	5	14	10	11	1	9	0	1	4	3	9	2
1409	18	4	0	10	102	3	9	3	9	7	8	1	6	0	1	3	2	6	1
1410	21	5	65	143	296	7	10	1	14	20	19	7	12	6	12	20	12	10	8
1411	10	2	2	194	230	1	6	7	15	14	9	2	10	1	15	11	5	11	3
1412	18	4	0	2	113	0	9	4	14	10	9	1	10	0	1	4	3	9	2
1413	17	3	0	1	91	0	8	3	13	9	8	1	9	0	1	4	2	9	2
1414	21	4	36	483	84	5	10	2	7	8	1	1	8	2	2	9	5	7	4
1415	20	3	38	54	90	2	6	0	16	9	6	2	7	1	1	8	6	8	7
1416	56	18	0	1113	189	0	29	0	32	39	21	6	17	1	4	10	8	22	4
1417	65	14	2	1411	353	46	36	0	22	26	22	0	28	1	6	22	21	35	11
1418	52	11	0	1199	185	42	29	0	15	22	22	4	13	1	4	14	9	25	7
1419	10	2	2	211	172	1	4	10	19	12	10	5	9	1	15	10	7	12	3
1420	18	4	0	10	96	0	8	6	18	10	10	3	10	0	1	4	4	10	2
1421	17	3	0	8	77	0	7	4	16	9	9	2	9	0	1	4	4	9	2
1422	11	3	61	41	132	5	4	3	11	14	6	3	7	3	7	9	4	7	3
1423	11	2	2	194	290	5	7	16	17	18	12	6	9	1	14	11	5	10	3
1424	21	4	0	2	133	6	11	3	17	12	11	2	10	0	1	5	3	11	2
1425	7	1	5	180	26	0	3	1	2	2	1	0	5	0	6	1	1	10	1
1426	15	3	0	38	190	1	6	5	12	16	9	5	8	1	2	5	4	10	2
1427	26	9	7	499	198	2	12	1	14	21	9	4	8	3	8	11	8	11	4
1428	27	10	7	550	191	3	12	1	14	21	9	4	7	3	8	11	8	10	4
1429	16	5	13	172	172	3	6	1	12	15	7	2	8	4	12	11	5	7	4
1430	24	8	6	519	146	1	12	1	14	19	8	3	7	3	7	8	5	9	3
1431	15	3	31	434	237	74	8	4	6	14	1	4	8	10	9	11	6	7	5
1432	16	5	53	55	238	97	7	3	10	16	6	3	8	2	12	13	6	10	4
1433	17	3	0	6	191	0	8	2	15	10	9	3	9	0	2	6	4	11	2
1434	16	3	0	5	157	0	7	2	15	9	9	3	9	0	1	5	3	10	2
1435	20	4	0	28	132	3	10	24	15	12	12	3	12	0	2	5	5	11	4
1436	13	3	0	32	131	3	7	28	9	9	8	3	8	0	2	3	5	8	3
1437	19	4	0	23	68	2	8	10	14	9	9	2	9	0	1	4	2	9	2
1438	17	7	35	14	124	11	5	14	7	7	6	3	6	1	3	4	4	6	2

Desserts & Sweets

Food #	Food Description & Amount	wt gm	wt oz	calo-ries	%cal fat	prot gm	carbo gm	fiber gm
1439	Rhubarb cobbler [1 cup]	217	7.7	545	24%	5	102	2.9
1440	Rhubarb pie, two-crust [1/8 of 9"dia]	150	5.3	448	47%	5	56	2.3
1441	Rhubarb pie, one crust [1/8 of 9"dia]	137	4.8	338	39%	3	49	2.2
1442	Rhubarb pie, individual size or tart [1 tart]	120	4.2	385	48%	4	46	1.9
1443	Shoo-fly pie [1/8 of 9"dia]	114	4.0	397	29%	4	68	1.0
1444	Sour cream raisin pie [1/8 of 9"dia]	144	5.1	523	58%	8	50	2.1
1445	Squash pie [1/8 of 9"dia]	154	5.4	293	38%	6	40	2.1
1446	Strawberry pie, one crust [1/8 of 9"dia]	168	5.9	385	38%	4	58	3.3
1447	Strawberry pie, individual size or tart [1 tart]	120	4.2	319	43%	3	43	2.3
1448	Strawberry cream pie [1/8 of 9"dia]	144	5.1	294	48%	2	38	1.7
1449	Strawberry cream pie, individual size or tart [1 tart]	117	4.1	281	51%	2	33	1.4
1450	Strawberry-rhubarb pie [1/8 of 9"dia]	150	5.3	424	46%	5	54	2.6
1451	Sweet potato pie [1/8 of 9"dia]	154	5.4	295	43%	6	36	1.5
1452	Tofu pie with fruit and graham cracker crust [1/8 of 9"dia]	144	5.1	311	52%	8	33	1.8
1453	Toll house pie (include chocolate-chip cookie pie) [1/8 of 9"dia]	114	4.0	610	65%	7	52	2.4
1454	Vanilla cream pie (Include butterscotch pie) [1/8 of 9"dia]	144	5.1	400	47%	7	47	0.9
1455	Vanilla wafer dessert base [1 cup]	129	4.6	685	61%	5	65	0.1
Frozen Desserts								
1500	Baked Alaska [1/8 of Baked Alaska]	103	3.6	254	35%	5	37	0.1
1501	Fruit juice bar with cream, frozen (Include Dole Fruit and Cream Bars) [1 bar]	65	2.3	86	14%	1	19	0.1
1502	Fruit juice bar, frozen, sweetened with low calorie sweetener, flavors other than orange (Include Dole No Sugar Added Fruit Juice Bar) [1 bar]	54	1.9	24	1%	0	6	0.1
1503	Fruit juice bar, frozen, flavors other than orange (Include Dole Fruit 'N Juice Bar) [1 bar]	74	2.6	61	1%	1	15	0.0
1504	Fruit juice bar, frozen, orange flavor (Include Dole Fruit 'N Juice Bar) [1 bar]	74	2.6	68	0%	0	17	0.1
1505	Gelatin, frozen, whipped, on a stick (Include Jell-O Gelatin Pops) [1 pop]	53	1.9	31	0%	1	7	0.0
1506	Ices, fruit [1 cup]	193	6.8	247	0%	1	63	0.0
1507	Popsicle filled with ice cream, all flavors (Include Disney Cream Pop) [1 pop]	59	2.1	68	29%	1	12	0.0
1508	**Popsicle [1 double stick]**	**128**	**4.5**	**92**	**0%**	**0**	**24**	**0.0**
1509	Popsicle, sweetened with low-cal sweetener [1 double stick]	128	4.5	35	3%	1	5	0.0
1510	Rice dessert bar, frozen, flavors other than chocolate, non-dairy, carob covered [1 bar]	113	4.0	256	54%	3	31	4.3
1511	Rice, frozen dessert, nondairy, flavors other than chocolate (Include Rice Dream) [1 cup]	172	6.1	259	36%	3	40	2.1
1512	Snow cone, slurps [1 cup]	193	6.8	247	0%	1	63	0.0
1513	Sorbet, fruit, citrus [1 cup]	200	7.1	184	0%	1	46	0.2
1514	Sorbet, fruit, noncitrus [1 cup]	200	7.1	164	1%	2	40	0.0
1515	Tofu yogurt [1 cup]	262	9.2	254	17%	9	43	0.5
1516	Tofu, frozen dessert, chocolate (Include Tofutti) [1 cup]	193	6.8	423	61%	7	48	7.1
1517	Tofu, frozen dessert, flavors other than chocolate (Include Tofutti) [1 cup]	193	6.8	503	63%	9	45	1.4
Puddings								
1550	Barfi or Burfi, Indian dessert, made from milk and/or cream and/or Ricotta cheese [1 cubic inch]	21	0.7	59	38%	1	8	0.1
1551	Basbousa (semolina dessert dish) [1 piece (3x2½")]	82	2.9	220	35%	4	33	0.6
1552	Chantilly Cream [1 cup]	120	4.2	380	83%	3	15	0.0
1553	Coconut custard, Puerto Rican style (Include Flan de coco) [1 cup]	245	8.6	695	34%	20	98	0.8
1554	Coconut pudding [1 cup]	255	9.0	272	21%	8	47	0.4
1555	Corn custard, fresh, Puerto Rican style (Include Mazamorra, Mundo Nuevo) [1 cup]	280	9.9	1114	56%	11	130	10.0
1556	Cornmeal coconut dessert, Puerto Rican style (Include Harina de maiz con coco) [1 cup]	262	9.2	768	63%	8	72	7.3
1557	Cornstarch coconut dessert, Puerto Rican style (Include Tembleque) [1 cup]	250	8.8	702	72%	5	52	5.3
1558	Cornstarch pudding, with milk base (Include Diet Care) [1 cup]	255	9.0	138	3%	9	25	0.0
1559	Crème Brulèe (½ cup)	142	5.0	500	76%	4	27	0.0
1560	**Custard [1 cup]**	**244**	**8.6**	**234**	**33%**	**12**	**27**	**0.0**
1561	Danish dessert pudding [1 cup]	274	9.7	406	0%	0	103	1.2
1562	Diplomat pudding, Puerto Rican style (Include Budin Diplomatico) [1 cup]	256	9.0	731	29%	18	112	1.3

Food #	fat gm	sat fat gm	choles mg	sodium mg	potass mg	% of Daily Value													
						vit A	vit E	vit C	thia- min	ribo- flavin	nia- cin	vit B-6	fol- ate	vit B-12	cal- cium	phos- phorus	magne- sium	iron	zinc
1439	14	3	2	239	356	7	7	10	16	13	11	2	10	1	21	11	6	11	3
1440	23	5	0	3	107	0	10	3	20	13	12	2	13	0	12	6	5	13	3
1441	15	3	0	3	105	1	7	4	13	9	8	1	8	0	15	4	5	9	2
1442	21	4	0	2	85	0	9	2	17	11	11	1	11	0	9	5	4	11	2
1443	13	3	37	141	543	2	5	0	15	11	10	11	10	1	9	6	21	19	3
1444	34	12	81	87	329	17	11	2	17	19	10	5	11	4	10	14	6	13	4
1445	12	3	67	51	243	25	5	5	11	15	6	5	8	4	9	11	5	7	4
1446	16	3	0	2	194	0	7	82	14	12	9	4	11	0	2	5	4	10	2
1447	15	3	0	2	132	0	7	51	13	10	8	2	9	0	1	4	3	9	2
1448	16	7	33	11	129	10	4	55	6	7	4	2	6	1	3	4	3	5	2
1449	16	6	23	8	101	7	5	39	8	8	5	2	7	1	2	4	2	6	2
1450	22	4	0	3	134	0	9	33	18	13	12	2	13	0	6	6	5	12	3
1451	14	3	58	54	231	94	6	15	10	18	6	9	8	4	10	11	5	7	4
1452	18	3	31	240	180	15	8	23	5	9	3	4	5	1	9	11	19	23	5
1453	44	10	49	269	219	23	16	1	14	12	7	6	9	2	4	12	14	13	7
1454	21	6	89	374	181	12	6	1	13	18	7	4	9	7	13	15	5	8	5
1455	47	10	50	664	102	37	24	0	16	17	14	3	16	2	5	10	3	12	2
1500	10	4	59	126	146	11	2	1	6	15	3	2	4	5	8	8	3	5	3
1501	1	1	5	20	64	1	0	13	0	3	1	1	1	1	3	1	0	1	0
1502	0	0	0	2	9	0	0	31	0	1	0	1	0	0	0	0	1	0	0
1503	0	0	0	3	39	0	0	12	1	1	1	1	1	0	0	0	1	1	0
1504	0	0	0	6	74	2	0	32	0	1	1	1	4	0	1	1	1	2	0
1505	0	0	0	22	1	0	0	0	0	0	0	0	0	0	0	1	0	0	0
1506	0	0	0	42	6	0	0	3	0	0	0	0	0	0	0	0	0	2	0
1507	2	1	9	20	40	2	0	0	1	3	0	0	0	1	2	2	1	0	1
1508	0	0	0	15	5	0	0	0	0	0	0	0	0	0	0	0	0	0	0
1509	0	0	0	6	33	0	0	0	0	0	1	0	0	0	0	0	0	1	0
1510	15	7	0	100	110	0	12	0	7	5	10	9	3	0	4	9	10	3	4
1511	10	1	0	73	125	0	12	27	11	3	11	10	3	0	1	13	15	4	6
1512	0	0	0	42	6	0	0	3	0	0	0	0	0	0	0	0	0	2	0
1513	0	0	0	16	200	5	0	86	1	4	2	2	11	0	2	3	4	5	0
1514	0	0	0	8	106	1	0	32	1	2	2	3	3	0	1	1	2	2	1
1515	5	1	0	92	123	1	3	11	10	3	3	3	4	0	31	10	26	15	5
1516	29	6	0	478	527	0	14	0	3	5	2	3	4	0	5	19	29	24	11
1517	35	5	0	510	124	0	15	1	7	3	2	6	6	0	5	12	13	12	6
1550	3	1	8	11	27	2	0	0	0	2	0	0	0	1	3	3	1	0	1
1551	8	2	2	72	125	1	5	0	7	10	5	1	5	2	10	9	5	5	3
1552	35	22	130	57	91	40	2	1	1	10	0	1	1	3	6	6	2	0	1
1553	26	16	291	318	708	22	4	4	8	53	2	9	9	12	49	51	14	8	16
1554	6	4	18	525	373	11	1	3	6	21	1	12	3	13	27	37	9	2	6
1555	69	60	0	64	1125	3	7	22	21	6	21	8	22	0	5	41	39	31	17
1556	54	47	0	35	642	1	6	8	16	7	15	7	18	0	4	25	24	28	12
1557	56	50	0	37	624	0	6	9	4	0	9	4	8	0	4	24	22	22	11
1558	1	0	5	260	467	12	0	4	7	23	1	6	3	17	33	27	8	1	7
1559	42	25	315	50	140	35	4	0	2	10	0	4	6	10	10	15	4	4	4
1560	9	4	201	160	381	19	2	2	5	32	1	6	6	13	28	28	8	4	9
1561	0	0	0	7	56	0	0	3	1	1	0	1	0	0	1	1	1	3	1
1562	24	7	423	345	394	32	9	6	15	45	8	10	14	17	24	33	9	20	12

Desserts & Sweets

Food #	Food Description & Amount	wt gm	wt oz	calo- ries	%cal fat	prot gm	carbo gm	fiber gm
1563	Egg dessert, custard-like, made with water and sugar, Puerto Rican style (Include Tocino del cielo, Heaven's delight) [1 cup]	265	9.3	882	25%	15	155	0.0
1564	Fruit dessert with cream and/or pudding and nuts (Include Watergate salad) [1 cup]	178	6.3	360	44%	3	52	1.3
1565	**Gelatin dessert** (Include Jell-O) [1 cup]	**240**	**8.5**	**142**	**0%**	**3**	**34**	**0.0**
1566	Gelatin dessert with apples, grapes, celery (with/without other fruits, vegetables) [1 cup]	240	8.5	151	3%	2	37	1.7
1567	Gelatin dessert with apples, grapes, celery, walnuts (with/without other fruits, vegetables, nuts) [1 cup]	240	8.5	186	25%	3	34	1.6
1568	Gelatin dessert with bananas, grapes (with/without other fruits) [1 cup]	240	8.5	159	3%	3	39	1.4
1569	Gelatin dessert with bananas, grapes, cream cheese (with/without other fruits) [1 cup]	239	8.4	190	21%	3	37	1.4
1570	Gelatin dessert with bananas, grapes, whipped non-dairy topping (with/without other fruits) [1 cup]	227	8.0	196	23%	2	38	1.3
1571	Gelatin dessert with bananas, grapes, walnuts, whipped non-dairy topping (with/without other fruits, nuts) [1 cup]	227	8.0	235	35%	3	38	1.5
1572	Gelatin dessert with cream cheese [1 cup]	239	8.4	192	29%	4	31	0.0
1573	Gelatin dessert with sour cream [1 cup]	227	8.0	212	45%	4	27	0.0
1574	Gelatin dessert with strawberries, bananas, pineapple, sour cream (with/without other fruits) [1 cup]	249	8.8	271	21%	3	54	2.5
1575	Gelatin dessert with whipped non-dairy topping [1 cup]	227	8.0	177	21%	3	33	0.0
1576	Gelatin dessert, dietetic (low-cal sweetener) [1 cup]	240	8.5	18	0%	3	2	0.0
1577	Gelatin dessert, dietetic (low-cal sweetener), with apples, grapes, walnuts (with/without other fruits, vegetables, nuts) [1 cup]	240	8.5	120	43%	3	16	1.8
1578	Gelatin dessert, dietetic (low-cal sweetener), with bananas, grapes (with/without other fruit)	240	8.5	87	5%	3	20	1.6
1579	Gelatin dessert, dietetic (low-cal sweetener), with bananas, grapes, whipped dietetic non-dairy topping (with/without other fruit) [1 cup]	249	8.8	88	17%	2	20	1.4
1580	Gelatin dessert, dietetic (low-cal sweetener), with bananas, grapes, cream cheese (with/without other fruit) [1 cup]	239	8.4	128	31%	3	22	1.8
1581	Gelatin dessert, dietetic (low-cal sweetener), with cream cheese [1 cup]	239	8.4	128	79%	5	2	0.0
1582	Gelatin dessert, dietetic (low-cal sweetener), with sour cream [1 cup]	227	8.0	105	74%	4	4	0.0
1583	Gelatin dessert, dietetic (low-cal sweetener), with strawberries, bananas, pineapple, sour cream (with/without other fruit) [1 cup]	249	8.8	195	24%	14	26	2.6
1584	Gelatin dessert, dietetic (low-cal sweetener), with whipped dietetic non-dairy topping [1 cup]	227	8.0	24	40%	2	3	0.0
1585	Gelatin powder, dietetic (low-cal sweetener), dry [2Tbs]	18	0.6	62	0%	10	6	0.0
1586	Gelatin powder, sweetened with sugar, dry [2Tbs]	24	0.8	91	0%	2	22	0.0
1587	Gelatin-vegetable (carrots, celery, green pepper, radishes) salad [1 cup]	243	8.6	127	1%	3	30	0.9
1588	Gelatin (dietetic)-vegetable (carrots, celery, green pepper, radishes) salad [1 cup]	243	8.6	14	7%	1	3	0.9
1589	Haupia (coconut pudding) [1 cup]	213	7.5	580	68%	4	50	4.2
1590	Indian Pudding [1 cup]	237	8.4	311	25%	10	48	1.5
1591	Lime souffle (and other citrus fruit souffles) [1 cup]	120	4.2	386	42%	10	49	1.3
1592	Mexican bread pudding (Include Capirotada) [1 cup]	204	7.2	561	39%	8	80	2.6
1593	Mexican bread pudding, lower fat (Include Capirotada) [1 cup]	250	8.8	636	26%	12	111	3.6
1594	Milk dessert or milk candy, Puerto Rican style (Include Dulce de leche) [½ cup]	155	5.5	482	16%	8	96	0.0
1595	**Mousse, chocolate** [1 cup]	**170**	**6.0**	**361**	**66%**	**7**	**27**	**1.0**
1596	Mousse, chocolate, lowfat, made from dry mix, water added [1 cup]	216	7.6	770	19%	27	148	11.9
1597	Mousse, not chocolate (Include fruit mousse) [1 cup]	170	6.0	353	68%	2	29	1.4
1598	Pineapple custard, Puerto Rican style (Include Flan de pina) [1 cup]	260	9.2	413	25%	15	63	0.3
1599	Pudding pops, chocolate [1 pop]	57	2.0	87	28%	2	14	0.2
1600	Pudding pops, flavors other than chocolate [1 pop]	57	2.0	91	25%	2	15	0.0
1601	Pudding roll-up, chocolate [2 roll-ups]	28	1.0	107	28%	1	21	1.0
1602	Pudding roll-up, flavors other than chocolate [2 roll-ups]	28	1.0	110	26%	1	21	0.0
1603	**Pudding, bread** (Include with raisins) [1 cup]	**200**	**7.1**	**310**	**28%**	**11**	**46**	**1.8**
1604	Pudding, canned, chocolate [4-oz can]	113	4.0	150	27%	3	26	1.1
1605	Pudding, canned, chocolate and non-chocolate flavors combined [4-oz can]	113	4.0	149	26%	3	25	0.6

Food #	fat gm	sat fat gm	choles mg	sodium mg	potass mg	% of Daily Value													
						vit A	vit E	vit C	thia-min	ribo-flavin	nia-cin	vit B-6	fol-ate	vit B-12	cal-cium	phos-phorus	magne-sium	iron	zinc
1563	24	7	1001	65	100	46	8	0	7	34	0	15	21	32	11	39	2	16	17
1564	17	10	0	260	179	4	2	16	9	2	2	6	3	0	3	16	8	3	3
1565	0	0	0	101	2	0	0	0	0	0	0	0	0	0	0	5	1	0	0
1566	0	0	0	76	165	1	2	13	4	2	1	4	2	0	2	5	2	2	1
1567	5	1	0	71	186	1	2	11	5	3	1	6	3	0	2	7	5	2	2
1568	0	0	0	65	247	1	1	14	4	4	2	15	3	0	1	5	4	2	1
1569	4	3	12	95	248	5	2	14	4	5	2	14	3	1	2	6	4	2	1
1570	5	4	0	61	219	2	1	12	3	4	2	13	2	0	1	4	4	2	1
1571	9	4	0	60	247	2	2	12	5	4	2	14	3	0	2	6	7	2	2
1572	6	4	19	145	23	7	1	0	0	2	0	1	1	1	2	7	1	2	1
1573	11	7	22	101	74	10	1	1	1	5	0	1	1	2	6	8	2	0	1
1574	6	4	13	74	295	6	1	62	6	7	3	12	6	1	5	7	6	4	2
1575	4	4	0	93	5	1	0	0	0	0	0	0	0	0	1	5	1	0	0
1576	0	0	0	119	1	0	0	0	0	0	0	0	0	0	0	7	1	0	0
1577	6	1	0	80	202	1	2	12	6	3	1	6	3	0	2	8	5	2	2
1578	1	0	0	74	271	1	2	16	4	5	2	16	3	0	1	6	4	2	1
1579	2	1	0	94	242	1	1	14	4	4	2	14	2	0	1	6	4	1	1
1580	4	3	12	97	310	5	2	16	4	6	2	19	3	1	2	6	5	2	1
1581	11	7	35	198	39	12	1	0	0	4	0	1	1	2	3	9	1	2	2
1582	9	7	3	109	84	0	0	1	1	5	0	1	2	3	6	9	2	0	2
1583	5	4	2	479	340	1	1	61	6	8	3	12	7	2	6	32	7	5	2
1584	1	1	0	119	5	0	0	0	0	0	0	0	0	0	0	6	1	0	0
1585	0	0	0	390	3	0	0	0	0	1	0	0	1	0	0	23	0	0	0
1586	0	0	0	61	2	0	0	0	0	0	0	0	0	0	0	3	0	0	0
1587	0	0	0	97	113	28	1	26	2	2	1	3	3	0	1	5	2	1	1
1588	0	0	0	35	111	28	1	26	2	1	1	3	3	0	1	2	2	1	1
1589	44	39	0	29	481	0	4	9	3	0	7	3	7	0	3	19	17	17	8
1590	9	5	89	129	709	10	1	1	12	28	7	14	10	6	30	24	24	13	8
1591	18	3	308	92	170	14	4	10	10	22	1	7	8	10	4	18	7	8	11
1592	24	9	28	463	359	4	12	2	14	13	11	3	9	2	18	16	14	14	8
1593	18	6	24	602	493	3	10	2	19	18	15	5	12	2	25	22	19	20	10
1594	9	5	34	125	354	6	1	2	3	22	1	2	2	2	30	24	7	2	6
1595	26	15	241	74	252	29	3	1	4	20	1	5	6	12	17	22	9	6	8
1596	16	5	11	312	1985	37	7	6	18	62	7	12	10	38	75	83	62	36	32
1597	27	16	98	29	220	31	2	31	2	7	2	8	3	2	5	6	4	1	2
1598	11	4	482	145	309	22	4	20	8	34	2	14	15	15	8	21	7	11	9
1599	3	1	1	94	128	2	0	0	1	6	0	1	0	5	8	6	3	1	1
1600	3	1	1	60	79	3	0	0	2	7	0	1	1	4	7	6	2	0	1
1601	3	1	1	43	99	0	2	0	1	3	0	1	1	2	3	3	3	3	2
1602	3	1	1	50	41	0	2	0	0	3	0	0	0	0	3	2	8	1	1
1603	10	3	126	294	445	15	4	2	12	27	7	7	9	7	23	22	9	12	7
1604	5	1	3	146	203	1	0	3	2	10	2	2	1	0	10	9	6	3	3
1605	4	1	6	149	166	1	0	2	2	10	2	1	0	1	10	8	4	2	3

Desserts & Sweets

Food #	Food Description & Amount	wt gm	wt oz	calo-ries	%cal fat	prot gm	carbo gm	fiber gm
1606	Pudding, canned, chocolate, fat free (Include Swiss Miss Fat Free Chocolate Pudding Snacks) [4-oz can]	113	4.0	98	3%	2	23	0.5
1607	Pudding, canned, chocolate, low calorie [4-oz can]	113	4.0	73	20%	4	11	0.1
1608	Pudding, canned, chocolate, reduced fat (Include Jell-O Light) [4-oz can]	113	4.0	98	7%	2	22	0.2
1609	Pudding, canned, flavors other than chocolate [4-oz can]	113	4.0	147	25%	3	25	0.1
1610	Pudding, canned, flavors other than chocolate, fat free [4-oz can]	113	4.0	99	1%	2	23	0.0
1611	Pudding, canned, flavors other than chocolate, low calorie [4-oz can]	113	4.0	70	18%	4	11	0.0
1612	Pudding, canned, flavors other than chocolate, reduced fat (Include Jell-O Light, Ultra Slim Fast) [4-oz can]	113	4.0	104	14%	2	20	0.0
1613	Pudding, canned, tapioca [4-oz can]	113	4.0	134	28%	2	22	0.1
1614	Pudding, canned, tapioca, fat free [4-oz can]	113	4.0	98	1%	2	23	0.1
1615	Pudding, chocolate, home recipe made with whole milk [1 cup]	261	9.2	268	18%	8	49	0.8
1616	Pudding, chocolate, low calorie, made from dry mix and 2% fat milk (Include D-Zerta) [1 cup]	250	8.8	162	20%	9	25	0.2
1617	Pudding, chocolate, made from dry mix and whole milk [1 cup]	261	9.2	271	18%	8	50	0.9
1618	Pudding, flavors other than chocolate, home recipe made with whole milk [1 cup]	261	9.2	262	16%	7	49	0.0
1619	Pudding, flavors other than chocolate, low calorie, made from dry mix and 2% fat milk (Include D-Zerta) [1 cup]	260	9.2	161	18%	8	24	0.0
1620	Pudding, flavors other than chocolate, made from dry mix and whole milk [1 cup]	264	9.3	272	16%	8	51	0.0
1621	Puerto Rican bread pudding (Budin de pan) [1 cup]	175	6.2	473	31%	14	68	1.7
1622	Puerto Rican custard (Flan) [1 cup]	240	8.5	399	24%	12	65	0.0
1623	Puerto Rican pumpkin pudding (Flan de calabaza) [1 cup]	262	9.2	598	41%	13	78	1.0
1624	Pumpkin pudding [1 cup]	265	9.3	243	20%	7	43	0.2
1625	Rice dessert (rice, pineapple, marshmallows, whipped cream, sugar) (Include glorified rice) [1 cup]	155	5.5	277	47%	3	35	0.8
1626	Rice flour cream, Puerto Rican style (Majarete, manjar blanco) [1 cup]	250	8.8	395	19%	10	70	0.5
1627	Rice flour pudding, with nuts (Indian dessert) [1 cup]	250	8.8	359	20%	9	63	0.6
1628	**Rice pudding** [1 cup]	**225**	**7.9**	**302**	**11%**	**8**	**60**	**1.0**
1629	Spanish custard, Puerto Rican style (Natilla Espanol) [1 cup]	243	8.6	448	34%	13	62	0.0
1630	Tapioca pudding, chocolate, made from dry mix and whole milk [1 cup]	165	5.8	188	18%	6	35	1.7
1631	**Tapioca pudding, vanilla, made from dry mix and whole milk [1 cup]**	**165**	**5.8**	**177**	**16%**	**5**	**33**	**0.0**
1632	Tapioca pudding, vanilla, made from home recipe [1 cup]	205	7.2	238	25%	10	35	0.0
1633	Vanilla wafer pudding (vanilla pudding, vanilla wafers, bananas) [1 cup]	187	6.6	280	24%	6	49	1.6
1634	Yokan, Japanese bean dessert [2 slices]	56	2.0	97	0%	1	24	0.4
1635	Zabaglione [1 cup]	60	2.1	157	31%	3	17	0.0
	Pastries							
1650	Blintz, cheese-filled [1 blintz]	70	2.5	136	39%	7	14	0.2
1651	Blintz, fruit-filled [1 blintz]	70	2.5	124	32%	4	17	0.5
1652	Baklava (Include Kadayif) [1 piece (2"x2"x1½")]	78	2.8	336	61%	5	29	1.8
1653	Cheese puffs (Include cheese straws) [5 puffs/straws]	30	1.1	80	66%	3	4	0.1
1654	**Churro** (Include Mexican crueller) [1 churro]	**26**	**0.9**	**116**	**57%**	**1**	**12**	**0.2**
1655	Cream puff, no filling or icing [1 cream puff]	27	1.0	98	64%	2	6	0.2
1656	Crepe suzette [1 crepe with sauce]	66	2.3	159	51%	4	16	0.4
1657	Crepe, dessert type, chocolate-filled [1 crepe]	78	2.8	119	34%	4	16	0.7
1658	Crepe, dessert type, blueberry-filled (Include other fruit) [1 crepe]	78	2.8	145	35%	4	21	1.0
1659	Crepe, dessert type, ice cream-filled [1 crepe]	78	2.8	161	43%	5	18	0.3
1660	**Crisp, apple,** apple dessert (Include apple betty) [1 cup]	**246**	**8.7**	**402**	**20%**	**4**	**79**	**4.6**
1661	Crisp, blueberry [1 cup]	246	8.7	632	36%	5	101	5.1
1662	Crisp, cherry [1 cup]	246	8.7	704	35%	6	113	2.8
1663	Crisp, peach [1 cup]	246	8.7	508	28%	4	92	4.1
1664	Crisp, rhubarb [1 cup]	246	8.7	556	26%	3	106	3.9
1665	Cruller [1 cruller (3¼"dia)]	49	1.7	206	49%	2	24	0.7

Food #	fat gm	sat fat gm	choles mg	sodium mg	potass mg	% of Daily Value													
						vit A	vit E	vit C	thia-min	ribo-flavin	nia-cin	vit B-6	fol-ate	vit B-12	cal-cium	phos-phorus	magne-sium	iron	zinc
1606	0	0	1	240	125	3	0	1	1	5	0	1	1	2	7	6	3	2	2
1607	2	1	6	216	282	6	0	1	2	10	1	2	1	4	13	19	6	2	3
1608	1	0	5	163	185	6	1	0	2	7	0	1	0	2	8	7	5	9	3
1609	4	1	8	153	128	1	0	0	2	9	1	1	0	2	10	8	2	1	2
1610	0	0	1	251	99	4	0	1	1	5	0	1	1	2	7	6	2	0	2
1611	1	1	6	263	170	6	0	1	2	10	0	2	1	4	13	18	4	0	3
1612	2	1	6	118	120	7	1	1	2	7	0	2	1	5	9	7	3	0	2
1613	4	1	1	133	118	0	0	1	2	7	2	5	1	2	9	9	2	1	2
1614	0	0	1	251	99	4	0	1	1	5	0	1	1	2	8	6	2	1	2
1615	5	3	18	264	430	11	1	3	6	26	1	5	3	13	29	25	13	5	8
1616	4	2	12	477	625	14	1	4	6	23	1	5	3	14	29	42	13	5	7
1617	5	3	19	508	442	11	1	4	6	24	1	5	3	14	28	44	13	5	8
1618	5	3	18	420	350	11	1	3	6	21	1	5	3	13	27	21	8	1	6
1619	3	2	13	605	391	14	0	4	6	23	1	5	3	15	30	43	8	1	7
1620	5	3	19	594	357	11	1	3	5	21	1	4	2	11	28	38	8	1	6
1621	16	6	127	474	421	15	5	2	18	34	12	6	13	5	30	28	10	14	9
1622	11	5	256	146	279	14	2	1	3	29	1	5	6	8	21	24	6	5	8
1623	27	7	297	324	491	47	15	11	14	35	8	8	15	11	10	22	7	15	9
1624	5	3	15	365	452	17	3	8	6	20	2	5	4	11	24	20	8	3	6
1625	15	9	53	21	104	16	1	13	9	4	5	5	9	1	3	5	4	5	3
1626	8	5	33	121	406	8	1	4	16	24	1	7	17	12	30	26	10	9	9
1627	8	4	26	96	341	6	2	2	13	20	7	5	12	6	24	22	10	8	7
1628	4	2	15	94	417	9	1	3	6	18	3	7	2	6	23	21	9	4	7
1629	17	8	430	124	370	25	4	3	8	33	1	10	11	24	31	36	8	7	12
1630	4	2	13	77	315	7	0	2	4	15	1	3	2	7	19	18	11	5	6
1631	3	2	13	263	243	8	0	2	4	15	1	3	2	8	19	15	5	1	4
1632	7	3	157	125	298	14	2	2	5	25	1	5	5	13	22	22	6	4	7
1633	7	3	83	216	369	6	2	8	7	19	5	18	7	6	12	14	8	5	4
1634	0	0	0	23	17	0	0	0	0	1	0	0	0	0	0	1	1	1	0
1635	5	2	221	10	44	10	2	0	2	7	0	3	6	9	3	9	1	4	4
1650	6	2	68	223	75	8	2	0	5	10	3	2	5	6	7	10	2	4	3
1651	4	1	53	93	78	7	2	1	3	8	2	2	3	3	3	6	2	5	2
1652	23	9	36	293	144	12	7	2	13	9	7	2	6	0	3	9	9	10	3
1653	6	2	38	83	25	6	2	0	2	5	1	1	2	2	4	4	1	2	2
1654	7	2	2	7	8	1	3	0	3	2	2	0	2	0	0	1	0	2	0
1655	7	2	53	150	26	8	3	0	4	6	2	1	3	2	1	3	1	3	1
1656	9	4	83	74	86	8	2	5	6	10	3	2	5	4	5	7	2	4	2
1657	4	2	56	87	127	6	1	1	5	12	2	2	3	4	8	9	3	4	3
1658	6	1	60	72	89	8	3	7	5	9	3	2	4	3	4	6	2	4	2
1659	8	3	85	81	138	10	2	1	6	14	3	3	5	6	8	10	3	4	4
1660	9	2	0	343	239	7	4	9	14	10	10	5	8	0	7	6	4	10	3
1661	25	5	0	722	180	26	17	27	19	14	12	4	14	0	13	22	4	10	3
1662	27	5	2	836	219	25	14	5	14	15	10	7	18	2	15	32	5	19	3
1663	16	3	0	202	535	23	12	17	12	11	14	3	8	0	7	6	9	13	3
1664	16	3	0	202	323	17	9	9	11	9	8	3	8	0	28	5	9	12	2
1665	11	2	18	268	62	1	6	0	7	7	5	1	6	2	2	13	2	5	2

Desserts & Sweets

Food #	Food Description & Amount	wt gm	wt oz	calo-ries	%cal fat	prot gm	carbo gm	fiber gm
1666	Danish pastry (Include fruit and/or spice, pecan swirls, snail Danish, pastry with icing, Babka, bear claw) [1 pastry (5"dia)]	94	3.3	379	50%	7	42	1.2
1667	Danish pastry, with cheese [1 pastry (5"dia)]	112	4.0	419	53%	9	42	1.1
1668	Danish pastry, with cheese, very lowfat [1 slice (3¾x1¾x¾")]	32	1.1	95	2%	3	21	0.4
1669	Danish pastry, with fruit [1 pastry (4"dia)]	71	2.5	263	45%	4	34	1.3
1670	Danish pastry, with nuts [1 pastry (4"dia)]	65	2.3	280	53%	5	30	1.3
1671	**Doughnut, cake type** (including coconut, sugar-coated, glazed, plain cruller) [1 doughnut (3"dia)]	42	1.5	177	49%	2	21	0.6
1672	Doughnut, cake type, chocolate (including glazed) [1 doughnut (3"dia)]	42	1.5	175	43%	2	24	0.9
1673	Doughnut, cake type, chocolate covered [1 doughnut (3"dia)]	53	1.9	251	59%	3	25	1.1
1674	Doughnut, cake type, chocolate covered, dipped in peanuts (Include peanut stick) [1 doughnut (3"dia)]	53	1.9	214	48%	3	26	1.0
1675	Doughnut, cake type, chocolate, with chocolate icing [1 doughnut (3"dia)]	53	1.9	219	47%	3	28	1.1
1676	Doughnut, chocolate cream-filled [1 doughnut]	65	2.3	220	49%	4	25	0.8
1677	Doughnut, custard-filled (Include Long John cream-filled doughnut) [1 doughnut]	65	2.3	235	61%	4	20	0.5
1678	Doughnut, custard-filled, with icing [1 doughnut]	70	2.5	245	36%	3	37	0.5
1679	Doughnut, eggless, carob-covered, raised or yeast [1 doughnut]	78	2.8	288	55%	5	33	6.7
1680	Doughnut, French cruller (including sugar-coated, glazed) [1 cruller (3"dia)]	49	1.7	202	40%	2	29	0.6
1681	Doughnut, jelly [1 doughnut]	65	2.3	221	50%	4	25	0.6
1682	Doughnut, oriental (Include Okinawan donut) [2 doughnuts]	36	1.3	151	42%	2	20	0.4
1683	**Doughnut, raised or yeast,** glazed or honey-dipped (Include doughboys, doughnut holes, malasadas) [1 doughnut (3"dia)]	60	2.1	242	51%	4	27	0.7
1684	Doughnut, raised or yeast, chocolate covered [1 doughnut (3"dia)]	71	2.5	276	46%	4	36	1.1
1685	Doughnut, raised or yeast, chocolate [1 doughnut (3"dia)]	50	1.8	198	51%	3	22	1.5
1686	Doughnut, raised or yeast, chocolate, with chocolate icing [1 doughnut (3"dia)]	71	2.5	277	47%	4	36	2.4
1687	Doughnut, wheat (Include glazed) [1 doughnut]	42	1.5	151	48%	3	18	0.9
1688	Doughnut, wheat, chocolate covered [1 doughnut (3"dia)]	71	2.5	287	42%	4	39	2.2
1689	**Eclair,** custard-filled cream puff, chocolate icing [1 eclair (5"x2"x1¾")]	102	3.6	267	54%	7	25	0.6
1690	Eclair, custard-filled cream puff, no icing [1 eclair (5"x2 x1¾")]	90	3.2	232	54%	6	21	0.4
1691	Empanada, fruit-filled [1 cup]	142	5.0	590	49%	6	71	2.1
1692	Empanada, pumpkin (Include squash empanada, sweet potato empanada) [1 cup]	132	4.7	327	39%	5	46	2.6
1693	Fritter or fried puff, unfilled, without syrup, Puerto Rican style (Include Bunuelos de viento, wheat flour turnover, Pastelillo de harina de trigo) [2 puffs]	55	1.9	193	49%	3	22	0.3
1694	Fritter, apple [2 fritters]	48	1.7	174	57%	3	16	0.7
1695	**Fritter, banana** [2 fritters (2" long)]	68	2.4	223	56%	3	23	1.3
1696	Fritter, berry [2 fritters]	48	1.7	156	58%	3	14	0.9
1697	Fritter, wheat flour, no syrup [2 fritters]	44	1.6	198	78%	3	8	0.3
1698	Ladoo, round ball, Asian-Indian dessert [1 ball (1¾"dia)]	63	2.2	246	55%	4	26	3.2
1699	Meringues [2 meringues]	44	1.6	143	0%	3	33	0.0
1700	Moon Cake, oriental pastry made with bean or lotus seed paste filling (baked) [1 Moon Cake]	138	4.9	459	11%	9	92	3.6
1701	Moon Cake, oriental pastry made with bean paste and salted egg yolk filling (baked) [1 Moon Cake]	138	4.9	467	23%	12	77	3.0
1702	Pastry, Chinese, made with rice flour (Include nine-layer Chinese steamed rice and syrup pudding) [1 piece]	56	2.0	135	22%	1	25	0.6
1703	Pastry, flour and water only, fried (Include Taco Bell Cinnamon Crispa) [3 crispas]	30	1.1	135	35%	2	20	1.0
1704	Pastry, cookie type, fried [1 pastry]	46	1.6	174	59%	3	16	0.4
1705	Pastry, fruit-filled (Include hamantaschen) [1 pastry]	78	2.8	265	51%	3	31	3.1
1706	Pastry, Italian, with cheese (Include cannoli) [1 pastry]	85	3.0	233	40%	8	27	0.7
1707	Pastry, puff (Include angel wings, flaky pastry, patty shell) [2 puffs]	22	0.8	123	62%	2	10	0.3
1708	Pastry, puff, custard or cream filled (Include cream horn, Napoleon) [2 puffs]	114	4.0	467	66%	6	34	1.0
1709	Pop-Tart (Include all flavors), Kellogg's [1 Pop-Tart]	52	1.8	210	23%	2	37	1.0
1710	Pop-Tart, Low Fat (Include all flavors), Kellogg's [1 Pop-Tart]	50	1.8	190	14%	2	39	0.8

Food #	fat gm	sat fat gm	choles mg	sodium mg	potass mg	% of Daily Value													
						vit A	vit E	vit C	thia-min	ribo-flavin	nia-cin	vit B-6	fol-ate	vit B-12	cal-cium	phos-phorus	magne-sium	iron	zinc
1666	21	5	28	349	118	1	10	0	19	15	13	2	15	3	7	10	4	10	5
1667	25	8	50	504	110	7	10	0	14	17	11	2	17	4	4	12	4	10	6
1668	0	0	0	88	39	0	0	0	6	6	4	1	5	1	1	3	1	3	1
1669	13	3	15	251	59	1	4	5	12	9	7	1	6	1	3	6	3	7	3
1670	16	4	30	236	62	1	6	2	10	9	7	3	13	2	6	7	5	7	4
1671	10	2	16	229	53	1	5	0	6	6	4	1	5	2	2	11	2	5	2
1672	8	2	24	143	50	1	3	0	1	2	1	1	4	1	9	7	4	5	2
1673	16	4	31	227	60	2	8	0	4	3	3	1	4	3	2	11	5	7	2
1674	11	2	15	218	85	1	5	0	6	6	5	2	5	2	2	13	4	5	3
1675	12	3	16	231	85	1	5	0	6	7	4	1	5	2	3	13	5	6	2
1676	12	3	5	188	78	1	5	0	13	8	7	2	6	1	4	6	3	6	3
1677	16	4	16	201	52	1	5	0	15	6	7	1	10	1	2	5	3	7	3
1678	10	3	4	161	61	1	4	0	10	6	6	1	5	1	3	5	3	5	2
1679	18	4	0	79	217	0	10	0	9	8	12	7	6	0	7	15	14	10	7
1680	9	2	5	169	38	0	4	0	6	7	4	1	4	1	1	6	1	4	1
1681	12	3	17	190	51	1	5	1	14	5	7	1	10	1	2	6	3	6	3
1682	7	2	25	77	31	1	3	0	6	6	4	1	4	1	5	4	1	5	1
1683	14	3	4	205	65	1	6	0	15	8	9	2	6	1	3	6	3	7	3
1684	14	4	4	184	94	2	5	0	13	8	7	2	6	1	3	7	6	7	4
1685	11	3	3	163	89	0	5	0	12	7	7	2	5	1	2	6	6	7	4
1686	14	4	3	179	138	1	5	0	12	8	8	2	6	1	3	9	10	9	5
1687	8	1	8	149	62	1	4	0	6	6	4	2	2	2	2	4	2	3	2
1688	13	4	19	103	128	1	6	0	8	7	7	3	5	2	5	10	8	7	4
1689	16	4	130	344	119	19	7	1	8	16	4	3	7	6	6	11	4	7	4
1690	14	3	121	307	104	18	7	0	7	15	4	3	6	5	6	10	3	6	4
1691	32	6	0	101	91	0	16	0	20	13	13	2	13	0	7	8	4	15	3
1692	14	3	34	10	184	107	8	3	16	13	11	3	12	1	4	7	6	16	3
1693	10	3	65	99	32	10	4	0	4	7	3	1	4	2	1	4	1	4	2
1694	11	2	40	19	68	3	5	1	5	7	3	2	4	2	3	4	2	4	2
1695	14	3	40	32	193	4	6	5	6	9	4	12	5	2	3	5	4	4	2
1696	10	2	34	28	59	3	5	4	5	7	3	1	3	2	2	4	1	3	2
1697	17	4	70	110	35	11	8	0	5	8	3	1	4	2	1	4	1	4	2
1698	15	2	0	6	129	0	9	1	4	2	1	3	15	0	2	6	5	6	4
1699	0	0	0	49	44	0	0	0	0	8	0	0	0	1	0	0	1	0	0
1700	6	1	69	117	153	3	3	1	24	19	14	3	27	2	2	11	7	16	5
1701	12	3	353	738	150	16	5	0	22	24	12	7	29	11	5	21	6	18	9
1702	3	0	0	5	50	0	2	0	2	0	3	4	1	0	1	3	4	2	2
1703	5	1	0	135	38	0	3	0	10	5	5	1	8	0	4	4	2	6	1
1704	11	3	52	44	56	6	5	1	6	7	4	1	6	2	3	5	2	4	2
1705	15	2	15	6	148	2	5	2	11	8	6	5	6	0	1	6	5	8	4
1706	10	5	35	48	90	7	3	0	9	12	5	2	7	3	12	11	3	7	5
1707	8	1	0	56	14	0	2	0	5	3	4	0	3	0	0	1	1	3	1
1708	34	9	53	187	97	12	6	0	15	15	12	2	8	2	5	8	4	10	4
1709	6	2	0	180	50	10	3	0	10	10	10	10	10	0	0	2	2	10	2
1710	3	1	0	230	30	10	3	0	10	10	10	10	10	0	0	6		10	1

Desserts & Sweets

Food #	Food Description & Amount	wt gm	wt oz	calo-ries	%cal fat	prot gm	carbo gm	fiber gm
1711	Sopaipilla with syrup or honey [2 sopaipillas (1½"square)]	24	0.8	86	39%	1	12	0.3
1712	Sopaipilla, no syrup or honey [2 sopaipillas (1½"square)]	20	0.7	73	49%	1	8	0.3
1713	Strudel, apple [2"square]	64	2.3	175	37%	2	26	1.4
1714	Strudel, berry [2"square]	64	2.3	161	23%	2	30	1.6
1715	Strudel, cheese and pineapple (with/without other fruit) [2"square]	64	2.3	141	35%	4	19	0.6
1716	Strudel, cheese [2"square]	64	2.3	196	38%	6	24	0.4
1717	Strudel, cherry [2"square]	64	2.3	179	32%	3	29	1.1
1718	Strudel, peach [2"square]	64	2.3	127	22%	2	24	1.3
1719	Strudel, pineapple [2"square]	64	2.3	159	20%	2	31	0.8
1720	Tamale, sweet (including with sugar and spices) [2 tamales]	68	2.4	176	44%	2	24	2.1
1721	Tamale, sweet, with bananas, pineapple, raisins [2 tamales]	98	3.5	198	38%	2	31	2.6
1722	**Turnover or dumpling, apple [1 turnover]**	**82**	**2.9**	**290**	**46%**	**3**	**37**	**1.2**
1723	Turnover or dumpling, berry [1 turnover]	78	2.8	279	45%	3	36	1.6
1724	Turnover or dumpling, cherry [1 turnover]	78	2.8	240	44%	3	31	1.0
1725	Turnover or dumpling, lemon [1 turnover]	78	2.8	238	47%	3	29	0.6
1726	Turnover or dumpling, peach [1 turnover]	78	2.8	256	44%	3	34	1.4
1727	Turnover, guava [1 turnover]	78	2.8	234	48%	2	28	2.6
1728	Turnover, pumpkin [1 turnover]	78	2.8	196	52%	4	20	1.3
	Jams, Sweeteners, Toppings							
1750	Apple butter (Include fruit butters) [2Tbs]	35	1.2	65	1%	0	17	0.5
1751	Aspartame sweetener (Include Equal) [1 individual packet]	1	0.0	4	0%	0	1	0.0
1752	Aspartame-sugar blend, sugar substitute [1 individual packet (½ tsp)]	2	0.1	8	0%	0	2	0.0
1753	Bean paste, sweetened (Include Japanese red beans) [2Tbs]	40	1.4	84	1%	2	19	2.1
1754	Cane and corn syrup blend [2Tbs]	41	1.4	112	0%	0	30	0.0
1755	Carob syrup (carob powder in corn syrup) [2Tbs]	37	1.3	82	1%	0	24	3.0
1756	Chocolate sauce (milk-based) [2Tbs]	34	1.2	85	15%	1	18	0.5
1757	**Chocolate syrup**, thin type [2Tbs]	**38**	**1.3**	**82**	**4%**	**1**	**22**	**0.7**
1758	Chocolate-flavored hazelnut spread (Include Nutella) [2Tbs]	31	1.1	154	52%	2	19	1.0
1759	Corn syrup (Include Karo brand, light or dark) [2Tbs]	41	1.4	116	0%	0	31	0.0
1760	Fructose sweetener [1 individual packet]	3	0.1	11	0%	0	3	0.0
1761	Fruit sauce (all fruits) [2Tbs]	42	1.5	89	27%	0	17	0.1
1762	Fruit syrup (Include fruit-flavored pancake syrup) [2Tbs]	39	1.4	105	0%	0	28	0.0
1763	Green papaya preserve, Puerto Rican style (Include Dulce de lechoza) [2Tbs]	19	0.7	58	0%	0	15	0.3
1764	Guava paste [2Tbs]	38	1.3	107	0%	0	28	0.4
1765	Hard sauce [2Tbs]	21	0.7	96	48%	0	13	0.0
1766	**Honey (Include pear honey, raw honey) [2Tbs]**	**42**	**1.5**	**129**	**0%**	**0**	**35**	**0.1**
1767	Icing, chocolate [2Tbs]	34	1.2	136	25%	0	27	0.5
1768	Icing, white (including flavored) (Include creme filling) [2Tbs]	40	1.4	163	24%	0	32	0.0
1769	**Jam, preserves**, all flavors [2Tbs]	**40**	**1.4**	**97**	**1%**	**0**	**26**	**0.5**
1770	Jams, preserves, marmalades, sweetened with fruit juice concentrate, all flavors (Include Polaner All Fruit) [2Tbs]	40	1.4	73	3%	0	18	1.0
1771	Jams, preserves, marmalades, low sugar (all flavors) [2Tbs]	36	1.3	51	2%	0	13	0.6
1772	Jams, preserves, marmalades, dietetic, all flavors, sweetened with artificial sweetener [2Tbs]	40	1.4	4	25%	0	21	1.0
1773	**Jellies**, all flavors [2Tbs]	**38**	**1.3**	**102**	**0%**	**0**	**27**	**0.4**
1774	Jellies, reduced sugar, all flavors [2Tbs]	38	1.3	67	0%	0	17	0.3
1775	Jellies, dietetic, all flavors, sweetened with low-cal sweetener [2Tbs]	38	1.3	12	0%	0	22	0.3
1776	Maple syrup (100% maple) (Include Maple Cream) [2Tbs]	39	1.4	103	1%	0	26	0.0
1777	Molasses [2Tbs]	41	1.4	109	0%	0	28	0.0
1778	Orange Marmalade (Include other flavors) [2Tbs]	40	1.4	98	0%	0	27	0.1
1779	Raisin sauce [2Tbs]	31	1.1	41	36%	0	7	0.2
1780	Saccharin (Include Necta Sweet) [1 tablet (½ grain)]	0	0.0	0	0%	0	0	0.0
1781	Saccharin-based liquid sweetener (Include Fasweet, Sweet n'Low, Sweet 10) [1 tsp]	5	0.2	0	0%	0	0	0.0

Food #	fat gm	sat fat gm	choles mg	sodium mg	potass mg	vit A	vit E	vit C	thia-min	ribo-flavin	nia-cin	vit B-6	fol-ate	vit B-12	cal-cium	phos-phorus	magne-sium	iron	zinc
						for % of Daily Value													

Food #	fat gm	sat fat gm	choles mg	sodium mg	potass mg	vit A	vit E	vit C	thia-min	ribo-flavin	nia-cin	vit B-6	fol-ate	vit B-12	cal-cium	phos-phorus	magne-sium	iron	zinc
1711	4	1	0	28	13	0	2	0	4	3	3	0	2	0	2	2	1	3	1
1712	4	1	0	32	11	0	2	0	4	3	3	0	3	0	2	2	1	3	1
1713	7	1	18	172	62	1	4	2	2	1	1	1	2	2	1	2	1	1	1
1714	4	1	11	82	58	4	3	8	7	6	5	1	4	0	2	3	2	5	1
1715	5	3	28	61	88	6	1	4	6	7	3	2	3	1	7	6	3	4	3
1716	8	4	42	93	66	9	2	1	6	9	4	1	5	2	9	9	2	5	4
1717	6	1	9	74	104	7	2	5	7	5	4	3	4	0	2	4	4	5	2
1718	3	1	9	61	104	5	3	5	5	5	5	1	3	0	2	2	2	4	1
1719	4	1	10	63	59	4	2	5	7	5	4	2	4	0	1	2	2	4	1
1720	9	2	0	2	56	0	4	0	13	7	8	3	6	0	3	4	5	9	2
1721	8	2	0	2	136	0	4	3	14	8	8	7	6	0	4	4	7	9	2
1722	15	3	0	4	56	0	6	1	11	8	8	1	7	0	1	3	2	7	1
1723	14	3	0	3	55	0	7	5	12	8	8	1	7	0	1	3	2	7	2
1724	12	2	0	8	59	3	5	1	10	7	6	1	6	0	1	3	2	9	1
1725	12	3	48	13	32	3	5	3	9	7	5	1	7	2	1	4	1	6	2
1726	12	2	0	1	91	1	6	3	11	8	8	1	7	0	1	3	2	7	2
1727	13	3	0	13	120	3	7	80	10	7	7	3	6	0	1	3	2	6	2
1728	11	3	34	35	156	62	5	2	8	11	5	2	6	1	8	9	4	7	3
1750	0	0	0	1	32	0	0	0	0	0	0	1	0	0	0	0	0	0	0
1751	0	0	0	0	0	0	0	0	0	0	0	0	0	0	0	0	0	0	0
1752	0	0	0	0	0	0	0	0	0	0	0	0	0	0	0	0	0	0	0
1753	0	0	0	1	150	0	0	0	3	1	1	2	6	0	1	3	3	4	2
1754	0	0	0	37	14	0	0	0	2	1	0	0	0	0	0	0	1	4	0
1755	0	0	0	3	62	0	0	0	0	2	1	1	1	0	3	1	1	1	1
1756	1	1	4	19	50	2	0	0	1	3	1	0	1	1	2	3	2	2	1
1757	0	0	0	36	84	0	0	0	0	1	1	0	0	0	1	5	6	4	2
1758	9	1	0	12	118	0	6	0	2	3	1	2	1	1	4	5	7	3	2
1759	0	0	0	50	2	0	0	0	0	0	0	0	0	0	0	0	0	0	0
1760	0	0	0	0	0	0	0	0	0	0	0	0	0	0	0	0	0	0	0
1761	3	1	0	32	45	4	1	7	1	1	0	1	1	0	0	0	1	1	0
1762	0	0	0	15	7	0	0	2	0	0	0	0	0	0	0	0	0	0	0
1763	0	0	0	3	46	0	0	8	0	0	0	0	0	0	1	0	1	1	0
1764	0	0	0	1	26	0	0	28	0	0	0	1	0	0	0	0	0	0	0
1765	5	3	14	52	2	5	0	0	0	0	0	0	0	0	0	0	0	0	0
1766	0	0	0	2	22	0	0	0	0	1	0	1	0	0	0	0	0	1	1
1767	4	1	0	42	47	4	2	0	0	1	0	0	0	0	1	2	2	2	1
1768	4	1	0	51	7	4	2	0	0	0	0	0	0	0	1	0	0	0	0
1769	0	0	0	16	31	0	0	6	0	1	0	0	3	0	1	0	0	1	0
1770	0	0	0	10	205	0	0	25	1	2	1	3	1	0	1	2	3	3	1
1771	0	0	0	0	38	0	0	17	0	1	0	1	1	0	0	0	1	1	0
1772	0	0	0	0	28	0	0	0	0	0	0	0	1	0	0	0	1	1	0
1773	0	0	0	14	24	0	0	1	0	1	0	0	0	0	0	0	1	0	0
1774	0	0	0	1	27	0	0	0	0	0	0	1	0	0	0	0	1	0	0
1775	0	0	0	0	25	0	0	0	0	0	0	1	0	0	0	0	0	0	0
1776	0	0	0	4	80	0	0	0	0	0	0	0	0	0	3	0	1	3	11
1777	0	0	0	15	600	0	0	0	1	0	2	14	0	0	8	1	25	11	1
1778	0	0	0	22	15	0	0	3	0	0	0	0	4	0	2	0	0	0	0
1779	2	0	0	20	27	2	1	0	0	0	0	0	0	0	0	0	0	1	0
1780	0	0	0	0	1	0	0	0	0	0	0	0	0	0	0	0	0	0	0
1781	0	0	0	1	5	0	0	0	0	0	0	0	0	0	0	0	0	0	0

Desserts & Sweets

Food #	Food Description & Amount	wt gm	wt oz	calo-ries	%cal fat	prot gm	carbo gm	fiber gm
1782	Sugar, brown [2Tbs]	28	1.0	103	0%	0	27	0.0
1783	Sugar, brown, liquid [2Tbs]	42	1.5	109	0%	0	28	0.0
1784	Sugar, caramelized [2Tbs]	30	1.1	113	0%	0	29	0.0
1785	Sugar, cinnamon [1 tsp]	4	0.1	16	0%	0	4	0.1
1786	Sugar, maple [2Tbs]	18	0.6	64	1%	0	16	0.0
1787	Sugar, raw [2Tbs]	24	0.9	92	0%	0	24	0.0
1788	Sugar, white, powdered, confectioner's [2Tbs]	15	0.5	58	0%	0	15	0.0
1789	Sugar, white, granulated or lump (Include rock sugar, rock candy) [2Tbs]	25	0.9	98	0%	0	25	0.0
1790	Sugar Twin [1 individual packet]	1	0.0	3	0%	0	1	0.0
1791	Sugar Twin, brown [1 tsp]	0	0.0	1	0%	0	0	0.0
1792	Sweet Magic [1 individual packet]	1	0.0	0	0%	0	1	0.0
1793	Sweet'ner, Sweet n' Low [1 individual packet]	1	0.0	4	0%	0	1	0.0
1794	Sweet potato paste [1 cubic inch]	22	0.8	67	0%	0	17	0.1
1795	Syrup, brown sugar and water [2Tbs]	30	1.1	37	0%	0	10	0.0
1796	Syrup, buttered blends (Include Mrs. Butterworth, Log Cabin with butter) [2Tbs]	39	1.4	115	5%	0	30	0.0
1797	Syrup, corn and maple (2% maple) (Include pancake syrup, Log Cabin Brand) [2Tbs]	39	1.4	104	0%	0	27	0.0
1798	Syrup, dietetic [2Tbs]	30	1.1	12	0%	0	15	0.0
1799	Syrup, fruit flavored, used for milk beverages [2Tbs]	40	1.4	106	0%	0	28	0.0
1800	Syrup, pancake [2Tbs]	40	1.4	106	0%	0	28	0.0
1801	Syrup, reduced calorie [2Tbs]	30	1.1	49	0%	0	13	0.0
1802	Syrup, sorghum [2Tbs]	41	1.5	119	0%	0	31	0.0
1803	Syrup, white sugar and water syrup [2Tbs]	30	1.1	38	0%	0	10	0.0
1804	Topping, butterscotch or caramel [2Tbs]	42	1.5	122	7%	0	31	0.0
1805	Topping, chocolate, thick, fudge type [2Tbs]	42	1.5	148	23%	2	27	1.2
1806	Topping, chocolate, hard coating (Include Smuckers Magic Shell Topping) [2Tbs]	33	1.2	182	74%	2	16	2.7
1807	Topping, chocolate flavor, fat free [2Tbs]	40	1.4	102	5%	1	27	1.4
1808	Topping, chocolate, dietetic (apple juice and molasses base) [2Tbs]	28	1.0	16	24%	1	4	0.9
1809	Topping, chocolate with cereal (Include Nestle's Candy Tops Crunch Ice Cream Topping) [2Tbs]	35	1.2	217	71%	2	16	0.6
1810	Topping, fruit (jam-type) [2Tbs]	42	1.5	108	0%	0	28	0.4
1811	Topping, marshmallow [2Tbs]	38	1.3	118	1%	1	30	0.0
1812	Topping, peanut butter, thick, fudge type [2Tbs]	42	1.5	123	27%	3	24	1.8
1813	Topping, pineapple, unsweetened (Include Sorrell Ridge Brand) [2Tbs]	40	1.4	24	1%	0	6	0.3
1814	Topping, walnuts (or other nuts) in syrup [2Tbs]	42	1.5	173	49%	2	23	0.7
1815	Vanilla sauce (Include rum sauce) [2Tbs]	33	1.2	49	47%	0	6	0.0
	Candy							
	Candy comes in so many sizes, the values are given for 1 oz (28 gm). Use the candy wrapper to find the weight of your candy; multiply the values accordingly. For nutrients not on your label, get them from a candy in this section. Find the closest match using the descriptions and the %Cal fat that you calculate from info on your label (see pages 16 and 18 on how to do this).							
1850	100 Grand Bar [1 oz]	28	1.0	132	35%	1	20	0.4
1851	3 Musketeers Bar [1 oz]	28	1.0	118	28%	1	22	0.5
1852	Almonds, chocolate covered [1 oz]	28	1.0	160	73%	5	9	1.6
1853	Almonds, sugar-coated (Include Jordan almonds) [1 oz]	28	1.0	129	37%	2	20	1.3
1854	Almonds, yogurt-covered [1 oz]	28	1.0	156	63%	4	12	0.9
1855	Andes Mint Wafers [1 oz]	28	1.0	153	54%	2	17	0.0
1856	Baby Ruth [1 oz]	28	1.0	136	40%	2	18	0.8
1857	Bar None (Include Sweet Escapes Triple Chocolate Wafer Bar) [1 oz]	28	1.0	142	56%	2	15	0.7
1858	Butterfinger (Include Butterfinger BB's, Bittyfingers) [1 oz]	28	1.0	136	35%	4	19	0.7
1859	Butterscotch chips/morsels [1 oz]	28	1.0	147	50%	1	19	0.0
1860	Butterscotch hard candy [1 oz]	28	1.0	112	8%	0	27	0.0
1861	Caramel with nuts and cereal, chocolate covered [1 oz]	28	1.0	139	45%	2	17	0.7
1862	Caramel with nuts, chocolate covered (Include Turtles, Reese's NutRageous, Goo Goo Cluster, Peanut Chews, Toffifay) [1 oz]	28	1.0	140	38%	3	18	1.2

Food #	fat gm	sat fat gm	choles mg	sodium mg	potass mg	% of Daily Value													
						vit A	vit E	vit C	thia-min	ribo-flavin	nia-cin	vit B-6	fol-ate	vit B-12	cal-cium	phos-phorus	magne-sium	iron	zinc
1782	0	0	0	11	95	0	0	0	0	0	0	0	0	0	2	1	2	3	0
1783	0	0	0	11	100	0	0	0	0	0	0	0	0	0	2	1	2	3	0
1784	0	0	0	12	104	0	0	0	0	0	0	0	0	0	3	1	2	3	0
1785	0	0	0	0	1	0	0	0	0	0	0	0	0	0	0	0	0	1	0
1786	0	0	0	2	49	0	0	0	0	0	0	0	0	0	2	0	1	2	7
1787	0	0	0	10	84	0	0	0	0	0	0	0	0	0	2	1	2	3	0
1788	0	0	0	0	0	0	0	0	0	0	0	0	0	0	0	0	0	0	0
1789	0	0	0	0	1	0	0	0	0	0	0	0	0	0	0	0	0	0	0
1790	0	0	0	5	1	0	0	0	0	0	0	0	0	0	1	0	0	0	0
1791	0	0	0	2	0	0	0	0	0	0	0	0	0	0	0	0	0	0	0
1792	0	0	0	57	1	0	0	0	0	0	0	0	0	0	0	0	0	0	0
1793	0	0	0	4	45	0	0	0	0	0	0	0	0	0	0	0	0	0	0
1794	0	0	0	1	12	11	0	2	0	1	0	1	0	0	0	0	0	0	0
1795	0	0	0	5	34	0	0	0	0	0	0	0	0	0	1	0	1	1	0
1796	1	0	2	53	2	1	0	0	0	0	0	0	0	0	0	0	0	0	0
1797	0	0	0	24	2	0	0	0	0	0	0	0	0	0	0	0	0	0	1
1798	0	0	0	6	0	0	0	0	0	0	0	0	0	0	0	0	0	0	0
1799	0	0	0	1	0	0	0	0	0	0	0	0	0	0	0	0	0	0	0
1800	0	0	0	24	2	0	0	0	0	0	0	0	0	0	0	0	0	0	1
1801	0	0	0	60	1	0	0	0	0	0	0	0	0	0	0	1	0	0	0
1802	0	0	0	3	412	0	0	0	3	4	0	14	0	0	6	2	10	9	1
1803	0	0	0	1	0	0	0	0	0	0	0	0	0	0	0	0	0	0	0
1804	1	1	0	46	5	0	0	0	0	0	0	0	0	0	0	0	0	0	0
1805	4	2	1	147	153	0	4	0	2	6	1	1	0	1	3	6	5	3	2
1806	15	8	0	28	131	0	4	0	1	1	1	1	1	0	1	6	11	6	4
1807	1	0	0	66	120	0	0	0	1	2	1	0	0	0	1	4	6	4	2
1808	0	0	0	2	114	0	0	0	0	1	0	1	0	0	1	2	5	3	1
1809	17	6	5	36	85	0	7	0	1	4	1	1	1	2	4	5	3	1	2
1810	0	0	0	13	57	0	0	24	0	0	0	0	0	0	1	0	0	2	1
1811	0	0	0	17	2	0	0	0	0	0	0	0	0	0	0	0	0	0	0
1812	4	1	0	12	187	0	2	0	1	3	5	2	2	1	3	7	8	5	4
1813	0	0	0	0	49	0	0	6	3	0	1	1	0	0	1	0	1	1	0
1814	9	1	0	18	89	0	1	1	5	3	1	4	2	0	2	5	7	2	3
1815	3	0	0	31	2	3	1	0	0	0	0	0	0	0	0	0	0	0	0
1850	5	3	5	59	64	1	1	0	5	7	5	5	5	1	3	4	3	0	2
1851	4	2	3	55	38	1	0	0	1	2	0	0	0	1	2	3	2	1	1
1852	13	3	2	9	182	0	14	0	3	9	3	1	2	1	7	12	15	5	5
1853	5	0	0	6	72	0	2	0	1	5	1	1	1	0	3	5	7	3	2
1854	11	4	0	15	140	0	10	0	2	8	3	1	2	2	6	10	10	3	3
1855	9	6	6	26	81	0	2	0	1	5	1	1	1	4	6	5	1	0	1
1856	6	3	1	64	112	0	2	0	2	2	4	1	2	0	1	4	6	0	2
1857	9	5	3	26	100	1	2	0	3	3	4	1	2	1	3	5	5	2	2
1858	5	3	0	56	107	0	1	0	2	1	3	1	2	0	1	4	6	1	2
1859	8	7	0	27	53	0	2	0	2	0	0	0	0	1	1	1	0	0	0
1860	1	0	3	104	1	1	0	0	0	0	0	0	0	0	0	0	0	0	0
1861	7	3	4	48	87	1	2	0	6	6	7	5	6	1	3	5	5	1	3
1862	6	1	0	7	126	0	3	1	1	3	7	2	7	0	2	5	6	3	4

Desserts & Sweets

Food #	Food Description & Amount	wt gm	wt oz	calo-ries	%cal fat	prot gm	carbo gm	fiber gm
1863	Caramel, chocolate covered (Include Black Cow, Caramello, Chew-Its, Marathon Bar, Milk Duds, Pom Poms, Sugar Momma, Riesen Chocolate Chew, Russell Stover Chocolate Heart) [1 oz]	28	1.0	117	29%	1	21	0.5
1864	Caramel, chocolate-flavored (Include Tootsie Roll) [1 oz]	28	1.0	102	6%	1	25	0.2
1865	Caramel, flavor other than chocolate (Include Kraft Royals, Caramel Creams, Sugar Babies, Sugar Daddy, Jersey's, Pearson Caramel Nips) [1 oz]	28	1.0	108	19%	1	22	0.3
1866	Caramel, with nuts [1 oz]	28	1.0	116	31%	2	20	0.5
1867	Carob chips [1 oz]	28	1.0	153	52%	2	16	1.1
1868	Chewing gum, candy-coated (Include Chiclets, gum balls) [1 oz, about 20 chiclets]	28	1.0	97	1%	0	27	0.0
1869	Chewing gum, sugarless, uncoated (Include chewing gum with non-nutritive sweeteners) [1 oz, about 10-15 sticks]	28	1.0	76	1%	0	27	0.0
1870	**Chewing gum, uncoated [1 oz, about 10-15 sticks]**	**28**	**1.0**	**86**	**1%**	**0**	**27**	**0.0**
1871	Chocolate chips/morsels, semi-sweet (Include Toll House morsels) [1 oz]	28	1.0	136	56%	1	18	1.7
1872	Chocolate discs, sugar-coated (Include Nonpareils, Oompas) [1 oz]	28	1.0	139	39%	1	20	0.7
1873	Chocolate with fondant and caramel (Include Sky Bar) [1 oz]	28	1.0	131	41%	1	20	0.7
1874	Chocolate, dark, bittersweet (Include Hershey's Special Dark) [1 oz]	28	1.0	156	53%	1	17	1.4
1875	**Chocolate, milk, plain or flavored (Include Hershey Bar or Symphony Bar, Hershey Kiss or Star, Hershey's Hugs or Nuggets, Nestle Bar, Dove Milk Chocolate Bar, chocolate coins or Easter bunnies or eggs) [1 oz]**	**28**	**1.0**	**145**	**54%**	**2**	**17**	**1.0**
1876	Chocolate, milk, with almonds (Include Hershey with Almonds, Nestle Chocolate Bar with Almonds, Hershey Kisses or Nuggets with Almonds) [1 oz]	28	1.0	149	59%	3	15	1.8
1877	Chocolate, milk, with cereal (Include Nestle Crunch Bar, Krackel Bar, Malted Milk Balls, Whoppers, Hershey's Cookies 'n' Mint) [1 oz]	28	1.0	141	48%	2	18	0.7
1878	Chocolate, milk, with fruit and nuts (Include Cadbury's Fruit and Nut Bar, Chunky with Fruit and Nuts) [1 oz]	28	1.0	129	48%	2	17	1.3
1879	Chocolate, milk, with nuts, not almond or peanuts (Include Cadbury's Hazelnut with Chocolate, Brach's Bridge Mix, Chunky with pecans) [1 oz]	28	1.0	152	61%	2	15	1.1
1880	Chocolate, milk, with peanuts (Include Mr. Goodbar, Chunky with peanuts) [1 oz]	28	1.0	155	58%	3	15	1.0
1881	Chocolate, white, with almonds (Include Nestle Alpine White with Almonds [1 oz]	28	1.0	155	58%	2	15	0.3
1882	Chocolate, white, with cereal (Include Hershey's Cookies 'n' Crème, Nestle White Crunch) [1 oz]	28	1.0	146	48%	2	18	0.0
1883	**Chocolate-flavored sprinkles (Include Jimmies) [1 oz]**	**28**	**1.0**	**143**	**54%**	**1**	**19**	**0.9**
1884	Coconut candy, chocolate covered (Include Mounds, Almond Joy, Bounty, chocolate covered coconut Easter bunny) [1 oz]	28	1.0	135	47%	1	17	1.7
1885	Coconut candy, no chocolate covering (Include Rainbow coconut, Russell Stover Bon-bon) [1 oz]	28	1.0	113	28%	0	21	0.4
1886	Coconut candy, Puerto Rican style (coconut milk and sugar) [1 oz]	28	1.0	116	30%	0	21	0.4
1887	Date candy (dates, figs, raisins, pecans candied orange peel, lemon juice) (Include Fruit Nut Bar) [1 oz]	28	1.0	106	41%	1	17	2.4
1888	Easter egg, candy coated chocolate (Include Cadbury's Mini Eggs) [1 bag Cadbury Mini Eggs 1 oz]	28	1.0	139	39%	1	20	0.7
1889	Espresso coffee beans, chocolate-covered [20 beans]	28	1.0	25	32%	1	4	0.1
1890	Fruit leather (Include Fruit Roll-Up, Fruit Wrinkles, Fun Fruits, Fruit Snacks, Fruit By The Foot, Fruit String Thing, Fruit Jammers) [1 oz]	28	1.0	99.2	8%	0	24	1.0
1891	Fruit peel (orange, lemon, or grapefruit), candied [1 oz]	28	1.0	89.6	1%	0	23	1.9
1892	Fruit snack candy, with added vitamin C (Include Brach's Hi-C Gummy Fruits and Fruit Snacks) [1 oz]	28	1.0	106	8%	0	24	1.0
1893	Fudge, brown sugar (penuche) [1 oz]	28	1.0	114	25%	1	22	0.3
1894	Fudge, caramel and nut, chocolate-coated (Include Oh Henry! Bar, Butternut Bar, Powerhouse Bar, Clark Bun Bar) [1 oz]	28	1.0	122	35%	3	18	1.0
1895	**Fudge, chocolate [1 oz]**	**28**	**1.0**	**108**	**20%**	**0**	**23**	**0.2**
1896	Fudge, chocolate, chocolate-coated (Include Mary Sue's Butter Fudge) [1 oz]	28	1.0	119	32%	1	21	0.4
1897	Fudge, chocolate, chocolate-coated, with nuts [1 oz]	28	1.0	128	41%	1	19	0.5
1898	Fudge, chocolate, with nuts [1 oz]	28	1.0	121	34%	1	21	0.4

Food #	fat gm	sat fat gm	choles mg	sodium mg	potass mg	vit A	vit E	vit C	thia-min	ribo-flavin	nia-cin	vit B-6	fol-ate	vit B-12	cal-cium	phos-phorus	magne-sium	iron	zinc
						% of Daily Value													
1863	4	3	3	59	72	1	1	0	0	3	0	1	0	0	4	4	2	1	1
1864	1	0	0	7	29	0	0	0	0	1	0	0	0	0	1	1	2	1	1
1865	2	2	2	69	61	0	0	0	0	3	0	0	0	0	4	3	1	0	1
1866	4	2	2	62	70	0	1	0	1	3	0	1	1	0	4	4	2	1	1
1867	9	8	1	30	179	0	2	0	2	3	1	2	2	5	9	4	3	2	7
1868	0	0	0	2	1	0	0	0	0	0	0	0	0	0	0	0	0	0	0
1869	0	0	0	2	0	0	0	0	0	0	0	0	0	0	1	0	0	0	0
1870	0	0	0	2	1	0	0	0	0	0	0	0	0	0	0	0	0	0	0
1871	9	5	0	3	103	0	1	0	1	2	1	0	0	0	1	4	8	5	3
1872	6	4	4	17	75	2	1	0	1	4	0	0	0	1	3	4	3	2	2
1873	6	4	4	27	79	1	1	0	1	4	0	0	0	1	4	4	3	1	2
1874	9	6	0	2	85	0	0	0	1	1	1	0	0	0	1	4	8	4	3
1875	9	5	6	23	109	2	1	0	1	5	0	1	1	2	5	6	4	2	3
1876	10	5	5	21	126	0	2	0	1	7	1	1	1	3	6	7	6	3	3
1877	8	5	5	41	97	0	1	0	1	5	1	1	1	2	5	5	3	1	2
1878	7	3	2	13	140	0	2	0	2	4	2	2	1	2	4	5	5	3	2
1879	10	5	5	19	115	1	3	0	3	5	1	1	1	2	5	7	6	3	4
1880	10	4	2	42	127	1	3	0	3	4	5	1	3	1	3	7	6	2	3
1881	10	5	5	22	101	0	5	0	1	6	2	1	1	3	6	7	4	1	2
1882	8	5	5	67	74	3	2	4	5	8	4	4	5	3	5	5	1	2	2
1883	9	7	0	1	79	0	0	0	0	1	0	0	0	0	0	2	4	3	1
1884	7	6	1	42	70	0	1	0	1	1	0	1	0	0	0	3	4	3	2
1885	4	3	0	35	35	0	0	0	0	0	0	1	0	0	0	1	1	1	1
1886	4	3	0	3	43	0	0	1	0	0	1	0	1	0	0	2	1	2	1
1887	5	0	0	7	160	0	1	1	5	2	1	2	1	0	2	3	4	3	3
1888	6	4	4	17	75	2	1	0	1	4	0	0	0	1	3	4	3	2	2
1889	1	1	1	8	378	0	0	0	0	1	6	0	0	0	2	1	8	3	1
1890	1	0	0	17	83	0	0	3	1	0	0	4	1	0	1	1	1	2	0
1891	0	0	0	30	15	0	0	0	0	0	0	0	0	0	0	0	0	0	0
1892	1	0	0	90	46	0	0	57	1	2	0	4	1	0	1	1	1	1	0
1893	3	0	1	19	101	1	1	0	2	1	0	1	0	0	3	2	3	3	2
1894	5	2	3	67	92	0	1	0	0	3	4	1	2	2	3	5	4	1	2
1895	2	1	4	18	29	1	0	0	0	1	0	0	0	0	1	2	2	1	1
1896	4	3	5	19	53	1	0	0	1	2	0	0	0	1	2	3	3	1	1
1897	6	3	5	19	64	1	1	0	1	3	0	1	1	1	3	4	4	1	2
1898	5	2	4	17	45	1	0	0	1	1	0	1	1	0	1	3	3	1	1

Desserts & Sweets

Food #	Food Description & Amount	wt gm	wt oz	calo-ries	%cal fat	prot gm	carbo gm	fiber gm
1899	Fudge, divinity [1 oz]	28	1.0	113	17%	1	24	0.2
1900	Fudge, peanut butter (Include chocolate fudge with peanut butter) [1 oz]	28	1.0	120	35%	2	19	0.4
1901	Fudge, peanut butter, with nuts [1 oz]	28	1.0	130	44%	2	17	0.5
1902	Fudge, vanilla or fruit-flavored [1 oz]	28	1.0	105	13%	0	23	0.0
1903	Fudge, vanilla or fruit-flavored, with nuts [1 oz]	28	1.0	118	29%	1	21	0.2
1904	Fun Fruits Creme Supremes (frosted fruit leather) [1 oz]	28	1.0	132	41%	1	19	0.4
1905	Gumdrops (Include Gummi Bears or other shapes, Jelly Beans, Hot Tamales, Jujubes, Jujy Fruits, Mike and Ike, Mint Leaves, Chuckles, Dots, Jellied Fruit Slices, Good and Fruity, Brach's Rocks, spice drops or sticks, Life Savers Gummi Savers) [1 oz]	28	1.0	109	0%	0	28	0.0
1906	Gumdrops, chocolate covered (Include Chocolate Jelly, Chocolate-Covered Jelly Rings) [1 oz]	28	1.0	120	18%	1	25	0.3
1907	Gumdrops, dietetic or low calorie [1 oz]	28	1.0	46	1%	0	25	5.1
1908	Halvah, chocolate covered [1 oz]	28	1.0	144	53%	3	16	1.2
1909	Halvah, plain [1 oz]	28	1.0	143	52%	3	16	1.3
1910	Hard candy (Include Breath Savers or Mints, Certs, Bottle Caps, Blow-Pop, Candy Cane or Buttons, Cinnamon or Conversation Hearts, Cotton Candy, Cough drops, Jawbreakers, Jolly Rancher, Life Savers, Lollipops, Pop Rocks, Smarties, Tic Tac, Sweet or Sour Tarts) [1 oz]	28	1.0	106	0%	0	28	0.0
1911	Honey-combed hard candy with peanut butter (Include Chick-o-Stick, Clark's Peanut Butter Log, Peanut Pillows, Zagnut) [1 oz]	28	1.0	131	40%	3	19	0.7
1912	Honey-combed hard candy with peanut butter, chocolate covered (Include Clark Bar, Fifth Avenue) [1 oz]	28	1.0	139	39%	3	19	0.6
1913	Kit Kat (Include Take Five) [1 oz]	28	1.0	146	45%	2	18	0.5
1914	Ladoo, round ball, Asian-Indian dessert [1 oz]	28	1.0	111	55%	2	12	1.4
1915	Licorice (Include Good and Plenty, Twizzlers, Twizzlers Nib) [1 oz]	28	1.0	104	1%	0	26	0.0
1916	M&M's Almond Chocolate Candies [1 oz]	28	1.0	149	48%	2	17	0.9
1917	M&M's Peanut Butter Chocolate Candies [1 oz]	28	1.0	145	45%	3	17	0.8
1918	M&M's Peanut Chocolate Candies (Peanut M&Ms) [1 oz]	28	1.0	146	46%	3	17	1.0
1919	M&M's Plain Chocolate Candies [1 oz]	28	1.0	139	39%	1	20	0.7
1920	Mars Bar (chocolate almond bar) [1 oz]	28	1.0	132	44%	2	18	0.6
1921	Marshmallow (marshmallow animals, Brach's Circus Peanuts) [1 oz]	28	1.0	90.2	1%	1	23	0.0
1922	Marshmallow, candy-coated (Include candy-coated marshmallow Easter egg) [1 oz]	28	1.0	97.2	0%	0	25	0.0
1923	Marshmallow, chocolate covered (Include Mallo Cup, Chocolate covered marshmallow Easter egg) [1 oz]	28	1.0	106	25%	1	21	0.5
1924	Marshmallow, coconut-coated [1 oz]	28	1.0	94.1	15%	1	20	0.2
1925	Mexican chocolate [1 oz]	28	1.0	121	33%	1	22	1.1
1926	Milky Way Bar [1 oz]	28	1.0	120	34%	1	20	0.4
1927	Milky Way II [1 oz]	28	1.0	94	38%	1	21	0.4
1928	Milky Way Midnight [1 oz]	28	1.0	127	33%	1	21	0.6
1929	Mints and buttercreams, chocolate covered (Include Junior Mints, Peppermint Pattie, Thin Mints, Cadbury's creme egg, chocolate-covered cherries, Chocolate Jots, Mint Jots, Irish Cream Mints, Brach's Mints) [1 oz]	28	1.0	104	23%	1	23	0.3
1930	Mints and Candy Corn (Include Mentos, Delson Merri-Mints) [1 oz]	28	1.0	101	0%	0	26	0.0
1931	Nougat, chocolate covered (Include Charleston Chew) [1 oz]	28	1.0	115	28%	1	21	0.3
1932	Nougat, plain (Include Italian nougat candy) [1 oz]	28	1.0	103	14%	1	23	0.1
1933	Nougat, with caramel, chocolate covered (Include Zero Bar) [1 oz]	28	1.0	120	34%	1	20	0.4
1934	Nut roll, fudge, nougat, or caramel and nuts (Include Big Hunk, PayDay) [1 oz]	28	1.0	128	45%	3	16	1.0
1935	Nuts, carob-coated (Include peanuts, cashews, walnuts, almonds) [1 oz]	28	1.0	158	66%	4	10	1.6
1936	Nuts, chocolate covered, not almonds or peanuts [1 oz]	28	1.0	162	72%	3	11	1.2
1937	P.B. Max Peanut Butter Snack [1 oz]	28	1.0	160	58%	4	14	1.2
1938	Peanut Bar, chocolate covered [1 oz]	28	1.0	147	57%	4	14	1.4
1939	Peanut Bar, Planters [1 oz]	28	1.0	142	52%	4	15	1.5
1940	Peanut brittle [1 oz]	28	1.0	128	38%	2	20	0.6

Food #	fat gm	sat fat gm	choles mg	sodium mg	potass mg	vit A	vit E	vit C	thia-min	ribo-flavin	nia-cin	vit B-6	fol-ate	vit B-12	cal-cium	phos-phorus	magne-sium	iron	zinc
1899	2	0	0	14	24	0	0	0	1	1	0	1	1	0	0	2	2	1	1
1900	5	1	3	47	58	1	2	0	1	1	5	2	1	0	1	3	3	1	2
1901	6	2	3	46	71	1	3	0	1	1	5	3	2	0	1	4	4	1	2
1902	2	1	5	19	14	1	0	0	0	1	0	0	0	0	1	1	0	0	0
1903	4	1	4	17	32	1	0	0	1	1	0	1	1	0	1	2	2	1	1
1904	6	3	4	22	82	0	1	1	1	3	1	2	1	2	4	3	1	1	1
1905	0	0	0	12	1	0	0	0	0	0	0	0	0	0	0	0	0	1	0
1906	2	1	2	15	32	0	0	0	0	1	0	0	0	1	2	2	1	1	1
1907	0	0	0	2	0	0	0	0	0	0	0	0	0	0	0	0	0	0	0
1908	8	3	2	10	63	0	3	0	4	2	2	1	2	1	3	8	8	4	6
1909	8	1	0	5	45	0	4	0	5	1	3	1	3	0	1	9	10	5	8
1910	0	0	0	11	1	0	0	0	0	0	0	0	0	0	0	0	0	0	0
1911	6	2	1	89	70	0	3	0	1	1	7	2	2	0	0	4	4	1	2
1912	6	2	2	47	84	0	2	0	3	2	5	1	3	1	2	4	5	2	2
1913	7	5	2	21	82	1	1	0	3	9	4	2	10	1	5	7	3	1	2
1914	7	1	0	3	58	0	4	0	2	1	0	2	7	0	1	3	2	3	2
1915	0	0	0	7	10	0	0	0	0	0	0	0	0	0	0	0	0	2	0
1916	8	3	2	30	107	1	6	0	1	6	2	1	1	1	4	7	8	3	3
1917	7	2	4	36	111	0	3	0	1	3	5	3	4	2	3	8	6	2	3
1918	7	3	3	14	98	1	2	0	3	4	3	1	3	1	3	5	4	2	3
1919	6	4	4	17	75	2	1	0	1	4	0	0	0	1	3	4	3	2	2
1920	7	2	3	48	92	1	1	0	1	5	1	1	1	1	5	6	5	2	2
1921	0	0	0	13	1	0	0	0	0	0	0	0	0	0	0	0	0	0	0
1922	0	0	0	9	1	0	0	0	0	0	0	0	0	0	0	0	0	0	0
1923	3	2	0	11	26	0	0	0	0	1	0	0	0	0	1	3	2	1	
1924	2	1	0	24	17	0	0	0	0	0	0	1	0	0	0	1	1	1	1
1925	4	2	0	1	113	0	0	0	1	2	3	0	0	0	1	4	7	3	2
1926	5	2	4	68	68	2	1	0	1	4	0	1	1	2	4	5	2	1	1
1927	4	3	6	75	74	1	1	0	1	3	0	0	1	1	3	3	2	1	1
1928	5	2	4	65	81	1	0	0	0	2	0	1	1	0	2	4	4	1	2
1929	3	2	0	7	48	0	0	0	0	1	1	0	0	0	0	3	4	2	1
1930	0	0	0	11	5	0	0	0	0	0	0	0	0	0	0	0	0	0	0
1931	4	2	2	49	37	1	0	0	1	2	1	1	0	1	2	2	1	1	1
1932	2	1	0	60	9	0	0	0	1	2	1	1	0	0	0	0	0	1	0
1933	5	2	4	68	68	2	1	0	1	4	0	1	1	2	4	5	2	1	1
1934	6	1	2	66	89	1	3	0	2	2	8	2	3	0	2	6	5	1	5
1935	12	5	0	17	193	0	8	0	5	5	6	3	6	2	7	8	9	4	6
1936	13	4	3	12	133	1	5	0	7	4	1	3	2	1	5	10	11	4	5
1937	10	2	1	96	109	0	5	0	3	2	7	2	2	0	2	6	6	3	3
1938	9	3	2	38	113	0	3	0	2	3	8	2	4	1	3	8	7	2	6
1939	8	1	0	75	113	0	4	0	3	1	12	2	5	0	1	9	8	2	7
1940	5	1	4	128	59	1	2	0	4	1	5	1	5	0	1	3	4	2	2

Desserts & Sweets

Food #	Food Description & Amount	wt gm	wt oz	calories	%cal fat	prot gm	carbo gm	fiber gm
1941	Peanut Butter Boppers [1-oz]	28	1.0	151	58%	3	14	0.8
1942	Peanut butter chips/morsels [1 oz]	28	1.0	141	54%	5	13	0.3
1943	Peanut butter, chocolate covered (Include Peanut Butter Meltaway Crispy Bar, Chocolate-covered peanut butter Easter egg, peanut butter candy or treats) [1 oz]	28	1.0	143	51%	3	16	0.9
1944	Peanut Munch Bar [1 oz]	28	1.0	148	58%	4	13	1.6
1945	**Peanuts, chocolate covered** (Include Goobers, Peanut Clusters) [1 oz]	28	1.0	147	58%	4	14	1.2
1946	Peanuts, sugar-coated (Include Boston Baked Beans, Squirrel Nuts) [1 oz]	28	1.0	148	58%	4	13	1.6
1947	Peanuts, yogurt covered [1 oz]	28	1.0	154	61%	4	12	1.1
1948	Pecans, sugared (sugar and egg white coating) [1 oz]	28	1.0	154	76%	2	10	1.5
1949	Pineapple candy, Puerto Rican style (pineapple, sugar, lemon peel) [1 oz]	28	1.0	93.3	0%	0	24	0.4
1950	Pralines [1 oz]	28	1.0	114	25%	1	22	0.3
1951	Raisins, carob covered [1 oz]	28	1.0	114	30%	1	20	1.1
1952	**Raisins, chocolate covered** (Include Raisinets, Raisin Clusters) [1 oz]	28	1.0	111	34%	1	19	1.2
1953	Raisins, yogurt covered [1 oz]	28	1.0	111	27%	1	21	0.7
1954	Reese's Peanut Butter Cup [1 oz]	28	1.0	153	52%	3	15	0.9
1955	Reese's Pieces [1 oz]	28	1.0	139	39%	4	17	0.8
1956	Rolo [1 oz]	28	1.0	117	44%	1	15	0.2
1957	Sesame Crunch (Sahadi) [1 oz]	28	1.0	147	58%	3	14	2.2
1958	Sixlets [1 oz]	28	1.0	139	39%	1	20	0.7
1959	Skittles [1 oz]	28	1.0	115	10%	0	26	0.0
1960	**Snickers** Bar [1 oz]	28	1.0	136	46%	2	17	0.7
1961	Snickers Peanut Butter Bar [1 oz]	28	1.0	158	57%	4	13	1.1
1962	Sugar-free candy, chocolate covered (Include Dietetic Chocolate TV Mix or Chocolate Wafers or Covered Raisins or Fruit and Nut Bar or Crunch Bar or Peanut Butter Cups, or Milk Almond Bar) [1 oz]	28	1.0	156	65%	4	12	2.0
1963	Sugar-free Caramels, all flavors (Include Estee Caramels) [1 oz]	28	1.0	120	30%	1	20	0.2
1964	Sugar-free hard candy (Include diet licorice, Sweet 'n Low sugar-free hard candy) [1 oz]	28	1.0	106	0%	0	26	0.0
1965	Sugar-free mints [1 oz]	28	1.0	106	0%	0	26	0.0
1966	Taffy (Include Starburst, Bit-O-Honey, Fruit Chews, Kits, Salt-water taffy, Bonkers!, Laffy Taffy, Air Heads, Tangy Taffy, Now and Later, Peanut Kisses, Mighty Bite, Mary Jane) [1 oz]	28	1.0	112	19%	0	24	0.0
1967	Toblerone, milk chocolate with honey and almond nougat [1 oz]	28	1.0	139	49%	2	18	0.8
1968	Toffee, chocolate covered (Include Heath Bar, Skor, Heath Sensations, Sweet Escapes Chocolate Toffee Crisp Bar) [1 oz]	28	1.0	120	31%	1	21	0.5
1969	Toffee, chocolate-coated, with nuts (Include Almond Roca) [3 pieces]	28	1.0	125	38%	2	19	0.7
1970	Toffee, plain or mint [1 oz]	28	1.0	110	19%	1	22	0.3
1971	**Truffles** [1 oz]	28	1.0	135	64%	2	12	0.7
1972	Twix Chocolate Fudge Cookie Bars (Include Twix Cookies-n-Creme Bars) [1 oz]	28	1.0	156	54%	2	16	0.9
1973	Twix Cookie Bars [1 oz]	28	1.0	141	44%	1	19	0.3
1974	Twix Peanut Butter Cookie Bars [1 oz]	28	1.0	150	55%	3	15	1.0
1975	Wax candy, liquid filled (Include Pop Bottles, Super Sips wax tubes) [1 oz liquid]	28	1.0	35.7	0%	0	9	0.0
1976	Whatchamacallit (Include Sweet Escapes Caramel Peanut Butter Crispy Bar) [1 oz]	28	1.0	126	39%	3	17	0.6
Your Additions								

Food #	fat gm	sat fat gm	choles mg	sodium mg	potass mg	vit A	vit E	vit C	thia-min	ribo-flavin	nia-cin	vit B-6	fol-ate	vit B-12	cal-cium	phos-phorus	magne-sium	iron	zinc
1941	10	3	2	133	102	1	7	2	3	4	10	4	4	1	2	6	5	2	3
1942	8	4	0	71	143	0	3	0	1	3	12	3	7	0	3	9	8	3	4
1943	8	3	2	55	105	1	4	0	1	2	7	2	2	1	2	6	5	2	3
1944	10	1	0	44	115	0	4	0	2	2	11	2	6	0	2	9	8	2	8
1945	9	4	3	12	142	0	2	0	2	3	6	3	1	2	3	6	6	2	4
1946	10	1	0	44	115	0	4	0	2	2	11	2	6	0	2	9	8	2	8
1947	10	5	0	16	135	0	5	0	6	4	8	3	8	2	4	8	6	3	4
1948	13	1	0	5	79	0	2	1	9	2	1	2	2	0	1	6	6	2	7
1949	0	0	0	1	49	0	0	5	2	1	1	2	0	0	1	0	2	1	0
1950	3	0	1	19	101	1	1	0	2	1	0	1	0	0	3	2	3	3	2
1951	4	3	0	15	199	0	1	1	2	2	1	3	1	2	4	3	2	3	3
1952	4	2	1	10	146	0	1	0	2	3	1	2	0	1	2	4	3	3	1
1953	3	3	0	13	158	0	1	1	2	3	1	2	1	1	3	4	2	2	1
1954	9	3	1	90	100	1	4	0	5	3	7	2	6	1	2	6	6	2	3
1955	6	5	1	42	65	0	2	0	2	2	4	1	2	1	2	4	3	1	1
1956	6	3	5	50	70	1	1	0	1	4	0	0	0	1	4	4	3	1	2
1957	9	1	0	6	124	0	1	0	10	3	5	8	5	0	20	13	18	7	7
1958	6	4	4	17	75	2	1	0	1	4	0	0	0	1	3	4	3	2	2
1959	1	0	0	5	1	0	0	32	0	0	0	0	0	0	0	0	0	0	0
1960	7	3	4	75	96	1	1	0	4	3	5	2	5	1	3	5	5	1	3
1961	10	2	1	76	114	0	0	0	2	2	8	2	5	1	3	6	6	2	3
1962	11	6	1	31	172	0	4	1	4	8	3	3	4	3	9	9	9	2	5
1963	4	1	0	48	91	0	2	0	1	5	0	1	0	2	3	4	2	1	1
1964	0	0	0	0	0	0	0	0	0	0	0	0	0	0	0	0	0	0	0
1965	0	0	0	0	0	0	0	0	0	0	0	0	0	0	0	0	0	0	0
1966	2	1	0	30	9	0	1	19	0	1	0	0	0	0	0	1	0	0	0
1967	8	5	5	29	94	1	1	0	1	4	1	1	1	2	5	5	4	2	2
1968	4	3	3	58	74	1	1	0	1	4	0	1	0	0	4	4	2	1	1
1969	5	3	3	51	89	1	1	0	2	4	2	1	2	1	4	5	3	1	2
1970	2	2	2	71	62	0	0	0	0	3	0	1	0	0	4	3	1	0	1
1971	10	6	14	20	85	4	1	0	1	4	0	1	0	2	4	5	3	2	2
1972	9	1	2	75	88	0	2	0	3	3	2	1	1	2	4	4	3	2	2
1973	7	3	1	55	57	1	1	0	3	4	2	0	0	1	3	3	2	1	1
1974	9	3	1	77	101	1	1	0	2	2	6	2	2	1	2	5	5	1	3
1975	0	0	0	1	0	0	0	0	0	0	0	0	0	0	0	0	0	0	0
1976	5	3	3	58	88	1	1	0	9	10	10	8	1	2	3	5	4	1	2

Meringue Pie with Fruit is a heavenly dessert that not only counts as a fruit portion in the Food Guide Pyramid but, compared to most desserts, is low in fat and added sugar. It's easy to make, and absolutely delicious when fresh fruit is in peak season (though frozen fruit can substitute). If the fruit needs sweetening, add sugar or a liqueur that complements the fruit. Go for eye appeal as well, e.g., sliced yellow peaches that have a touch of red at their edge combined with fresh raspberries, strawberries combined with blueberries.

Meringue Pie with Fruit

5 egg whites	1½ cups sugar
½ tsp cream of tartar	1 cup (½ pint) whipping cream
¼ tsp salt	3-4 cups fresh strawberries (or other fruit)
1 tsp vanilla	Grand Marnier liqueur (or other liqueur)

Preheat the oven to 400° Beat egg whites until frothy. Add cream of tartar, salt, and vanilla. While continuing to beat, add the sugar gradually. Beat for 10 minutes more, so the sugar dissolves completely and the meringue won't "weep." Spread the meringue into a lightly buttered or oiled 10″ glass pie pan. Put the meringue in the preheated oven; immediately turn off the oven; and leave overnight (i.e., until the oven loses its heat)—no peeking!

Whip the cream until it forms soft peaks (sugar and vanilla can be added, but the meringue can provide enough sweetness). Cover the meringue with the whipped cream and refrigerate for at least 3 hours (so the cream can soften the top of the meringue).

Cut the strawberries in half or quarters and mix in some Grand Marnier liqueur. Serve each piece of pie with a generous portion of strawberries.

* * * * * * * * * * *

Another fruit dessert, and a way to use apples that have lost their crispness.:

Apple Crisp

4 cups sliced apples	½ cup flour	¾ tsp cinnamon
2/3 cup brown sugar	½ cup oats	¾ tsp nutmeg
1/3 cup butter (cut into chunks)		

The amounts don't have to be precise, and you don't have to peel the apples. (You can also use or combine other fruits, e.g., apricots, blueberries, strawberries.) If using a food processor, use the slicer blade to slice the quartered and cored apples, and put the apples into a glass or non-stick pan about 8″ square. Change the blade to a chopper, and put in the remaining ingredients. Blend until crumbly and put on top of apples. Bake at 375° for 30-35 minutes. Serve in scoops with a little milk, whipped cream, or vanilla ice cream on top.

Fruits and Vegetables

Fruits *2000*

Vegetables *2350*

Your Additions

End-of-Section Recipes
Carrot-Custard Soufflé
Blueberry Muffins

Fruits & Vegetables

Food #	Food Description & Amount	wt gm	wt oz	calories	%cal fat	prot gm	carbo gm	fiber gm
	Fruits							
2000	Acerola, raw [½ cup]	49	1.7	16	8%	0	4	0.5
2001	Ambrosia (oranges, bananas, coconut, sugar) [1 cup]	193	6.8	250	38%	3	41	6.4
2002	**Apple** [1 apple (2¾"dia, about 3 per lb)]	**138**	**4.9**	**81**	**5%**	**0**	**21**	**3.7**
2003	Apple, baked, unsweetened [1 apple with liquid]	161	5.7	102	5%	0	26	4.7
2004	Apple, baked, with sugar (Include scalloped apples) [1 apple with liquid]	171	6.0	173	3%	0	45	4.4
2005	Apple, cooked or canned, with syrup [1 cup, slices]	204	7.2	137	6%	0	34	4.1
2006	Apple, candied or caramel-covered (Include caramel apples) [1 apple]	184	6.5	243	14%	2	54	4.3
2007	Apple-cabbage-mayonnaise salad [1 cup]	161	5.7	217	72%	1	17	3.6
2008	Apple chips [15 chips]	33	1.2	152	42%	0	24	3.2
2009	Apple, dried, cooked, unsweetened [1 cup]	255	9.0	145	1%	1	39	5.1
2010	Apple, dried, cooked, with sugar [1 cup]	280	9.9	244	1%	1	65	5.1
2011	Apple, dried, uncooked, plain or flavored [5 rings]	32	1.1	78	1%	0	21	2.8
2012	Apple, dried, uncooked, low sodium [5 rings]	32	1.1	78	1%	0	21	2.8
2013	Apple, fried (apples, margarine, sugar) [1 cup]	179	6.3	268	37%	0	46	4.5
2014	Apple, pickled (apples, sugar, vinegar, with/without spices) [1 apple]	29	1.0	38	2%	0	10	0.5
2015	Apple rings, fried [4 rings]	76	2.7	97	40%	0	16	2.0
2016	Apple salad with dressing (Include Waldorf salad) [1 cup]	137	4.8	192	60%	2	21	3.2
2017	Applesauce, stewed apples, unsweetened or sweetened with low-cal sweetener [1 cup]	244	8.6	105	1%	0	28	2.9
2018	Applesauce, stewed apples, with sugar (Include apple pie filling) [1 cup]	255	9.0	194	2%	0	51	3.1
2019	Applesauce with other fruits [1 cup]	256	9.0	156	3%	1	40	2.8
2020	**Apricot**, raw [2 apricots]	**70**	**2.5**	**34**	**7%**	**1**	**8**	**1.7**
2021	Apricot, cooked or canned in heavy syrup, drained solids [2 whole apricots]	76	2.7	63	1%	0	16	1.7
2022	Apricot, cooked or canned (including home canned), in heavy syrup [2 whole apricots with liquid]	106	3.7	88	1%	1	23	1.7
2023	Apricot, cooked or canned, in light syrup [2 whole apricots with liquid]	106	3.7	67	1%	1	17	1.7
2024	Apricot, cooked or canned, juice pack [2 whole apricots with liquid]	90	3.2	43	1%	1	11	1.4
2025	Apricot, cooked or canned, unsweetened, water pack [2 whole apricots with liquid]	90	3.2	24	5%	1	6	1.4
2026	Apricot, dried, uncooked [8 halves]	28	1.0	67	2%	1	17	2.5
2027	Apricot, dried, cooked, unsweetened [1 cup]	250	8.8	213	2%	3	55	8.0
2028	Apricot, dried, cooked, with sugar [1 cup]	270	9.5	304	1%	3	78	7.8
2029	Avocado, raw, California (rough black skin) [1 avocado]	173	6.1	306	86%	4	12	8.5
2030	Avocado, raw, Florida (smooth green skin) [1 avocado]	304	10.7	340	71%	5	27	16.8
2031	**Banana**, yellow, common, raw [1 fruit (7½"long)]	**114**	**4.0**	**105**	**5%**	**1**	**27**	**2.7**
2032	Banana, yellow, boiled [1 fruit]	91	3.2	84	5%	1	21	2.2
2033	Banana, yellow, fried in margarine [1 fruit]	91	3.2	181	51%	1	24	2.4
2034	Banana, yellow, fried with cheese, Puerto Rican style (Include guineos nifios con queso) [1 banana (4"x1½"x1½")]	40	1.4	85	53%	1	10	1.0
2035	Banana, baked (banana, sugar, lemon juice) [1 banana (7"long)]	128	4.5	167	4%	1	43	3.4
2036	Banana, batter-dipped, fried (banana, pancake mix, soybean oil) [1 fruit]	136	4.8	341	59%	3	35	2.7
2037	Banana chips [1 cup]	92	3.2	338	16%	3	76	6.1
2038	Banana, chocolate-covered with peanuts [1 banana]	145	5.1	331	50%	7	43	5.1
2039	Banana flakes, dehydrated [1 cup]	100	3.5	346	5%	4	88	7.5
2040	Banana whip (bananas, egg white, sugar, lemon juice, salt) [1 cup]	130	4.6	179	2%	6	40	2.1
2041	Banana, apple, raw (Include apple banana) [1 fruit]	73	2.6	67	5%	1	17	1.8
2042	Banana, Chinese, raw (Include Cavendish, dwarf or finger banana) [1 fruit (5"long)]	63	2.2	58	5%	1	15	1.5
2043	Banana, green, cooked in salt water [1 fruit]	54	1.9	50	5%	1	13	1.3
2044	Banana, green, fried in corn oil [4 slices]	92	3.2	159	49%	1	22	2.3
2045	Banana, red, fried [1 fruit (7"long)]	94	3.3	194	53%	1	24	2.1
2046	Banana, red, ripe (Include guineo morado) [1 fruit (7"long)]	104	3.7	94	2%	1	24	2.1

Food #	fat gm	sat fat gm	choles mg	sodium mg	potass mg	vit A	vit E	vit C	thia-min	ribo-flavin	nia-cin	vit B-6	fol-ate	vit B-12	cal-cium	phos-phorus	magne-sium	iron	zinc
2000	0	0	0	3	72	4	0	1370	1	2	1	0	2	0	1	1	2	1	0
2001	11	9	0	7	580	2	2	74	8	7	4	29	11	0	4	6	11	6	3
2002	0	0	0	0	159	1	1	13	2	1	1	3	1	0	1	1	2	1	0
2003	1	0	0	0	179	1	2	13	2	1	1	4	1	0	1	1	2	2	0
2004	1	0	0	0	170	1	2	12	1	2	1	4	1	0	1	1	2	2	0
2005	1	0	0	6	143	1	0	1	1	1	1	4	0	0	1	1	2	3	1
2006	4	3	3	102	253	1	2	14	2	6	1	4	2	0	7	6	4	2	2
2007	17	3	13	131	239	3	9	37	3	2	1	11	7	1	4	2	3	3	1
2008	7	1	0	32	150	0	8	1	1	2	1	3	0	0	0	1	1	3	1
2009	0	0	0	51	268	1	0	4	1	3	2	6	0	0	1	2	3	5	1
2010	0	0	0	51	268	1	0	4	1	3	2	6	0	0	1	2	3	5	1
2011	0	0	0	28	144	0	1	2	0	3	1	2	0	0	0	1	1	2	0
2012	0	0	0	0	144	0	0	2	0	3	1	2	0	0	0	1	1	2	0
2013	11	2	0	121	178	11	7	11	2	2	1	4	1	0	2	1	2	2	0
2014	0	0	0	0	28	0	0	2	0	0	0	0	0	0	0	0	1	0	0
2015	4	1	0	47	80	4	3	5	1	1	0	2	0	0	1	1	1	1	0
2016	13	2	5	153	208	2	5	11	4	2	1	6	4	1	3	5	6	3	2
2017	0	0	0	5	183	1	0	5	2	4	2	3	0	0	1	2	2	2	0
2018	0	0	0	8	156	0	0	7	2	4	2	3	0	0	1	2	2	5	1
2019	1	0	0	15	138	0	2	24	2	5	2	4	1	0	2	2	2	5	1
2020	0	0	0	1	207	18	2	12	1	2	2	2	2	0	1	1	1	2	1
2021	0	0	0	3	109	14	3	4	1	1	1	2	0	0	1	1	1	1	1
2022	0	0	0	4	148	13	3	5	1	1	2	3	0	0	1	1	2	2	1
2023	0	0	0	4	146	14	3	5	1	1	2	3	0	0	1	1	2	2	1
2024	0	0	0	4	149	15	3	7	1	1	2	2	0	0	1	2	2	2	1
2025	0	0	0	3	173	12	3	5	1	1	2	2	0	0	1	1	2	2	1
2026	0	0	0	3	386	20	1	1	0	2	4	2	1	0	1	3	3	7	1
2027	0	0	0	8	1223	59	4	7	1	4	12	14	0	0	4	10	11	23	4
2028	0	0	0	8	1200	58	4	7	1	5	12	14	0	0	4	10	10	23	4
2029	30	4	0	21	1097	5	11	23	12	12	17	24	29	0	2	7	18	11	5
2030	27	5	0	15	1484	9	9	40	22	22	29	43	40	0	3	12	29	9	9
2031	1	0	0	1	451	1	1	17	3	7	3	33	5	0	1	2	8	2	1
2032	0	0	0	1	324	1	1	10	2	5	2	24	2	0	1	2	7	2	1
2033	10	2	0	116	367	10	6	11	3	6	2	26	2	0	1	2	7	2	1
2034	5	1	3	38	156	1	3	4	1	3	1	11	1	1	3	3	3	1	1
2035	1	0	0	2	512	1	1	22	3	8	3	39	4	0	1	3	10	2	2
2036	22	3	3	160	347	1	15	10	10	13	8	24	6	1	2	13	8	8	2
2037	6	4	0	3	1212	3	0	9	10	12	11	18	3	0	2	6	22	5	3
2038	18	7	0	6	592	1	6	15	6	11	16	32	10	0	3	15	23	8	11
2039	2	1	0	3	1491	3	0	12	12	14	14	22	4	0	2	7	27	6	4
2040	0	0	0	83	387	1	1	16	2	18	2	24	3	1	1	2	8	2	1
2041	0	0	0	1	289	1	1	11	2	4	2	21	3	0	0	1	5	1	1
2042	0	0	0	1	249	1	1	10	2	4	2	18	3	0	0	1	5	1	1
2043	0	0	0	1	192	0	0	6	1	3	1	14	1	0	0	1	4	1	1
2044	9	1	0	1	335	1	7	10	2	5	2	24	2	0	1	2	7	2	1
2045	11	2	0	133	350	14	7	12	3	2	3	27	2	0	1	2	8	5	1
2046	0	0	0	1	385	4	1	17	3	2	3	30	5	0	1	2	8	5	1

Fruits & Vegetables

Food #	Food Description & Amount	wt gm	wt oz	calo-ries	%cal fat	prot gm	carbo gm	fiber gm
2047	Banana, white, ripe (Include guineo blanco maduro) [1 fruit]	119	4.2	109	5%	1	28	2.9
2048	Blackberries, raw (Include dewberries, youngberries, marionberries) [1 cup]	144	5.1	75	7%	1	18	7.6
2049	Blackberries, cooked or canned, in heavy syrup (Include dewberries, youngberries, marionberries) [1 cup]	256	9.0	236	1%	3	59	8.7
2050	Blackberries, frozen [1 cup]	143	5.0	92	6%	2	22	7.2
2051	Blueberries, raw [1 cup]	145	5.1	81	6%	1	20	3.9
2052	Blueberries, cooked or canned, in heavy syrup (Include home canned) [1 cup]	256	9.0	225	3%	2	56	3.8
2053	Blueberries, cooked or canned, unsweetened, water pack [1 cup]	244	8.6	92	6%	1	23	4.4
2054	Blueberries, frozen [1 cup]	230	8.1	117	11%	1	28	6.2
2055	Blueberries, frozen, sweetened [1 cup]	230	8.1	186	1%	1	50	4.8
2056	Boysenberries, raw [1 cup]	144	5.1	75	7%	1	18	7.6
2057	Boysenberries, cooked or canned in heavy syrup [1 cup]	256	9.0	225	1%	3	57	6.7
2058	Boysenberries, frozen [1 cup]	143	5.0	72	5%	2	17	5.6
2059	Breadfruit, cooked, salt added (Include pana) [1 cup]	252	8.9	289	2%	3	76	13.8
2060	Breadfruit, fried in corn oil (Include tostones) [1 cup]	170	6.0	379	50%	2	52	9.4
2061	Calamondin, raw [4 fruit (1"dia)]	76	2.7	33	4%	0	9	1.7
2062	Cantaloupe, raw (Include muskmelon) [¼ melon]	169	6.0	59	7%	1	14	1.4
2063	Cantaloupe, frozen (balls) [1 cup]	173	6.1	61	7%	2	14	1.4
2064	Carambola, cooked with sugar (Include starfruit) [1 cup]	205	7.2	109	6%	1	27	5.9
2065	Cassaba melon, raw (Include crenshaw melon) [1 cup]	170	6.0	44	3%	2	11	1.4
2066	Cherries, sweet, raw (Queen Anne, Bing) [10 cherries]	68	2.4	49	12%	1	11	1.6
2067	Cherries, frozen [1 cup]	155	5.5	71	9%	1	17	2.5
2068	Cherries, maraschino [10 cherries]	43	1.5	50	2%	0	13	0.4
2069	Cherries, sour, red, cooked, unsweetened [1 cup, pitted]	244	8.6	88	3%	2	22	2.7
2070	Cherries, sour, red, raw [1 cup, pitted]	155	5.5	78	5%	2	19	2.5
2071	Cherries, sweet, cooked or canned, drained solids [1 cup, pitted]	179	6.3	149	2%	1	38	2.1
2072	Cherries, sweet, cooked or canned (including home canned), in heavy syrup [1 cup, pitted]	253	8.9	210	2%	2	54	3.8
2073	Cherries, sweet, cooked or canned, in light syrup [1 cup, pitted]	252	8.9	169	2%	2	44	3.8
2074	Cherries, sweet, cooked or canned, juice pack [1 cup, pitted]	250	8.8	135	0%	2	35	3.8
2075	Cherries, sweet, cooked, unsweetened, water pack [1 cup, pitted]	248	8.7	114	3%	2	29	3.7
2076	Carambola (starfruit), raw [1 medium (3½" long)]	91	3.2	30	10%	0	7	2.5
2077	Cranberries, cooked or canned (Include cranberry sauce) [1 cup]	277	9.8	418	1%	1	108	2.8
2078	Cranberries, dried [1 cup]	110	3.9	363	3%	0	95	9.7
2079	Cranberries, raw [1 cup, chopped]	110	3.9	54	4%	0	14	4.6
2080	Cranberry salad (cranberry, pineapple, celery, walnuts, sugar, gelatin) [1 cup]	253	8.9	348	30%	5	61	4.5
2081	Cranberry-orange relish (cranberry, orange, sugar), uncooked [1 cup]	275	9.7	470	1%	1	124	7.5
2082	Currants, dried [1 cup]	144	5.1	408	1%	6	107	9.8
2083	Currants, raw [1 cup]	112	4.0	63	3%	2	15	4.8
2084	Dates [10 dates]	83	2.9	228	1%	2	61	6.2
2085	Dewberries, raw [1 cup]	144	5.1	75	7%	1	18	7.6
2086	Elderberries, cooked or canned in syrup [1 cup]	256	9.0	304	3%	1	78	13.1
2087	Elderberries, raw [1 cup]	145	5.1	106	6%	1	27	10.2
2088	Figs, raw [1 medium (2¼"dia)]	50	1.8	37	4%	0	10	1.7
2089	Figs, cooked or canned (including home canned), in heavy syrup [1 fig with liquid]	28	1.0	25	1%	0	6	0.6
2090	Figs, cooked or canned, in light syrup [1 cup]	252	8.9	174	1%	1	45	4.5
2091	Figs, cooked or canned, unsweetened, water pack [4 figs with liquid]	108	3.8	57	2%	0	15	2.4
2092	Figs, dried, cooked, unsweetened [1 cup]	259	9.1	280	4%	3	71	12.4
2093	Figs, dried, cooked, with sugar [1 cup]	270	9.5	358	3%	3	92	11.8

Food #	fat gm	sat fat gm	choles mg	sodium mg	potass mg	% of Daily Value													
						vit A	vit E	vit C	thia-min	ribo-flavin	nia-cin	vit B-6	fol-ate	vit B-12	cal-cium	phos-phorus	magne-sium	iron	zinc
2047	1	0	0	1	471	1	1	18	4	7	3	34	6	0	1	2	9	2	1
2048	1	0	0	0	282	2	3	50	3	3	3	4	12	0	5	3	7	5	3
2049	0	0	0	8	253	6	6	12	5	6	4	5	17	0	5	4	11	9	3
2050	1	0	0	1	200	2	3	7	3	4	9	4	12	0	4	4	8	6	2
2051	1	0	0	9	129	1	5	31	5	4	3	3	2	0	1	1	2	1	1
2052	1	0	0	8	102	2	9	5	6	8	1	5	1	0	1	3	3	5	1
2053	1	0	0	12	131	1	5	18	4	4	3	3	1	0	1	2	2	2	1
2054	1	0	0	2	124	2	8	10	5	5	6	7	4	0	2	3	3	2	1
2055	0	0	0	2	138	1	5	4	3	7	3	7	4	0	1	2	1	5	1
2056	1	0	0	0	282	2	3	50	3	3	3	4	12	0	5	3	7	5	3
2057	0	0	0	8	230	1	6	26	4	4	3	5	22	0	5	3	7	6	3
2058	0	0	0	1	199	1	2	7	5	3	5	4	23	0	4	4	6	7	2
2059	1	0	0	5	1238	1	10	102	16	4	11	12	6	0	5	8	17	8	2
2060	21	3	0	4	847	1	22	65	11	3	8	9	3	0	3	6	12	6	2
2061	0	0	0	1	119	7	1	39	5	1	1	3	4	0	1	1	2	0	1
2062	0	0	0	15	522	54	1	119	4	2	5	10	7	0	2	3	5	2	2
2063	0	0	0	16	535	53	1	116	4	2	5	10	7	0	2	3	5	2	2
2064	1	0	0	4	320	9	3	62	3	3	4	10	5	0	1	4	5	3	2
2065	0	0	0	20	357	1	1	45	7	2	3	10	7	0	1	1	3	4	2
2066	1	0	0	0	152	1	0	8	2	2	1	1	1	0	1	1	2	1	0
2067	1	0	0	2	192	13	1	4	5	3	1	5	2	0	2	2	3	5	1
2068	0	0	0	21	54	0	0	0	0	0	0	0	0	0	1	1	0	1	0
2069	0	0	0	17	239	18	1	9	3	6	2	5	5	0	3	2	4	19	1
2070	0	0	0	5	268	20	1	26	3	4	3	3	3	0	2	2	3	3	1
2071	0	0	0	5	265	4	0	11	3	5	4	3	2	0	2	4	4	3	1
2072	0	0	0	8	367	4	1	15	4	6	5	4	3	0	2	5	6	5	2
2073	0	0	0	8	373	4	1	16	4	6	5	4	3	0	2	5	6	5	2
2074	0	0	0	8	328	3	1	10	3	4	5	4	3	0	4	6	8	8	2
2075	0	0	0	2	325	4	1	9	4	6	5	4	3	0	3	4	6	5	1
2076	0	0	0	2	148	4	1	32	2	1	2	5	3	0	0	1	2	1	1
2077	0	0	0	80	72	1	1	9	3	3	1	2	1	0	1	2	2	3	1
2078	1	0	0	3	96	0	2	1	1	6	0	3	0	0	2	1	2	3	1
2079	0	0	0	1	78	1	0	25	2	1	1	4	0	0	1	1	1	1	1
2080	12	1	0	30	300	1	2	28	12	5	3	12	6	0	5	8	13	6	5
2081	0	0	0	3	201	2	1	97	6	4	2	6	5	0	5	3	4	4	2
2082	0	0	0	12	1284	1	0	11	15	12	12	21	4	0	12	18	15	26	6
2083	0	0	0	1	308	1	0	77	3	3	1	4	2	0	4	5	4	6	2
2084	0	0	0	2	541	0	0	0	5	5	9	8	3	0	3	3	7	5	2
2085	1	0	0	0	282	2	3	50	3	3	3	4	12	0	5	3	7	5	3
2086	1	0	0	12	473	8	6	79	7	6	4	19	1	0	7	7	2	17	2
2087	1	0	0	9	406	9	5	87	7	5	4	17	2	0	6	6	2	13	1
2088	0	0	0	1	116	1	1	2	2	1	1	3	1	0	2	1	2	1	1
2089	0	0	0	0	28	0	1	0	0	1	1	1	0	0	1	0	1	0	0
2090	0	0	0	3	257	1	7	4	4	6	6	9	1	0	7	3	6	4	2
2091	0	0	0	1	111	0	3	2	2	2	2	4	1	0	3	1	3	2	1
2092	1	0	0	13	780	4	0	19	2	17	8	17	1	0	16	8	16	14	4
2093	1	0	0	13	742	4	0	18	2	16	8	16	1	0	15	7	15	13	3

Fruits & Vegetables

Food #	Food Description & Amount	wt gm	wt oz	calo-ries	%cal fat	prot gm	carbo gm	fiber gm
2094	Fruit cocktail or mix, raw, made with fresh fruit (no citrus fruits) [1 cup]	175	6.2	101	5%	1	26	3.5
2095	Fruit cocktail or mix, raw, made with fresh fruit (including citrus fruits) [1 cup]	175	6.2	99	5%	1	25	3.3
2096	Fruit cocktail or mix, frozen [1 cup]	215	7.6	112	7%	2	27	5.6
2097	Fruit cocktail, canned, in heavy syrup [1 cup]	248	8.7	181	1%	1	47	2.5
2098	Fruit cocktail, canned in heavy syrup, drained solids [1 cup]	214	7.5	156	1%	1	40	3.9
2099	Fruit cocktail, canned, in light syrup [1 cup]	242	8.5	138	1%	1	36	2.4
2100	**Fruit cocktail, canned, juice pack [1 cup]**	237	8.4	109	0%	1	28	2.4
2101	Fruit cocktail, canned, unsweetened, water pack [1 cup]	245	8.6	78	1%	1	21	2.5
2102	Fruit mixture, dried (including three or more of: apples, apricots, dates, papaya, peaches, pears, pineapples, prunes, raisins) [1 cup]	136	4.8	330	2%	3	87	10.6
2103	Fruit salad, mixed, fresh, with dressing [1 cup]	188	6.6	115	14%	1	26	3.7
2104	Fruit salad (no citrus fruit) with cream substitute [1 cup]	175	6.2	148	20%	1	32	3.0
2105	Fruit salad (no citrus fruit) with cream [1 cup]	182	6.4	165	36%	1	28	3.3
2106	Fruit salad (no citrus fruit) with marshmallows [1 cup]	171	6.0	187	8%	1	46	2.7
2107	Fruit salad (no citrus fruit) with pudding [1 cup]	182	6.4	173	15%	3	35	0.8
2108	Fruit salad (no citrus fruit) with salad dressing or mayonnaise [1 cup]	188	6.6	184	40%	1	30	3.5
2109	Fruit salad (including citrus fruit) with cream [1 cup]	182	6.4	132	39%	1	21	2.7
2110	Fruit salad (including citrus fruit) with cream substitute [1 cup]	175	6.2	114	25%	1	22	2.6
2111	Fruit salad (including citrus fruit) with marshmallows [1 cup]	171	6.0	155	8%	1	37	2.4
2112	Fruit salad (including citrus fruit) with pudding [1 cup]	182	6.4	168	16%	3	34	1.1
2113	Fruit salad (including citrus fruit) with salad dressing or mayonnaise [1 cup]	188	6.6	152	47%	1	22	3.0
2114	Fruit salad, Puerto Rican style (Include Ensalada de frutas tropicales) [1 cup]	247	8.7	141	4%	2	36	3.8
2115	Genip, raw [10 small]	50	1.8	39	2%	1	10	2.1
2116	Gooseberries, cooked or canned [1 cup]	252	8.9	184	2%	2	47	6.0
2117	Gooseberries, raw [1 cup]	150	5.3	66	12%	1	15	6.5
2118	**Grapefruit, raw (Include chironja) [½ medium (4"dia)]**	128	4.5	41	3%	1	10	1.4
2119	Grapefruit, canned or frozen, in light syrup [1 cup]	254	9.0	152	2%	1	39	1.0
2120	Grapefruit, canned or frozen, unsweetened, water pack [1 cup]	244	8.6	88	3%	1	22	1.0
2121	Grapefruit and orange sections, raw [1 cup]	217	7.7	84	3%	2	21	3.6
2122	Grapefruit and orange sections, cooked, canned, or frozen, unsweetened, water pack [1 cup]	244	8.6	65	3%	1	16	2.8
2123	Grapefruit and orange sections, cooked, canned, or frozen, in light syrup [1 cup]	254	9.0	152	1%	1	39	2.5
2124	Grapes, American type, slip skin, raw (Include Concord grapes) [about 10 grapes]	24	0.8	16	5%	0	4	0.2
2125	**Grapes, European type, adherent skin, raw (Include tokay, emperor, thompson, red flame grapes) [10 grapes]**	50	1.8	36	7%	0	9	0.5
2126	Grapes, seedless, cooked or canned (including home canned), in heavy syrup [1 cup]	256	9.0	187	1%	1	50	1.0
2127	Grapes, seedless, cooked or canned, unsweetened, water pack [1 cup]	245	8.6	98	2%	1	25	2.5
2128	Guacamole with tomatoes (avocado, tomato, onion, garlic, parsley, lemon juice, salt) [1 cup]	233	8.2	273	80%	4	16	8.8
2129	**Guacamole (avocado, onion, lemon juice, salt) (Include avocado dip) [1 cup]**	233	8.2	369	85%	5	17	11.5
2130	Guava, canned in heavy syrup [1 cup]	310	10.9	300	4%	2	75	11.9
2131	Guava, raw [1 guava]	90	3.2	46	11%	1	11	4.9
2132	**Honeydew melon, raw [1 wedge (1/8 of 6½"dia melon)]**	160	5.6	56	3%	1	15	1.0
2133	Honeydew, frozen (balls) [1 cup]	230	8.1	81	3%	1	21	1.4
2134	Huckleberries, raw [1 cup]	145	5.1	81	6%	1	20	3.9
2135	Jackfruit, cooked or canned [4 pieces]	88	3.1	83	3%	1	21	1.4
2136	Jackfruit, raw [1 cup, sliced]	165	5.8	155	3%	2	40	2.6
2137	Jobo, raw [1 fruit]	75	2.6	65	3%	1	17	1.1
2138	Juneberry, raw [1 cup]	165	5.8	92	6%	1	23	4.5

Food #	fat gm	sat fat gm	choles mg	sodium mg	potass mg	vit A	vit E	vit C	thia-min	ribo-flavin	nia-cin	vit B-6	fol-ate	vit B-12	cal-cium	phos-phorus	magne-sium	iron	zinc
2094	1	0	0	1	328	3	2	24	5	5	4	10	3	0	1	2	5	2	1
2095	1	0	0	1	309	1	2	49	4	4	2	12	4	0	2	2	4	2	1
2096	1	0	0	1	356	9	3	20	5	6	7	4	6	0	3	3	5	4	2
2097	0	0	0	15	218	5	2	8	3	3	5	6	2	0	1	3	3	4	1
2098	0	0	0	13	193	7	3	7	3	3	4	5	2	0	1	3	3	3	1
2099	0	0	0	15	215	5	2	8	3	3	5	6	2	0	1	3	3	4	1
2100	0	0	0	9	225	7	2	11	2	2	5	6	1	0	2	3	4	3	1
2101	0	0	0	10	230	6	2	9	3	2	4	6	2	0	1	3	4	3	1
2102	1	0	0	24	1082	33	5	9	4	13	13	13	1	0	6	11	13	20	5
2103	2	1	4	3	328	4	2	28	5	5	4	9	4	0	2	3	5	2	1
2104	3	2	1	22	353	1	1	24	5	5	3	19	4	1	2	3	7	3	2
2105	7	4	18	7	359	6	1	25	6	6	3	19	4	0	2	3	7	3	1
2106	2	1	0	23	305	1	1	22	5	4	3	17	4	0	1	2	6	3	1
2107	3	2	11	283	199	4	1	4	3	9	2	4	2	5	10	20	4	2	3
2108	8	2	5	47	375	2	4	27	6	5	3	22	5	0	1	3	7	3	1
2109	6	4	15	18	260	5	1	82	8	4	3	5	5	0	4	3	5	2	1
2110	3	2	1	21	257	2	1	79	8	4	3	5	5	1	4	3	5	2	1
2111	1	1	0	23	218	1	1	72	7	3	3	5	4	0	3	2	4	2	1
2112	3	2	11	293	218	4	1	20	4	9	2	4	2	5	12	21	4	1	3
2113	8	2	5	51	274	2	4	95	8	3	3	8	7	0	4	2	5	2	1
2114	1	0	0	3	496	6	3	108	11	6	4	21	10	0	4	3	9	3	2
2115	0	0	0	3	117	0	0	4	2	1	2	3	2	0	1	1	2	2	0
2116	1	0	0	5	194	4	3	42	3	8	2	2	2	0	4	2	4	5	2
2117	1	0	0	2	297	4	2	69	4	3	2	6	2	0	4	4	4	3	1
2118	0	0	0	0	178	2	1	73	3	2	2	3	3	0	2	1	3	1	1
2119	0	0	0	5	328	0	2	90	6	3	3	3	5	0	4	3	6	6	1
2120	0	0	0	5	322	0	2	89	6	3	3	2	5	0	4	2	6	6	1
2121	0	0	0	0	342	3	2	154	8	4	3	5	10	0	5	2	5	1	1
2122	0	0	0	2	264	3	1	114	6	3	2	4	6	0	4	2	4	1	1
2123	0	0	0	4	316	2	2	116	8	3	3	4	7	0	5	2	5	3	1
2124	0	0	0	0	46	0	0	2	1	1	0	1	0	0	0	0	0	0	0
2125	0	0	0	1	93	0	1	9	3	2	1	3	0	0	1	1	1	1	0
2126	0	0	0	13	264	2	6	4	5	3	2	8	2	0	3	4	4	13	1
2127	0	0	0	15	262	2	6	4	5	3	2	8	2	0	2	4	4	13	1
2128	24	4	0	21	1096	13	8	47	14	13	17	25	27	0	2	8	17	11	5
2129	35	6	0	23	1374	14	10	32	16	16	22	32	36	0	3	9	22	13	6
2130	1	0	0	9	564	13	8	337	6	6	12	14	4	0	4	6	6	4	4
2131	1	0	0	3	256	7	3	275	3	3	5	6	3	0	2	2	2	2	1
2132	0	0	0	16	434	1	1	66	8	2	5	5	2	0	1	2	3	1	1
2133	0	0	0	23	623	1	1	95	12	2	7	7	3	0	1	2	4	1	1
2134	1	0	0	9	129	1	5	31	5	4	3	3	2	0	1	1	2	1	1
2135	0	0	0	3	240	2	0	7	1	5	2	4	2	0	3	3	8	3	2
2136	0	0	0	5	500	5	1	18	3	11	3	9	6	0	6	6	15	6	5
2137	0	0	0	2	203	3	2	61	5	2	2	4	3	0	1	3	2	4	1
2138	1	0	0	10	147	2	6	36	5	5	3	3	3	0	1	2	2	2	1

Fruits & Vegetables

Food #	Food Description & Amount	wt gm	wt oz	calories	%cal fat	prot gm	carbo gm	fiber gm
2139	Kiwi fruit, raw [1 fruit]	76	2.7	46	6%	1	11	2.6
2140	Kumquat, cooked or canned, in syrup [4 kumquats]	56	2.0	50	1%	0	13	2.4
2141	Kumquat, raw [4 kumquats]	76	2.7	48	1%	1	12	5.0
2142	**Lemon, raw [1 fruit (2" dia)]**	**58**	**2.0**	**17**	**9%**	**1**	**5**	**1.6**
2143	Lime, raw [1 fruit (2" dia)]	67	2.4	20	6%	0	7	1.9
2144	Loganberries, cooked or canned in heavy syrup [1 cup]	256	9.0	225	1%	3	57	6.7
2145	Loganberries, frozen [1 cup]	147	5.2	81	5%	2	19	7.2
2146	Loganberries, raw [1 cup]	144	5.1	79	5%	2	19	7.1
2147	Loquats, raw [4 loquats]	64	2.3	30	4%	0	8	1.1
2148	Lychee, cooked or canned, in sugar or syrup [4 lychees with liquid]	84	3.0	76	3%	0	19	0.7
2149	Lychee, dried (Include lychee nuts) [10 nuts]	25	0.9	69	4%	1	18	1.2
2150	Lychee, raw or frozen [1 lychee]	40	1.4	26	6%	0	7	0.5
2151	Mamey, raw (Include mamea apple) [1 portion (¼ of fruit)]	212	7.5	108	9%	1	26	6.3
2152	**Mango, raw [1 mango]**	**207**	**7.3**	**135**	**4%**	**1**	**35**	**3.7**
2153	Mango, cooked [4 oz]	112	4.0	73	4%	1	19	2.0
2154	Mango, pickled [4 slices]	112	4.0	150	1%	0	39	1.4
2155	Mango, dried [10 strips (3¼"x¾"x1/8")]	50	1.8	157	2%	1	41	2.6
2156	Mulberries, raw [1 cup]	140	4.9	60	8%	2	14	2.4
2157	Nectarine, cooked in heavy syrup [1 cup]	262	9.2	250	3%	2	63	3.0
2158	Nectarine, raw [1 fruit (2½"dia)]	136	4.8	67	8%	1	16	2.2
2159	**Orange, raw [1 orange (3"dia)]**	**184**	**6.5**	**86**	**2%**	**2**	**22**	**4.4**
2160	Orange peel [2Tbs]	12	0.4	12	2%	0	3	1.3
2161	Orange, sections, canned, juice pack [1 cup]	204	7.2	92	3%	2	23	3.4
2162	Orange, mandarin, canned or frozen, drained [1 cup]	189	6.7	72	1%	2	18	2.3
2163	Orange, mandarin, canned or frozen, in light syrup [1 cup]	252	8.9	154	1%	1	41	1.8
2164	Orange, mandarin, canned or frozen, juice pack [1 cup]	249	8.8	92	1%	2	24	1.7
2165	Papaya, cooked or canned, in sugar or syrup [1 cup]	132	4.7	101	1%	1	26	1.6
2166	**Papaya, raw [1 medium (5"long x 4"dia)]**	**288**	**10.2**	**112**	**3%**	**2**	**28**	**5.2**
2167	Papaya, dried [4 strips]	92	3.2	238	3%	4	60	11.0
2168	Papaya, green, cooked [1 cup]	132	4.7	24	3%	1	6	1.6
2169	Passion fruit, raw [4 fruit]	72	2.5	70	6%	2	17	7.5
2170	**Peach, raw [1 peach (2¾"dia)]**	**157**	**5.5**	**68**	**2%**	**1**	**17**	**3.1**
2171	Peach, cooked or canned in heavy syrup, drained solids [2 halves]	146	5.1	112	2%	1	29	2.5
2172	Peach, cooked or canned (including home canned), in heavy syrup [2 halves with liquid]	196	6.9	145	1%	1	39	2.5
2173	Peach, cooked or canned, in light or medium syrup [2 halves with liquid]	196	6.9	106	1%	1	29	2.5
2174	Peach, cooked or canned, juice pack [2 halves with liquid]	196	6.9	86	1%	1	23	2.5
2175	Peach, cooked or canned, unsweetened, water pack [2 halves with liquid]	196	6.9	47	2%	1	12	2.5
2176	Peach, dried, cooked, unsweetened [1 cup]	258	9.1	199	3%	3	51	7.0
2177	Peach, dried, cooked, with sugar [1 cup]	270	9.5	278	2%	3	72	6.5
2178	Peach, dried, uncooked [4 halves]	52	1.8	124	3%	2	32	4.3
2179	Peach, frozen, unsweetened [1 cup, sliced]	250	8.8	107	2%	2	28	5.0
2180	Peach, frozen, with sugar [1 cup, sliced]	250	8.8	235	1%	2	60	4.5
2181	Peach, pickled [1 fruit]	88	3.1	105	0%	0	27	1.2
2182	Peach, spiced [1 cup]	248	8.7	186	1%	1	50	3.2
2183	**Pear, raw [1 medium pear]**	**166**	**5.9**	**98**	**6%**	**1**	**25**	**4.0**
2184	Pear, cooked or canned in heavy syrup, drained solids [1 half]	48	1.7	36	2%	0	9	1.2
2185	Pear, cooked or canned (including home canned), in heavy syrup [2 halves with liquid]	152	5.4	112	2%	0	29	2.4
2186	Pear, cooked or canned, in light syrup [2 halves with liquid]	152	5.4	87	0%	0	23	2.4
2187	Pear, cooked or canned, juice pack [2 halves with liquid]	152	5.4	76	1%	1	20	2.4

Food #	fat gm	sat fat gm	choles mg	sodium mg	potass mg	% of Daily Value													
						vit A	vit E	vit C	thia-min	ribo-flavin	nia-cin	vit B-6	fol-ate	vit B-12	cal-cium	phos-phorus	magne-sium	iron	zinc
2139	0	0	0	4	252	1	3	124	1	2	2	3	7	0	2	3	6	2	1
2140	0	0	0	3	64	1	0	16	2	2	1	1	1	0	2	1	1	1	0
2141	0	0	0	5	148	2	1	47	4	4	2	2	3	0	3	1	2	2	0
2142	0	0	0	1	80	0	0	51	2	1	0	2	2	0	2	1	1	2	0
2143	0	0	0	1	68	0	1	32	1	1	1	1	1	0	2	1	1	2	0
2144	0	0	0	8	230	1	6	26	4	4	3	5	22	0	5	3	7	6	3
2145	0	0	0	1	213	1	11	37	5	3	6	5	9	0	4	4	8	5	3
2146	0	0	0	1	209	1	11	37	5	3	6	5	9	0	4	4	8	5	3
2147	0	0	0	1	170	10	2	1	1	1	1	3	2	0	1	2	2	1	0
2148	0	0	0	1	84	0	1	45	0	2	1	2	1	0	0	2	1	1	0
2149	0	0	0	1	278	0	1	76	0	8	4	1	1	0	1	5	3	2	0
2150	0	0	0	0	68	0	1	48	0	2	1	2	1	0	0	1	1	1	0
2151	1	0	0	32	99	5	4	49	3	5	4	11	7	0	2	2	8	8	1
2152	1	0	0	4	323	81	8	96	8	7	6	14	7	0	2	2	5	1	1
2153	0	0	0	2	157	33	4	36	3	3	3	7	2	0	1	1	3	1	0
2154	0	0	0	2	140	28	3	33	3	3	2	5	3	0	1	1	3	1	0
2155	0	0	0	3	227	28	5	13	4	5	4	9	3	0	1	2	3	1	0
2156	1	0	0	14	272	0	2	85	3	8	4	2	2	0	5	5	6	14	1
2157	1	0	0	2	356	10	6	12	2	4	8	2	1	0	1	3	4	2	1
2158	1	0	0	0	288	10	4	12	2	3	7	2	1	0	1	2	3	1	1
2159	0	0	0	0	333	4	1	163	11	4	3	6	14	0	7	3	5	1	1
2160	0	0	0	0	25	1	0	27	1	1	1	1	1	0	2	0	1	1	0
2161	0	0	0	1	365	4	1	154	10	4	3	7	10	0	6	3	5	2	1
2162	0	0	0	9	255	25	4	107	11	3	4	4	2	0	2	2	5	3	7
2163	0	0	0	15	197	21	3	83	9	7	6	5	3	0	2	3	5	5	4
2164	0	0	0	12	331	21	4	142	14	4	6	5	3	0	3	2	7	4	8
2165	0	0	0	4	205	2	3	46	1	2	1	1	4	0	2	0	2	1	1
2166	0	0	0	9	740	8	11	297	5	5	5	3	27	0	7	1	7	2	1
2167	1	0	0	18	1566	9	23	126	8	10	9	5	29	0	15	3	15	3	3
2168	0	0	0	8	179	0	0	43	1	1	1	1	2	0	3	2	2	2	1
2169	1	0	0	20	251	5	3	36	0	6	5	4	3	0	1	5	5	6	0
2170	0	0	0	0	309	8	4	17	2	4	8	1	1	0	1	2	3	1	1
2171	0	0	0	9	137	7	6	7	1	2	4	1	1	0	0	2	2	2	1
2172	0	0	0	12	180	6	6	9	1	3	6	2	2	0	1	2	2	3	1
2173	0	0	0	10	190	7	6	8	1	3	6	2	2	0	1	2	2	4	1
2174	0	0	0	8	251	7	10	12	1	2	6	2	2	0	1	3	3	3	1
2175	0	0	0	6	194	10	6	9	1	2	5	2	2	0	0	2	2	3	1
2176	1	0	0	5	826	5	0	16	1	3	20	5	0	0	2	10	8	19	3
2177	1	0	0	5	788	5	0	15	1	3	19	5	0	0	2	9	8	18	3
2178	0	0	0	4	518	11	0	4	0	6	11	2	0	0	1	6	5	12	2
2179	0	0	0	0	443	13	6	394	3	6	12	2	2	0	1	3	4	2	2
2180	0	0	0	15	325	7	7	393	2	5	8	2	2	0	1	3	3	5	1
2181	0	0	0	0	134	3	1	6	1	2	3	1	0	0	0	1	2	1	1
2182	0	0	0	10	211	8	7	22	2	5	7	2	2	0	1	2	4	4	1
2183	1	0	0	0	208	0	3	11	2	4	1	1	3	0	2	2	2	2	1
2184	0	0	0	2	32	0	1	1	0	1	1	0	0	0	0	0	0	1	0
2185	0	0	0	8	99	0	3	3	1	2	2	1	0	0	1	1	2	2	1
2186	0	0	0	8	100	0	3	2	1	1	1	1	0	0	1	1	2	2	1
2187	0	0	0	6	146	0	3	4	1	1	1	1	0	0	1	2	3	2	1

Fruits & Vegetables

Food #	Food Description & Amount	wt gm	wt oz	calories	%cal fat	prot gm	carbo gm	fiber gm
2188	Pear, cooked or canned, unsweetened, water pack [2 halves with liquid]	152	5.4	44	1%	0	12	2.4
2189	Pear, dried, cooked, unsweetened [1 cup]	255	9.0	324	2%	2	86	16.3
2190	Pear, dried, cooked, with sugar [1 cup]	280	9.9	392	2%	2	104	16.2
2191	Pear, dried, uncooked [4 halves]	72	2.5	189	2%	1	50	5.4
2192	Pear, Japanese, raw [1 pear]	307	10.8	129	5%	2	33	11.1
2193	Pear salad with dressing [1 serving (lettuce, ½ pear, dressing)]	112	4.0	116	44%	1	18	2.2
2194	Pear, spiced, drained solids [1 pear]	45	1.6	42	4%	0	11	1.0
2195	Persimmon, raw [1 persimmon (2½"dia x 3½"high)]	168	5.9	118	2%	1	31	6.0
2196	**Pineapple**, raw [1 cup, diced]	**155**	**5.5**	**76**	**8%**	**1**	**19**	**1.9**
2197	Pineapple, cooked or canned, drained solids [2 slices (3"dia)]	70	2.5	42	2%	0	11	0.8
2198	Pineapple, cooked or canned (including home canned), in heavy syrup [2 slices (3"dia) with liquid]	98	3.5	76	1%	0	20	0.8
2199	Pineapple, cooked or canned, in light syrup [2 slices (3"dia) with liquid]	96	3.4	50	2%	0	13	0.8
2200	Pineapple, cooked or canned, juice pack [2 slices (3"dia) with liquid]	94	3.3	56	1%	0	15	0.8
2201	Pineapple, cooked or canned, unsweetened, water pack [2 slices (3"dia) with liquid]	94	3.3	30	3%	0	8	0.8
2202	Pineapple, dehydrated [4 pieces]	112	4.0	280	8%	2	71	6.9
2203	Pineapple chunk, chocolate covered [4 pieces]	40	1.4	71	79%	0	4	0.8
2204	Pineapple salad with cream cheese [1 serving (lettuce, 1 slice of pineapple, cream cheese)]	66	2.3	89	54%	1	10	0.4
2205	Pineapple salad with dressing [1 serving (lettuce, 1 cup diced pineapple, dressing)]	184	6.5	141	38%	1	24	2.0
2206	Plantain, ripe, raw [1 fruit]	203	7.2	248	3%	3	65	4.7
2207	Plantain chips [2 oz]	56	2.0	291	58%	1	33	4.3
2208	Plantain, green, boiled or baked [1 small]	152	5.4	176	1%	1	47	3.5
2209	Plantain, green, fried in corn oil, salted, Puerto Rican style (Include Tostones) [4 small tostones]	80	2.8	193	45%	1	29	2.1
2210	Plantain, ripe, boiled (Include baked ripe plantain) [1 small]	208	7.3	241	1%	2	65	4.8
2211	Plantain, ripe, candied (margarine-sugar-wine syrup), Puerto Rican style (Include Platano en almibar) [½ plantain with syrup]	140	4.9	365	26%	1	70	1.8
2212	Plantain, ripe, fried in soybean oil, Puerto Rican style (Include Platano maduro frito) [½ plantain (2 slices, 4"x¾")]	76	2.7	191	47%	1	27	2.0
2213	Plantain, ripe, fritters, Puerto Rican style (Include Pionono) [1 pionono (2"x2½"x¾")]	58	2.0	244	63%	7	17	1.4
2214	Plantain, ripe, rolled in flour, fried in soybean oil [2 pieces (2½"long)]	90	3.2	220	44%	2	33	2.2
2215	**Plum**, raw [2 plums (2½"dia)]	**132**	**4.7**	**73**	**10%**	**1**	**17**	**2.0**
2216	Plum, cooked or canned, heavy syrup, drained solids [2 plums]	62	2.2	55	1%	0	14	0.9
2217	Plum, cooked or canned (including home canned), in heavy syrup [2 plums with liquid]	92	3.2	82	1%	0	21	0.9
2218	Plum, cooked or canned, in light syrup [2 plums with liquid]	92	3.2	58	1%	0	15	0.9
2219	Plum, cooked or canned, juice pack [2 plums with liquid]	92	3.2	53	0%	0	14	0.9
2220	Plum, cooked or canned, unsweetened, water pack [2 plums with liquid]	92	3.2	38	0%	0	10	0.9
2221	Plum, Japanese, dried with rock salt (Include umeboshi) [10 dried plums]	30	1.1	102	2%	1	27	2.8
2222	Pomegranate, raw [1 pomegranate (3½" dia)]	154	5.4	105	4%	1	26	0.9
2223	Prune, dried, cooked, unsweetened [4 prunes]	36	1.3	39	2%	0	10	2.4
2224	Prune, dried, cooked, with sugar (Include Ciruelas) [4 prunes]	36	1.3	45	2%	0	12	1.4
2225	Prune, dried, uncooked [4 prunes]	28	1.0	67	2%	1	18	2.0
2226	Prune whip (prunes, egg white, sugar, lemon juice, salt) [1 cup]	130	4.6	191	1%	6	44	5.9
2227	Quince, raw [1 quince]	92	3.2	52	2%	0	14	1.7
2228	**Raisins** (Include cinnamon-coated raisins) [1 cup]	**145**	**5.1**	**435**	**1%**	**5**	**115**	**5.8**
2229	Raisins, cooked [1 cup]	295	10.4	646	1%	4	169	5.5
2230	Raspberries, black, raw (Include black caps) [1 cup]	134	4.7	66	10%	1	16	9.1
2231	Raspberries, cooked or canned (including home canned), in heavy syrup [1 cup]	256	9.0	233	1%	2	60	8.4
2232	Raspberries, cooked or canned, unsweetened, water pack [1 cup]	243	8.6	80	10%	1	19	11.1

Food #	fat gm	sat fat gm	choles mg	sodium mg	potass mg	% of Daily Value													
						vit A	vit E	vit C	thia-min	ribo-flavin	nia-cin	vit B-6	fol-ate	vit B-12	cal-cium	phos-phorus	magne-sium	iron	zinc
2188	0	0	0	3	81	0	3	3	1	1	0	1	0	0	1	1	2	2	1
2189	1	0	0	8	658	1	0	17	1	3	4	4	0	0	4	7	10	14	3
2190	1	0	0	8	686	1	0	18	1	3	5	5	0	0	4	8	11	15	3
2191	0	0	0	4	384	0	0	8	0	6	5	3	0	0	2	4	6	8	2
2192	1	0	0	0	371	0	5	19	2	2	3	3	6	0	1	3	6	0	0
2193	6	1	4	114	123	2	4	6	1	2	1	1	3	1	1	2	2	2	1
2194	0	0	0	0	46	0	1	2	0	1	0	0	0	0	0	0	1	1	0
2195	0	0	0	2	270	36	3	21	3	2	1	8	3	0	1	3	4	1	1
2196	1	0	0	2	175	0	1	40	10	3	3	7	4	0	1	1	5	3	1
2197	0	0	0	1	87	0	0	11	5	1	1	3	1	0	1	0	3	1	0
2198	0	0	0	1	102	0	0	12	6	1	1	4	1	0	1	1	4	2	1
2199	0	0	0	1	101	0	0	12	6	1	1	4	1	0	1	1	4	2	1
2200	0	0	0	1	115	0	0	15	6	1	1	3	1	0	1	1	3	1	1
2201	0	0	0	1	119	0	0	12	6	1	1	3	1	0	1	0	4	2	1
2202	2	0	0	6	646	1	2	29	25	11	11	22	8	0	4	4	20	12	3
2203	6	1	0	2	64	0	4	30	0	2	0	1	1	0	1	1	1	1	0
2204	5	3	17	46	74	6	1	6	3	3	1	2	2	1	2	2	2	2	1
2205	6	1	4	112	194	2	3	42	10	4	3	7	5	1	1	2	6	4	1
2206	1	0	0	8	1013	23	2	62	7	6	7	30	11	0	1	7	19	7	2
2207	19	16	0	3	300	0	10	6	3	1	2	7	2	0	1	3	11	4	3
2208	0	0	0	8	707	14	1	28	5	5	6	18	10	0	0	4	12	5	1
2209	10	1	0	5	409	8	7	20	3	3	3	12	3	0	0	3	9	3	1
2210	0	0	0	10	967	19	1	38	6	6	8	25	14	0	0	6	17	7	2
2211	10	2	0	124	377	17	6	17	2	3	3	11	2	0	1	3	8	3	1
2212	10	1	0	3	386	7	7	18	2	2	3	12	2	0	0	3	8	3	1
2213	17	4	58	194	351	7	9	14	7	8	7	11	3	6	1	8	7	5	6
2214	11	1	0	4	411	8	8	19	5	4	4	12	4	0	0	4	9	4	1
2215	1	0	0	0	227	4	3	21	4	7	3	5	1	0	1	1	2	1	1
2216	0	0	0	12	58	2	2	0	1	1	1	1	0	0	1	1	1	3	0
2217	0	0	0	17	84	2	2	1	1	2	1	1	1	0	1	1	1	4	0
2218	0	0	0	18	86	2	2	1	1	2	1	1	1	0	1	1	1	4	0
2219	0	0	0	1	142	9	2	4	1	3	2	1	1	0	1	1	2	2	1
2220	0	0	0	1	116	8	2	4	1	2	2	1	1	0	1	1	1	1	0
2221	0	0	0	986	317	5	1	0	2	3	5	11	0	0	2	3	5	6	2
2222	0	0	0	5	399	0	3	16	3	3	2	8	2	0	0	1	1	3	1
2223	0	0	0	1	120	1	0	2	1	2	1	4	0	0	1	1	2	2	1
2224	0	0	0	1	112	1	0	2	1	2	1	4	0	0	1	1	2	2	1
2225	0	0	0	1	209	6	1	2	2	3	3	4	0	0	1	2	3	4	1
2226	0	0	0	80	347	2	0	9	1	17	3	10	0	1	2	4	6	6	2
2227	0	0	0	4	181	0	2	23	1	2	1	2	1	0	1	2	2	4	0
2228	1	0	0	17	1089	0	3	8	15	8	6	18	1	0	7	14	12	17	3
2229	1	0	0	24	929	0	3	5	11	7	5	15	1	0	7	13	12	16	3
2230	1	0	0	0	204	2	2	56	3	7	6	4	9	0	3	2	6	4	4
2231	0	0	0	8	241	1	4	37	3	5	6	5	7	0	3	2	8	6	3
2232	1	0	0	2	223	2	2	47	3	8	7	4	5	0	4	2	8	5	5

Fruits & Vegetables

Food #	Food Description & Amount	wt gm	wt oz	calories	%cal fat	prot gm	carbo gm	fiber gm
2233	Raspberries, frozen, unsweetened [1 cup]	250	8.8	123	10%	2	29	17.0
2234	Raspberries, frozen, with sugar [1 cup]	250	8.8	258	1%	2	65	11.0
2235	**Raspberries**, red, raw [1 cup]	**123**	**4.3**	**60**	**10%**	**1**	**14**	**8.4**
2236	Rhubarb, cooked or canned, drained solids [1 cup]	240	8.5	278	0%	1	75	4.8
2237	Rhubarb, cooked or canned (including home canned), in heavy syrup (Include rhubarb sauce) [1 cup]	240	8.5	278	0%	1	75	4.8
2238	Rhubarb, cooked or canned, in light syrup [1 cup]	240	8.5	220	1%	1	56	3.5
2239	Rhubarb, cooked or canned, unsweetened [1 cup]	240	8.5	50	9%	2	11	4.3
2240	Rhubarb, frozen, with sugar [1 cup]	240	8.5	278	0%	1	75	4.8
2241	Rhubarb, raw [1 cup, diced]	122	4.3	26	9%	1	6	2.2
2242	Sapodilla, raw [1 sapodilla]	170	6.0	141	12%	1	34	9.0
2243	Soursop (annona muricata), raw [1 cup, pulp]	225	7.9	149	4%	2	38	7.4
2244	**Strawberries**, raw [6 strawberries (1¼"dia)]	**108**	**3.8**	**32**	**11%**	**1**	**8**	**2.5**
2245	Strawberries, cooked or canned, in syrup [1 cup]	254	9.0	234	3%	1	60	4.3
2246	Strawberries, cooked or canned, unsweetened, water pack [1 cup]	242	8.5	49	11%	1	11	3.7
2247	Strawberries, frozen, unsweetened [1 cup]	221	7.8	77	3%	1	20	4.6
2248	Strawberries, frozen, with sugar [1 cup]	255	9.0	222	1%	1	60	4.8
2249	Strawberries, raw, with sugar [1 cup, sliced]	174	6.1	83	7%	1	20	3.8
2250	Strawberry, chocolate covered [4 pieces]	76	2.7	136	79%	1	8	1.6
2251	Sweetsop, raw (Include annona squamosa, sugar-apple) [1 fruit (2¾"dia)]	155	5.5	146	3%	3	37	6.8
2252	Tamarind pulp, dried, sweetened (Include Pulpitas) [1 cup, pieces, without seeds]	220	7.8	558	2%	6	146	10.1
2253	Tamarind, raw [10 tamarind]	20	0.7	48	2%	1	13	1.0
2254	Tangelo, raw [1 fruit (2¾"dia)]	114	4.0	54	2%	1	13	2.7
2255	Tangerine, raw (Include mandarin orange, satsuma orange) [1 fruit (2½"dia)]	98	3.5	43	4%	1	11	2.3
2256	**Watermelon**, raw [1 cup, diced]	**152**	**5.4**	**49**	**12%**	**1**	**11**	**0.8**
2257	Watermelon, pickled [5 squares or cubes]	50	1.8	51	1%	1	13	0.6
2258	Wi-apple, raw [1 cup]	125	4.4	63	5%	1	16	2.5
2259	Youngberries, raw [1 cup]	144	5.1	75	7%	1	18	7.6
	Vegetables							
2350	Alfalfa sprouts, raw [1 cup]	33	1.2	10	21%	1	1	0.8
2351	Algae, dried (Include spirulina) [2Tbs]	16	0.6	47	18%	7	6	0.7
2352	Artichoke salad (artichokes in olive oil) [1 cup]	130	4.6	155	64%	4	13	6.4
2353	Artichoke, globe (French), canned [1 cup, hearts]	168	5.9	84	3%	6	19	9.0
2354	**Artichoke**, globe (French), cooked, from fresh without salt [1 medium globe]	**120**	**4.2**	**60**	**3%**	**4**	**13**	**6.5**
2355	Artichoke, globe (French), cooked, from frozen [1 cup, hearts]	168	5.9	76	10%	5	15	7.7
2356	Artichokes, stuffed with mixture of breadcrumbs, celery, onion, parmesan cheese, olive oil, parsley, salt [1 stuffed globe]	251	8.9	400	33%	15	55	8.4
2357	Artichoke, Jerusalem, raw (Include sunchoke) [1 cup]	150	5.3	114	0%	3	26	2.4
2358	Arugula, raw (Include Rocket lettuce, Roquette lettuce) [1 cup]	20	0.7	5	24%	1	1	0.3
2359	Asparagus, canned [1 cup]	242	8.5	46	31%	5	6	3.9
2360	**Asparagus**, cooked, from fresh without salt [1 cup]	**180**	**6.3**	**43**	**12%**	**5**	**8**	**2.9**
2361	Asparagus, cooked, from frozen [1 cup]	180	6.3	50	14%	5	9	2.9
2362	Asparagus, from canned, creamed or with cheese sauce [1 cup]	235	8.3	178	63%	10	9	2.8
2363	Asparagus, from fresh, creamed or with cheese sauce [1 cup]	235	8.3	216	60%	12	12	2.6
2364	Asparagus, from frozen, creamed or with cheese sauce [1 cup]	235	8.3	222	59%	13	13	2.6
2365	Asparagus, raw [1 cup]	134	4.7	31	8%	3	6	2.8
2366	Bamboo shoots, canned or cooked with salt [1 cup, slices]	120	4.2	33	10%	3	6	2.7
2367	Bamboo shoots, fried [1 cup]	156	5.5	100	51%	5	11	4.4
2368	Bean salad, yellow and/or green string beans (Include three bean salad) [1 cup]	150	5.3	140	49%	4	15	5.3
2369	Bean sprouts, canned [1 cup]	125	4.4	15	5%	2	3	1.0

Food #	fat gm	sat fat gm	choles mg	sodium mg	potass mg	% of Daily Value													
						vit A	vit E	vit C	thia-min	ribo-flavin	nia-cin	vit B-6	fol-ate	vit B-12	cal-cium	phos-phorus	magne-sium	iron	zinc
2233	1	0	0	0	342	3	4	73	5	13	11	7	15	0	5	3	11	8	8
2234	0	0	0	3	285	2	4	69	3	7	3	4	16	0	4	4	8	9	3
2235	1	0	0	0	187	2	2	51	2	7	6	4	8	0	3	1	6	4	4
2236	0	0	0	2	207	1	2	9	2	3	2	2	2	0	33	2	7	3	1
2237	0	0	0	2	230	2	2	13	3	3	2	2	3	0	35	2	7	3	1
2238	0	0	0	4	210	2	1	15	4	4	2	2	4	0	38	2	9	3	1
2239	0	0	0	10	622	2	2	22	3	4	3	3	2	0	20	3	7	3	2
2240	0	0	0	2	230	2	2	13	3	3	2	2	3	0	35	2	7	3	1
2241	0	0	0	5	351	1	1	16	2	2	2	1	2	0	10	2	4	1	1
2242	2	0	0	20	328	1	1	42	0	2	2	3	6	0	4	2	5	8	1
2243	1	0	0	32	626	0	3	77	11	7	10	7	8	0	3	6	12	8	2
2244	0	0	0	1	179	0	1	102	1	4	1	3	5	0	2	2	3	2	1
2245	1	0	0	10	218	1	1	134	4	5	1	6	18	0	3	3	5	7	2
2246	1	0	0	4	269	0	1	146	2	6	2	5	7	0	2	3	4	3	2
2247	0	0	0	4	327	1	2	152	3	5	5	3	9	0	4	3	6	9	2
2248	0	0	0	5	250	1	2	172	3	10	4	4	6	0	3	3	4	8	1
2249	1	0	0	2	275	0	1	156	2	7	5	5	7	0	2	3	4	4	1
2250	12	2	0	3	121	0	7	57	1	3	1	2	3	0	1	2	2	2	1
2251	0	0	0	14	383	0	3	94	11	10	7	16	5	0	4	5	8	5	1
2252	1	1	0	56	1244	0	5	2	40	16	17	6	3	0	15	22	46	31	1
2253	0	0	0	6	126	0	0	1	6	2	2	1	1	0	1	2	5	3	0
2254	0	0	0	0	206	2	1	101	7	3	2	3	9	0	5	2	3	1	1
2255	0	0	0	1	154	9	1	50	7	1	1	3	5	0	1	1	3	1	2
2256	1	0	0	3	176	6	1	24	8	2	2	11	1	0	1	1	4	1	1
2257	0	0	0	1	49	0	0	5	1	1	1	2	0	0	1	1	1	1	0
2258	0	0	0	3	198	8	5	105	4	1	8	6	4	0	1	3	4	2	0
2259	1	0	0	0	282	2	3	50	3	3	3	4	12	0	5	3	7	5	3
2350	0	0	0	2	26	1	0	5	2	2	1	1	3	0	1	2	2	2	2
2351	1	0	0	130	209	1	3	2	19	26	8	3	9	0	4	2	14	24	3
2352	11	1	0	113	422	2	5	20	5	5	6	7	15	0	5	10	18	9	4
2353	0	0	0	529	591	3	1	28	7	7	8	9	21	0	8	14	25	12	5
2354	0	0	0	114	425	2	1	20	5	5	6	7	15	0	5	10	18	9	4
2355	1	0	0	89	444	3	1	14	7	16	8	7	50	0	4	10	13	5	4
2356	15	4	7	753	645	5	6	29	28	20	23	11	28	1	31	26	26	29	11
2357	0	0	0	6	644	0	1	10	20	5	10	6	5	0	2	12	6	28	1
2358	0	0	0	5	74	5	0	5	1	1	0	1	1	0	3	1	2	2	1
2359	2	0	0	695	416	13	3	67	9	14	12	13	55	0	4	10	6	25	6
2360	1	0	0	20	288	10	2	32	15	13	10	11	66	0	4	10	5	7	5
2361	1	0	0	7	392	15	8	73	8	11	9	2	61	0	4	10	6	6	7
2362	12	6	24	771	382	17	5	48	9	19	9	11	40	4	22	22	7	19	10
2363	14	7	30	361	359	18	5	29	16	23	10	11	59	4	27	26	8	8	11
2364	15	7	30	350	449	23	9	64	10	21	9	3	55	4	28	26	9	7	12
2365	0	0	0	3	366	8	9	29	13	10	8	9	43	0	3	8	6	6	2
2366	0	0	0	5	593	0	4	7	10	5	3	13	2	0	2	7	1	3	9
2367	6	1	0	68	1078	5	9	11	18	8	6	23	3	0	3	12	2	6	15
2368	8	1	0	520	247	2	6	7	5	6	4	2	14	0	4	8	7	8	4
2369	0	0	0	175	34	0	0	1	2	5	1	2	3	0	2	4	3	3	2

Fruits & Vegetables

Food #	Food Description & Amount	wt gm	wt oz	calo- ries	%cal fat	prot gm	carbo gm	fiber gm
2370	Bean sprouts, raw (Include soybeans, mung beans) [1 cup]	104	3.7	31	5%	3	6	1.9
2371	Bean sprouts, cooked, from fresh without salt [1 cup]	124	4.4	58	38%	6	6	1.0
2372	Beans, lima and corn, cooked, with salt (Include succotash) [1 cup]	192	6.8	179	9%	8	38	7.9
2373	Beet greens, cooked, with salt [1 cup]	144	5.1	39	7%	4	8	4.2
2374	Beet greens, raw [1 cup]	38	1.3	7	3%	1	2	1.4
2375	Beets with Harvard sauce (sugar, vinegar, margarine, cornstarch, salt) [1 cup]	246	8.7	291	25%	3	56	3.5
2376	Beets, canned [1 cup, slices]	170	6.0	53	4%	2	12	2.9
2377	Beets, canned, low sodium [1 cup]	170	6.0	48	2%	1	11	2.0
2378	**Beets**, cooked, from fresh or frozen, unsalted [1 cup, slices]	170	6.0	75	4%	3	17	3.4
2379	Beets, raw [1 cup]	136	4.8	58	4%	2	13	3.8
2380	Bittermelon, cooked without salt (Include Balsam pear) [1 cup]	124	4.4	24	9%	1	5	2.5
2381	Bittermelon leaves, horseradish leaves, jute leaves, or radish leaves, cooked without salt [1 cup]	123	4.3	51	8%	5	10	2.4
2382	Broccoflower, cooked without salt [1 cup, fresh]	82	2.9	26	9%	2	5	2.7
2383	Broccoflower, raw [1 cup]	64	2.3	20	9%	2	4	2.0
2384	Broccoli casserole (broccoli, noodles, and cream sauce) [1 cup]	228	8.0	312	47%	9	34	3.6
2385	Broccoli casserole (broccoli, rice, cheese, and mushroom sauce) [1 cup]	228	8.0	284	41%	12	31	2.4
2386	Broccoli salad with cauliflower, cheese, bacon bits, and dressing [1 cup]	154	5.4	428	79%	10	17	2.9
2387	Broccoli, batter-dipped and fried [1 cup]	85	3.0	122	65%	3	9	2.2
2388	**Broccoli**, cooked without salt [1 cup]	184	6.5	52	11%	5	9	5.3
2389	Broccoli, cooked, from fresh, with cheese sauce [1 cup]	228	8.0	230	60%	13	13	4.3
2390	Broccoli, cooked, from fresh, with mushroom sauce [1 cup]	228	8.0	138	51%	6	14	3.6
2391	Broccoli, cooked, from frozen [1 cup, frozen, chopped]	184	6.5	52	4%	6	10	5.5
2392	Broccoli, cooked, from frozen, with cheese sauce [1 cup]	228	8.0	213	57%	13	13	4.7
2393	Broccoli, cooked, from frozen, with cream sauce [1 cup]	228	8.0	174	52%	8	16	4.3
2394	Broccoli, cooked, from frozen, with mushroom sauce [1 cup]	228	8.0	132	47%	6	14	4.0
2395	Broccoli, cooked, with cheese sauce [1 cup]	228	8.0	230	60%	13	13	4.3
2396	Broccoli, cooked, with cream sauce [1 cup]	228	8.0	174	52%	8	16	4.3
2397	Broccoli, cooked, with mushroom sauce [1 cup]	228	8.0	132	47%	6	14	4.0
2398	Broccoli, raw [1 cup, chopped]	88	3.1	25	11%	3	5	2.6
2399	**Brussels sprouts**, cooked, from fresh without salt [1 cup]	155	5.5	60	12%	4	13	4.0
2400	Brussels sprouts, cooked, from frozen [1 cup]	155	5.5	65	8%	6	13	6.4
2401	Brussels sprouts, creamed, cooked from fresh [1 cup]	228	8.0	198	52%	7	20	3.5
2402	Brussels sprouts, creamed, cooked from frozen [1 cup]	228	8.0	203	50%	9	20	5.4
2403	Brussels sprouts, raw [1 cup]	88	3.1	38	6%	3	8	3.3
2404	Buckwheat sprouts, raw [1 cup]	140	4.9	277	6%	10	60	1.5
2405	Burdock, cooked without salt (Include gobo) [1 cup]	125	4.4	110	1%	3	26	2.3
2406	Cabbage, Chinese, raw (Include bok choy, napa, pa-tsai) [1 cup]	76	2.7	10	14%	1	2	0.8
2407	Cabbage, Chinese, cook without salt [1 cup]	170	6.0	24	12%	2	4	4.0
2408	Cabbage, Chinese, raw, with French dressing [1 cup]	76	2.7	66	74%	1	4	2.0
2409	Cabbage, green, raw [1 cup, chopped]	89	3.1	22	10%	1	5	2.0
2410	**Cabbage**, green, cooked without salt [1 cup]	150	5.3	33	18%	2	7	3.5
2411	Cabbage, creamed [1 cup]	200	7.1	158	58%	5	13	2.7
2412	Cabbage, red, raw [1 cup, chopped]	89	3.1	24	9%	1	5	1.8
2413	Cabbage, red, cooked without salt [1 cup]	150	5.3	32	9%	2	7	3.0
2414	Cabbage, savoy, cooked without salt [1 cup]	145	5.1	39	3%	3	9	4.5
2415	**Cabbage salad or coleslaw** [1 cup]	184	6.5	271	81%	2	14	3.5
2416	Cabbage salad or coleslaw with apples, raisins, mayonnaise [1 cup]	132	4.7	255	71%	2	20	2.8
2417	Cabbage salad or coleslaw with pineapple, mayonnaise [1 cup]	132	4.7	133	49%	1	18	1.9
2418	Cactus, cooked without salt (Include nopal) [1 cup]	149	5.3	22	3%	2	5	3.0

| Food # | fat gm | sat fat gm | choles mg | sodium mg | potass mg | % of Daily Value | | | | | | | | | | | | | |
						vit A	vit E	vit C	thia-min	ribo-flavin	nia-cin	vit B-6	fol-ate	vit B-12	cal-cium	phos-phorus	magne-sium	iron	zinc
2370	0	0	0	6	155	0	0	23	6	8	4	5	16	0	1	6	5	5	3
2371	2	0	0	12	261	0	0	21	10	6	6	5	16	0	4	9	10	6	6
2372	2	0	0	86	509	4	2	19	9	8	13	9	16	0	3	13	11	9	6
2373	0	0	0	347	1309	73	1	60	11	24	4	10	5	0	16	6	24	15	5
2374	0	0	0	76	208	23	2	19	3	5	1	2	1	0	5	2	7	7	1
2375	8	2	0	224	571	8	6	10	3	5	3	6	34	0	3	7	12	9	4
2376	0	0	0	330	252	0	2	11	1	4	1	5	12	0	3	3	7	17	2
2377	0	0	0	36	241	1	2	8	1	4	1	5	12	0	2	3	7	6	3
2378	0	0	0	131	519	1	2	10	3	4	3	6	34	0	3	6	10	7	4
2379	0	0	0	106	442	1	1	11	3	3	2	5	37	0	2	5	8	6	3
2380	0	0	0	7	396	1	3	68	4	4	2	3	16	0	1	4	5	3	6
2381	0	0	0	14	639	56	2	81	11	21	7	44	25	0	18	9	28	16	5
2382	0	0	0	18	228	1	0	99	4	5	3	8	8	0	3	5	4	3	3
2383	0	0	0	15	192	1	0	94	3	4	2	7	9	0	2	4	3	3	3
2384	16	6	52	129	235	29	7	47	14	12	9	7	19	3	10	15	10	13	7
2385	13	6	23	667	437	23	7	76	13	21	10	11	20	5	27	28	11	10	11
2386	37	9	41	500	265	13	18	72	7	8	3	18	15	6	17	16	7	5	7
2387	9	1	15	64	242	10	10	89	5	8	4	5	10	1	7	7	5	5	3
2388	1	0	0	48	537	26	10	229	7	12	5	13	23	0	8	11	11	9	5
2389	15	7	31	404	537	30	11	180	8	22	5	12	20	5	32	28	12	9	11
2390	8	2	3	675	429	17	10	143	6	13	6	9	15	2	10	12	8	8	6
2391	0	0	0	44	331	35	8	123	7	9	4	12	20	0	9	10	9	6	4
2392	13	6	28	366	379	38	9	103	8	18	5	12	18	4	31	25	11	7	9
2393	10	3	6	359	388	31	10	92	9	16	5	11	17	4	18	17	10	6	5
2394	7	2	3	622	310	24	8	84	6	11	6	9	14	2	11	12	8	6	6
2395	15	7	31	404	537	30	11	180	8	22	5	12	20	5	32	28	12	9	11
2396	10	3	6	359	388	31	9	92	9	16	5	11	12	4	18	17	10	6	5
2397	7	2	3	622	310	24	7	84	6	11	6	9	10	2	11	12	8	6	6
2398	0	0	0	24	286	14	5	137	4	6	3	7	16	0	4	6	6	4	2
2399	1	0	0	33	491	11	4	160	11	7	5	14	23	0	6	9	8	10	3
2400	1	0	0	36	504	9	3	118	11	10	4	22	39	0	4	8	9	6	4
2401	11	3	7	386	559	15	8	132	14	17	6	13	21	5	17	17	10	10	6
2402	11	3	7	389	569	13	7	97	13	19	5	20	34	5	15	17	11	7	6
2403	0	0	0	22	342	8	3	125	8	5	3	10	13	0	4	6	5	7	2
2404	2	0	0	22	237	0	0	6	21	13	22	19	13	0	4	28	29	17	15
2405	0	0	0	5	450	0	1	5	3	4	2	17	6	0	6	12	12	5	3
2406	0	0	0	49	192	23	0	57	2	3	2	7	12	0	3	4	4	3	1
2407	0	0	0	36	497	31	1	67	4	6	3	16	20	0	14	5	5	6	2
2408	5	1	0	183	160	9	4	28	2	2	1	7	13	0	5	2	2	1	1
2409	0	0	0	16	219	1	0	48	3	2	1	4	10	0	4	2	3	3	1
2410	1	0	0	12	146	2	1	50	6	5	2	8	8	0	5	2	3	1	1
2411	10	3	6	331	248	6	4	38	8	13	3	8	7	4	14	11	5	3	3
2412	0	0	0	10	183	0	0	85	3	2	1	9	5	0	5	4	3	2	1
2413	0	0	0	12	210	0	1	86	3	2	2	11	5	0	6	4	4	3	2
2414	0	0	0	39	300	13	1	60	6	2	2	12	20	0	5	5	10	3	2
2415	24	4	18	199	383	47	13	70	5	4	3	16	15	1	7	5	6	6	2
2416	20	3	15	157	336	3	11	43	4	3	2	13	9	1	5	4	4	5	2
2417	7	1	5	160	211	3	3	41	5	2	2	5	8	1	4	2	4	3	1
2418	0	0	0	30	291	7	0	13	1	4	2	5	1	0	24	2	18	4	2

Fruits & Vegetables

Food #	Food Description & Amount	wt gm	wt oz	calo-ries	%cal fat	prot gm	carbo gm	fiber gm
2419	Cactus, raw [1 cup]	118	4.2	19	7%	2	4	2.7
2420	Caesar salad (with romaine lettuce) [1 cup]	108	3.8	167	75%	5	6	1.4
2421	Calabasa (Include Spanish pumpkin), cooked without salt [1 cup, cubed]	166	5.9	56	7%	2	13	4.8
2422	Carrot chips, dried [15 chips]	15	0.5	51	4%	1	12	3.5
2423	Carrots in tomato sauce [1 cup]	176	6.2	209	45%	1	31	1.7
2424	Carrots, canned [1 cup, sliced]	146	5.1	37	7%	1	8	2.2
2425	Carrots, canned, creamed [1 cup]	228	8.0	185	55%	5	16	2.1
2426	Carrots, canned, glazed [1 cup]	161	5.7	189	56%	1	21	2.1
2427	Carrots, canned, low sodium [1 cup, sliced]	146	5.1	34	5%	1	8	2.6
2428	Carrots, canned, with cheese sauce [1 cup]	228	8.0	233	61%	10	14	2.2
2429	**Carrots, cooked, from fresh, without salt [1 cup, sliced]**	**156**	**5.5**	**70**	**4%**	**2**	**16**	**5.1**
2430	Carrots, cooked, from fresh, creamed [1 cup]	228	8.0	206	48%	5	23	4.4
2431	Carrots, cooked, from fresh, glazed [1 cup]	161	5.7	217	49%	2	28	4.6
2432	Carrots, cooked, from fresh, with cheese sauce [1 cup]	228	8.0	255	53%	10	21	4.9
2433	Carrots, cooked, from frozen, creamed [1 cup]	228	8.0	199	51%	5	20	4.5
2434	Carrots, cooked, from frozen [1 cup, sliced]	146	5.1	53	3%	2	12	5.1
2435	Carrots, cooked, from frozen, glazed [1 cup]	161	5.7	205	51%	2	25	4.9
2436	Carrots, cooked, from frozen, with cheese sauce [1 cup]	228	8.0	249	56%	11	17	5.0
2437	**Carrots, raw [1 medium (5½"x1")]**	**50**	**1.8**	**21**	**4%**	**1**	**5**	**1.5**
2438	Carrot-raisin salad (with mayonnaise) [1 cup]	175	6.2	419	64%	3	40	4.3
2439	Casabe, cassava bread [1 piece (6"dia)]	100	3.5	304	2%	3	72	3.4
2440	Cassava, cooked without salt (Include yuca blanca, manioc, yucca, tapioca plant) [4 pieces]	80	2.8	129	2%	1	31	1.5
2441	Cassava Pasteles, Puerto Rican style (Include Pasteles de yuca) [1 pastel (6"x2"x½")]	145	5.1	374	60%	10	28	1.7
2442	Cassava with creole sauce, Puerto Rican style (Include Yuca al mojo) [1 serving (2 pieces with sauce)]	230	8.1	305	23%	3	57	4.0
2443	Cauliflower, batter-dipped, fried (Include breaded, fried) [2 flowerets]	52	1.8	106	68%	2	7	1.0
2444	Cauliflower, canned [1 cup]	180	6.3	41	18%	3	7	4.8
2445	**Cauliflower, cooked, from fresh, without salt [1 cup, pieces]**	**125**	**4.4**	**29**	**18%**	**2**	**5**	**3.4**
2446	Cauliflower, cooked, from frozen [1 cup]	180	6.3	34	10%	3	7	4.9
2447	Cauliflower, creamed or with cheese sauce [1 cup]	228	8.0	249	64%	12	12	3.7
2448	Cauliflower, canned, creamed [1 cup]	228	8.0	247	64%	12	12	3.7
2449	Cauliflower, cooked from fresh, creamed [1 cup]	228	8.0	249	64%	12	12	3.7
2450	Cauliflower, cooked from frozen, creamed [1 cup]	228	8.0	202	62%	10	11	4.2
2451	Cauliflower, raw [1 cup]	100	3.5	25	8%	2	5	2.5
2452	Celeriac, cooked without salt (Include Puerto Rican apio) [1 cup, pieces]	155	5.5	69	6%	2	15	2.9
2453	Celery, cooked without salt [1 cup, diced]	150	5.3	27	8%	1	6	2.4
2454	Celery, creamed [1 cup]	228	8.0	175	58%	5	14	2.2
2455	**Celery, raw [2 small stalks (5"long)]**	**34**	**1.2**	**5**	**8%**	**0**	**1**	**0.6**
2456	Celery, stuffed with cheese [1 small stalk (5"long)]	32	1.1	39	78%	1	1	0.4
2457	Chard, cooked without salt [1 cup, stalk and leaves]	145	5.1	29	4%	3	6	3.0
2458	Chard, raw [1 cup]	36	1.3	7	9%	1	1	0.6
2459	Chives, dried or dehydrated [2Tbs]	2	0.1	6	22%	1	1	0.5
2460	Chives, raw [2Tbs]	6	0.2	2	22%	0	0	0.2
2461	Christophine, cooked without salt (Include chayote) [1 cup]	160	5.6	33	6%	1	8	3.0
2462	Christophine, creamed, Puerto Rican style (Chayote a la crema) [½ chayote (4½"x3½"x1½"), without shell]	107	3.8	154	27%	2	27	1.6
2463	**Cilantro, raw (Include coriander leaves, chinese parsley) [1 cup]**	**16**	**0.6**	**4**	**18%**	**0**	**1**	**0.4**
2464	Cress, canned [1 cup]	135	4.8	31	23%	3	5	0.9
2465	Cobb salad with dressing [1 cup]	129	4.6	179	74%	8	5	2.3

Food #	fat gm	sat fat gm	choles mg	sodium mg	potass mg	vit A	vit E	vit C	thia-min	ribo-flavin	nia-cin	vit B-6	fol-ate	vit B-12	cal-cium	phos-phorus	magne-sium	iron	zinc
2419	0	0.	0	26	376	5	0	26	1	3	3	4	1	0	19	2	17	4	2
2420	14	3	39	266	251	20	7	32	7	10	7	3	26	3	10	9	3	8	4
2421	0	0	0	8	342	366	6	12	3	5	3	5	5	0	4	6	10	13	2
2422	0	0	0	41	381	159	2	4	5	4	5	8	2	0	3	5	4	3	2
2423	10	1	0	176	239	80	9	49	3	2	3	8	3	0	2	3	6	6	1
2424	0	0	0	353	261	201	2	6	2	3	4	8	3	0	4	4	3	5	3
2425	11	3	7	670	384	175	6	7	6	14	6	9	5	5	15	13	6	6	5
2426	12	2	0	478	304	204	8	6	2	3	4	8	3	0	5	4	4	6	3
2427	0	0	0	50	231	141	2	5	2	2	3	8	3	0	5	3	3	4	3
2428	16	8	33	722	372	204	5	7	5	15	5	10	5	5	30	23	7	7	10
2429	0	0	0	103	354	383	2	6	4	5	4	19	5	0	5	5	5	5	3
2430	11	3	7	443	445	316	6	6	8	15	5	18	6	5	16	14	8	6	5
2431	12	2	0	232	371	354	8	5	3	5	4	17	5	0	6	5	6	6	3
2432	15	7	32	463	443	364	5	6	6	17	5	20	7	5	30	23	9	7	10
2433	11	3	7	445	358	223	6	7	7	14	5	10	5	5	16	13	7	5	5
2434	0	0	0	86	231	258	2	7	3	3	3	9	4	0	4	4	4	4	2
2435	12	2	0	222	274	259	8	6	3	3	3	9	4	0	6	4	5	5	2
2436	16	7	33	465	343	260	5	7	6	16	4	11	6	5	31	23	8	6	10
2437	0	0	0	17	161	140	1	8	3	2	2	4	2	0	1	2	2	1	1
2438	30	4	22	249	600	265	17	22	10	5	6	22	5	2	5	9	7	8	2
2439	1	0	0	27	515	0	1	49	10	5	8	8	10	0	3	5	10	3	4
2440	0	0	0	11	197	0	1	18	4	2	3	3	4	0	1	2	4	1	2
2441	25	5	35	371	404	6	11	44	17	10	12	10	5	5	4	13	7	5	10
2442	8	1	0	354	538	10	6	66	9	6	8	12	9	0	4	6	10	5	4
2443	8	2	5	96	103	2	5	20	4	5	3	3	5	1	4	8	2	3	2
2444	1	0	0	563	254	0	0	132	5	6	4	15	20	0	3	6	4	3	2
2445	1	0	0	19	178	0	0	92	4	4	3	11	14	0	2	4	3	2	2
2446	0	0	0	32	250	0	0	94	4	6	3	8	18	0	3	4	4	4	2
2447	18	8	36	441	320	12	4	98	7	18	4	14	17	5	32	26	7	5	10
2448	18	8	36	832	319	12	4	98	7	18	4	13	17	5	31	26	7	5	10
2449	18	8	36	441	320	12	4	98	7	18	4	14	17	5	32	26	7	5	10
2450	14	7	29	361	316	10	3	80	7	16	3	8	17	4	26	21	7	5	8
2451	0	0	0	30	303	0	0	77	4	4	3	11	14	0	2	4	4	2	2
2452	0	0	0	155	441	0	2	14	4	5	5	12	2	0	7	17	8	6	3
2453	0	0	0	137	426	2	2	15	4	4	2	6	8	0	6	4	5	4	1
2454	11	3	7	480	515	7	6	14	8	15	4	7	9	5	17	13	7	5	4
2455	0	0	0	30	98	0	0	4	1	1	1	1	2	0	1	1	1	1	0
2456	3	2	10	85	77	4	1	3	1	2	0	1	2	1	3	4	1	1	1
2457	0	0	0	260	796	46	9	44	3	7	3	6	3	0	8	5	31	18	3
2458	0	0	0	77	136	12	2	18	1	2	1	2	1	0	2	2	7	4	1
2459	0	0	0	1	59	8	0	16	1	1	1	1	4	0	2	1	2	2	1
2460	0	0	0	0	18	3	0	6	0	0	0	0	2	0	1	0	1	1	0
2461	0	0	0	3	198	1	1	15	2	3	4	6	27	0	3	3	5	3	8
2462	5	1	47	88	161	5	2	8	4	6	3	4	17	3	5	6	4	4	6
2463	0	0	0	9	82	10	1	9	1	2	1	1	2	0	1	1	1	1	0
2464	1	0	0	380	473	103	3	51	5	13	5	11	12	0	8	6	9	6	1
2465	15	4	72	256	376	14	6	20	7	11	10	10	16	5	6	11	6	6	5

Fruits & Vegetables

Food #	Food Description & Amount	wt gm	wt oz	calo-ries	%cal fat	prot gm	carbo gm	fiber gm
2466	Collards, canned [1 cup]	162	5.7	42	12%	3	8	4.5
2467	Collards, cooked, from fresh, without salt [1 cup, fresh]	128	4.5	33	12%	3	6	3.6
2468	Collards, cooked, from frozen [1 cup, frozen]	170	6.0	61	10%	5	12	4.8
2469	Collards, raw [1 cup]	186	6.6	56	13%	5	11	6.7
2470	Corn fritter [1 cup]	107	3.8	405	50%	8	43	2.2
2471	Corn with cream sauce [1 cup]	228	8.0	291	42%	8	39	3.4
2472	Corn with peppers, red or green, cooked without salt (Include Mexican style corn) [1 cup]	178	6.3	179	11%	6	42	4.7
2473	Corn, canned, with cream sauce, made with milk [1 cup]	228	8.0	261	46%	7	32	2.5
2474	Corn, cooked, from fresh, with cream sauce, made with milk [1 cup]	228	8.0	291	42%	8	39	3.4
2475	Corn, cooked, from frozen, with cream sauce, made with milk [1 cup]	228	8.0	259	44%	8	33	2.9
2476	Corn, dried, cooked [2 oz]	56	2.0	75	45%	1	11	0.9
2477	Corn, raw [1 cup]	154	5.4	132	12%	5	29	4.2
2478	Corn, scalloped or pudding (Include corn souffle) [1 cup]	214	7.5	260	38%	10	34	3.3
2479	Corn, white, canned [1 cup]	164	5.8	133	11%	4	30	3.3
2480	Corn, white, cooked, from fresh, without salt [1 medium ear (6¾" to 7½" long)]	100	3.5	108	11%	3	25	2.7
2481	Corn, white, cooked, from frozen [1 cup]	164	5.8	131	5%	5	32	3.9
2482	Corn, white, canned, cream style [1 cup]	256	9.0	184	5%	4	46	3.1
2483	Corn, yellow, canned, low sodium [1 cup]	164	5.8	177	11%	5	41	4.6
2484	Corn, yellow, canned [1 cup]	164	5.8	133	11%	4	30	3.3
2485	**Corn, yellow, cooked, from fresh, without salt [1 medium ear (6¾" to 7½" long)]**	**100**	**3.5**	**108**	**11%**	**3**	**25**	**2.8**
2486	Corn, yellow, cooked, from frozen [1 cup]	164	5.8	131	5%	5	32	3.9
2487	Corn, yellow, from canned, cream style [1 cup]	256	9.0	184	5%	4	46	3.1
2488	Cowpeas with snap beans, cooked [1 cup]	138	4.9	126	4%	4	26	6.7
2489	Cress, cooked, from fresh [1 cup]	135	4.8	31	23%	3	5	0.9
2490	Cress, raw [1 cup]	50	1.8	16	20%	1	3	0.6
2491	Cucumber-carrot-mushroom namasu (marinade of vinegar, sugar, ginger root) [1 cup]	155	5.5	52	3%	1	13	1.3
2492	Cucumber salad without oil (cucumber, onions, vinegar, sugar) [1 cup]	159	5.6	48	3%	1	12	1.1
2493	Cucumber salad with oil (cucumber, onion, vinegar, soybean oil, sugar, salt) [1 cup]	159	5.6	179	78%	1	11	1.0
2494	Cucumber salad (cucumbers with sour cream) [1 cup]	133	4.7	68	74%	1	4	0.8
2495	Cucumber, cooked without salt [1 cup]	180	6.3	29	9%	2	6	1.8
2496	**Cucumber, raw [1 small (6½" long)]**	**158**	**5.6**	**19**	**12%**	**1**	**4**	**1.1**
2497	Dandelion greens, cooked without salt [1 cup, chopped]	105	3.7	35	16%	2	7	3.0
2498	Dandelion greens, raw [1 cup]	55	1.9	25	14%	1	5	1.9
2499	Dasheen, boiled (Include malanga) [1 cup, pieces]	190	6.7	285	2%	4	67	10.4
2500	Dasheen, fried (Include malanga) [1 cup, pieces]	123	4.3	306	31%	1	52	7.7
2501	Eggplant in tomato sauce, cooked [1 cup]	231	8.1	67	6%	3	16	4.3
2502	Eggplant, batter-dipped, fried [1 cup]	220	7.8	329	65%	5	26	5.2
2503	Eggplant, cooked without salt [1 eggplant]	538	19.0	151	7%	4	36	13.5
2504	Eggplant, raw [1 eggplant, peeled (yield from 1.25 lb)]	458	16.2	119	6%	5	28	11.5
2505	Endive, chicory, escarole, or romaine, raw [1 cup, mixed greens]	40	1.4	7	12%	1	1	1.2
2506	Escarole, cooked without salt (Include endive) [1 cup]	130	4.6	29	11%	2	6	5.2
2507	Escarole, creamed [1 cup]	200	7.1	173	57%	6	14	5.1
2508	Fern shoots, cooked without salt (Include fiddleheads) [1 cup]	142	5.0	57	2%	0	16	5.3
2509	Flowers or blossoms of sesbania, squash, or lily [1 cup]	104	3.7	16	5%	1	3	0.9
2510	Fried stuffed potatoes, Puerto Rican style (Rellenos de papas) [1 fritter (4"x2"x¾")]	95	3.4	167	51%	5	16	1.3
2511	**Garlic, raw [4 cloves]**	**12**	**0.4**	**18**	**3%**	**1**	**4**	**0.3**
2512	Garlic, cooked without salt [4 cloves]	8	0.3	12	3%	1	3	0.2
2513	Ginger, raw [¼ cup sliced fresh ginger]	24	0.8	17	1%	0	4	0.5
2514	Greek Salad [1 cup]	105	3.7	106	62%	7	3	1.0
2515	Green peppers and onions, cooked, fat added [1 cup]	144	5.1	80	38%	2	12	1.9

Food #	fat gm	sat fat gm	choles mg	sodium mg	potass mg	% of Daily Value													
						vit A	vit E	vit C	thia-min	ribo-flavin	nia-cin	vit B-6	fol-ate	vit B-12	cal-cium	phos-phorus	magne-sium	iron	zinc
2466	1	0	0	448	418	50	5	49	4	10	5	10	37	0	19	4	7	4	5
2467	0	0	0	12	333	40	4	39	3	8	4	8	30	0	15	3	5	3	4
2468	1	0	0	85	427	102	3	75	5	12	5	10	32	0	36	5	13	11	3
2469	1	0	0	37	314	71	14	109	7	14	7	15	77	0	27	2	4	2	2
2470	23	5	72	318	203	6	9	6	18	20	14	3	17	3	13	16	6	16	5
2471	14	4	8	426	461	9	6	13	21	17	11	6	15	5	14	23	13	6	7
2472	2	0	0	28	429	5	1	37	24	7	13	7	19	0	0	17	13	6	5
2473	13	3	8	649	400	8	6	17	8	18	9	5	15	5	14	19	10	8	6
2474	14	4	8	426	461	9	6	13	21	17	11	6	15	5	14	23	13	6	7
2475	13	3	8	412	346	9	6	7	12	17	10	10	11	5	14	18	9	4	6
2476	4	1	0	138	98	4	2	7	1	3	3	1	6	0	1	3	2	2	1
2477	2	0	0	23	416	4	0	17	21	5	13	4	18	0	0	14	14	4	5
2478	11	3	155	140	420	17	4	11	9	21	11	15	13	7	9	21	9	6	7
2479	2	0	0	530	320	0	0	22	3	8	10	4	19	0	1	11	8	8	4
2480	1	0	0	17	249	0	0	10	14	4	8	3	12	0	0	10	8	3	3
2481	1	0	0	8	241	0	0	8	9	7	11	11	13	0	1	9	8	3	4
2482	1	0	0	730	343	0	1	19	4	8	12	8	27	0	1	13	11	5	9
2483	2	0	0	28	408	4	0	17	24	7	13	5	19	0	0	17	13	6	5
2484	2	0	0	351	320	3	1	22	3	8	10	4	19	0	1	11	8	8	4
2485	1	0	0	17	249	2	0	10	14	4	8	3	12	0	0	10	8	3	3
2486	1	0	0	8	241	4	0	8	9	7	11	11	13	0	1	9	8	3	4
2487	1	0	0	730	343	3	1	19	4	8	12	8	27	0	1	13	11	5	9
2488	1	0	0	5	561	11	1	7	9	12	9	4	41	0	17	7	17	9	9
2489	1	0	0	11	477	104	3	52	5	13	5	11	12	0	8	6	9	6	1
2490	0	0	0	7	303	47	1	58	3	8	3	6	10	0	4	4	5	4	1
2491	0	0	0	8	221	46	1	11	3	4	4	3	4	0	2	4	5	2	2
2492	0	0	0	3	206	2	0	10	2	1	1	3	4	0	2	3	5	3	2
2493	15	2	0	329	186	2	10	10	2	1	1	3	4	0	2	3	5	3	1
2494	6	3	11	16	196	6	1	5	2	3	1	4	4	1	5	4	4	1	1
2495	0	0	0	4	288	4	1	16	3	3	2	4	5	0	3	4	6	3	3
2496	0	0	0	3	234	1	0	7	2	1	1	6	6	0	2	3	5	1	1
2497	1	0	0	46	244	123	9	32	9	11	3	8	3	0	15	4	6	11	2
2498	0	0	0	42	218	77	5	32	7	8	2	7	4	0	10	4	5	9	2
2499	1	0	0	27	1355	0	20	12	13	3	7	32	9	0	10	19	20	7	4
2500	11	2	0	23	726	0	7	10	9	2	4	24	5	0	3	11	11	6	3
2501	0	0	0	787	732	13	6	30	11	6	10	14	7	0	2	6	9	8	3
2502	24	5	36	66	465	2	11	4	13	12	10	9	12	2	6	10	8	9	4
2503	1	0	0	16	1334	3	1	12	27	6	16	23	19	0	3	12	17	10	5
2504	1	0	0	14	994	4	0	13	16	9	14	19	22	0	3	10	16	7	4
2505	0	0	0	10	137	12	1	12	2	2	1	1	13	0	3	2	2	2	1
2506	0	0	0	35	477	33	2	11	8	7	3	1	39	0	8	4	6	7	8
2507	11	3	7	386	605	36	7	12	12	18	5	3	39	5	20	14	9	9	11
2508	0	0	0	7	7	3	4	71	0	25	25	13	5	0	1	1	2	1	3
2509	0	0	0	6	110	18	0	9	1	2	2	3	11	0	4	4	7	5	1
2510	10	2	31	76	443	1	5	17	8	5	9	12	3	2	1	7	5	5	4
2511	0	0	0	2	48	0	0	6	2	1	0	7	0	0	2	2	1	1	1
2512	0	0	0	1	32	0	0	3	1	0	0	5	0	0	1	1	1	1	1
2513	0	0	0	3	100	0	0	2	0	0	1	2	1	0	0	1	3	1	1
2514	7	3	119	410	181	13	3	10	5	18	5	8	11	10	12	12	5	6	6
2515	3	1	0	40	234	6	3	76	5	2	2	12	5	0	2	4	4	3	2

Fruits & Vegetables

Food #	Food Description & Amount	wt gm	wt oz	calo-ries	%cal fat	prot gm	carbo gm	fiber gm
2516	Green plantain with cracklings, Puerto Rican style (Mofongo) [1 ball (3"dia)]	64	2.3	229	63%	6	17	1.2
2517	Greens, canned [1 cup]	170	6.0	42	12%	3	8	4.7
2518	Greens, cooked, from fresh, without salt [1 cup]	146	5.1	36	12%	3	7	4.1
2519	Greens, cooked, from frozen [1 cup]	161	5.7	52	12%	5	9	4.5
2520	Hominy, white, canned [1 cup]	165	5.8	119	11%	2	24	4.1
2521	Horseradish (marong-gay), pods, cooked without salt [1 cup]	118	4.2	42	5%	2	10	5.0
2522	Jai, Monk's Food (mushrooms, lily roots, bean curd, water chestnuts) [1 cup]	188	6.6	179	23%	10	29	5.6
2523	**Jicama, raw (Include yambean) [1 cup]**	130	4.6	49	2%	1	11	6.4
2524	Kale, canned [1 cup, canned]	163	5.7	45	13%	3	9	3.2
2525	Kale, cooked, from fresh, without salt [1 cup]	130	4.6	36	13%	2	7	2.6
2526	Kale, cooked, from frozen [1 cup]	130	4.6	39	15%	4	7	2.6
2527	Kohlrabi, cooked without salt [1 cup]	165	5.8	48	3%	3	11	1.8
2528	Kohlrabi, creamed [1 cup]	187	6.6	149	52%	5	15	1.3
2529	Kohlrabi, raw [1 cup]	135	4.8	36	3%	2	8	4.9
2530	Lambsquarter, cooked without salt [1 cup]	180	6.3	58	20%	6	9	3.8
2531	Leek, cooked with margarine [1 cup]	171	6.0	163	39%	3	24	3.1
2532	Leek, raw [1 leek]	89	3.1	54	4%	1	13	1.6
2533	Lettuce salad with egg, cheese, tomato, and/or carrots, with or without other vegetables, no dressing (Include McDonald's Garden Salad; McDonald's Side Salad) [1 salad]	236	8.3	122	56%	8	7	2.8
2534	**Lettuce, Boston (Include deer tongue lettuce, native lettuce, red leaf lettuce) [1 cup, shredded or chopped]**	55	1.9	7	15%	1	1	0.6
2535	Lettuce, cooked without salt [1 cup]	81	2.9	10	14%	1	2	1.1
2536	Lettuce, manoa [1 cup]	50	1.8	7	14%	1	1	0.8
2537	**Lettuce, iceberg, raw [1 cup, shredded or chopped]**	55	1.9	7	14%	1	1	0.8
2538	Lettuce salad with assorted vegetables, no tomatoes, carrots, or dressing [1 cup]	74	2.6	11	10%	1	2	0.9
2539	Lettuce salad with assorted vegetables including tomatoes and/or carrots, no dressing (Include Burger King Side Salad, Hardee's Side Salad) [1 cup]	73	2.6	13	12%	1	3	1.1
2540	Lettuce salad with avocado, tomato, and/or carrots, with or without other vegetables, no dressing [1 cup]	87	3.1	45	63%	1	4	2.1
2541	Lettuce salad with cheese, tomato and/or carrots, with or without other vegetables, no dressing (Include Burger King Garden Salad) [1 cup]	77	2.7	79	64%	5	3	1.0
2542	Lettuce salad with egg, tomato, and/or carrots, with or without other vegetables, no dressing [1 cup]	88	3.1	47	47%	3	3	1.1
2543	Lettuce, wilted, with bacon dressing [1 cup]	125	4.4	103	76%	3	4	1.9
2544	Lima beans, raw [1 cup]	156	5.5	176	7%	11	31	7.6
2545	Lima beans, canned, low sodium, no fat [1 cup]	174	6.1	124	4%	7	23	6.3
2546	Lima beans, canned [1 cup]	174	6.1	213	2%	12	41	9.2
2547	Lima beans, canned, with mushroom sauce [1 cup]	228	8.0	247	27%	10	36	6.5
2548	Lima beans, canned, creamed or with cheese sauce [1 cup]	228	8.0	338	33%	18	39	7.9
2549	Lima beans, cooked, from fresh, without salt [1 cup]	170	6.0	209	2%	12	40	9.0
2550	Lima beans, cooked, from fresh, with mushroom sauce [1 cup]	228	8.0	247	27%	10	36	6.6
2551	Lima beans, cooked, from fresh, creamed or with cheese sauce [1 cup]	228	8.0	340	33%	18	40	7.9
2552	**Lima beans, cooked, from frozen [1 cup]**	180	6.3	185	3%	11	34	10.6
2553	Lima beans, cooked, from frozen, with mushroom sauce [1 cup]	228	8.0	220	31%	9	30	7.2
2554	Lima beans, from frozen, creamed or with cheese sauce [1 cup]	228	8.0	308	35%	18	33	8.9
2555	Lotus root, cooked [1 cup]	120	4.2	79	1%	2	19	3.7
2556	Luffa (Chinese okra), cooked [1 cup]	178	6.3	57	5%	3	13	4.5
2557	**Mixed salad greens, raw [1 cup, shredded or chopped]**	55	1.9	9	13%	1	2	1.2
2558	Mixed vegetables (corn, lima beans, peas, green beans, and carrots), canned, low sodium [1 cup]	182	6.4	66	5%	3	13	5.6
2559	Mixed vegetables (corn, lima beans, peas, green beans, and carrots), canned [1 cup]	182	6.4	86	5%	5	17	5.5

Food #	fat gm	sat fat gm	choles mg	sodium mg	potass mg	vit A	vit E	vit C	thia-min	ribo-flavin	nia-cin	vit B-6	fol-ate	vit B-12	cal-cium	phos-phorus	magne-sium	iron	zinc
2516	16	4	15	276	326	5	6	12	9	4	8	10	2	5	0	8	6	3	4
2517	1	0	0	439	394	86	6	77	5	9	4	12	33	0	19	5	8	6	3
2518	0	0	0	28	341	74	6	67	4	7	4	11	29	0	16	4	7	6	3
2519	1	0	0	45	420	109	7	66	5	9	5	7	18	0	27	5	10	12	3
2520	1	0	0	347	15	0	0	0	0	1	0	0	0	0	2	6	7	6	12
2521	0	0	0	51	539	1	0	191	4	5	3	7	9	0	2	6	12	3	3
2522	5	1	0	28	641	1	1	19	11	19	17	19	12	0	10	18	31	29	17
2523	0	0	0	5	195	0	2	44	2	2	1	3	4	0	2	2	4	4	1
2524	1	0	0	500	369	120	5	111	6	7	4	11	5	0	12	5	7	8	3
2525	1	0	0	30	296	96	4	89	5	5	3	9	4	0	9	4	6	7	2
2526	1	0	0	20	417	83	1	55	4	9	4	6	5	0	18	4	6	7	2
2527	0	0	0	35	561	1	9	149	4	2	3	13	5	0	4	7	8	4	3
2528	9	2	6	308	487	5	10	97	7	10	4	10	5	4	12	13	8	4	4
2529	0	0	0	27	473	1	2	140	5	2	3	10	5	0	3	6	6	3	0
2530	1	0	0	52	518	175	8	111	12	28	8	16	6	0	46	8	10	7	4
2531	7	1	0	109	282	8	9	24	6	3	3	19	19	0	10	6	11	19	1
2532	0	0	0	18	160	1	3	18	4	2	2	10	14	0	5	3	6	10	1
2533	8	4	87	151	417	34	3	28	7	13	3	7	23	5	16	16	7	7	7
2534	0	0	0	3	141	5	1	7	2	2	1	1	10	0	2	1	2	1	1
2535	0	0	0	7	128	3	1	4	2	1	1	1	10	0	2	2	2	2	1
2536	0	0	0	4	121	7	1	11	2	2	1	1	10	0	2	1	1	2	1
2537	0	0	0	5	87	2	1	4	2	1	1	1	8	0	1	1	1	2	1
2538	0	0	0	15	132	1	1	5	2	1	1	2	6	0	2	2	2	1	1
2539	0	0	0	13	149	18	1	12	3	2	1	2	7	0	1	2	2	2	1
2540	3	1	0	15	263	35	2	14	4	3	3	5	9	0	1	3	4	3	1
2541	6	3	17	115	152	36	1	11	3	5	1	3	6	2	13	10	3	2	4
2542	2	1	91	42	176	38	1	12	3	8	2	4	8	4	2	5	2	3	2
2543	9	3	10	99	306	19	2	27	6	6	4	4	12	2	7	5	4	9	3
2544	1	0	0	12	729	5	4	61	23	9	11	16	13	0	5	21	23	27	8
2545	1	0	0	7	496	3	2	25	3	4	5	5	7	0	5	12	15	16	7
2546	1	0	0	408	986	6	1	29	16	10	9	17	11	0	6	22	32	24	9
2547	7	2	3	896	767	5	4	21	13	12	9	12	9	2	9	20	24	18	10
2548	12	6	30	681	957	14	2	26	16	20	9	16	11	5	29	37	31	22	14
2549	1	0	0	29	969	6	1	29	16	10	9	16	11	0	5	22	31	23	9
2550	7	2	3	638	770	5	4	21	13	12	9	12	9	2	9	20	24	18	10
2551	12	6	30	358	961	15	2	26	16	20	9	16	11	5	29	37	31	22	14
2552	1	0	0	73	737	3	3	28	9	6	8	11	8	0	5	16	20	17	6
2553	7	2	3	681	577	3	4	27	8	10	9	8	7	2	7	13	12	11	7
2554	12	6	30	387	726	12	4	24	9	16	8	11	9	5	28	31	21	15	11
2555	0	0	0	54	436	0	0	55	10	1	2	13	2	0	3	9	7	6	3
2556	0	0	0	9	573	10	4	48	16	6	8	17	20	0	11	10	25	4	7
2557	0	0	0	14	174	15	1	15	3	3	1	2	16	0	3	2	3	4	2
2558	0	0	0	47	251	92	1	12	4	4	4	7	8	0	4	7	7	7	6
2559	0	0	0	271	530	212	4	14	5	5	5	7	10	0	5	8	7	11	5

Fruits & Vegetables

Food #	Food Description & Amount	wt gm	wt oz	calo-ries	%cal fat	prot gm	carbo gm	fiber gm
2560	Mixed vegetables (corn, lima beans, peas, green beans, and carrots), cooked, from frozen [1 cup]	182	6.4	107	2%	5	24	8.0
2561	Mixed vegetables (green beans, broccoli, onions, mushrooms), cooked [1 cup]	129	4.6	36	6%	2	8	3.4
2562	Mixed vegetables, stew type (including potatoes, carrots, onions, celery) cooked [1 cup]	160	5.6	77	2%	2	17	3.5
2563	Mushroom, Oriental, dried (Include shiitake) [1 cup]	145	5.1	80	4%	2	21	3.0
2564	Mushrooms, batter-dipped, fried [4 small]	32	1.1	71	68%	1	5	0.4
2565	Mushrooms, canned [1 cup]	156	5.5	37	11%	3	8	3.7
2566	**Mushrooms, cooked, from fresh or frozen, without salt [1 cup]**	156	5.5	42	16%	3	8	3.4
2567	Mushrooms, from canned or frozen, creamed [1 cup]	217	7.7	171	56%	6	15	3.1
2568	Mushrooms, cooked from fresh, creamed [1 cup]	217	7.7	174	56%	6	15	2.8
2569	Mushrooms, raw [1 cup, pieces]	70	2.5	18	15%	1	3	0.8
2570	Mushrooms, stuffed [2 stuffed caps]	48	1.7	138	48%	5	13	0.9
2571	Mustard cabbage, cooked without salt [1 cup]	170	6.0	20	12%	3	3	2.7
2572	Mustard greens, canned [1 cup, canned]	153	5.4	23	14%	3	3	3.0
2573	Mustard greens, cooked, from fresh, without salt [1 cup, fresh]	140	4.9	21	14%	3	3	2.8
2574	Mustard greens, cooked, from frozen [1 cup]	150	5.3	29	12%	3	5	4.2
2575	Mustard greens, raw [1 cup]	56	2.0	15	7%	2	3	1.8
2576	Okra, batter- or cornmeal-dipped, fried in corn oil [1 cup]	92	3.2	175	64%	2	14	2.2
2577	Okra, canned [1 cup]	167	5.9	53	5%	3	12	4.1
2578	Okra, cooked, from fresh [1 cup]	160	5.6	51	5%	3	12	4.0
2579	Okra, cooked, from frozen [1 cup]	184	6.5	52	10%	4	11	5.2
2580	**Onion rings, batter-dipped, fried in corn oil [10 small rings (1½"dia)]**	48	1.7	73	59%	1	7	0.8
2581	Onion rings, from fresh, batter-dipped, baked or fried [10 medium rings (2½" dia)]	60	2.1	108	62%	1	9	1.0
2582	Onion rings, from frozen, batter-dipped, baked or fried [10 medium rings (2½"dia)]	60	2.1	108	63%	1	9	0.9
2583	Onion, dehydrated [2Tbs]	7	0.2	24	1%	1	6	0.6
2584	Onions, creamed [1 cup]	228	8.0	188	45%	5	22	2.2
2585	Onions, from fresh, creamed [1 cup]	228	8.0	188	45%	5	22	2.2
2586	Onions, mature, cooked or sauteed, from fresh, fat added [1 cup]	215	7.6	126	30%	3	21	2.9
2587	Onions, mature, cooked or sauteed, from frozen, fat added [1 cup]	215	7.6	91	37%	2	14	3.4
2588	**Onions, mature, cooked, from fresh, without salt [1 cup]**	210	7.4	92	4%	3	21	2.9
2589	Onions, mature, cooked, from frozen [1 cup]	210	7.4	59	2%	2	14	3.4
2590	Onions, mature, raw (Include red onions) [1 cup, chopped]	160	5.6	61	4%	2	14	2.9
2591	Onions, pearl, canned [1 cup]	185	6.5	81	4%	2	19	2.6
2592	Onions, pearl, cooked, from fresh [1 cup]	185	6.5	81	4%	3	19	2.6
2593	Onions, pearl, cooked, from frozen [1 cup]	185	6.5	52	2%	1	12	2.6
2594	Onions, young green, cooked, from fresh, without salt [1 cup]	219	7.7	74	5%	4	17	6.0
2595	Onions, young green, raw [1 cup, chopped]	100	3.5	32	5%	2	7	2.6
2596	Palm hearts, cooked without salt [1 cup]	146	5.1	150	2%	4	39	2.2
2597	Parsley, cooked without salt [10 sprigs]	12	0.4	4	20%	0	1	0.4
2598	**Parsley, raw [1 cup]**	60	2.1	22	20%	2	4	2.0
2599	Parsnips, cooked without salt [1 cup, pieces]	156	5.5	126	3%	2	30	6.2
2600	Parsnips, creamed [1 cup]	228	8.0	252	40%	6	34	5.3
2601	Pea salad with cheese (peas, cheese, mayonnaise, egg, onion, pimento, salt) [1 cup]	214	7.5	571	76%	19	18	5.6
2602	Pea salad (peas, mayonnaise, egg, onion, pimento, salt) [1 cup]	214	7.5	501	76%	11	21	6.9
2603	Peas and carrots, canned [1 cup]	160	5.6	85	5%	5	16	5.0
2604	Peas and carrots, canned, low sodium [1 cup]	160	5.6	61	6%	3	14	5.3
2605	Peas and carrots, cooked, from fresh [1 cup]	160	5.6	110	3%	6	22	7.4
2606	Peas and carrots, cooked, from frozen [1 cup]	160	5.6	77	8%	5	16	5.0
2607	Peas and carrots, canned, creamed [1 cup]	244	8.6	230	46%	8	24	4.5
2608	Peas and carrots, cooked from fresh, creamed [1 cup]	244	8.6	252	42%	9	28	6.5

Food #	fat gm	sat fat gm	choles mg	sodium mg	potass mg	% of Daily Value													
						vit A	vit E	vit C	thia-min	ribo-flavin	nia-cin	vit B-6	fol-ate	vit B-12	cal-cium	phos-phorus	magne-sium	iron	zinc
2560	0	0	0	64	308	78	2	10	9	13	8	7	9	0	5	9	10	8	6
2561	0	0	0	17	223	9	3	31	4	8	6	6	10	0	5	6	6	6	3
2562	0	0	0	66	366	103	1	16	7	3	6	12	5	0	3	4	4	6	2
2563	0	0	0	6	170	0	1	1	4	15	11	12	8	0	0	4	5	4	13
2564	5	1	1	51	71	0	4	1	3	7	5	1	2	0	1	5	1	3	1
2565	0	0	0	663	201	0	1	0	8	2	12	5	5	0	2	10	6	7	7
2566	1	0	0	3	555	0	1	10	8	28	35	7	7	0	1	14	5	15	9
2567	11	3	7	854	306	5	5	1	11	12	12	6	5	5	13	17	8	7	8
2568	11	3	7	344	579	5	5	9	10	32	29	8	7	5	12	20	7	13	10
2569	0	0	0	3	259	0	0	4	5	18	14	3	4	0	0	7	2	5	3
2570	7	2	6	298	209	5	3	5	10	15	13	3	5	2	10	11	4	8	5
2571	0	0	0	58	631	44	1	74	4	6	4	14	17	0	16	5	5	10	2
2572	0	0	0	428	307	46	10	64	4	6	3	7	28	0	11	6	6	6	1
2573	0	0	0	22	283	42	9	59	4	5	3	7	26	0	10	6	5	5	1
2574	0	0	0	38	209	67	9	35	4	5	2	8	26	0	15	4	5	9	2
2575	0	0	0	14	198	30	4	65	3	4	2	5	26	0	6	2	4	5	1
2576	13	2	2	122	190	4	10	17	12	8	7	6	11	1	6	12	9	7	3
2577	0	0	0	394	535	10	4	45	15	5	7	16	19	0	10	9	24	4	6
2578	0	0	0	8	515	9	4	43	14	5	7	15	18	0	10	9	23	4	6
2579	1	0	0	6	431	9	4	37	12	13	7	4	67	0	18	8	23	7	8
2580	5	1	1	46	61	0	3	3	3	3	2	2	2	0	1	4	1	2	1
2581	7	1	1	71	72	0	5	3	4	4	3	2	3	0	2	6	1	3	1
2582	8	1	1	75	66	1	5	4	4	4	3	2	3	0	2	6	1	4	1
2583	0	0	0	1	114	0	0	9	2	0	0	6	3	0	2	2	2	1	1
2584	9	2	6	305	370	5	4	14	8	11	3	11	7	4	13	13	7	3	4
2585	9	2	6	305	370	5	4	14	8	11	3	11	7	4	13	13	7	3	4
2586	4	1	0	51	351	4	3	18	6	3	2	14	8	0	5	7	6	3	3
2587	4	1	0	63	222	4	3	13	3	3	1	7	7	0	5	2	4	4	1
2588	0	0	0	6	349	0	1	18	6	3	2	14	8	0	5	7	6	3	3
2589	0	0	0	21	220	1	1	13	3	3	1	7	7	0	4	2	4	4	1
2590	0	0	0	5	251	0	1	17	4	2	1	9	8	0	3	5	4	2	2
2591	0	0	0	514	305	0	1	16	5	3	2	12	7	0	4	6	5	2	3
2592	0	0	0	6	307	0	1	16	5	3	2	12	7	0	4	6	5	2	3
2593	0	0	0	15	187	0	1	16	2	2	1	6	6	0	5	0	4	3	1
2594	0	0	0	35	573	8	1	51	7	10	6	7	26	0	16	8	11	18	6
2595	0	0	0	16	276	4	0	31	4	5	3	3	16	0	7	4	5	8	3
2596	0	0	0	20	2637	1	2	17	4	15	6	53	7	0	3	20	4	14	36
2597	0	0	0	6	60	6	1	16	1	1	1	0	3	0	2	1	1	4	1
2598	0	0	0	34	332	31	4	133	3	3	4	3	23	0	8	3	8	21	4
2599	0	0	0	16	573	0	5	34	9	5	6	7	23	0	6	11	11	5	3
2600	11	3	7	372	623	6	9	29	12	15	7	8	20	5	17	19	13	6	5
2601	48	14	144	619	349	25	18	60	19	23	11	23	19	11	34	37	12	13	19
2602	42	7	125	450	381	17	22	74	22	17	13	27	21	6	5	20	12	14	13
2603	0	0	0	397	280	88	2	18	8	6	5	6	12	0	3	8	5	7	6
2604	0	0	0	6	160	92	2	17	7	5	5	7	7	0	4	7	6	7	6
2605	0	0	0	45	406	161	2	25	18	11	11	18	18	0	5	13	12	10	9
2606	1	0	0	109	253	124	2	22	24	6	9	7	10	0	4	8	6	8	5
2607	12	3	7	719	407	81	7	17	12	17	7	8	12	0	16	18	8	8	8
2608	12	3	8	419	514	142	7	23	20	21	12	18	17	5	17	22	14	11	11

Fruits & Vegetables

Food #	Food Description & Amount	wt gm	wt oz	calo-ries	%cal fat	prot gm	carbo gm	fiber gm
2609	Peas and carrots, cooked from frozen, creamed [1 cup]	244	8.6	223	48%	8	24	4.5
2610	**Peas and corn**, cooked without salt[1 cup]	162	5.7	156	7%	7	33	6.7
2611	Peas and onions, cooked [1 cup]	180	6.3	81	4%	5	16	4.0
2612	Peas and potatoes, cooked [1 cup]	158	5.6	134	2%	6	28	6.0
2613	Peas with mushroom sauce [1 cup]	244	8.6	215	34%	9	28	7.1
2614	Peas with mushrooms, cooked [1 cup]	159	5.6	108	4%	7	20	7.7
2615	Peas, canned, with mushroom sauce [1 cup]	244	8.6	196	37%	8	24	5.5
2616	Peas, cooked, from fresh, with mushroom sauce [1 cup]	244	8.6	215	34%	9	28	7.1
2617	Peas, cooked, from frozen, with mushroom sauce [1 cup]	244	8.6	208	35%	9	26	7.1
2618	Peas, cowpeas, field peas, or blackeye peas, canned [1 cup]	180	6.3	173	4%	6	36	8.9
2619	Peas, cowpeas, field peas, or blackeye peas, cooked, from fresh (not dried) [1 cup]	165	5.8	160	4%	5	34	8.3
2620	Peas, cowpeas, field peas, or blackeye peas, cooked, from frozen (not dried) [1 cup]	170	6.0	224	5%	14	40	10.9
2621	Peas, canned, creamed [1 cup]	244	8.6	249	42%	10	27	6.0
2622	Peas, cooked from fresh, creamed [1 cup]	244	8.6	272	39%	11	31	7.7
2623	Peas, cooked from frozen, creamed [1 cup]	244	8.6	264	40%	11	29	7.7
2624	Peas, green, canned, low sodium [1 cup]	170	6.0	90	5%	5	17	5.4
2625	Peas, green, canned [1 cup]	170	6.0	117	5%	8	21	7.0
2626	Peas, green, cooked, from fresh, without salt [1 cup]	160	5.6	134	2%	9	25	8.8
2627	**Peas**, green, cooked, from frozen [1 cup]	160	5.6	125	3%	8	23	8.8
2628	Peas, green, raw [1 cup]	146	5.1	118	4%	8	21	7.4
2629	Pepper, banana, raw [1 medium (4½"long)]	46	1.6	12	15%	1	2	1.6
2630	Pepper, Jalapeno [2 peppers]	90	3.2	36	5%	2	9	1.4
2631	Pepper, poblano, raw [1 pepper]	64	2.3	17	6%	1	4	1.2
2632	Pepper, Serrano, raw [4 peppers]	24	0.9	8	12%	0	2	0.9
2633	Pepper, sweet, green, raw [1 small]	74	2.6	20	6%	1	5	1.3
2634	Pepper, sweet, red, raw [1 small]	74	2.6	20	6%	1	5	1.5
2635	Peppers, green, cooked [1 cup]	136	4.8	38	6%	1	9	1.6
2636	Peppers, hot, canned [1 cup, chopped]	136	4.8	57	4%	3	13	2.1
2637	Peppers, hot, cooked, from fresh, without salt [1 cup, chopped]	136	4.8	57	4%	3	13	2.1
2638	Peppers, hot, cooked, from frozen [1 cup, chopped]	136	4.8	57	4%	3	13	2.1
2639	Peppers, red, cooked without salt [1 cup]	136	4.8	38	6%	1	9	1.6
2640	Pigeon peas, canned [1 cup]	153	5.4	169	11%	9	30	9.4
2641	Pigeon peas, cooked, from fresh, without salt [1 cup]	153	5.4	170	11%	9	30	9.5
2642	Pimientos, cooked without salt [1 cup]	184	6.5	52	12%	2	11	4.3
2643	Pinacbet (bitter melon, eggplant, tomato, onion, olive oil, garlic, oregano, salt) [1 cup]	214	7.5	156	64%	2	14	3.6
2644	Poi [1 cup]	240	8.5	269	1%	1	65	1.0
2645	Poke greens, cooked without salt [1 cup]	155	5.5	31	18%	4	5	2.3
2646	Potato, baked, peel eaten [1 potato (2½"x4½")]	202	7.1	220	1%	5	51	4.8
2647	**Potato, baked**, peel not eaten [1 potato (2½"x4½")]	161	5.7	150	1%	3	35	2.4
2648	Potato, boiled without salt, with peel [1 medium (2½"dia, raw)]	142	5.0	124	1%	3	29	2.6
2649	Potato, boiled without salt, without peel [1 medium (2½"dia, raw)]	122	4.3	105	1%	2	24	2.2
2650	Potato, canned, without peel, low sodium [1 canned potato (1"dia)]	35	1.2	21	3%	0	5	0.8
2651	Potato, cooked, with cheese (Include au gratin potatoes) [1 cup]	244	8.6	341	45%	12	36	2.6
2652	Potato, dry, powdered [1 cup, dry flakes]	55	1.9	195	1%	5	45	3.8
2653	**Potato, french fries**, deep fried from frozen (including fast food orders) [1 large fast food order]	176	6.2	544	47%	7	68	5.6
2654	Potato, french fries, deep fried from fresh (including fried with skins) [1 large portion]	176	6.2	477	45%	7	61	5.4
2655	Potato, french fries, oven baked from frozen [1 large portion]	176	6.2	352	34%	6	55	5.6
2656	Potato, french fries, breaded or battered (Include Jack-in-the-Box Curly Fries, Arby's Curly Fries) [1 large fast food order]	179	6.3	336	48%	4	40	3.2

Food #	fat gm	sat fat gm	choles mg	sodium mg	potass mg	% of Daily Value													
						vit A	vit E	vit C	thia-min	ribo-flavin	nia-cin	vit B-6	fol-ate	vit B-12	cal-cium	phos-phorus	magne-sium	iron	zinc
2609	12	3	7	472	383	112	6	20	26	17	10	8	11	5	16	17	9	9	7
2610	1	0	0	16	421	7	1	27	26	10	15	11	22	0	2	18	14	10	9
2611	0	0	0	67	211	6	1	21	18	7	9	8	9	0	3	6	6	9	3
2612	0	0	0	190	473	5	1	29	19	8	13	19	14	0	3	12	12	8	8
2613	8	2	3	686	436	9	5	31	23	17	16	14	20	2	9	20	14	13	13
2614	0	0	0	112	326	9	1	23	26	13	16	9	20	0	3	14	10	14	10
2615	8	2	3	982	319	11	5	21	12	12	8	5	14	2	8	14	7	9	10
2616	8	2	3	686	436	9	5	31	23	17	14	14	20	2	8	20	14	13	13
2617	8	2	3	790	309	9	4	22	25	13	12	8	19	2	8	17	11	13	11
2618	1	0	0	511	747	14	1	7	12	16	13	6	57	0	23	9	23	11	12
2619	1	0	0	7	690	13	1	6	11	14	12	5	52	0	21	8	21	10	11
2620	1	0	0	9	638	1	2	7	29	6	6	8	60	0	4	21	21	20	16
2621	11	3	7	720	405	17	6	23	15	18	7	7	17	5	15	20	10	9	9
2622	12	3	7	383	538	14	7	34	29	24	16	17	24	5	16	27	17	14	14
2623	12	3	7	498	397	15	6	24	31	20	12	10	22	5	16	23	14	14	12
2624	1	0	0	15	170	6	2	28	13	7	7	6	12	0	3	9	7	10	8
2625	1	0	0	428	294	13	2	26	13	8	6	5	18	0	3	11	7	9	8
2626	0	0	0	5	434	10	2	38	28	14	16	17	25	0	4	19	16	14	13
2627	0	0	0	139	269	11	1	26	30	9	12	9	23	0	4	14	12	14	10
2628	1	0	0	7	356	9	2	97	26	11	15	12	24	0	4	16	12	12	12
2629	0	0	0	6	118	2	1	63	2	1	3	8	3	0	1	1	2	1	1
2630	0	0	0	6	306	52	2	364	5	5	4	13	5	0	2	4	6	6	2
2631	0	0	0	1	113	4	1	95	3	1	2	8	4	0	1	1	2	2	1
2632	0	0	0	2	74	2	1	18	1	1	2	6	1	0	0	1	1	1	0
2633	0	0	0	1	131	5	2	110	3	1	2	9	4	0	1	1	2	2	1
2634	0	0	0	1	131	42	2	234	3	1	2	9	4	0	1	1	2	2	1
2635	0	0	0	3	226	8	3	169	5	2	3	16	5	0	1	2	3	3	1
2636	0	0	0	10	482	10	3	487	8	7	6	18	7	0	3	7	9	9	3
2637	0	0	0	9	434	10	3	458	7	7	6	18	6	0	2	6	8	9	3
2638	0	0	0	9	434	10	3	458	7	7	6	18	6	0	2	6	8	9	3
2639	0	0	0	3	226	51	3	388	5	2	3	16	5	0	1	2	3	3	1
2640	2	1	0	377	693	2	1	71	35	15	16	4	38	0	6	18	15	13	8
2641	2	1	0	8	698	2	1	72	36	15	16	4	38	0	6	18	15	13	8
2642	1	0	0	32	356	60	5	319	3	8	7	24	3	0	1	4	3	21	3
2643	11	2	0	14	573	9	8	113	9	6	6	13	13	0	2	7	8	6	4
2644	0	0	0	29	439	0	1	16	21	6	13	33	13	0	4	9	14	12	4
2645	1	0	0	28	285	135	4	212	7	23	9	9	3	0	8	5	5	10	2
2646	0	0	0	16	844	0	0	43	14	4	17	35	6	0	2	12	14	15	4
2647	0	0	0	8	630	0	0	34	11	2	11	24	4	0	1	8	10	3	3
2648	0	0	0	6	538	0	0	31	10	2	10	21	4	0	1	6	8	2	3
2649	0	0	0	6	400	0	0	15	8	1	8	16	3	0	1	5	6	2	2
2650	0	0	0	2	80	0	0	3	2	0	2	3	0	0	0	1	1	2	1
2651	17	7	32	282	998	18	4	41	11	17	13	21	7	3	28	28	13	9	11
2652	0	0	0	59	596	0	0	77	38	4	17	21	6	0	1	8	9	4	2
2653	28	9	1	287	1253	1	1	16	16	4	20	23	15	4	3	23	15	13	6
2654	24	5	0	20	1838	0	11	89	16	7	24	42	8	0	2	16	18	14	9
2655	13	2	0	53	736	0	1	30	13	3	18	27	5	0	1	14	10	12	5
2656	18	3	3	480	447	1	11	16	16	11	15	18	7	1	3	18	8	9	4

Fruits & Vegetables

Food #	Food Description & Amount	wt gm	wt oz	calo-ries	%cal fat	prot gm	carbo gm	fiber gm
2657	Potato, hash brown, from dry mix [1 cup]	156	5.5	340	47%	5	44	3.1
2658	Potato, hash brown, from fresh [1 cup]	156	5.5	326	60%	4	33	3.1
2659	**Potato, hash brown**, from frozen [1 cup]	**145**	**5.1**	**316**	**47%**	**5**	**41**	**2.9**
2660	Potato, home fries, with onions (Include Cottage style potatoes, German fried potatoes, Potatoes O'Brien) [1 cup]	194	6.8	270	47%	3	34	3.3
2661	Potato, home fries, with green or red peppers and onions [1 cup]	145	5.1	127	13%	2	26	2.7
2662	**Potato, mashed**, made from fresh with milk and margarine [1 cup]	**210**	**7.4**	**227**	**32%**	**4**	**36**	**3.1**
2663	Potato, mashed, made from dry flakes, with milk and margarine [1 cup]	210	7.4	191	48%	4	22	1.7
2664	Potato, mashed, made with milk, margarine, and cheese [1 cup]	210	7.4	264	39%	7	34	2.8
2665	Potato, mashed, made with milk, fat, and egg (Include Pillsbury twice baked potatoes, Betty Crocker twice baked potatoes) [1 cup]	235	8.3	638	50%	17	66	5.2
2666	Potato, mashed, made with milk, fat, egg, and cheese (Include Betty Crocker Twice Baked Cheese & Potato Mix) [1 cup]	235	8.3	461	64%	19	25	3.7
2667	Potato, patty (Include potato croquettes) [1 cup]	196	6.9	374	57%	8	34	3.4
2668	Potato, puffs (Include Ore Ida Crispy Crowns) [1 cup]	128	4.5	284	44%	4	39	4.1
2669	Potato, raw (peel not eaten) [1 potato (2½"x4½")]	202	7.1	160	1%	4	36	3.2
2670	Potatoes, roasted without salt [1 cup]	122	4.3	173	1%	5	39	3.5
2671	**Potatoes, scalloped** (Include creamed potatoes) [1 cup]	**226**	**8.0**	**226**	**29%**	**7**	**35**	**2.5**
2672	Potatoes, scalloped, with ham (with or without cheese) [1 cup]	232	8.2	252	29%	13	32	2.3
2673	Potatoes, stewed, Mexican style (Include Papas guisadas) [1 cup]	231	8.1	342	53%	4	37	3.8
2674	Potatoes, stewed, Puerto Rican style (Include Papas guisadas) [1 medium]	163	5.7	186	26%	4	30	2.9
2675	Potatoes, stewed with tomatoes [1 cup]	236	8.3	189	49%	3	23	2.7
2676	Potatoes, stewed with tomatoes, Mexican style (Include Papas guisadas con tomate) [1 cup]	231	8.1	200	48%	3	24	2.9
2677	Potato, sticks (include french fry shaped) [20 sticks]	6	0.2	31	59%	0	3	0.2
2678	Potato, stuffed with ham, broccoli and cheese sauce, baked, peel eaten (Include Weight Watchers) [1 entree (11 oz)]	312	11.0	222	16%	16	31	3.4
2679	Potato, stuffed, baked, peel eaten, stuffed with bacon and cheese [1 potato (2½"x4½"raw)]	264	9.3	419	33%	13	58	5.3
2680	Potato, stuffed, baked, peel eaten, stuffed with broccoli and cheese sauce [1 potato (2½"x4½"raw)]	290	10.2	343	23%	9	60	6.5
2681	Potato, stuffed, baked, peel eaten, stuffed with cheese [1 potato (2½"x4½"raw)]	254	9.0	375	28%	11	57	5.2
2682	Potato, stuffed, baked, peel eaten, stuffed with chicken, broccoli and cheese sauce (Include Weight Watchers) [1 entree (11 oz)]	312	11.0	399	23%	25	53	5.8
2683	Potato, stuffed, baked, peel eaten, stuffed with chili [1 potato (2½"x4½"raw)]	350	12.3	421	21%	11	76	9.9
2684	Potato, stuffed, baked, peel eaten, stuffed with meat in cream sauce [1 potato (2½"x4½"raw)]	274	9.7	360	27%	11	56	5.3
2685	Potato, stuffed, baked, peel eaten, stuffed with sour cream [1 potato (2½"x4½"raw)]	284	10.0	405	38%	7	57	5.2
2686	Potato, stuffed, baked, peel not eaten, stuffed with bacon and cheese [1 potato (2½"x4½"raw)]	215	7.6	340	41%	12	39	2.6
2687	Potato, stuffed, baked, peel not eaten, stuffed with broccoli and cheese sauce [1 potato (2½"x4½"raw)]	241	8.5	262	30%	7	41	3.8
2688	Potato, stuffed, baked, peel not eaten, stuffed with cheese [1 potato (2½"x4½"raw)]	206	7.3	296	36%	9	39	2.6
2689	Potato, stuffed, baked, peel not eaten, stuffed with chicken, broccoli and cheese sauce (Include Weight Watchers) [1 entree (11 oz)]	292	10.3	356	28%	25	39	3.6
2690	Potato, stuffed, baked, peel not eaten, stuffed with chili [1 potato (2½"x4½"raw)]	295	10.4	329	27%	9	54	6.8
2691	Potato, stuffed, baked, peel not eaten, stuffed with meat in cream sauce [1 potato (2½"x4½"raw)]	225	7.9	281	34%	9	38	2.7
2692	Potato, stuffed, baked, peel not eaten, stuffed with sour cream [1 potato (2½"x4½"raw)]	236	8.3	327	48%	5	39	2.5
2693	Potato from Puerto Rican beef stew (with gravy) [1 medium potato]	160	5.6	119	11%	4	23	2.1
2694	Potato from Puerto Rican chicken fricassee (with sauce) [1 medium potato]	163	5.7	136	23%	3	24	2.1

Food #	fat gm	sat fat gm	choles mg	sodium mg	potass mg	vit A	vit E	vit C	thia-min	ribo-flavin	nia-cin	vit B-6	fol-ate	vit B-12	cal-cium	phos-phorus	magne-sium	iron	zinc
2657	18	7	0	53	680	0	1	16	12	2	19	10	3	0	2	11	7	13	3
2658	22	8	0	37	501	0	1	15	8	2	16	22	3	0	1	7	8	7	3
2659	17	7	0	49	632	0	1	15	11	2	18	9	2	0	2	10	6	12	3
2660	14	2	0	7	638	0	9	31	11	2	12	25	4	0	1	8	9	3	3
2661	2	0	0	26	442	3	1	37	8	2	8	19	4	0	2	6	7	3	2
2662	8	2	2	108	613	9	4	22	12	5	11	24	4	2	5	10	10	3	4
2663	10	2	4	160	340	11	5	34	18	6	8	10	3	3	7	9	6	2	3
2664	11	4	13	297	611	12	4	20	11	9	11	23	4	5	14	17	10	4	7
2665	35	17	305	1875	1034	33	7	84	45	30	22	32	11	12	17	31	17	9	10
2666	33	17	229	910	463	28	8	26	14	26	6	5	9	14	41	38	11	7	14
2667	24	6	148	467	489	9	10	15	13	16	11	19	9	5	6	14	8	8	6
2668	14	7	0	955	486	0	0	15	17	5	14	15	5	0	4	6	6	11	3
2669	0	0	0	12	1097	0	0	66	12	4	15	26	6	0	1	9	11	9	5
2670	0	0	0	13	1187	0	0	57	11	4	15	27	6	0	2	10	11	9	6
2671	7	2	8	115	953	10	3	39	10	13	12	19	6	2	12	16	11	8	6
2672	8	3	23	490	960	9	3	36	22	16	18	24	5	5	12	21	12	9	11
2673	20	5	9	12	979	0	8	40	8	4	13	24	5	0	2	10	10	8	5
2674	5	2	8	223	546	1	1	27	12	3	11	22	4	1	2	8	8	3	4
2675	10	1	0	14	672	4	8	42	7	4	9	15	5	0	2	7	8	6	3
2676	11	3	5	15	718	4	5	45	7	4	9	17	5	0	2	7	8	6	3
2677	2	1	0	15	74	0	1	5	0	0	1	1	1	0	0	1	1	1	0
2678	4	2	27	671	722	14	3	46	29	17	17	28	9	10	20	28	13	12	14
2679	15	7	26	545	1046	11	3	48	20	14	21	41	7	8	20	29	18	19	12
2680	9	3	9	178	1078	13	5	97	18	10	20	42	12	1	11	20	18	19	8
2681	12	6	20	430	1000	11	3	47	16	12	18	40	7	6	20	27	17	18	11
2682	10	3	55	200	1091	12	5	86	19	13	52	54	11	4	11	30	20	20	11
2683	10	3	14	510	1396	8	5	59	21	10	23	51	12	0	7	28	27	36	17
2684	11	3	21	233	997	6	4	45	18	10	23	39	7	11	5	20	16	21	13
2685	17	9	27	98	999	16	4	48	17	10	18	38	8	3	10	18	16	17	6
2686	15	7	26	540	794	11	3	37	16	12	15	29	5	8	19	25	14	5	11
2687	9	3	9	169	826	13	5	87	14	8	14	29	10	1	10	16	14	6	6
2688	12	6	20	424	753	11	3	36	12	10	12	28	4	6	19	23	13	5	9
2689	11	4	60	210	943	13	6	83	17	12	50	46	10	5	10	29	18	9	11
2690	10	3	14	507	1110	8	5	46	17	8	16	36	9	0	5	23	22	20	15
2691	11	3	21	222	752	6	4	34	14	8	17	27	5	11	3	16	12	8	11
2692	17	9	28	90	751	16	3	37	13	8	12	26	6	3	8	14	12	4	4
2693	1	1	2	327	383	0	0	13	8	2	9	14	3	1	1	6	5	4	6
2694	3	1	1	347	405	7	0	13	7	3	8	14	3	1	2	6	5	3	5

Fruits & Vegetables

Food #	Food Description & Amount	wt gm	wt oz	calories	%cal fat	prot gm	carbo gm	fiber gm
2695	Potato from Puerto-Rican style stuffed pot roast (with gravy) [1 medium potato]	137	4.8	102	11%	3	20	1.8
2696	Potato only from Puerto Rican mixed dishes [1 medium potato]	127	4.5	109	1%	2	25	2.3
2697	Potato pancake [2 pancakes (2¾"dia, 1/8" thick)]	44	1.6	85	48%	2	9	0.8
2698	Potato pudding [1 cup]	228	8.0	282	57%	8	25	2.4
2699	Potato puffs, cheese-filled [1 cup]	70	2.5	334	63%	6	27	1.8
2700	Potato salad [1 cup]	193	6.8	277	50%	3	34	3.1
2701	Potato skins, chips, plain or flavored (Include Tato Skins) [1 oz]	28	1.0	156	62%	2	14	1.0
2702	Potato skins, with adhering flesh, baked [skin from round potato (2½"dia)]	29	1.0	43	1%	1	10	1.4
2703	Potato skins, with adhering flesh, fried [skin from round potato (2½"dia)]	34	1.2	140	27%	2	24	3.4
2704	Potato skins, with adhering flesh, fried, with cheese [skin from round potato (2½"dia)]	28	1.0	114	37%	3	16	2.2
2705	Potato skins, with adhering flesh, fried, with cheese and bacon [skin from round potato (2½"dia)]	42	1.5	164	44%	5	18	2.5
2706	Puerto Rican pasteles (Include Pasteles de masa) [1 pastel (5½"x2¼"x¼")]	149	5.3	313	55%	11	26	4.1
2707	Pumpkin fritters, Puerto Rican style [2 fritters (2"dia)]	70	2.5	170	34%	2	28	0.6
2708	Pumpkin, canned [1 cup]	245	8.6	83	7%	3	20	7.1
2709	Pumpkin, cooked, from fresh or frozen, without salt [1 cup]	245	8.6	49	3%	2	12	2.7
2710	Radicchio, raw [1 cup, shredded]	40	1.4	9	10%	1	2	0.4
2711	Radish, Japanese, cooked without salt (Include daikon) [1 cup]	147	5.2	28	5%	1	6	2.5
2712	**Radish**, raw [4 small]	8	0.3	2	24%	0	0	0.1
2713	Ratatouille [1 cup]	214	7.5	152	72%	2	11	3.2
2714	Rutabaga, cooked without salt [1 cup, pieces]	170	6.0	66	5%	2	15	3.1
2715	Rutabaga, raw [1 small]	192	6.8	69	5%	2	16	4.8
2716	Salsify, cooked without salt (Include vegetable oyster) [1 cup]	135	4.8	92	2%	4	21	4.2
2717	**Sauerkraut**, canned [1 cup]	142	5.0	27	7%	1	6	3.6
2718	Sauerkraut, canned, low sodium [1 cup]	142	5.0	27	5%	1	6	3.6
2719	Seaweed, dried (Include sea moss, kelp) [½ cup]	8	0.3	22	12%	2	4	0.4
2720	Seaweed, prepared with soy sauce [1 cup]	96	3.4	41	9%	4	8	0.7
2721	Seaweed, raw or blanched [1 cup]	80	2.8	31	6%	2	7	0.7
2722	Sequin, cooked (Include Portuguese squash) [1 cup]	180	6.3	36	14%	2	8	2.5
2723	Seven-layer salad (lettuce salad made wiith onion, celery, green pepper, peas, mayonnaise, cheese, eggs, and/or bacon) [1 cup]	119	4.2	197	65%	5	13	1.6
2724	**Snow peas**, raw (Include pea pods) [1 cup]	145	5.1	61	4%	4	11	3.8
2725	Snow peas, cooked, from fresh or frozen, without salt [1 cup]	160	5.6	67	5%	5	11	4.5
2726	Snow peas, cooked, from frozen [1 cup]	160	5.6	83	7%	6	14	5.0
2727	Spinach and cheese casserole (Include spinach casserole) [1 cup]	200	7.1	271	48%	15	21	3.0
2728	Spinach and chickpeas, fat added [1 cup]	245	8.6	195	44%	10	21	8.5
2729	Spinach salad (spinach, mushrooms, eggs, croutons), no dressing [1 cup]	74	2.6	108	40%	5	11	1.6
2730	Spinach souffle [1 cup]	100	3.5	125	60%	5	7	0.9
2731	**Spinach, raw** [1 cup]	30	1.1	7	14%	1	1	0.8
2732	Spinach, canned [1 cup, canned]	214	7.5	49	20%	6	7	5.1
2733	Spinach, cooked, from fresh [1 cup, fresh]	180	6.3	41	10%	5	7	4.3
2734	Spinach, cooked, from frozen [1 cup, frozen, chopped]	205	7.2	57	7%	6	11	6.2
2735	Spinach, cooked, from frozen [1 cup, frozen, leaf]	190	6.7	53	7%	6	10	5.7
2736	Spinach, canned, with cheese sauce [1 cup]	200	7.1	157	59%	9	10	3.4
2737	Spinach, cooked, from fresh, with cheese sauce [1 cup]	200	7.1	170	58%	9	10	3.2
2738	Spinach, cooked, from frozen, with cheese sauce [1 cup]	200	7.1	172	55%	9	12	4.0
2739	Spinach, canned, creamed [1 cup]	200	7.1	137	55%	6	11	3.2
2740	Spinach, cooked, from fresh, creamed [1 cup]	200	7.1	148	55%	7	12	3.0
2741	Spinach, cooked, from frozen, creamed [1 cup]	200	7.1	150	52%	7	14	3.8
2742	Sprouts (1:1 mix of alfalfa and mung sprouts) [1 cup]	56	2.0	16	15%	2	3	1.2

Food #	fat gm	sat fat gm	choles mg	sodium mg	potass mg	vit A	vit E	vit C	thia-min	ribo-flavin	nia-cin	vit B-6	fol-ate	vit B-12	cal-cium	phos-phorus	magne-sium	iron	zinc
						\multicolumn{14}{c}{% of Daily Value}												
2695	1	1	1	280	328	0	0	11	7	2	7	12	2	1	1	5	5	3	5
2696	0	0	0	6	417	0	0	16	8	1	8	17	3	0	1	5	6	2	2
2697	4	1	31	12	250	1	2	12	3	3	4	6	2	1	1	4	3	3	2
2698	18	7	151	511	499	20	5	15	10	18	7	17	6	9	12	17	8	4	6
2699	23	7	12	604	545	4	8	7	7	9	8	5	1	1	13	23	9	4	6
2700	15	2	11	211	599	3	8	40	11	2	11	28	5	1	2	8	9	4	4
2701	11	3	0	184	282	0	5	4	4	2	4	2	0	0	1	4	4	2	1
2702	0	0	0	4	141	0	0	6	2	1	3	7	1	0	1	2	3	6	1
2703	4	1	0	9	338	0	2	12	4	3	8	15	2	0	1	5	6	15	2
2704	5	2	6	42	224	2	2	8	3	3	5	10	2	0	5	6	4	10	2
2705	8	3	13	154	289	2	2	11	7	5	8	13	2	2	6	10	5	12	4
2706	19	7	37	234	593	5	4	29	17	9	11	18	12	4	5	16	11	8	8
2707	6	2	6	1	199	8	2	6	6	6	4	2	4	0	1	4	2	5	2
2708	1	0	0	383	503	538	9	16	4	8	4	7	7	0	6	9	14	19	3
2709	0	0	0	2	564	26	9	19	5	11	5	5	5	0	4	7	6	8	4
2710	0	0	0	9	121	0	3	5	0	1	1	1	6	0	1	2	1	1	2
2711	0	0	0	31	319	0	0	40	2	2	1	3	8	0	4	3	6	3	1
2712	0	0	0	2	19	0	0	3	0	0	0	0	1	0	0	0	0	0	0
2713	12	2	0	79	474	6	6	32	7	4	5	10	7	0	4	6	8	5	2
2714	0	0	0	34	554	10	1	53	9	4	6	9	6	0	8	10	10	5	4
2715	0	0	0	38	647	11	2	80	12	5	7	10	10	0	9	11	11	6	4
2716	0	0	0	22	382	0	1	10	5	14	3	15	5	0	6	8	6	4	3
2717	0	0	0	939	241	0	0	31	2	2	1	9	8	0	4	3	5	12	2
2718	0	0	0	437	241	0	0	35	2	2	1	6	9	0	4	3	5	12	2
2719	0	0	0	43	93	0	1	1	6	9	2	1	6	0	3	1	9	10	2
2720	0	0	0	1061	147	15	3	12	4	14	7	3	24	0	10	6	16	11	5
2721	0	0	0	71	147	11	2	15	2	13	3	3	30	0	7	5	17	17	6
2722	1	0	0	2	346	5	1	17	5	4	5	6	9	0	5	7	11	4	5
2723	14	4	55	330	155	8	5	16	7	7	3	5	10	4	7	9	3	4	5
2724	0	0	0	6	290	2	2	145	15	7	4	12	15	0	6	8	9	17	3
2725	0	0	0	6	384	2	2	128	14	7	4	12	12	0	7	9	10	18	4
2726	1	0	0	8	347	3	1	59	7	11	5	14	14	0	9	9	11	21	5
2727	15	6	185	1032	442	67	5	20	12	30	7	10	24	8	30	26	16	18	12
2728	10	5	20	458	1034	164	7	32	15	29	6	27	81	0	28	18	47	44	14
2729	5	1	77	227	242	18	3	11	8	17	8	5	17	4	5	8	7	8	4
2730	8	2	98	129	175	30	4	6	5	14	2	4	11	6	10	10	6	5	4
2731	0	0	0	24	167	20	2	14	2	3	1	3	15	0	3	1	6	5	1
2732	1	0	0	58	740	188	9	48	2	17	4	11	50	0	27	9	41	27	7
2733	0	0	0	126	839	147	6	29	11	25	4	22	66	0	24	10	39	36	9
2734	0	0	0	176	611	159	7	42	8	20	4	15	55	0	30	10	35	17	10
2735	0	0	0	163	566	148	6	39	8	19	4	14	51	0	28	9	33	16	9
2736	10	4	16	297	562	125	8	31	4	19	4	8	33	3	32	17	28	19	8
2737	11	5	18	381	700	111	7	22	11	27	4	17	48	4	34	20	31	27	11
2738	11	4	18	394	489	108	7	27	8	22	4	11	37	4	35	18	25	13	10
2739	8	2	5	295	552	115	9	30	5	18	4	8	31	3	25	13	27	17	6
2740	9	2	6	373	678	101	7	20	11	25	5	16	45	4	26	15	29	25	8
2741	9	2	6	385	483	98	7	26	9	21	4	10	34	4	27	14	24	12	8
2742	0	0	0	3	61	1	0	10	3	4	2	2	6	0	1	4	3	3	3

Fruits & Vegetables

Food #	Food Description & Amount	wt gm	wt oz	calo-ries	%cal fat	prot gm	carbo gm	fiber gm
2743	Squash fritter or cake [2 fritters]	48	1.7	163	54%	3	16	1.2
2744	Squash, spaghetti, cooked without salt [1 cup]	155	5.5	42	9%	1	10	2.2
2745	Squash, summer, raw (Include zucchini, yellow squash, green squash) [1 cup, sliced]	113	4.0	23	9%	1	5	2.1
2746	**Squash, summer**, cooked, from fresh [1 cup, diced]	210	7.4	42	14%	2	9	2.9
2747	Squash, summer, cooked, from frozen [1 cup, diced]	210	7.4	43	7%	3	9	2.8
2748	Squash, summer, canned [1 cup, diced]	210	7.4	27	5%	1	6	2.9
2749	Squash, summer, cooked, from fresh, creamed [1 cup]	217	7.7	156	57%	5	14	2.0
2750	Squash, summer, cooked, from frozen, creamed [1 cup]	217	7.7	148	54%	5	14	2.0
2751	Squash, summer, canned, creamed [1 cup]	217	7.7	135	57%	4	11	2.1
2752	Squash, summer, casserole, with tomato and cheese [1 cup]	217	7.7	148	65%	6	9	2.5
2753	Squash, summer, casserole, with cheese sauce [1 cup]	217	7.7	191	48%	7	19	2.4
2754	Squash, summer, casserole, with rice and tomato sauce [1 cup]	233	8.2	107	5%	3	24	2.8
2755	Squash, summer, and onions, cooked without salt [1 cup]	185	6.5	53	8%	2	12	2.6
2756	Squash, summer, souffle [1 cup]	136	4.8	168	64%	6	10	1.1
2757	Squash, summer, breaded or battered, baked [1 cup]	220	7.8	156	12%	5	30	3.0
2758	Squash, summer, breaded or battered, fried (Include zucchini pancakes) [1 cup]	220	7.8	366	68%	4	26	2.6
2759	Squash, winter, raw (Include pumpkin squash, acorn squash, butternut squash, hubbard squash) [1 cup cubes]	140	4.9	52	6%	2	12	2.1
2760	**Squash, winter**, baked [1 cup, cubes]	205	7.2	80	15%	2	18	5.7
2761	Squash, winter, baked, fat and sugar added [1 cup, cubes]	214	7.5	158	28%	2	30	5.5
2762	Squash, winter, mashed [1 cup]	240	8.5	94	15%	2	21	6.7
2763	Squash, winter, mashed, fat added [1 cup]	245	8.6	133	40%	2	21	6.7
2764	Squash, winter, mashed, fat and sugar added [1 cup]	257	9.1	190	28%	2	36	6.6
2765	Squash, winter, baked with cheese [1 cup]	224	7.9	331	56%	7	32	5.4
2766	Squash, winter, souffle [1 cup]	157	5.5	127	27%	5	19	3.4
2767	Starchy vegetables, Puerto Rican style, including green or ripe plantains, tannier, yam, white sweet potato (viandas) [1 cup]	195	6.9	265	1%	2	65	6.0
2768	Starchy vegetables, Puerto Rican style, including yam, white sweet potato, tannier, no plantain (viandas) [1 cup]	190	6.7	271	1%	2	65	6.3
2769	String beans, green, and potatoes, cooked, with onion, pork fat, salt [1 cup]	143	5.0	110	23%	2	20	3.3
2770	String beans, green, and potatoes, cooked, with salt [1 cup]	138	4.9	82	3%	2	19	3.6
2771	String beans, green, raw [1 cup]	110	3.9	34	3%	2	8	3.7
2772	String beans, green, canned [1 cup, canned]	135	4.8	27	5%	2	6	2.6
2773	String beans, green, canned, low sodium (Include pole beans, Italian beans, snap beans, french cut beans) [1 cup]	135	4.8	27	5%	2	6	2.6
2774	**String beans, green**, cooked, from fresh, without salt [1 cup, fresh]	125	4.4	44	7%	2	10	4.0
2775	String beans, green, cooked, from frozen [1 cup, frozen]	135	4.8	38	5%	2	9	4.1
2776	String beans, green, cooked szechwan-style with garlic, sesame, chinese hot oil [1 cup]	185	6.5	114	42%	4	16	6.5
2777	String beans, green, canned, creamed or with cheese sauce [1 cup]	228	8.0	235	62%	11	12	2.7
2778	String beans, green, cooked, from fresh, creamed or with cheese sauce [1 cup]	228	8.0	264	59%	12	17	4.4
2779	String beans, green, cooked, from frozen, creamed or with cheese sauce [1 cup]	228	8.0	246	60%	12	15	4.2
2780	String beans, green, canned, with mushroom sauce [1 cup]	228	8.0	134	54%	4	13	2.3
2781	String beans, green, cooked, from fresh, with mushroom sauce [1 cup]	228	8.0	153	50%	4	17	3.5
2782	String beans, green, cooked, from frozen, with mushroom sauce [1 cup]	228	8.0	143	51%	4	15	3.5
2783	String beans, green, with almonds, cooked [1 cup]	122	4.3	194	68%	7	13	4.9
2784	String beans, green, with chickpeas, cooked [1 cup]	134	4.7	87	12%	5	16	5.8
2785	String beans, green, with mushroom sauce (Include green bean casserole) [1 cup]	228	8.0	143	51%	4	15	3.5
2786	String beans, green, with onions, cooked, with margarine [1 cup]	151	5.3	88	39%	2	13	3.5
2787	String beans, green, with onions, cooked without salt [1 cup]	146	5.1	46	5%	2	10	3.9
2788	String beans, green, with pinto or Shellie beans, cooked, with salt [1 cup]	136	4.8	41	6%	2	8	4.6
2789	String beans, green, with spaetzel, cooked without salt [1 cup]	147	5.2	80	9%	4	17	4.1

Food #	fat gm	sat fat gm	choles mg	sodium mg	potass mg	% of Daily Value													
						vit A	vit E	vit C	thia-min	ribo-flavin	nia-cin	vit B-6	fol-ate	vit B-12	cal-cium	phos-phorus	magne-sium	iron	zinc
2743	10	2	30	80	162	10	4	3	8	8	6	2	6	1	6	6	2	6	2
2744	0	0	0	28	181	2	1	9	4	2	6	8	3	0	3	2	4	3	2
2745	0	0	0	2	220	2	0	28	5	2	3	6	7	0	2	4	6	3	2
2746	1	0	0	2	403	6	1	19	6	5	5	7	11	0	6	8	13	4	5
2747	0	0	0	8	465	7	2	18	5	5	4	7	5	0	4	7	10	6	4
2748	0	0	0	11	202	3	1	9	2	3	4	4	5	0	3	4	7	8	4
2749	10	3	6	316	385	9	5	13	8	13	5	6	8	4	14	14	11	4	6
2750	9	2	6	294	427	9	5	13	7	12	4	6	5	4	12	12	9	5	5
2751	9	2	6	288	256	6	4	7	5	11	4	4	5	4	11	11	7	7	5
2752	11	4	13	417	560	19	5	33	8	9	5	10	7	2	16	15	11	6	6
2753	10	4	15	343	391	10	3	14	12	14	8	7	12	4	20	18	12	8	8
2754	1	0	0	638	506	11	4	26	12	6	11	12	14	0	4	9	12	9	6
2755	0	0	0	3	337	3	1	17	5	4	4	8	8	0	5	7	9	3	4
2756	12	3	118	152	235	17	5	5	6	15	3	5	7	5	9	12	6	5	5
2757	2	0	5	300	444	7	2	19	21	19	15	8	14	2	6	27	11	15	5
2758	28	4	5	265	392	6	19	16	18	17	13	7	11	1	5	24	10	13	4
2759	0	0	0	6	490	57	1	29	9	2	6	6	8	0	4	4	7	5	1
2760	1	0	0	2	896	73	1	33	12	3	7	7	14	0	3	4	4	4	4
2761	5	1	0	50	905	73	3	31	11	3	7	7	14	0	4	4	5	5	4
2762	2	0	0	2	1049	85	1	38	14	3	8	9	17	0	3	5	5	4	4
2763	6	1	0	54	1049	90	3	38	14	3	8	9	17	0	4	5	5	4	4
2764	6	1	0	60	1087	88	3	38	14	3	8	9	17	0	5	5	6	6	4
2765	20	6	12	437	820	79	8	28	19	11	13	8	17	1	17	13	7	11	7
2766	4	1	119	43	564	47	1	18	10	12	5	6	12	4	5	9	4	6	5
2767	0	0	0	21	877	4	1	37	10	5	7	20	10	0	2	8	12	5	3
2768	0	0	0	24	845	0	2	37	12	4	6	18	9	0	3	9	11	5	4
2769	3	1	2	175	419	3	1	19	8	4	6	12	7	0	3	5	7	5	3
2770	0	0	0	163	432	5	0	20	8	5	7	11	7	0	4	5	8	6	3
2771	0	0	0	7	230	7	2	30	6	7	4	4	10	0	4	4	7	6	2
2772	0	0	0	354	147	5	1	10	1	4	1	2	10	0	4	3	4	7	3
2773	0	0	0	3	147	5	1	11	1	4	1	2	11	0	4	3	4	7	3
2774	0	0	0	4	374	8	1	20	6	7	4	4	10	0	6	5	8	9	3
2775	0	0	0	12	170	5	1	9	3	7	3	4	8	0	7	4	8	7	4
2776	5	1	0	506	400	12	4	42	10	12	8	7	14	1	8	8	13	11	4
2777	16	8	34	758	275	16	4	11	5	18	3	5	13	5	32	23	9	9	10
2778	17	8	36	423	527	21	4	22	10	21	6	6	13	5	35	27	13	12	11
2779	16	8	34	413	298	17	4	10	7	20	4	6	10	5	35	25	12	9	12
2780	8	2	3	970	218	5	4	9	3	10	4	3	9	2	8	8	5	8	6
2781	8	2	3	720	410	8	4	18	7	12	7	4	9	3	10	10	8	10	6
2782	8	2	3	702	236	5	4	9	4	12	5	4	7	2	11	9	8	8	7
2783	15	1	0	6	488	6	19	16	7	16	7	4	10	0	11	18	26	12	8
2784	1	0	0	13	226	4	1	7	4	7	3	5	13	0	6	8	10	9	7
2785	8	2	3	702	236	5	4	9	4	12	5	4	7	2	11	9	8	8	7
2786	4	1	0	45	350	9	2	19	6	6	3	7	9	0	5	6	7	7	3
2787	0	0	0	11	196	5	1	11	4	7	2	5	8	0	6	5	8	6	4
2788	0	0	0	454	148	3	0	7	3	4	1	3	6	0	4	4	5	7	2
2789	1	0	10	6	360	8	1	19	9	8	6	4	14	0	6	7	9	11	4

Fruits & Vegetables

Food #	Food Description & Amount	wt gm	wt oz	calo-ries	%cal fat	prot gm	carbo gm	fiber gm
2790	String beans, green, with tomatoes or tomato-based sauce, cooked, with salt [1 cup]	148	5.2	49	7%	2	11	3.8
2791	String beans, yellow, canned [1 cup]	135	4.8	27	5%	2	6	1.8
2792	String beans, yellow, cooked, from fresh, without salt [1 cup]	125	4.4	44	7%	2	10	4.1
2793	String beans, yellow, cooked, from frozen [1 cup]	135	4.8	38	5%	2	9	4.1
2794	String beans, yellow, canned, creamed or with cheese sauce [1 cup]	228	8.0	235	62%	11	12	1.9
2795	String beans, yellow, cooked, from fresh, creamed or with cheese sauce [1 cup]	228	8.0	264	59%	12	17	4.5
2796	String beans, yellow, cooked, from frozen, creamed or with cheese sauce [1 cup]	228	8.0	246	60%	12	15	4.2
2797	Sweet potato and pumpkin casserole, Puerto Rican style [1 cup]	266	9.4	631	27%	8	112	5.9
2798	Sweet potato leaves, cooked (Include squash leaves, pumpkin leaves, chrysanthemum leaves, bean leaves, swamp cabbage) [1 cup leaves]	64	2.3	15	8%	1	3	1.4
2799	Sweet potato, baked, peel eaten [1 small]	77	2.7	95	1%	2	22	3.1
2800	**Sweet potato, baked, peel not eaten [1 small]**	60	2.1	62	1%	1	15	1.8
2801	Sweet potato, boiled, with peel [1 small]	78	2.8	82	3%	1	19	1.4
2802	Sweet potato, boiled, without peel [1 small]	76	2.7	80	3%	1	18	1.4
2803	Sweet potato, candied [1 piece (½ medium potato)]	104	3.7	156	22%	1	30	2.6
2804	**Sweet potato, canned in syrup [1 cup, pieces]**	196	6.9	174	2%	2	41	4.9
2805	Sweet potato, canned without syrup [1 cup, pieces]	200	7.1	182	2%	3	42	3.6
2806	Sweet potato, casserole or mashed from fresh (Include sweet potato pudding) [1 cup]	247	8.7	276	21%	5	51	3.6
2807	Sweet potato, casserole or mashed, from dried flakes [1 cup]	255	9.0	305	22%	4	56	6.7
2808	Sweet potato, fried [1 cup]	205	7.2	417	39%	4	61	4.5
2809	Sweet potato with fruit [1 cup]	254	9.0	288	2%	2	72	3.4
2810	Sweet potato, Puerto Rican, boiled [1 cup, diced]	140	4.9	147	3%	2	34	2.5
2811	Sweet potato, Puerto Rican, fried [1 small]	227	8.0	792	32%	7	129	19.0
2812	Sweet potato, Puerto Rican, roasted or baked [1 cup]	200	7.1	255	23%	3	47	5.8
2813	Tannier, cooked (Include yautia) [1 cup]	190	6.7	293	2%	4	69	10.7
2814	Tannier fritters, Puerto Rican style (Include Frituras de yautia) [2 fritters (2½"x1½"x½")]	40	1.4	95	43%	3	11	1.6
2815	Tannier fritters, stuffed, Puerto Rican style (Include Alcapurrias) [2 small (4"x1"x½")]	48	1.7	189	69%	6	10	1.2
2816	Taro chips [10 chips]	23	0.8	115	45%	1	16	1.7
2817	Taro leaves, cooked [1 cup]	145	5.1	75	16%	9	12	6.6
2818	Taro, baked [1 cup]	132	4.7	192	2%	3	45	7.0
2819	Thistle leaves, cooked [1 cup]	180	6.3	41	23%	3	7	1.3
2820	Tomato aspic [1 cup]	227	8.0	64	2%	6	12	0.8
2821	Tomato paste [1 cup]	262	9.2	215	6%	10	51	10.7
2822	Tomato puree [1 cup]	250	8.8	100	4%	4	24	5.0
2823	**Tomatoes, raw (Include plum tomatoes, Italian tomatoes) [1 medium (2½"dia)]**	123	4.3	26	14%	1	6	1.4
2824	Tomatoes, broiled, from fresh, without salt [1 medium]	105	3.7	28	14%	1	6	1.4
2825	Tomatoes, canned, low sodium [1 cup]	240	8.5	46	6%	2	10	2.4
2826	Tomatoes, dried [1 cup]	54	1.9	139	10%	8	30	6.6
2827	Tomatoes, fried, from fresh [1 cup, or 2 medium tomatoes]	180	6.3	300	68%	5	21	1.9
2828	Tomatoes, scalloped, from fresh [1 cup]	235	8.3	248	51%	4	28	2.8
2829	Tomatoes, scalloped, from canned [1 cup]	235	8.3	231	53%	4	25	2.8
2830	Tomatoes, stewed, from fresh [1 cup]	255	9.0	185	32%	5	29	3.0
2831	**Tomatoes, stewed, canned [1 cup]**	255	9.0	71	4%	2	17	2.6
2832	Tomatoes and celery, cooked [1 cup]	244	8.6	46	6%	2	11	2.7
2833	Tomatoes and corn, cooked [1 cup]	242	8.5	107	10%	4	25	3.4
2834	Tomatoes and lima beans, cooked [1 cup]	242	8.5	150	3%	8	30	6.7
2835	Tomatoes and okra, cooked [1 cup]	217	7.7	53	5%	3	12	3.5
2836	Tomatoes and onion, cooked [1 cup]	237	8.4	73	11%	3	16	2.6
2837	Tomatoes and onion, cooked with margarine [1 cup]	242	8.5	108	40%	3	16	2.6
2838	Tomatoes with corn and okra, cooked [1 cup]	212	7.5	86	9%	4	20	3.6

Food #	fat gm	sat fat gm	choles mg	sodium mg	potass mg	% of Daily Value													
						vit A	vit E	vit C	thia-min	ribo-flavin	nia-cin	vit B-6	fol-ate	vit B-12	cal-cium	phos-phorus	magne-sium	iron	zinc
2790	0	0	0	324	481	12	3	27	7	7	6	7	9	0	5	5	8	9	3
2791	0	0	0	339	147	1	1	10	1	4	1	2	10	0	4	3	4	7	3
2792	0	0	0	4	374	1	1	20	6	7	4	4	10	0	6	5	8	9	3
2793	0	0	0	12	170	1	1	9	3	7	3	4	8	0	7	4	8	7	4
2794	16	8	34	743	275	13	5	11	5	18	3	5	13	5	32	23	9	9	10
2795	17	8	36	423	527	13	5	22	10	21	6	6	13	5	35	27	13	12	11
2796	16	8	34	413	298	13	4	10	7	20	4	6	10	5	35	25	12	9	12
2797	19	10	100	138	832	274	12	57	12	29	11	24	12	3	8	18	12	17	9
2798	0	0	0	36	281	24	2	13	2	6	2	4	6	0	3	3	5	8	1
2799	0	0	0	10	306	131	1	28	4	6	4	12	4	0	2	5	5	8	2
2800	0	0	0	6	209	131	1	25	3	4	2	7	3	0	2	3	3	2	1
2801	0	0	0	10	144	133	1	22	3	6	2	10	2	0	2	2	2	2	1
2802	0	0	0	10	140	130	1	22	3	6	2	9	2	0	2	2	2	2	1
2803	4	1	0	90	222	62	3	17	2	3	2	3	2	0	3	3	4	6	1
2804	0	0	0	86	363	112	2	34	3	5	4	5	3	0	3	5	6	9	2
2805	0	0	0	106	624	160	2	88	5	7	7	19	8	0	4	10	11	10	2
2806	6	2	3	105	434	348	4	58	8	20	7	25	6	3	9	9	6	6	5
2807	7	2	4	203	412	371	5	44	4	9	4	27	6	2	10	10	7	8	5
2808	18	4	0	33	460	426	10	71	9	21	8	31	7	0	5	7	6	8	4
2809	0	0	0	74	279	186	1	31	4	10	4	15	3	0	4	4	4	6	3
2810	0	0	0	18	258	239	1	40	5	12	4	17	4	0	3	4	4	4	3
2811	29	6	0	42	3780	0	14	106	28	8	12	64	20	0	8	25	24	14	7
2812	7	1	0	94	672	425	5	79	9	14	6	23	11	0	6	11	10	5	4
2813	1	0	0	27	1390	0	21	13	13	3	7	33	9	0	11	20	20	8	4
2814	5	1	30	92	242	2	5	2	2	3	1	6	2	1	8	8	4	2	2
2815	14	3	19	188	277	2	8	7	7	4	6	8	2	4	1	7	4	3	5
2816	6	1	0	79	174	0	4	2	3	0	1	5	1	0	1	3	5	2	1
2817	1	0	0	5	1044	82	12	93	21	46	12	12	37	0	18	10	19	21	5
2818	0	0	0	19	1014	0	14	10	10	2	5	23	8	0	7	14	14	5	3
2819	1	0	0	14	635	139	4	69	7	17	7	14	17	0	11	9	12	8	2
2820	0	0	0	644	414	10	5	70	6	4	6	10	10	0	2	4	5	6	2
2821	1	0	0	231	2455	64	38	185	27	29	42	50	15	0	9	21	33	28	14
2822	0	0	0	85	1065	32	21	43	12	8	21	19	7	0	4	10	15	17	4
2823	0	0	0	11	273	8	2	39	5	3	4	5	5	0	1	3	3	3	1
2824	0	0	0	12	291	7	2	40	5	4	4	5	3	0	1	3	4	3	1
2825	0	0	0	24	545	14	3	57	7	4	9	11	5	0	7	5	7	7	3
2826	2	0	0	1131	1851	5	0	35	19	16	24	9	9	0	6	19	26	27	7
2827	23	5	42	138	357	10	11	40	13	13	9	6	9	2	10	11	6	9	3
2828	14	3	0	300	641	27	9	78	16	12	12	11	9	0	4	9	9	11	3
2829	14	3	0	596	516	25	9	49	13	9	12	10	7	0	10	7	8	11	3
2830	7	1	0	219	757	22	6	91	18	12	14	12	9	0	5	10	11	13	3
2831	0	0	0	564	607	14	3	48	8	5	9	2	3	0	8	5	8	10	3
2832	0	0	0	337	566	13	3	52	7	5	8	11	6	0	8	5	7	7	3
2833	1	0	0	423	509	10	2	48	6	7	11	9	15	0	5	9	9	9	4
2834	1	0	0	227	885	12	2	50	14	8	10	16	9	0	7	16	23	18	7
2835	0	0	0	197	567	13	3	54	12	5	9	14	12	0	9	7	16	6	5
2836	1	0	0	22	601	14	3	74	10	7	7	12	8	0	2	8	8	6	2
2837	5	1	0	22	602	17	4	74	10	7	7	12	8	0	2	8	8	6	2
2838	1	0	0	268	513	10	3	46	9	6	10	11	16	0	7	9	14	7	5

Fruits & Vegetables

Food #	Food Description & Amount	wt gm	wt oz	calories	%cal fat	prot gm	carbo gm	fiber gm
2839	Tomatoes, green, raw [1 small]	91	3.2	22	8%	1	5	1.0
2840	Tomatoes, green, fried in batter [1 cup]	180	6.3	355	68%	6	24	1.8
2841	Tomatoes, green, pickled [1 tomato (2¼"dia)]	74	2.6	27	6%	1	6	0.9
2842	Turnips, raw [1 cup]	130	4.6	35	3%	1	8	2.3
2843	Turnips, cooked, from fresh [1 cup, pieces]	155	5.5	33	3%	1	8	3.1
2844	Turnips, cooked, from frozen [1 cup, pieces]	155	5.5	36	9%	2	7	3.1
2845	Turnips, creamed, cooked from fresh, creamed [1 cup]	226	8.0	174	56%	5	15	2.7
2846	Turnips, creamed, cooked from frozen, creamed [1 cup]	226	8.0	177	56%	6	15	2.7
2847	Turnips, creamed, cooked from canned [1 cup]	226	8.0	174	56%	5	15	2.7
2848	**Turnip greens**, cooked, from fresh, without salt [1 cup, fresh]	**144**	**5.1**	**29**	**10%**	**2**	**6**	**5.0**
2849	Turnip greens, cooked, from frozen, without salt [1 cup, frozen]	165	5.8	50	13%	6	8	5.6
2850	Turnip greens, canned [1 cup]	159	5.6	32	10%	2	7	5.5
2851	Turnip greens with roots, cooked, from fresh [1 cup]	163	5.7	33	7%	1	8	4.4
2852	Turnip greens with roots, cooked, from frozen [1 cup]	163	5.7	28	8%	3	5	2.9
2853	**Vegetable combo (including carrots, broccoli, and/or dark-green leafy)**, cooked, with butter sauce [1 cup]	**196**	**6.9**	**176**	**52%**	**4**	**19**	**4.1**
2854	Vegetable combo (of above vegetables), cooked, with cheese sauce [1 cup]	228	8.0	142	19%	8	24	6.7
2855	Vegetable combo (of above vegetables), cooked, with cream sauce [1 cup]	228	8.0	197	53%	7	18	4.3
2856	Vegetable combo (of above vegetables), cooked, with pasta [1 cup]	137	4.8	107	5%	5	22	3.8
2857	Vegetable combo (of above vegetables), cooked, with sauce and pasta (Include Birdseye New England Style Mixed Vegetables) [1 cup]	197	6.9	203	34%	6	29	4.9
2858	Vegetable combo (of above vegetables), cooked, with soy-based sauce (Include stir-fry vegetables) [1 cup]	185	6.5	85	5%	5	18	4.3
2859	Vegetable combo, cooked, plain (broccoli, carrots, corn, cauliflower) [1 cup]	141	5.0	56	4%	3	12	4.2
2860	**Vegetable combo (no carrots, broccoli, or dark-green leafy)**, cooked, with cheese sauce [1 cup]	**228**	**8.0**	**177**	**17%**	**9**	**31**	**6.9**
2861	Vegetable combo (of above vegetables), cooked, with cream sauce [1 cup]	228	8.0	259	42%	9	30	5.8
2862	Vegetable combo (of above vegetables), cooked, with soy-based sauce [1 cup]	185	6.5	117	5%	5	25	4.7
2863	Vegetable combo (of above vegetables), cooked, with pasta [1 cup]	137	4.8	130	5%	5	27	3.9
2864	Vegetable combo (of above vegetables), cooked, with sauce and pasta [1 cup]	197	6.9	223	30%	7	34	5.0
2865	Vegetable combo, asian mix (broccoli, peas, mushrooms, bamboo shoots, water chestnuts, red and green peppers), cooked, plain [1 cup]	127	4.5	48	5%	3	10	3.3
2866	Vegetable mixture, dried (Include Salad Crunchies) [2Tbs]	12	0.4	45	26%	2	7	2.4
2867	Vegetable stew without meat [1 cup]	239	8.4	135	16%	6	23	3.8
2868	Vegetable sticks, breaded (including corn, carrots, and green beans) [1 cup]	116	4.1	240	35%	5	36	3.6
2869	Vegetable tempura (assortment of carrots, asparagus, mushrooms, green beans, eggplant, squash) [1 cup]	63	2.2	102	56%	3	9	1.0
2870	Water chestnuts [1 cup]	158	5.6	79	1%	1	20	4.0
2871	Watercress, cooked [1 cup]	137	4.8	15	8%	3	2	2.1
2872	Watercress, raw [1 cup, chopped]	34	1.2	4	8%	1	0	0.5
2873	Winter melon, cooked (Include Chinese melon, Togan) [1 cup]	175	6.2	23	14%	1	5	1.8
2874	Yam buns, Puerto Rican style (Include Bunuelos de name) [1 cup]	153	5.4	468	56%	5	46	5.3
2875	Yam, Puerto Rican (Include Name), cooked [1 cup]	140	4.9	162	1%	2	39	5.5
2876	Zucchini, summer squash, raw (See also Squash, summer) [1 cup, sliced]	113	4.0	16	9%	1	3	1.4
2877	Zucchini with tomato sauce or tomatoes, cooked (See also Squash, summer) [1 cup]	233	8.2	40	4%	2	10	2.9
Your Additions								

Food #	fat gm	sat fat gm	choles mg	sodium mg	potass mg	% of Daily Value													
						vit A	vit E	vit C	thia-min	ribo-flavin	nia-cin	vit B-6	fol-ate	vit B-12	cal-cium	phos-phorus	magne-sium	iron	zinc
2839	0	0	0	12	186	6	1	35	4	2	2	4	2	0	1	3	2	3	0
2840	27	6	51	167	317	10	13	43	14	14	8	6	8	3	13	13	5	10	3
2841	0	0	0	92	133	6	1	35	2	1	1	3	1	0	1	2	2	2	0
2842	0	0	0	87	248	0	0	46	3	2	3	6	5	0	4	4	4	2	2
2843	0	0	0	78	209	0	0	30	3	2	2	5	4	0	3	3	3	2	2
2844	0	0	0	56	282	0	0	10	4	3	4	5	3	0	5	4	5	8	2
2845	11	3	7	419	326	6	5	26	7	13	4	6	5	5	15	12	6	3	4
2846	11	3	7	401	385	6	5	9	8	13	4	6	5	5	16	13	8	9	4
2847	11	3	7	419	326	6	5	26	7	13	4	6	5	5	15	12	6	3	4
2848	0	0	0	42	292	79	8	66	4	6	3	13	43	0	20	4	8	6	1
2849	1	0	0	25	370	132	16	60	6	7	4	6	16	0	25	6	11	18	5
2850	0	0	0	454	321	87	9	72	5	7	3	14	47	0	22	5	9	7	1
2851	0	0	0	65	273	43	5	52	4	5	3	10	25	0	13	4	6	5	2
2852	0	0	0	24	101	84	1	26	3	7	2	5	9	0	15	3	5	12	1
2853	10	6	26	426	419	90	2	66	5	5	7	12	8	0	5	8	7	7	4
2854	3	1	7	291	535	119	4	107	16	14	10	15	18	2	14	17	12	10	7
2855	12	3	8	418	401	70	8	59	9	17	5	10	14	5	17	15	9	6	5
2856	1	0	0	38	256	56	2	52	13	7	8	8	16	0	3	8	7	8	4
2857	8	1	0	130	319	82	6	68	17	9	11	10	21	0	4	10	9	11	6
2858	0	0	0	1195	476	17	3	133	8	13	13	13	13	0	6	10	10	14	5
2859	0	0	0	42	227	85	3	47	5	5	4	9	12	0	4	6	5	4	3
2860	3	1	8	297	555	22	3	125	16	13	12	17	15	2	11	18	13	10	7
2861	12	3	8	441	464	11	6	18	15	18	9	10	13	5	16	19	12	10	8
2862	1	0	0	1012	426	13	2	94	10	9	12	14	12	0	3	11	9	9	4
2863	1	0	0	726	256	10	1	57	13	6	10	9	15	0	2	8	8	8	4
2864	7	1	0	1002	330	19	5	73	17	8	13	11	19	0	3	11	10	10	6
2865	0	0	0	14	358	12	4	78	7	9	7	10	10	0	4	7	6	7	4
2866	1	0	0	58	212	39	3	44	7	4	4	6	7	0	3	5	5	9	3
2867	2	1	3	538	608	62	1	37	11	6	11	13	7	1	3	10	8	9	10
2868	9	1	0	729	227	55	6	7	15	10	10	7	12	0	3	9	7	11	4
2869	6	1	41	20	111	15	6	4	6	7	4	2	6	1	1	4	2	4	2
2870	0	0	0	13	186	0	3	3	1	2	3	13	2	0	1	3	2	8	4
2871	0	0	0	56	452	61	5	69	7	9	1	8	2	0	16	8	7	2	1
2872	0	0	0	14	112	16	1	24	2	2	0	2	1	0	4	2	2	0	0
2873	0	0	0	187	9	0	2	31	4	0	3	3	2	0	3	3	4	4	7
2874	29	10	81	409	904	9	5	26	14	11	7	16	10	3	4	11	7	8	4
2875	0	0	0	11	938	0	1	28	9	2	4	16	6	0	2	7	6	4	2
2876	0	0	0	3	280	4	0	17	5	2	2	5	6	0	2	4	6	3	2
2877	0	0	0	142	560	9	2	33	7	5	6	10	8	0	5	7	10	6	3

Vegetables are a nutritional bargain (lots of nutrients for the calories), but many of us don't eat enough of them. One way to eat more is to simply have them available ready-to-eat, as in a bowlful of carrot sticks, cherry tomatoes, sugar peas, radishes, etc., in the refrigerator. A glass bowl at eye level is best, so the colorful veggies will catch the eye of the person looking for a snack. If you put out the bowl just before dinner when everyone's hungry, chances are the veggies will disappear in no time.

It's harder to get people to eat cooked vegetables. Here's a vegetable recipe that's tasty and easy to make. Unlike a classic soufflé, you don't have to beat the egg whites separately and fold them in. Unlike a classic custard, you don't have to put the dish in a pan of water in the oven.

Carrot Custard-Soufflé

2 cups cooked carrots	½ tsp salt
2 tsp lemon juice	¼ tsp cinnamon
¼ cup sugar	1 cup milk
1 Tbs flour	3 eggs

Preheat the oven to 350° Purée the carrots [in a food processor], then add the other ingredients and blend until smooth. Pour into a lightly buttered 2-quart dish. Bake, uncovered, for about 45 minutes (until a knife inserted 1″ from the edge comes out clean).

* * * * * * * * * * * *

These muffins are very easy to make, and you'll be amazed how much better they taste than what you buy ready-made, or make from a mix. Frozen blueberries work just as well as fresh, and are handier and less expensive.

Blueberry Muffins

1 egg	½ cup sugar
½ cup milk	2 tsp baking powder
¼ cup salad oil	¼ tsp salt
1½ cup flour	1-2 cups blueberries

Whisk egg; whisk in milk and oil. Sift in dry ingredients together (if you don't have a sifter, smash any lumps in the baking powder and mix dry ingredients together before adding). Mix gently until dry mixture is just moistened (it will be lumpy). Fold in blueberries. If using frozen berries, put them in frozen. Put batter into 12-muffin pan, either lightly oiled or with muffin papers. Bake at 400° for 20-25 minutes, until tops are light brown.

Grains, Beans, Nuts, and Seeds

Breads *3000*

Crackers, Pretzels, Chips *3250*

Pancakes and Waffles *3400*

Cooked Cereals *3450*

Ready-To-Eat Cereals *3550*

Rice, Pasta, and Noodles *3800*

Beans and Peas/Legumes *3850*

Nuts and Seeds *3900*

Your Additions

End-of-Section Recipes
Oatmeal Packets
Bread Packets

Grains, Beans, Nuts, Seeds

Food #	Food Description & Amount	wt gm	wt oz	calo-ries	%cal fat	prot gm	carbo gm	fiber gm
	Breads							
3000	Anisette toast (Include almond toast) [3 pieces]	33	1.2	139	20%	4	24	1.1
3001	**Bagel** (Include water bagels, flavored bagels, egg bagels, bialy) [1 bagel (4"dia)]	89	3.1	245	5%	9	48	2.0
3002	Bagel, with raisins [1 bagel (4"dia)]	89	3.1	244	6%	9	49	2.0
3003	Bagel, with blueberries (Include fruit other than raisins) [1 bagel (4"dia)]	89	3.1	246	6%	8	49	2.0
3004	Bagel, multigrain, with raisins [1 bagel (4"dia)]	89	3.1	237	4%	9	50	6.2
3005	Bagel, multigrain [1 bagel (4"dia)]	89	3.1	231	4%	10	47	6.5
3006	Bagel, oat bran [1 bagel (4"dia)]	89	3.1	227	4%	10	47	3.2
3007	Bagel, pumpernickel (Include rye) [1 bagel (4"dia)]	89	3.1	258	4%	8	53	4.3
3008	Bagel, wheat bran [1 bagel (4"dia)]	89	3.1	242	4%	9	51	4.6
3009	Bagel, whole wheat, 100% [1 bagel (4"dia)]	89	3.1	235	5%	10	50	8.3
3010	Bagel, whole wheat, 100%, with raisins [1 bagel (4"dia)]	89	3.1	217	4%	8	48	7.1
3011	Bagel, whole wheat, less than 100% [1 bagel (4"dia)]	89	3.1	257	4%	9	52	3.9
3012	Bagel, whole wheat, less than 100%, with raisins [1 bagel (4"dia)]	89	3.1	248	4%	8	52	3.7
3013	Bagel, whole wheat, less than 100%, with fruit and nuts (Include California Energy Bar) [1 bagel (4"dia)]	89	3.1	262	8%	9	53	4.1
3014	Bagel chip (Include all flavors) [2 chips]	28	1.0	119	22%	2	21	1.7
3015	Biscuit dough, raw [1 cup]	170	6.0	437	16%	11	81	2.7
3016	Biscuit dough, fried [1 piece]	43	1.5	144	38%	3	20	0.7
3017	Biscuit mix, dry [1 cup]	120	4.2	514	32%	10	76	2.5
3018	**Biscuit**, baking powder or buttermilk type, commercially baked (Include McDonald's and other fast foods) [1 biscuit]	72	2.5	262	41%	4	35	0.9
3019	Biscuit, baking powder or buttermilk type, made from home recipe [1 biscuit (3"dia)]	63	2.2	224	42%	4	28	0.9
3020	Biscuit, baking powder or buttermilk type, made from mix [1 biscuit (3"dia)]	63	2.2	204	33%	5	29	0.9
3021	Biscuit, baking powder or buttermilk type, made from refrigerated dough (Include crescent biscuit) [1 biscuit]	29	1.0	100	38%	2	14	0.5
3022	Biscuit, baking powder or buttermilk type, made from refrigerated dough, lowfat (Include Ballard Extra Lights) [1 biscuit (2"dia)]	21	0.7	63	16%	2	12	0.4
3023	Biscuit, cheese [1 biscuit (3"dia)]	63	2.2	237	45%	6	26	0.9
3024	Biscuit, cinnamon-raisin [1 biscuit (3"dia)]	64	2.3	227	34%	4	35	1.1
3025	Biscuit, whole wheat [1 biscuit (3"dia)]	63	2.2	198	34%	6	30	4.6
3026	Bread stick, soft (Include "crazy bread") [1 stick (7" long)]	32	1.1	113	22%	3	18	0.7
3027	Bread stick, soft, prepared with garlic and parmesan cheese [1 medium stick or slice]	47	1.7	191	39%	5	24	0.9
3028	**Bread stick**, hard (Include sesame sticks) [4 sticks (5" long)]	40	1.4	165	21%	5	27	1.2
3029	Bread stick, hard, low sodium [4 sticks (7" long)]	40	1.4	170	27%	5	26	0.7
3030	Bread stick, hard, whole wheat [4 sticks (8" long)]	32	1.1	130	22%	4	22	2.5
3031	Bread stuffing, moist type (made from mix or homemade) [1 cup]	200	7.1	355	44%	6	43	1.8
3032	Bread, banana (Include other fruit breads, Keebler Banana Elfin Loaves) [1 slice]	41	1.4	134	29%	2	22	0.5
3033	Bread, banana nut (Include other fruit-nut breads) [1 slice]	56	2.0	217	41%	3	30	1.0
3034	Bread, barley [1 slice]	26	0.9	74	10%	2	14	1.5
3035	Bread, batter [1 slice]	33	1.2	93	21%	3	15	0.5
3036	Bread, black [1 slice]	26	0.9	65	11%	2	12	1.7
3037	Bread, Boston Brown [1 slice]	45	1.6	88	7%	2	19	2.1
3038	Bread, bran (Include Granola, Branola, Honey Bran) [1 slice]	36	1.3	89	12%	3	17	1.4
3039	Bread, bran, with raisins [1 slice]	36	1.3	91	11%	3	19	1.4
3040	Bread, buckwheat [1 slice]	27	1.0	72	13%	2	14	0.9
3041	Bread, caressed, Puerto Rican style (Pan sobao) [1 slice]	25	0.9	67	12%	2	12	0.6
3042	Bread, cheese (Include onion cheese) [1 slice]	26	0.9	71	17%	2	12	0.6
3043	**Bread, cinnamon** [1 slice]	26	0.9	69	12%	2	13	0.6
3044	Bread, corn and molasses (Include Anadama bread) [1 slice]	32	1.1	88	17%	2	16	0.7

Food #	fat gm	sat fat gm	choles mg	sodium mg	potass mg	% of Daily Value													
						vit A	vit E	vit C	thia-min	ribo-flavin	nia-cin	vit B-6	fol-ate	vit B-12	cal-cium	phos-phorus	magne-sium	iron	zinc
3000	3	1	7	73	135	0	0	3	5	5	2	2	8	0	1	3	2	2	1
3001	1	0	0	475	90	0	0	0	32	16	20	2	20	0	7	9	6	18	5
3002	2	0	0	287	135	1	0	1	23	15	14	3	20	0	2	7	5	19	4
3003	2	0	22	10	104	1	1	2	28	22	23	3	22	1	3	9	4	16	5
3004	1	0	0	8	373	0	2	0	20	14	17	9	17	0	3	18	15	15	8
3005	1	0	0	441	329	0	2	0	24	13	18	8	20	0	3	18	16	15	11
3006	1	0	0	451	182	0	1	0	20	18	13	9	18	0	1	15	13	15	12
3007	1	0	0	5	139	0	0	0	28	20	22	5	22	0	2	11	7	16	6
3008	1	0	0	582	195	4	1	0	30	25	29	9	26	0	2	16	12	25	11
3009	1	0	0	479	307	0	3	0	19	14	23	12	13	0	3	26	23	16	14
3010	1	0	0	385	310	0	2	0	16	11	19	11	11	0	3	22	20	14	11
3011	1	0	0	6	170	0	1	0	29	21	27	6	23	0	2	15	11	18	7
3012	1	0	0	6	203	0	1	0	26	19	23	6	20	0	2	13	10	16	7
3013	2	0	0	8	211	0	1	0	26	19	24	7	20	0	2	14	11	17	7
3014	3	1	0	168	67	0	2	0	4	3	3	3	5	0	0	6	4	3	2
3015	8	2	0	2122	270	0	5	0	51	22	28	2	36	0	3	68	6	25	4
3016	6	1	0	521	66	0	3	0	9	5	6	1	6	0	1	17	2	6	1
3017	18	5	1	1531	196	0	10	0	46	31	27	5	31	2	21	70	8	18	5
3018	12	2	1	757	161	0	7	0	20	12	12	2	11	2	4	31	3	13	2
3019	10	2	2	216	77	1	4	0	15	11	9	1	10	1	15	10	3	10	2
3020	7	2	3	579	119	1	4	0	14	13	9	2	8	2	12	29	4	7	3
3021	4	1	0	349	46	0	2	0	7	4	4	1	3	0	1	11	1	4	1
3022	1	0	0	305	39	0	1	0	6	3	4	0	4	0	0	10	1	4	1
3023	12	4	8	315	96	3	4	0	14	13	9	2	9	2	19	14	3	10	4
3024	8	2	2	166	116	1	4	1	12	9	7	2	7	1	12	9	3	9	2
3025	7	2	2	210	200	1	4	0	10	7	11	6	3	1	16	20	14	9	8
3026	3	1	0	142	34	0	1	0	11	8	9	1	8	0	1	3	2	7	2
3027	8	2	1	218	48	0	4	0	15	11	12	1	11	0	4	5	2	9	3
3028	4	1	0	263	50	0	2	0	16	13	11	1	12	0	1	5	3	10	2
3029	5	1	0	14	86	0	1	0	17	12	13	1	12	0	3	7	5	10	3
3030	3	1	0	185	92	0	1	0	11	7	10	3	7	0	1	9	8	8	5
3031	17	3	1	1085	148	15	9	0	18	13	15	4	14	1	6	8	6	12	4
3032	4	1	18	102	55	5	2	1	5	5	3	3	3	1	1	2	1	3	1
3033	10	2	28	104	98	1	4	2	8	7	5	6	6	1	6	6	4	6	2
3034	1	0	0	4	42	0	0	0	6	4	6	1	4	0	1	3	2	4	2
3035	2	1	13	11	51	1	1	0	8	8	5	1	7	1	2	4	2	5	2
3036	1	0	0	174	54	0	0	0	6	5	4	2	5	0	2	5	4	4	3
3037	1	0	0	284	143	0	0	0	0	3	3	2	1	0	3	5	7	5	2
3038	1	0	0	175	82	0	1	0	10	6	8	3	6	0	3	7	7	6	3
3039	1	0	0	155	100	0	1	0	9	6	7	3	6	0	3	6	7	6	3
3040	1	0	0	4	56	0	0	0	7	5	6	2	5	0	1	4	4	4	2
3041	1	0	0	135	30	0	0	0	8	5	5	1	6	0	2	2	2	4	1
3042	1	0	2	141	31	0	0	0	8	5	5	1	6	0	4	3	2	4	1
3043	1	0	0	140	31	0	0	0	8	5	5	1	6	0	3	2	2	4	1
3044	2	0	1	9	103	1	1	0	7	6	5	2	6	0	3	4	4	5	1

Grains, Beans, Nuts, Seeds

Food #	Food Description & Amount	wt gm	wt oz	calo-ries	%cal fat	prot gm	carbo gm	fiber gm
3045	Bread, cottonseed, toasted [1 slice]	41	1.4	129	18%	5	21	0.7
3046	Bread, cracked wheat (Include Honey Wheat bread, Roman Meal bread, Wheatberry bread, crushed wheat bread) [1 slice]	26	0.9	68	14%	2	12	1.1
3047	Bread, cracked wheat, made from home recipe or purchased at bakery [1 slice]	30	1.1	86	18%	3	15	1.1
3048	Bread, cracked wheat, reduced calorie, high fiber (Include Roman Light Wheat bread, Wonder Light Wheat bread, Arnold's Bakery Light Golden Wheat bread) [1 slice]	28	1.0	55	10%	3	12	3.4
3049	Bread, cracked wheat, with raisins [1 slice]	26	0.9	69	13%	2	13	1.1
3050	Bread, Cuban (Include Spanish bread, Portuguese bread) [1 slice]	20	0.7	55	10%	2	10	0.6
3051	Bread, dough, fried (Include Indian fried bread) [1 piece (7"dia)]	104	3.7	389	44%	7	47	1.6
3052	Bread, egg (Include Challah) [1 slice]	23	0.8	66	19%	2	11	0.5
3053	Bread, French or Vienna (Include Hawaiian sandwich bread) [1 slice (4¾"x4"x½")]	25	0.9	69	10%	2	13	0.8
3054	Bread, French or Vienna, whole wheat, less than 100%, made from home recipe or purchased at bakery [1 slice (4¾"x4"x½")]	25	0.9	69	10%	2	13	1.2
3055	Bread, garlic [1 slice (4¾"x4"x½")]	29	1.0	96	35%	2	13	0.8
3056	Bread, Irish soda [1 slice]	30	1.1	87	16%	2	17	0.7
3057	Bread, Italian, Grecian, Armenian (Include sesame bread) [1 slice]	20	0.7	54	12%	2	10	0.5
3058	Bread, Italian, reduced calorie and/or high fiber [1 slice]	20	0.7	39	14%	2	8	1.9
3059	Bread, lard, Puerto Rican style (Include Pan de manteca) [1 slice]	25	0.9	70	9%	2	14	0.5
3060	Bread, lowfat, 98% fat free [1 slice]	24	0.8	65	12%	2	12	0.6
3061	Bread, low gluten [1 slice]	30	1.1	73	17%	3	13	1.5
3062	Bread, milk and honey (including Arnold's) [1 slice]	28	1.0	73	7%	2	15	0.5
3063	Bread, multigrain [1 slice]	26	0.9	65	14%	3	12	1.7
3064	Bread, multigrain, reduced calorie, high fiber [1 slice]	26	0.9	53	10%	2	12	3.1
3065	Bread, multigrain, with raisins [1 slice]	26	0.9	66	10%	2	13	1.5
3066	Bread, Native water, Puerto Rican style (Include Pan de agua) [1 slice or bun]	25	0.9	69	10%	2	13	0.8
3067	Bread, Native, Puerto Rican style (Include Pan Criollo) [1 slice]	25	0.9	69	10%	2	13	0.8
3068	Bread, nut [1 slice]	49	1.7	167	40%	4	22	0.7
3069	Bread, oat bran [1 slice]	26	0.9	68	17%	3	11	1.3
3070	Bread, oat bran, reduced calorie, high fiber [1 slice]	29	1.0	58	14%	2	12	3.5
3071	Bread, oatmeal [1 slice]	25	0.9	67	15%	2	12	1.0
3072	Bread, onion [1 slice]	26	0.9	66	12%	2	12	0.6
3073	Bread, pita (including Greek, Syrian, Sahara, Arab breads) (Include flat bread, pocket bread) [1 pita (5"dia)]	45	1.6	124	4%	4	25	1.0
3074	Bread, pita, whole wheat, 100% (Include roti) [1 pita (5"dia)]	45	1.6	120	9%	4	25	3.3
3075	Bread, pita, whole wheat, less than 100% [1 pita (5"dia)]	45	1.6	123	5%	5	25	2.4
3076	Bread, potato [1 slice]	26	0.9	69	12%	2	13	0.6
3077	Bread, pumpernickel (Include with raisins) [1 slice]	26	0.9	65	11%	2	12	1.7
3078	Bread, pumpkin (Include with raisins and/or nuts) [1 slice]	60	2.1	179	21%	2	34	1.1
3079	Bread, puri or poori (Indian puffed bread) filled with coconut, fried [1 puri (5"dia)]	36	1.3	113	36%	3	16	1.9
3080	Bread, raisin (Include cinnamon-raisin bread) [1 slice]	26	0.9	71	14%	2	14	1.1
3081	Bread, reduced calorie, high fiber, white (including Fresh Horizons, New World, Less, Roman Light White Bread) [1 slice]	29	1.0	60	11%	3	13	2.8
3082	Bread, reduced calorie, high fiber, white, with fruit and/or nuts [1 slice]	29	1.0	60	12%	2	13	2.2
3083	Bread, rice [1 slice]	25	0.9	61	17%	2	11	1.2
3084	Bread, rye (Include corn rye) [1 slice]	26	0.9	67	11%	2	13	1.5
3085	Bread, rye, reduced calorie, high fiber [1 slice]	26	0.9	53	13%	2	11	3.1
3086	Bread, marble rye and pumpernickel [1 slice]	26	0.9	66	11%	2	12	1.6
3087	Bread, salt-rising [1 slice]	24	0.8	64	8%	2	13	0.4
3088	Bread, sour dough [1 slice (4¾"x4"x½")]	25	0.9	69	10%	2	13	0.8
3089	Bread, soy [1 slice]	26	0.9	69	13%	3	12	0.9

Food #	fat gm	sat fat gm	choles mg	sodium mg	potass mg	% of Daily Value													
						vit A	vit E	vit C	thia-min	ribo-flavin	nia-cin	vit B-6	fol-ate	vit B-12	cal-cium	phos-phorus	magne-sium	iron	zinc
3045	3	1	2	12	123	1	1	0	16	10	9	2	9	1	4	10	9	9	5
3046	1	0	0	138	52	0	0	0	7	4	5	1	5	0	3	4	3	5	2
3047	2	0	0	10	103	0	1	0	6	6	5	2	4	0	3	5	5	5	2
3048	1	0	0	143	35	0	0	0	8	5	5	2	5	0	2	3	2	5	2
3049	1	0	0	122	66	0	0	0	7	4	5	1	4	0	3	4	3	5	2
3050	1	0	0	122	23	0	0	0	7	4	5	0	5	0	1	2	1	3	1
3051	19	4	3	20	125	2	8	0	26	19	16	2	17	1	5	10	4	15	4
3052	1	0	12	113	26	1	1	0	7	6	6	1	6	0	2	2	1	4	1
3053	1	0	0	152	28	0	0	0	9	5	6	1	6	0	2	3	2	4	1
3054	1	0	0	4	55	0	1	0	6	5	6	2	5	0	1	4	3	4	2
3055	4	1	0	188	33	3	2	0	9	5	6	1	6	0	2	3	2	4	1
3056	2	0	6	67	80	1	1	1	6	5	4	1	4	0	2	3	2	4	1
3057	1	0	0	117	22	0	0	0	6	3	4	0	5	0	2	2	1	3	1
3058	1	0	0	117	15	0	1	0	5	3	3	1	5	0	2	2	1	3	1
3059	1	0	1	108	22	0	0	0	7	5	5	1	6	0	0	2	1	4	1
3060	1	0	0	140	26	0	0	0	8	4	5	1	6	0	3	2	2	4	1
3061	1	0	0	132	59	0	1	0	13	5	10	3	5	0	2	5	5	6	3
3062	1	0	0	5	36	0	0	0	8	6	5	1	7	0	1	3	1	5	1
3063	1	0	0	127	53	0	1	0	7	5	6	4	5	0	2	5	3	5	2
3064	1	0	3	133	45	0	0	0	7	4	5	2	5	0	2	6	6	4	4
3065	1	0	0	1	79	0	1	0	5	3	4	2	3	0	2	4	3	4	2
3066	1	0	0	152	28	0	0	0	9	5	6	1	6	0	1	3	2	4	1
3067	1	0	0	152	28	0	0	0	9	5	6	1	6	0	1	3	2	4	1
3068	7	1	28	108	73	2	2	0	8	8	4	2	6	1	8	8	4	6	3
3069	1	0	0	118	32	0	0	0	10	6	7	1	6	0	2	3	2	5	2
3070	1	0	0	102	30	0	0	0	7	3	5	1	5	0	2	4	3	5	2
3071	1	0	0	150	36	0	0	0	7	4	4	1	4	0	2	3	2	4	2
3072	1	0	0	131	32	0	0	0	8	5	5	1	6	0	3	2	2	4	1
3073	1	0	0	241	54	0	0	0	18	9	10	1	11	0	4	4	3	7	3
3074	1	0	0	239	77	0	1	0	10	2	6	5	4	0	1	8	8	7	5
3075	1	0	0	188	96	0	1	0	13	10	13	3	11	0	1	8	6	9	4
3076	1	0	0	140	31	0	0	0	8	5	5	1	6	0	3	2	2	4	1
3077	1	0	0	174	54	0	0	0	6	5	4	2	5	0	2	5	4	4	3
3078	4	1	26	79	86	33	3	1	6	6	4	2	5	1	3	4	2	6	1
3079	5	2	0	2	68	0	2	0	7	4	6	2	4	0	1	5	5	6	3
3080	1	0	0	101	59	0	1	0	6	6	5	1	6	0	2	3	2	4	1
3081	1	0	0	131	22	0	0	0	8	5	5	1	7	1	3	4	2	5	3
3082	1	0	0	95	49	0	0	0	6	4	4	1	5	1	2	3	2	4	2
3083	1	0	0	110	49	0	1	0	11	4	9	3	4	0	2	4	4	5	2
3084	1	0	0	172	43	0	0	0	8	5	5	1	6	0	2	3	3	4	2
3085	1	0	0	105	25	0	0	0	6	4	3	0	3	0	2	2	1	4	1
3086	1	0	0	173	49	0	0	0	7	5	4	1	5	0	2	4	3	4	2
3087	1	0	0	64	16	0	0	0	6	3	4	1	6	0	2	2	1	4	1
3088	1	0	0	152	28	0	0	0	9	5	6	1	6	0	2	3	2	4	1
3089	1	0	1	6	107	1	0	0	7	5	5	1	6	0	2	4	3	5	2

Grains, Beans, Nuts, Seeds

Food #	Food Description & Amount	wt gm	wt oz	calo- ries	%cal fat	prot gm	carbo gm	fiber gm
3090	Bread, Spanish coffee (Include Mallorca) [1 piece]	85	3.0	293	23%	6	50	1.6
3091	Bread, sprouted wheat [1 slice]	26	0.9	68	14%	2	12	1.1
3092	Bread, sunflower meal (Include sunflower seed bread) [1 slice]	27	1.0	75	17%	3	12	0.5
3093	Bread, sweet potato [1 slice]	25	0.9	74	19%	2	13	0.5
3094	Bread, triticale [1 slice]	25	0.9	63	13%	2	12	1.6
3095	Bread, very low sodium [1 slice]	26	0.9	69	12%	2	13	0.6
3096	Bread, walnut, whole wheat, (Include nut breads) [1 slice]	49	1.7	163	42%	4	21	2.1
3097	Bread, wheat germ [1 slice]	28	1.0	73	10%	3	14	0.6
3098	Bread, white and whole wheat (including half and half, Health Nut, Golden Meal, Country Grain) [1 slice]	26	0.9	67	14%	2	12	1.2
3099	**Bread, white** [1 slice]	**26**	**0.9**	**69**	**12%**	**2**	**13**	**0.6**
3100	Bread, white, made from home recipe or purchased at a bakery [1 slice]	32	1.1	92	18%	3	16	0.6
3101	**Bread, whole wheat**, 100% (Include dark bread, brown bread, Hollywood Dark bread, Honey Graham bread) [1 slice]	**26**	**0.9**	**64**	**15%**	**3**	**12**	**1.8**
3102	Bread, whole wheat, 100%, made from home recipe or purchased at bakery [1 slice]	30	1.1	82	21%	3	15	2.1
3103	Bread, whole wheat, 100%, with raisins [1 slice]	26	0.9	66	13%	2	13	1.7
3104	Bread, whole wheat, less than 100%, made from home recipe or purchased at bakery [1 slice]	30	1.1	83	17%	3	15	1.8
3105	Bread, zucchini (Include squash bread, carrot bread) [1 slice]	40	1.4	151	45%	2	19	0.6
3106	Brioche (Include Pan de Huevo) [1 piece]	77	2.7	269	35%	8	36	1.1
3107	**Coffee cake**, yeast type (with or without nuts) (Include coffee bread with icing) [1/8 of 8"dia]	**41**	**1.4**	**153**	**40%**	**3**	**21**	**1.0**
3108	Coffee cake, yeast type, made from home recipe or purchased at a bakery (with or without nuts) (Include coffee bread with icing) [1/8 of 8"dia]	41	1.4	140	24%	3	23	0.8
3109	Coffee cake, yeast type, very lowfat, no cholesterol, with fruit [1 piece (5"x¾"x1¼")]	33	1.2	94	2%	3	20	0.6
3110	Corn flour patties or tarts, fried [2 patties]	20	0.7	44	19%	1	8	0.9
3111	Corn pone (Include hoecake) [1 piece (1/8 of 9"dia x ¾" pone)]	61	2.2	129	22%	2	24	2.2
3112	Corn pone, fried [1 piece]	61	2.2	152	38%	2	22	2.1
3113	Cornstarch, dry (Include Uniopro Carboplex) [2Tbs]	16	0.6	61	0%	0	15	0.1
3114	**Cornbread**, made from mix [1 piece (2½"x2½"x1½")]	**65**	**2.3**	**152**	**29%**	**4**	**23**	**1.9**
3115	Cornbread, made from home recipe [1 piece (2½"x2½"x1½")]	65	2.3	184	30%	4	28	1.5
3116	Cornbread, made with egg substitute, made from home recipe [1 piece (2½"x2½"x1½")]	46	1.6	86	10%	3	16	1.4
3117	Cornbread, muffins, sticks, rounds, made from home recipe [1 muffin]	52	1.8	158	30%	4	24	1.3
3118	Cornbread muffins, sticks, rounds, made from mix [1 muffin]	52	1.8	159	25%	3	26	1.8
3119	Cornmeal bread, Dominican style (Include Arepa Dominicana) [1 piece (4"x2"x1¾")]	115	4.1	308	47%	7	35	4.1
3120	Cornbread stuffing [1 cup, moist type]	203	7.2	363	44%	6	44	5.9
3121	**Croissant** (Include Sara Lee Wheat 'n' Honey) [1 croissant]	**56**	**2.0**	**227**	**47%**	**5**	**26**	**1.5**
3122	Croissant, cheese [1 croissant]	42	1.5	174	45%	4	20	1.1
3123	Croissant, chocolate (Include Vie de France) [1 croissant]	56	2.0	234	53%	5	25	2.2
3124	Croissant, fruit (Include Sara Lee Apple, Strawberry, Cinnamon-Nut-Raisin) [1 croissant]	92	3.2	351	46%	7	40	2.4
3125	Croissant, nut (Include Vie de France) [1 croissant]	56	2.0	230	48%	5	25	1.5
3126	Croutons (Include seasoned bread crumbs) [1 cup]	30	1.1	140	35%	3	19	1.5
3127	Crumpet [1 medium (3¾"dia)]	45	1.6	80	5%	3	17	0.8
3128	**Flour, white** [1 cup]	**125**	**4.4**	**455**	**2%**	**13**	**95**	**3.4**
3129	Flour, whole wheat [1 cup]	120	4.2	407	5%	16	87	14.6
3130	Gordita/sope shell, plain, no filling, fried in oil [1 shell (3"dia)]	40	1.4	111	37%	2	16	2.0
3131	Gordita/sope shell, plain, no filling, grilled [1 shell (3"dia)]	42	1.5	88	9%	2	18	2.3
3132	Hush puppies (Include fried cornbread) [2 hush puppies]	44	1.6	148	36%	3	20	1.2
3133	Injera (Include Ethiopian bread) [1 injera (12"dia)]	127	4.5	173	6%	6	38	1.3
3134	Johnnycake [1 piece]	49	1.7	135	24%	4	21	1.6

Food #	fat gm	sat fat gm	choles mg	sodium mg	potass mg	% of Daily Value													
						vit A	vit E	vit C	thia-min	ribo-flavin	nia-cin	vit B-6	fol-ate	vit B-12	cal-cium	phos-phorus	magne-sium	iron	zinc
3090	7	1	32	12	82	1	3	0	25	17	15	2	19	1	1	8	3	14	5
3091	1	0	0	138	52	0	0	0	7	4	5	1	5	0	3	4	3	5	2
3092	1	0	1	6	34	1	1	0	10	5	6	1	5	0	2	4	3	4	2
3093	2	0	14	20	41	5	1	1	6	6	4	1	6	0	1	3	1	4	1
3094	1	0	0	148	52	0	1	0	7	4	5	2	4	0	2	4	4	4	3
3095	1	0	0	7	31	0	0	0	8	5	5	1	6	0	3	2	2	4	1
3096	8	1	28	109	119	2	3	0	5	5	5	4	3	1	8	11	8	5	5
3097	1	0	0	155	71	0	1	0	7	6	6	1	7	0	2	5	2	5	3
3098	1	0	0	138	48	0	1	0	7	4	5	2	5	0	2	4	4	5	2
3099	1	0	0	140	31	0	0	0	8	5	5	1	6	0	3	2	2	4	1
3100	2	0	1	7	47	1	1	0	9	7	6	1	7	0	2	4	2	5	1
3101	1	0	0	137	66	0	1	0	6	3	5	2	3	0	2	6	6	5	3
3102	2	0	0	4	115	0	1	0	5	3	5	4	3	0	2	7	7	5	4
3103	1	0	0	122	78	0	1	0	6	3	5	2	3	0	2	6	5	5	3
3104	2	0	0	104	94	0	1	0	6	4	6	3	5	0	1	6	6	5	3
3105	8	1	26	78	46	1	5	1	5	5	3	1	4	1	3	3	1	5	1
3106	10	2	73	117	93	11	5	1	19	19	15	2	15	3	3	9	4	12	4
3107	7	1	27	157	46	3	4	1	9	6	5	2	5	1	3	3	2	4	2
3108	4	1	10	9	61	1	1	0	10	9	7	2	9	1	2	5	2	6	2
3109	0	0	0	53	59	1	0	1	6	7	4	1	6	0	2	3	1	4	1
3110	1	0	0	1	28	0	0	0	7	4	4	2	3	0	1	2	3	4	1
3111	3	1	0	133	87	0	1	0	6	3	5	4	1	0	7	10	10	7	4
3112	6	1	0	125	82	0	3	0	5	3	5	4	1	0	7	9	9	6	4
3113	0	0	0	1	0	0	0	0	0	0	0	0	0	0	0	0	0	0	0
3114	5	2	22	356	105	3	2	0	8	9	5	3	6	2	7	19	3	5	3
3115	6	1	26	188	91	3	3	0	13	11	7	3	10	2	13	10	4	9	3
3116	1	0	2	202	92	2	0	2	8	7	4	3	6	1	4	5	3	4	2
3117	5	1	23	161	78	3	3	0	11	10	6	2	8	1	11	9	3	7	2
3118	4	1	27	271	36	2	2	0	9	10	5	2	8	2	4	15	5	8	2
3119	16	11	64	147	241	8	4	2	17	16	10	7	16	3	9	14	9	14	6
3120	18	4	0	924	126	17	9	3	16	11	13	4	49	0	5	7	7	11	3
3121	12	7	42	417	66	8	1	0	14	8	6	2	9	3	2	6	2	6	3
3122	9	4	27	233	55	7	1	0	15	8	5	2	8	2	2	5	3	5	3
3123	14	8	38	376	106	7	1	0	13	8	6	2	8	3	2	8	6	8	4
3124	18	10	62	617	123	11	1	3	22	12	9	3	13	4	3	9	4	10	4
3125	12	6	41	404	77	7	2	0	14	8	6	2	9	3	2	7	3	6	3
3126	5	2	1	371	54	0	2	0	10	7	7	1	7	0	3	4	3	5	2
3127	0	0	0	324	37	0	0	0	5	1	2	1	7	0	5	7	2	3	2
3128	1	0	0	3	134	0	0	0	65	36	37	3	48	0	2	14	7	32	6
3129	2	0	0	6	486	0	5	0	36	15	38	20	13	0	4	42	41	26	23
3130	5	1	0	2	63	0	3	0	15	8	9	4	6	0	3	5	6	9	3
3131	1	0	0	2	72	0	0	0	18	10	11	4	8	0	3	5	7	10	3
3132	6	1	20	294	63	2	2	0	10	9	6	2	8	1	12	8	3	7	2
3133	1	0	0	254	72	0	0	0	8	6	8	4	11	0	7	14	3	205	3
3134	4	1	36	154	106	3	1	0	12	11	6	4	11	2	5	7	4	6	3

Grains, Beans, Nuts, Seeds

Grains, Beans, Nuts, Seeds

Food #	Food Description & Amount	wt gm	wt oz	calories	%cal fat	prot gm	carbo gm	fiber gm
3135	Matzo, fritters [2 fritters]	30	1.1	109	57%	2	10	0.2
3136	Melba toast (Include flavors, Nutrisystem Crisp Toast, Bagel Chips) [5 slices]	25	0.9	98	7%	3	19	1.6
3137	Melba toast with wheat germ [5 slices]	25	0.9	97	11%	3	19	1.9
3138	**Muffin, bran, with raisins [1 muffin (3"dia)]**	**64**	**2.3**	**189**	**27%**	**3**	**33**	**4.9**
3139	Muffin, bran with fruit, lowfat (Include Jenny's Cuisine Banana Bran Muffin) [1 muffin (2¾"dia)]	58	2.0	136	19%	3	31	6.2
3140	Muffin, bran with fruit, no fat, no cholesterol (Include McDonald's Apple Bran) [1 muffin]	75	2.6	191	3%	8	40	3.1
3141	Muffin, buckwheat [1 muffin (3"dia)]	64	2.3	194	35%	5	28	1.8
3142	Muffin, carrot (Include with raisins) [1 muffin (3"dia)]	64	2.3	195	34%	4	29	1.1
3143	Muffin, cheese [1 muffin (3"dia)]	64	2.3	198	36%	6	26	0.7
3144	Muffin, chocolate [1 muffin (3"dia)]	64	2.3	214	42%	5	28	1.8
3145	Muffin, chocolate chip [1 muffin (3"dia)]	64	2.3	207	36%	5	29	1.1
3146	**Muffin, English** (Include sour dough) [1 muffin]	**58**	**2.0**	**136**	**7%**	**4**	**27**	**1.6**
3147	Muffin, English, bran (Include Branola) [1 muffin]	58	2.0	126	10%	5	25	2.7
3148	Muffin, English, bran, with raisins [1 muffin]	58	2.0	139	9%	5	29	2.8
3149	Muffin, English, cheese [1 muffin]	58	2.0	141	12%	5	25	1.5
3150	Muffin, English, multigrain [1 muffin]	58	2.0	136	7%	5	27	1.6
3151	Muffin, English, oat bran [1 muffin]	58	2.0	126	14%	5	25	2.6
3152	Muffin, English, oat bran, with raisins [1 muffin]	58	2.0	133	13%	5	28	2.6
3153	Muffin, English, pumpernickel [1 muffin]	58	2.0	130	12%	6	25	5.5
3154	Muffin, English, rye [1 muffin]	58	2.0	137	10%	5	26	2.5
3155	Muffin, English, cracked wheat (Include Roman Meal) [1 muffin]	58	2.0	129	8%	5	26	2.7
3156	Muffin, English, wheat or cracked wheat, with raisins [1 muffin]	58	2.0	146	9%	5	30	2.5
3157	Muffin, English, whole wheat, 100% [1 muffin]	58	2.0	118	9%	5	23	3.9
3158	Muffin, English, whole wheat, 100%, with raisins [1 muffin]	58	2.0	143	9%	5	30	4.4
3159	Muffin, English, whole wheat, less than 100% [1 muffin]	58	2.0	129	8%	5	26	2.7
3160	Muffin, English, whole wheat, less than 100%, with raisins [1 muffin]	58	2.0	146	9%	5	30	2.5
3161	**Muffin, English, with raisins [1 muffin]**	**58**	**2.0**	**141**	**10%**	**4**	**28**	**1.7**
3162	Muffin, English, with fruit other than raisins [1 muffin]	58	2.0	146	7%	5	29	1.8
3163	Muffin, fruit and/or nuts (Include blueberry, cranberry nut) [1 muffin (3"dia)]	64	2.3	177	21%	4	31	1.7
3164	Muffin, fruit, reduced fat, no cholesterol (Include Entenmann's) [1 muffin (3"dia)]	64	2.3	167	2%	4	38	2.2
3165	Muffin, multigrain, with fruit [1 muffin (3"dia)]	64	2.3	166	20%	6	30	4.3
3166	Muffin, multigrain, with nuts [1 muffin (3"dia)]	64	2.3	203	41%	6	27	3.9
3167	Muffin, oat bran with fruit and/or nuts [1 muffin (3"dia)]	64	2.3	186	30%	5	31	2.9
3168	Muffin, oat bran [1 muffin (3"dia)]	64	2.3	173	25%	4	31	2.9
3169	Muffin, oatmeal (Include Granola) [1 muffin (3"dia)]	64	2.3	153	23%	4	25	0.9
3170	Muffin, plain (Include Matzo Meal, spiced, poppy seed) [1 muffin (3"dia)]	64	2.3	196	32%	5	28	0.8
3171	Muffin, plain, no wheat, sugar free [1 muffin (3"dia)]	64	2.3	198	32%	4	30	2.1
3172	Muffin, pumpkin (Include with raisins, nuts) [1 muffin (3"dia)]	64	2.3	200	21%	3	38	1.2
3173	Muffin, white and whole wheat, 50-50 mix [1 muffin (3"dia)]	64	2.3	195	34%	5	28	2.1
3174	Muffin, whole wheat (Include graham) [1 muffin (3"dia)]	64	2.3	191	36%	5	28	3.4
3175	Muffin, zucchini (Include squash muffin; with nuts) [1 muffin (3"dia)]	64	2.3	242	45%	3	30	0.9
3176	Papad (Indian appetizer), grilled or broiled [4 papad]	36	1.3	125	8%	8	22	3.1
3177	Pannetone (Italian-style sweetbread) [1 slice]	27	1.0	87	23%	2	15	0.6
3178	**Popovers** (Include Dutch Baby, Yorkshire pudding) [1 popover]	**31**	**1.1**	**68**	**32%**	**3**	**9**	**0.3**
3179	Roll, cheese [1 roll]	41	1.4	125	25%	4	20	1.2
3180	Roll, diet [1 roll]	28	1.0	77	10%	2	15	0.8
3181	Roll, egg bread [1 roll]	28	1.0	86	19%	3	15	1.0
3182	Roll, French or Vienna [1 roll]	45	1.6	125	14%	4	23	1.4

Food #	fat gm	sat fat gm	choles mg	sodium mg	potass mg	vit A	vit E	vit C	thia-min	ribo-flavin	nia-cin	vit B-6	fol-ate	vit B-12	cal-cium	phos-phorus	magne-sium	iron	zinc
3135	7	2	43	75	19	2	3	0	2	4	1	1	2	1	1	2	1	3	1
3136	1	0	0	207	51	0	0	0	7	4	5	1	8	0	2	5	4	5	3
3137	1	0	0	202	60	0	1	0	3	3	3	2	8	0	3	6	4	3	3
3138	6	1	6	317	106	3	2	0	10	11	8	2	5	0	2	17	3	9	2
3139	3	0	8	165	129	0	2	0	8	6	6	3	5	1	7	11	7	7	3
3140	1	0	1	109	191	2	1	1	14	20	11	4	9	2	9	18	12	11	5
3141	8	2	27	151	146	2	3	0	10	9	8	5	6	2	12	13	11	8	5
3142	7	1	20	169	123	29	5	2	11	10	7	2	7	1	9	8	3	8	2
3143	8	3	30	213	96	4	3	0	12	13	7	2	8	2	14	12	3	8	4
3144	10	4	26	132	134	2	3	0	13	12	8	2	8	2	11	12	8	11	4
3145	8	3	26	129	101	2	3	0	12	12	8	1	8	2	10	10	4	9	4
3146	1	0	0	269	76	0	0	0	17	10	11	1	12	0	10	8	3	8	3
3147	1	0	0	33	122	4	1	0	18	18	17	6	19	0	5	9	6	17	7
3148	1	0	0	31	163	4	1	0	18	17	16	7	18	0	5	9	6	17	7
3149	2	1	3	274	75	1	0	0	16	10	11	1	11	1	12	9	3	8	3
3150	1	0	0	241	90	0	2	0	17	11	10	3	12	0	11	9	6	10	4
3151	2	0	0	10	126	0	1	0	19	14	12	3	16	0	6	13	8	11	4
3152	2	0	0	10	156	0	1	0	18	13	12	3	15	0	6	12	8	11	4
3153	2	0	0	10	181	0	2	0	11	12	12	6	14	0	6	17	13	11	10
3154	1	0	0	10	103	0	1	0	15	13	13	3	16	0	5	7	4	9	4
3155	1	0	0	222	108	0	1	0	17	10	10	3	8	0	10	7	6	9	4
3156	1	0	0	10	161	0	1	0	15	13	14	4	15	0	5	9	6	10	4
3157	1	0	0	369	122	0	1	0	12	5	10	5	7	0	15	16	10	8	6
3158	1	0	0	11	215	0	2	0	10	10	13	7	10	0	5	14	12	9	7
3159	1	0	0	222	108	0	1	0	17	10	10	3	8	0	10	7	6	9	4
3160	1	0	0	10	161	0	1	0	15	13	14	4	15	0	5	9	6	10	4
3161	2	0	0	259	121	0	0	0	15	10	10	2	12	0	9	4	2	8	4
3162	1	0	0	280	84	0	1	1	18	10	12	1	12	0	11	8	3	8	3
3163	4	1	19	286	79	1	2	1	6	5	4	1	7	6	4	13	3	6	2
3164	0	0	0	275	66	1	0	1	14	10	9	1	8	1	10	15	2	9	2
3165	4	1	45	176	268	3	3	1	11	11	8	8	6	2	14	19	16	12	7
3166	9	2	41	160	316	3	6	1	11	10	7	10	6	2	14	18	20	12	8
3167	6	1	0	227	330	0	5	1	11	4	1	6	8	0	4	23	24	14	8
3168	5	1	0	252	324	0	5	1	11	4	1	5	8	0	4	24	25	15	8
3169	4	1	23	165	80	2	1	0	12	10	7	1	8	1	12	10	3	8	3
3170	7	2	28	142	87	3	3	0	14	13	8	1	9	2	11	10	3	9	3
3171	7	2	25	196	280	3	3	2	6	5	5	11	2	2	14	14	7	5	3
3172	5	1	29	88	96	37	3	1	7	7	5	2	5	1	3	5	3	7	2
3173	7	2	26	188	121	2	3	0	10	10	8	3	6	2	14	13	7	8	4
3174	8	2	27	190	162	2	4	0	7	7	8	5	3	2	14	17	11	7	7
3175	12	2	42	124	73	2	7	2	9	8	5	2	7	1	4	5	2	7	2
3176	1	0	0	752	409	0	0	0	3	1	7	3	18	0	3	16	19	19	8
3177	2	1	19	28	54	2	0	0	7	7	5	1	7	1	2	4	1	4	1
3178	2	1	36	20	51	2	1	0	5	7	3	1	4	2	3	4	1	3	2
3179	4	1	3	216	54	1	1	0	13	8	8	1	9	0	6	6	2	7	2
3180	1	0	0	171	32	0	0	0	10	5	7	1	7	0	2	3	2	4	2
3181	2	0	14	153	29	1	1	0	10	9	5	1	7	1	2	3	2	5	2
3182	2	0	0	274	51	0	1	0	16	8	10	1	11	0	4	4	2	7	2

3000
Grains, Beans, Nuts, Seeds

Grains, Beans, Nuts, Seeds

Food #	Food Description & Amount	wt gm	wt oz	calo-ries	%cal fat	prot gm	carbo gm	fiber gm
3183	Roll, garlic [1 roll]	35	1.2	105	22%	3	18	1.0
3184	Roll, hoagie, submarine, or sandwich (Include steak roll, torpedo roll) [1 roll]	100	3.5	286	16%	9	50	2.7
3185	Roll, Mexican, bolillo [1 medium]	117	4.1	307	5%	10	61	2.2
3186	Roll, multigrain [1 roll]	28	1.0	74	21%	3	12	1.1
3187	Roll, oat bran [1 medium]	36	1.3	85	18%	3	14	1.5
3188	Roll, oatmeal [1 roll]	36	1.3	105	21%	3	17	1.0
3189	Roll, pumpernickel [1 roll]	36	1.3	100	9%	4	19	1.9
3190	Roll, rye [1 roll]	36	1.3	103	11%	4	19	1.8
3191	Roll, sour dough [1 roll]	45	1.6	123	10%	4	23	1.4
3192	Roll, sweet (Include butterhorn, Portuguese sweet bread) [1 roll]	55	1.9	205	40%	3	28	1.3
3193	**Roll, sweet, cinnamon bun, frosted [1 roll (2½"dia)]**	**55**	**1.9**	**209**	**36%**	**3**	**31**	**1.1**
3194	Roll, sweet, cinnamon bun, no frosting [1 roll (2½"dia)]	55	1.9	205	40%	3	28	1.3
3195	Roll, sweet, with fruit, frosted (Include hot cross buns) [1 roll (2½"dia)]	55	1.9	206	34%	3	32	1.1
3196	Roll, sweet, with fruit, no frosting (with/without jelly) (Include Mexican sweetbread, apple rolls, Kolaches, Lakvar, Kuchen) [1 roll (2½"dia)]	55	1.9	202	37%	3	29	1.4
3197	Roll, sweet, with fruit and nuts, frosted [1 roll (2½"dia)]	55	1.9	213	38%	3	31	1.1
3198	Roll, sweet, with fruit and nuts, no frosting [1 roll (2½"dia)]	39	1.4	149	42%	3	20	1.0
3199	Roll, sweet, with fruit, frosted, low calorie (Include Weight Watchers Apple Sweet Roll) [1 roll (2½"dia)]	55	1.9	151	19%	3	28	1.1
3200	Roll, sweet, Mexican, crumb topping (Include Pan de Huevo, Pan Dulce, Mexican sweet bread) [1 roll]	79	2.8	291	28%	5	48	1.1
3201	Roll, sweet, Mexican, Pan Dulce, no topping (Include Pan de Huevo) [1 roll]	69	2.4	214	18%	5	39	1.1
3202	Roll, sweet, Mexican, Pan Dulce, sugar topping (Include Pan de Huevo) [1 roll]	77	2.7	262	26%	5	44	1.0
3203	Roll, sweet, with nuts, frosted (Include caramel roll) [1 roll (2½"dia)]	39	1.4	147	38%	2	21	0.8
3204	Roll, sweet, with nuts, no frosting [1 roll (2½"dia)]	55	1.9	213	44%	3	27	1.5
3205	Roll, sweet, with raisins and icing, Mexican (Include Pan Dulce) [1 roll]	72	2.5	280	24%	5	49	1.2
3206	Roll, white, hard (Include Kaiser roll) [1 roll]	50	1.8	147	13%	5	26	1.2
3207	**Roll, white, soft (Include potato roll, onion roll, brown 'n' serve roll, hamburger bun, hot dog bun, crescent roll) [1 roll]**	**28**	**1.0**	**80**	**16%**	**2**	**14**	**0.8**
3208	Roll, white, soft, made from home recipe or purchased at a bakery [1 roll]	36	1.3	115	21%	3	19	0.6
3209	Roll, white, soft, reduced calorie, high fiber [1 roll]	43	1.5	84	9%	4	18	2.7
3210	Roll, whole wheat, 100% [1 roll]	36	1.3	96	16%	3	18	2.7
3211	Roll, whole wheat, 100%, made from home recipe or purchased at bakery [1 roll]	36	1.3	103	24%	4	17	2.4
3212	Roll, whole wheat, less than 100% [1 roll]	36	1.3	98	21%	3	17	1.4
3213	Roll, whole wheat, less than 100%, made from home recipe or purchased at bakery [1 roll]	36	1.3	106	23%	3	17	1.3
3214	**Scone [1 scone]**	**42**	**1.5**	**150**	**38%**	**4**	**19**	**0.6**
3215	Scone, whole wheat [1 scone]	42	1.5	144	42%	5	18	2.7
3216	Scone, with fruit [1 scone]	42	1.5	150	34%	4	21	0.7
3217	Spoonbread [1 cup]	187	6.6	309	38%	13	34	2.4
3218	Taco shell, corn (Include tostada shell) [2 shells (5"dia)]	26	0.9	122	43%	2	16	2.0
3219	Taco shell, flour (Include flour tostada shell, fried flour tortilla, taco salad shell) [1 shell (7"dia)]	34	1.2	173	47%	3	19	1.2
3220	Toaster muffin, fruit, toasted (including blueberry, apple spice) [1 muffin]	33	1.2	110	27%	2	19	0.6
3221	**Tortilla, corn [2 tortillas (6"dia)]**	**38**	**1.3**	**84**	**10%**	**2**	**18**	**2.0**
3222	Tortilla, flour [1 tortilla (8"dia)]	52	1.8	169	20%	5	29	1.7
3223	Tortilla, whole wheat (Include chapati, puri) [1 tortilla]	35	1.2	73	6%	3	20	1.9
3224	Whole wheat, cracked (including home ground) [1 cup]	120	4.2	392	4%	15	85	14.6
3225	Zwieback (Include rusk) [5 pieces]	35	1.2	149	20%	4	26	0.9

Food #	fat gm	sat fat gm	choles mg	sodium mg	potass mg	vit A	vit E	vit C	thia-min	ribo-flavin	nia-cin	vit B-6	fol-ate	vit B-12	cal-cium	phos-phorus	magne-sium	iron	zinc
3183	3	1	0	181	47	0	1	0	11	7	7	1	8	0	4	4	2	6	2
3184	5	1	0	560	141	0	5	0	32	18	20	2	32	1	14	9	5	18	4
3185	2	0	1	7	98	0	0	0	46	28	33	2	36	0	1	9	6	21	5
3186	2	0	0	128	42	0	1	0	9	5	6	1	7	0	3	3	3	6	2
3187	2	0	0	149	39	0	1	0	11	6	9	1	9	0	3	4	3	8	2
3188	2	1	7	7	52	1	1	0	10	7	6	1	6	0	1	5	3	5	3
3189	1	0	0	205	75	0	0	0	9	6	5	2	7	0	2	6	5	6	4
3190	1	0	0	321	65	0	1	0	9	6	7	1	8	0	1	6	5	5	2
3191	1	0	0	274	51	0	0	0	16	9	11	1	11	0	3	5	3	6	3
3192	9	2	36	211	61	4	5	2	12	9	7	3	7	1	4	4	2	5	2
3193	8	2	29	183	51	4	5	1	10	7	5	2	6	1	3	3	2	4	2
3194	9	2	36	211	61	4	5	2	12	9	7	3	7	1	4	4	2	5	2
3195	8	1	26	166	75	4	4	2	9	6	5	3	5	1	3	3	2	4	2
3196	8	2	34	196	86	3	5	2	11	8	6	3	7	1	4	4	2	5	2
3197	9	2	26	166	70	4	5	2	9	7	5	3	5	1	3	4	3	4	2
3198	7	1	23	136	62	2	4	1	8	6	4	3	5	1	3	3	2	4	2
3199	3	1	21	156	79	1	1	1	11	11	8	2	14	1	4	6	2	6	2
3200	9	2	26	75	57	7	4	0	15	13	10	1	12	1	1	6	2	10	2
3201	4	1	34	12	59	2	2	0	16	13	10	2	13	1	1	6	2	10	3
3202	8	2	33	55	79	5	3	0	15	13	10	2	13	1	2	6	3	11	3
3203	6	1	20	122	42	2	3	1	7	5	4	2	4	1	4	3	2	3	1
3204	11	2	34	199	69	3	5	2	13	8	6	3	7	1	4	5	3	5	3
3205	7	2	32	51	84	5	3	0	15	13	10	2	13	1	1	6	3	10	3
3206	2	0	0	272	54	0	0	0	16	10	11	1	12	0	5	5	3	9	3
3207	1	0	0	157	39	0	1	0	9	5	6	1	9	0	4	2	1	5	1
3208	3	1	13	33	55	3	1	0	10	9	6	1	8	1	2	5	2	6	2
3209	1	0	0	190	34	0	0	0	11	4	11	1	10	2	3	6	3	7	3
3210	2	0	0	172	98	0	1	0	6	3	7	4	3	0	4	8	8	5	5
3211	3	0	12	17	165	1	2	0	5	6	6	4	3	1	4	10	9	5	5
3212	2	1	0	122	48	0	1	0	10	6	7	2	5	0	6	4	4	7	2
3213	3	0	12	17	131	1	2	0	8	8	6	3	6	1	4	7	6	6	3
3214	6	2	49	171	49	7	2	0	10	10	6	1	7	2	8	7	2	7	2
3215	7	2	50	175	114	7	3	0	6	6	6	4	3	2	9	13	8	6	5
3216	6	2	44	153	78	6	2	0	9	9	6	2	6	2	7	7	2	7	2
3217	13	4	166	196	370	22	5	2	17	34	8	9	16	11	23	26	10	11	9
3218	6	1	0	95	47	1	3	0	4	1	2	5	7	0	4	6	7	4	2
3219	9	2	0	168	46	0	5	0	9	5	6	1	7	0	4	4	2	6	2
3220	3	1	2	168	29	2	1	0	4	5	3	0	4	0	0	6	1	1	1
3221	1	0	0	61	59	1	0	0	3	2	3	4	11	0	7	12	6	3	2
3222	4	1	0	249	68	0	2	0	18	9	9	1	16	0	7	6	3	10	2
3223	0	0	0	171	82	0	1	0	7	1	4	3	2	0	1	8	6	4	4
3224	2	0	0	2	414	0	6	0	24	7	30	16	8	0	3	33	38	20	21
3225	3	1	7	81	107	0	0	3	5	5	2	1	8	0	1	2	1	1	1

% of Daily Value

Grains, Beans, Nuts, Seeds

Food #	Food Description & Amount	wt gm	wt oz	calo-ries	%cal fat	prot gm	carbo gm	fiber gm
	Crackers, Pretzels, Chips							
3250	Cheese puffs and twists (Include **Cheetos**, Cheez Doodles, Funyuns, Bugles, Diggers, Flings, Planter's Sour Cream & Onion Puffs, Pizza Crunchies) [2 oz]	57	2.0	316	56%	4	31	0.6
3251	Cheese puffs and twists, lowfat (Include Ultra Slim Fast Cheese Curls) [1 oz]	28	1.0	121	25%	2	20	3.0
3252	Corn cake, puffed (including Quaker) [3 cakes]	28	1.0	108	6%	2	23	0.5
3253	**Corn chips**, salted (plain, flavored, or barbecued) (Include Fritos) [2 oz]	57	2.0	307	56%	4	32	2.8
3254	Corn chips, unsalted (Include plain, flavored, or barbecued) [2 oz]	57	2.0	308	53%	4	33	2.5
3255	Corn nuts (Include Frito Lay Toasted Corn Nuggets) [½ cup]	45	1.6	198	29%	4	33	3.1
3256	Cracker, animal (Include sweet crackers) [1 oz (about 10 crackers)]	28	1.0	125	28%	2	21	0.3
3257	**Cracker, butter** (Include bacon chips, Ritz crackers, Waverly Wafers, Nabisco Dip and Chip, Keebler Toasteds, sesame seed crackers, meal mates) [1 oz (about 10 crackers)]	28	1.0	141	45%	2	17	0.4
3258	Cracker, butter, low sodium [1 oz (about 10 crackers)]	28	1.0	141	45%	2	17	0.4
3259	Cracker, cheese, low sodium (Include low-salt Better Cheddars) [1 cup]	40	1.4	201	45%	4	23	1.0
3260	Cracker, cheese, reduced fat (Include Snackwell's and Cheez-its Reduced Fat) [1 cup]	48	1.7	199	16%	6	34	1.3
3261	**Cracker, cheese** (Include cheese sticks, Cheeblers, Cheez-its, Cheese Ritz, Better Cheddar crackers) [1 cup]	52	1.8	262	45%	5	30	1.2
3262	Cracker, corn (Include Stoned Corn Crackers) [1 cracker (1 square or 2 rectangular pieces)]	37	1.3	177	43%	3	23	1.7
3263	Cracker, Cuban [5 crackers]	25	0.9	100	15%	2	19	0.5
3264	Cracker, Cuca [1 cracker]	28	1.0	122	24%	3	20	0.8
3265	Cracker, cylindrical, peanut butter-filled (Include Combos) [10 combos]	29	1.0	151	54%	5	14	1.4
3266	**Cracker, graham** [2 large rectangular or 4 squares or 8 small rectangular pieces]	28	1.0	118	21%	2	22	0.8
3267	Cracker, graham, higher fat (Include Graham Bites) [1 cup,]	64	2.3	289	34%	4	45	1.2
3268	Cracker, graham, fat free [1 cup]	44	1.6	164	2%	4	37	1.7
3269	Cracker, graham, chocolate covered [2 crackers (2½"x2"x¼")]	26	0.9	126	43%	2	17	0.8
3270	Cracker, graham, sugar-honey coated, cinnamon crisps (Include Teddy Grahams) [2 large rectangular or 4 squares or 8 small rectangular pieces]	28	1.0	118	21%	2	22	0.8
3271	Crackers, graham, sandwich-type, with filling [10 sandwich crackers]	23	0.8	101	31%	1	17	0.3
3272	Cracker, graham, with raisins [2 large rectangular or 4 squares or 8 small rectangular pieces]	30	1.1	122	18%	2	24	0.9
3273	Cracker, high fiber (Include Wasa fiber-plus crisp bread) [2 crackers (4½"x2½"x1/8")]	22	0.8	73	2%	2	18	5.0
3274	**Cracker, matzo** [1 matzo]	30	1.1	119	3%	3	25	0.9
3275	Cracker, matzo, low sodium (Include with wheat germ) [1 matzo]	30	1.1	118	5%	3	24	1.1
3276	Cracker, milk (Include Milk Lunch New England Biscuit, Royal Lunch cracker) [2 crackers]	22	0.8	100	31%	2	15	0.4
3277	Cracker, mixed grain, salt free (Include Venus corn wafer, wheat wafer, rye wafer, cracked wheat wafer) [10 crackers]	30	1.1	138	36%	3	20	0.6
3278	Cracker, oat bran (Include Nabisco Oat Thin) [10 crackers]	20	0.7	87	27%	2	14	1.0
3279	Cracker, oatmeal [2 crackers]	22	0.8	103	34%	2	15	0.6
3280	Cracker, oyster (Include chowder cracker) [1 cup]	45	1.6	195	24%	4	32	1.4
3281	Cracker, rice (Include rice paper cracker) [10 crackers]	30	1.1	117	13%	2	23	0.4
3282	**Cracker, saltine** (Include soda cracker, Sea Toast, Uneeda Biscuit) [10 crackers]	30	1.1	130	24%	3	21	0.9
3283	Cracker, saltine, low sodium (Include oyster cracker, chowder cracker) [10 crackers]	30	1.1	130	24%	3	21	0.9
3284	Cracker, saltine, fat free, low sodium [10 crackers]	31	1.1	122	4%	3	26	0.8
3285	Cracker, saltine, whole wheat [1 cracker]	30	1.1	131	28%	3	21	1.8
3286	**Cracker, sandwich-type, peanut butter or cheese-filled** (Include rye-cheese cracker) [4 crackers]	32	1.1	154	43%	4	18	0.9
3287	Cracker, snack, lowfat, low sodium (Include Nabisco Harvest Crisps) [1 cup]	44	1.6	196	26%	3	33	1.3
3288	Cracker, snack, reduced fat (Include Ritz Reduced Fat cracker) [1 cup]	55	1.9	215	7%	4	45	0.9
3289	Cracker, snack, fat free (Include Snackwell's Fat Free Cracked Pepper Cracker) [1 cup]	43	1.5	164	3%	3	36	0.8

Food #	fat gm	sat fat gm	choles mg	sodium mg	potass mg	% of Daily Value													
						vit A	vit E	vit C	thia-min	ribo-flavin	nia-cin	vit B-6	fol-ate	vit B-12	cal-cium	phos-phorus	magne-sium	iron	zinc
3250	20	4	2	599	95	2	10	0	10	12	9	4	17	1	3	6	3	7	1
3251	3	1	0	360	80	12	10	10	10	10	10	10	10	10	10	10	3	2	4
3252	1	0	0	137	44	1	0	0	5	1	7	2	1	0	1	4	8	2	4
3253	19	3	0	359	81	1	3	0	1	5	3	7	3	0	7	11	11	4	5
3254	18	2	0	9	105	2	13	2	5	5	4	6	1	0	7	10	10	5	3
3255	6	1	0	247	125	0	2	0	1	3	4	5	0	0	0	12	13	4	5
3256	4	1	0	110	28	0	2	0	7	5	5	0	6	0	1	3	1	4	1
3257	7	1	0	237	37	0	4	0	8	6	6	1	5	0	3	6	2	6	1
3258	7	1	0	104	99	0	4	0	8	6	6	1	5	0	3	6	2	6	1
3259	10	4	5	183	42	1	1	0	15	10	9	11	8	3	6	9	4	11	3
3260	4	1	0	545	72	2	2	2	20	13	15	1	14	0	5	8	4	12	4
3261	13	5	7	517	75	2	2	0	20	13	12	14	10	4	8	11	5	14	4
3262	8	2	0	406	41	1	4	0	11	6	7	3	9	0	2	6	3	7	1
3263	2	0	0	60	64	0	1	0	1	0	1	1	1	0	2	2	3	2	1
3264	3	1	0	365	36	0	2	0	11	8	7	1	9	0	3	3	2	8	1
3265	9	1	1	225	97	0	5	0	10	5	10	2	9	0	2	5	6	7	3
3266	3	0	0	169	38	0	2	0	4	5	6	1	4	0	1	3	2	6	2
3267	11	3	0	321	173	0	1	0	3	16	8	2	5	0	6	21	4	12	3
3268	0	0	0	153	61	0	0	0	14	8	10	2	8	0	1	5	4	12	3
3269	6	3	0	76	54	0	1	0	2	3	3	1	1	0	2	3	4	5	2
3270	3	0	0	169	38	0	2	0	4	5	6	1	4	0	1	3	2	6	2
3271	3	1	0	90	45	1	1	0	1	4	2	0	1	0	2	5	1	3	1
3272	3	0	0	149	74	0	2	0	4	5	5	2	4	0	1	3	2	6	1
3273	0	0	0	175	109	0	1	0	6	4	2	3	2	0	1	7	7	7	4
3274	0	0	0	1	34	0	0	0	8	5	6	2	9	0	0	3	2	5	1
3275	1	0	0	1	52	0	2	0	10	6	6	3	10	0	0	5	4	6	4
3276	3	1	4	130	25	0	2	0	8	5	5	0	5	0	4	7	1	4	1
3277	6	1	0	3	65	0	1	0	10	6	7	2	5	0	1	6	4	7	2
3278	3	0	0	120	41	0	2	0	7	3	3	1	3	0	2	6	3	4	2
3279	4	1	0	62	53	0	2	0	6	3	3	1	3	0	1	3	3	4	1
3280	5	1	0	586	58	0	2	0	17	12	12	1	14	0	5	5	3	14	2
3281	2	0	0	1	33	0	1	0	1	1	2	2	1	0	1	3	2	1	2
3282	4	1	0	391	38	0	2	0	11	8	8	1	9	0	4	3	2	9	2
3283	4	1	0	191	217	0	2	0	11	8	8	1	9	0	4	3	2	9	2
3284	0	0	0	197	36	0	0	0	11	11	9	1	10	0	1	4	2	13	2
3285	4	1	0	311	64	0	2	0	10	6	8	2	5	0	1	6	5	7	3
3286	7	2	2	317	78	1	5	0	9	6	10	24	7	0	3	10	5	5	2
3287	6	1	0	129	60	0	3	0	14	6	9	2	7	0	4	10	4	12	3
3288	2	0	0	598	67	0	1	0	25	13	16	1	14	0	8	8	2	22	2
3289	0	0	0	437	50	0	0	0	20	9	13	1	11	0	8	13	2	17	2

Grains, Beans, Nuts, Seeds

Food #	Food Description & Amount	wt gm	wt oz	calo-ries	%cal fat	prot gm	carbo gm	fiber gm
3290	Cracker, toast, thin (rye, pumpernickel, white flour) (Include pizza thin, pumpernickel cracker, onion toast, Won-Ton Chip) [1 cup]	49	1.7	230	34%	4	34	2.8
3291	Cracker, toast, thin (rye, wheat, white flour), low sodium (Include Low Salt Wheat Thin) [1 cup]	49	1.7	238	33%	4	34	3.0
3292	Cracker, water biscuit [10 crackers]	40	1.4	166	27%	4	28	1.3
3293	Cracker, wheat (including toasted, cracked, or stoned wheat) (Include Wheatsworth cracker, Euphrates cracker, Wheatable cracker, Wheat Thin) [10 crackers]	40	1.4	189	39%	3	26	1.8
3294	Cracker, wheat, reduced fat [10 crackers]	14	0.5	60	25%	1	10	0.8
3295	Cracker, wheat, reduced fat (Include Wheat Thin) [10 crackers]	17	0.6	72	25%	2	12	1.0
3296	Cracker, 100% whole wheat (Include Triscuit, Wheatbury cracker, Wheatmeal English Biscuit, 100% stoned wheat wafer) [10 crackers]	40	1.4	177	35%	4	27	4.2
3297	Cracker, 100% whole wheat (or stoned wheat), low sodium (Include 100% stoned wheat wafer, Triscuits [10 crackers]	40	1.4	177	35%	4	27	4.2
3298	Cracker, 100% whole wheat, reduced fat (Include Triscuit) [10 crackers]	39	1.4	158	23%	5	28	5.1
3299	Cracker, whole wheat and bran (Include Wheat 'N Bran Triscuit) [10 crackers]	40	1.4	176	35%	4	27	4.4
3300	Crispbread, rye (Include Ry Krisp, Wasa rye crispbread, Finn rye crisp, Norwegian flatbread) [5 crackers (3½"x1¾"x¼")]	35	1.2	128	3%	3	29	5.8
3301	Crispbread, rye, low sodium [5 crackers (3½"x1¾"x¼")]	35	1.2	128	3%	3	29	5.8
3302	Crispbread, wheat (Include Armenian cracker bread, Lavosh, hardtack) [5 crackers]	30	1.1	122	2%	3	26	0.9
3303	Crispbread, wheat, low sodium (Include Low Sodium French Crisp Toast) [3 crackers]	26	0.9	103	2%	3	22	0.8
3304	Crispbread, white or rye, fat ingredient added (Include Wasa Extra Crisp) [5 crackers (5"x2")]	30	1.1	119	15%	3	22	2.1
3305	Multigrain, chips (all flavors) (Include Sun Chips) [1 cup (about 12 chips)]	25	0.9	129	45%	2	16	1.5
3306	Multigrain snack mix (pretzels, chex cereal, nuts) (Include Chex Party Mix) [1 cup]	45	1.6	193	28%	5	31	2.5
3307	Multigrain snack mix (bread sticks, sesame nuggets, pretzels, rye chips) [1 cup]	103	3.6	493	43%	9	61	2.5
3308	Onion-flavored rings [20 rings]	20	0.7	100	41%	2	13	0.8
3309	Party snack mix (corn puffs and chips, with pretzels, without nuts) (Include Keystone Party Mix) [1 cup]	40	1.4	202	47%	3	25	1.4
3310	Party snack mix, oriental-style (with peanuts, sesame sticks, chili rice crackers, fried green peas) [1 cup]	112	4.0	615	42%	19	58	14.8
3311	Party snack mix, wheat-based, high fiber (Include Spicer's flavored snacks) [1 cup]	46	1.6	177	29%	5	30	8.7
3312	Popcorn cake (Include Chicosan; puffed corn and rice cake) [3 cakes]	28	1.0	108	7%	3	22	0.8
3313	Popcorn, air-popped, plain [2 cups]	16	0.6	61	10%	2	12	2.4
3314	Popcorn, air-popped, buttered [2 cups]	26	0.9	126	52%	2	14	2.7
3315	Popcorn, buttered (including microwave butter popcorn) [2 cups]	28	1.0	146	57%	2	14	2.5
3316	Popcorn, flavored (including cheese-, butter-, barbecued-, sour cream and onion-flavored) [2 cups]	24	0.8	121	53%	2	12	2.4
3317	Popcorn, with parmesan cheese [2 cups]	52	1.8	258	51%	6	27	4.7
3318	Popcorn, lowfat, low sodium (Include Orville Redenbacher's Light Microwave popcorn) [1 pop-and-serve bag]	83	2.9	340	21%	10	60	11.8
3319	Popcorn, unbuttered (including microwave unbuttered popcorn) [2 cups]	28	1.0	140	51%	3	16	2.8
3320	Popcorn, unsalted (including Newman's Own Oldstyle Picture Show Microwave Popcorn Natural No-Salt Flavor) [1 pop-and-serve bag]	96	3.4	480	51%	9	55	9.6
3321	Popcorn, lowfat (including Betty Crocker Light Microwave Popcorn) [1 pop-and-serve bag]	74	2.6	303	21%	9	53	10.5
3322	Popcorn, caramel-coated, with nuts (Include Cracker Jacks, Fiddle Faddle, Crunch N' Munch) [1 cup]	42	1.5	168	18%	3	34	1.6
3323	Popcorn, caramel-coated (or sugar syrup coated) [1 cup]	35	1.2	151	27%	1	28	1.8
3324	Popcorn, caramel-coated, fat free (Include Louise's Caramel Fat-Free Popcorn) [1 cup]	33	1.2	117	4%	1	29	0.8

Food #	fat gm	sat fat gm	choles mg	sodium mg	potass mg	% of Daily Value													
						vit A	vit E	vit C	thia-min	ribo-flavin	nia-cin	vit B-6	fol-ate	vit B-12	cal-cium	phos-phorus	magne-sium	iron	zinc
3290	9	2	0	283	95	0	6	0	7	7	10	2	5	0	4	10	6	9	4
3291	9	2	0	130	61	0	7	0	9	5	7	2	5	0	1	5	5	8	3
3292	5	1	4	188	56	0	4	0	3	1	4	1	2	0	5	3	2	4	2
3293	8	2	0	318	73	0	5	0	13	8	10	3	4	0	2	9	6	10	4
3294	2	0	0	99	31	0	1	0	4	2	4	1	2	0	1	4	2	4	1
3295	2	0	0	121	37	0	1	0	5	3	4	1	3	0	2	5	3	5	2
3296	7	1	0	264	119	0	5	0	5	2	9	4	3	0	2	12	10	7	6
3297	7	1	0	99	119	0	5	0	5	2	9	4	3	0	2	12	10	7	6
3298	4	1	0	165	152	0	4	0	9	4	11	6	3	0	1	13	13	8	7
3299	7	1	0	260	124	0	5	0	5	3	9	4	3	0	2	12	11	7	6
3300	0	0	0	92	112	0	2	0	6	3	2	4	4	0	1	9	7	5	6
3301	0	0	0	92	112	0	2	0	6	3	2	4	4	0	1	9	7	5	6
3302	0	0	0	1	36	0	0	0	14	9	9	1	9	0	1	4	2	9	2
3303	0	0	0	83	30	0	0	0	12	7	7	1	8	0	0	3	2	7	1
3304	2	0	0	191	84	0	1	0	8	6	5	2	5	1	2	6	3	5	3
3305	7	0	0	105	34	1	5	0	2	1	1	2	2	0	0	2	2	1	1
3306	6	1	1	419	131	1	2	20	26	10	29	24	27	21	3	12	10	41	7
3307	23	4	1	1258	113	0	21	0	36	25	24	3	28	0	2	12	6	22	5
3308	5	1	0	196	29	0	1	1	3	4	3	1	6	0	1	1	1	4	0
3309	11	2	1	386	65	1	3	0	5	8	5	4	8	0	4	6	5	5	2
3310	29	4	0	463	367	0	31	1	23	11	17	4	11	0	6	29	33	15	20
3311	6	1	0	94	164	0	5	0	9	7	12	6	8	0	2	14	13	9	8
3312	1	0	0	81	92	0	0	0	1	3	8	3	1	0	0	8	11	3	7
3313	1	0	0	1	48	0	0	0	2	3	2	2	1	0	0	5	5	2	4
3314	7	4	17	67	56	6	0	0	2	3	2	2	1	0	0	6	6	3	4
3315	9	3	6	246	58	2	0	0	2	2	2	3	1	0	0	6	7	4	4
3316	7	2	2	201	57	1	3	0	2	3	2	2	1	0	2	6	5	2	4
3317	15	3	4	511	111	2	0	0	4	5	4	5	2	1	8	16	13	8	9
3318	8	1	0	407	200	1	3	0	19	5	9	7	4	0	1	22	31	11	21
3319	8	1	0	248	63	0	0	0	3	2	2	3	1	0	0	7	8	4	5
3320	27	5	0	3	216	1	18	0	8	8	7	10	4	0	1	24	26	15	17
3321	7	1	0	654	178	1	3	0	17	5	8	6	3	0	1	20	28	9	19
3322	3	0	0	124	149	0	2	0	1	3	4	4	2	0	3	5	8	9	3
3323	4	1	2	72	38	0	1	0	2	1	4	0	0	0	2	3	3	3	1
3324	0	0	0	94	36	0	0	0	1	1	1	1	0	0	1	2	2	1	1

Grains, Beans, Nuts, Seeds

Food #	Food Description & Amount	wt gm	wt oz	calo-ries	%cal fat	prot gm	carbo gm	fiber gm
3325	**Potato chips** (plain or flavored) [1 oz (about 10 rippled chips or 16 regular chips)]	28	1.0	150	58%	2	15	1.3
3326	Potato chips, unsalted (plain or flavored, unsalted) [1 oz]	28	1.0	150	58%	2	15	1.3
3327	Potato chips, reduced fat (Include Light Choice Ruffles) [1 oz]	28	1.0	132	40%	2	19	1.6
3328	Potato chips, reduced fat, unsalted (Include Michael Season's 40% less fat Potato Chips [1 oz]	28	1.0	132	40%	2	19	1.7
3329	Potato chips, fat free (Include Louise's Fat Free Potato Chips) [1 oz]	28	1.0	110	1%	3	23	2.1
3330	Potato chips, fat free, made with Olean (Include Wow! chips) [1 oz]	28	1.0	74	2%	2	17	1.1
3331	**Potato chips, restructured** (Include Pringles, Hearty Potato Krunch Twists) [1"stack (about 14 chips]	28	1.0	156	62%	2	14	1.0
3332	Potato chips, restructured, reduced fat and sodium (Include Pringles Right Crisps) [1"stack (about 14 chips]	28	1.0	140	46%	2	18	1.0
3333	Potato chips, restructured, baked (Include Mr. Phillips Tater Crisps, Baked Lay's) [1 oz]	28	1.0	133	35%	1	20	1.3
3334	Potato, chips, restructured, fat free, made with Olean (Include Pringles made with Olestra) [1" stack (about 14 chips)]	25	0.9	63	3%	1	14	1.6
3335	Potato based snacks, reduced fat, low sodium, all flavors (Include Nutri/System Flavor Crisps) [20 crisps]	14	0.5	65	44%	1	8	0.6
3336	**Pretzel, hard**, salted (plain or flavored) [1 oz]	28	1.0	107	8%	3	22	0.9
3337	Pretzel, hard, unsalted [1 oz]	28	1.0	107	8%	3	22	0.8
3338	Pretzel, baby [5 pretzels]	30	1.1	119	5%	3	25	0.7
3339	Pretzel, hard, oat bran [10 pretzels]	30	1.1	115	13%	4	22	1.2
3340	Pretzel, hard, multigrain [10 pretzels]	30	1.1	114	7%	4	24	2.9
3341	**Pretzel, soft** [1 pretzel]	55	1.9	190	8%	5	38	0.9
3342	Pretzel, cheese-filled (Include Combos) [10 combos]	30	1.1	129	34%	3	18	0.7
3343	Pretzel, chocolate-coated [2 pretzels]	22	0.8	92	24%	2	16	0.7
3344	Pretzel, yogurt-covered [10 pretzels (2"x1"x¼")]	42	1.5	191	32%	3	30	0.7
3345	**Rice cake**, puffed (including Arden, Chico San, Quaker, Spiral, rice cake with seeds and other grains) [3 cakes]	27	1.0	104	7%	2	22	1.1
3346	Puffed wheat cake (Include Quaker Wheat Cakes) [3 cakes]	27	1.0	98	5%	4	20	2.5
3347	Rice cake, cracker-type [10 mini rounds (1¾"dia)]	30	1.1	120	10%	2	25	1.3
3348	Rice paper [2 pieces (8½"dia)]	28	1.0	93	3%	1	21	0.6
3349	Shrimp chips (tapioca base) (Include shrimp crackers, prawn crackers, banh phong tom) [1 cup]	40	1.4	224	58%	3	21	0.2
3350	**Tortilla chips** (plain or flavored) (Include Tostitos, Doritos, Suncheros) [2 oz]	57	2.0	286	47%	4	36	3.7
3351	Tortilla chips, unsalted (plain or flavored) [2 oz]	57	2.0	290	47%	4	36	3.7
3352	Tortilla chips, light (baked with less oil), plain or flavored (Include Doritos Light) [2 oz]	57	2.0	263	30%	5	41	3.2
3353	Tortilla chips, lowfat, baked without fat (Include Baked Tostitos) [2 oz]	57	2.0	224	13%	6	46	3.0
3354	Tortilla chips, lowfat, baked without fat, unsalted [2 oz]	57	2.0	224	13%	6	46	3.0
3355	Tortilla chips, fat free, made with Olean (Include Doritos Wow! with Olestra) [2 oz]	57	2.0	182	11%	5	36	2.1
3356	Tortilla chips, with oat bran [2 oz]	57	2.0	278	47%	4	36	4.0
3357	Wheat-and-corn chips (Include wheat-cheese chips, Pizzarias Pizza Chips) [1 cup]	31	1.1	152	40%	3	20	1.0
3358	Wheat sticks, 100% whole wheat (with/without sesame seeds) [1 cup]	55	1.9	298	61%	6	26	1.5
	Pancakes & Waffles							
3400	Bread fritters, Puerto Rican style (Include Torrejas, Galician fritters) [2 fritters with syrup (4"x2½"x3¼")]	110	3.9	291	28%	5	48	0.8
3401	Crepe, plain (Include French pancake) [1 crepe (7"dia)]	50	1.8	113	45%	4	11	0.3
3402	Flour and milk patty [2 pancakes]	56	2.0	139	19%	5	25	4.0
3403	Flour and water patty (Include Chinese pancake) [2 pancakes]	56	2.0	116	2%	2	25	0.4
3404	French toast sticks, plain [2 sticks]	44	1.6	160	51%	3	18	0.8
3405	**French toast**, plain [1 slice]	65	2.3	160	35%	6	20	0.8
3406	Funnel cake [1 cake (6"dia)]	90	3.2	277	47%	7	29	0.9
3407	Pancake, buckwheat [1 pancake (5"dia)]	40	1.4	71	32%	3	10	1.0

Food #	fat gm	sat fat gm	choles mg	sodium mg	potass mg	vit A	vit E	vit C	thia-min	ribo-flavin	nia-cin	vit B-6	fol-ate	vit B-12	cal-cium	phos-phorus	magne-sium	iron	zinc
						% of Daily Value													
3325	10	3	0	166	357	0	5	15	3	3	5	9	3	0	1	5	5	3	2
3326	10	3	0	2	357	0	5	15	3	3	5	9	3	0	1	5	5	3	2
3327	6	1	0	138	488	0	3	12	4	4	10	9	2	0	1	5	6	2	0
3328	6	1	0	2	488	0	3	12	4	4	10	9	1	0	1	5	6	2	2
3329	0	0	0	180	456	0	0	4	20	2	9	11	3	0	1	5	5	6	1
3330	0	0	0	183	361	44	68	14	6	1	6	26	2	0	1	5	6	2	2
3331	11	3	0	184	282	0	5	4	4	2	4	2	0	0	1	4	4	2	1
3332	7	1	0	120	281	0	5	6	4	1	6	11	2	0	1	4	4	2	1
3333	5	1	0	257	202	0	2	0	6	1	6	7	0	0	4	8	3	1	1
3334	0	0	0	138	176	41	51	6	11	1	5	6	2	0	1	3	1	2	1
3335	3	0	1	77	102	0	5	1	2	1	2	3	1	0	2	2	2	1	1
3336	1	0	0	480	41	0	0	0	9	10	7	2	12	0	1	3	2	7	2
3337	1	0	0	81	41	0	0	0	9	10	7	2	6	0	1	3	2	7	2
3338	1	0	0	81	41	0	0	2	9	6	5	1	6	0	1	3	2	6	2
3339	2	0	0	219	58	0	1	0	4	3	3	1	6	0	1	6	4	3	2
3340	1	0	0	3	86	0	1	0	6	3	6	4	2	0	1	9	10	4	5
3341	2	0	2	772	48	0	0	0	15	9	12	1	2	0	1	4	3	12	3
3342	5	1	4	421	85	3	2	0	7	12	6	2	9	1	6	7	3	6	2
3343	2	1	1	277	47	0	0	0	5	7	4	1	7	0	2	3	2	4	1
3344	7	6	0	359	92	0	2	0	7	11	6	2	9	3	5	6	2	5	2
3345	1	0	0	88	78	0	1	0	1	3	11	2	1	0	0	10	9	2	5
3346	1	0	0	126	97	0	1	0	7	4	16	2	2	2	1	9	9	7	5
3347	1	0	0	21	128	0	1	0	1	3	12	2	2	0	0	11	10	2	6
3348	0	0	0	88	19	0	0	0	2	0	3	5	0	0	0	2	2	1	1
3349	14	3	23	31	30	0	14	0	0	2	1	0	2		2	3	1	4	1
3350	15	3	0	301	112	1	3	0	3	6	4	8	1	0	9	12	13	5	6
3351	15	2	0	138	107	2	8	2	5	5	4	7	1	0	9	13	12	5	5
3352	9	2	2	572	155	2	5	0	8	9	1	5	2	1	9	18	14	5	4
3353	3	0	0	239	155	2	5	0	8	9	1	5	2	0	9	18	14	5	4
3354	3	0	0	9	155	2	5	0	8	9	1	5	2	0	9	18	14	5	4
3355	2	1	1	451	226	65	96	0	12	11	8	11	2	3	8	14	14	3	6
3356	14	3	0	286	123	1	3	0	4	6	4	8	2	0	9	13	14	5	6
3357	7	1	1	285	51	0	4	0	10	7	6	1	7	0	2	4	2	6	2
3358	20	4	0	818	97	0	7	0	5	2	4	2	3	0	9	8	6	2	4
3400	9	2	49	183	97	3	3	0	8	11	6	2	5	3	6	7	3	5	3
3401	6	2	79	38	80	5	2	0	6	11	3	2	5	4	5	7	2	4	3
3402	3	1	2	14	170	1	3	0	8	6	9	5	3	1	4	14	12	7	7
3403	0	0	0	2	37	0	0	0	1	1	3	3	1	0	1	4	2	1	2
3404	9	1	23	156	40	0	4	0	5	5	5	4	6	0	2	4	2	5	2
3405	6	2	91	210	85	5	2	0	9	14	7	3	9	4	6	8	3	7	3
3406	14	3	63	117	155	6	8	1	16	19	9	3	11	4	13	14	4	10	4
3407	3	1	23	184	81	2	1	0	4	5	2	2	2	2	9	14	5	4	3

Grains, Beans, Nuts, Seeds

Food #	Food Description & Amount	wt gm	wt oz	calo-ries	%cal fat	prot gm	carbo gm	fiber gm
3408	Pancake, cornmeal [1 pancake (5"dia)]	40	1.4	81	26%	2	13	0.9
3409	Pancake, made with rice flour and dried peas (Include Indian pancake) [2 pancakes]	58	2.0	158	3%	5	33	3.9
3410	Pancake, Norwegian Lefse, potato and flour [1 lefse (6"dia)]	34	1.2	77	29%	1	12	0.7
3411	**Pancake, plain [1 pancake (5"dia)]**	40	1.4	92	13%	2	17	0.7
3412	Pancake, reduced calorie, high fiber [1 pancake (4"dia)]	32	1.1	59	17%	2	12	2.2
3413	Pancake, rye [1 pancake (5"dia)]	40	1.4	120	31%	3	18	1.2
3414	Pancake, sour dough [1 pancake (5"dia)]	40	1.4	88	26%	2	14	0.6
3415	Pancake, whole wheat [1 pancake (5"dia)]	40	1.4	93	40%	3	12	1.5
3416	Pancake, with fruit (Include blueberry pancake) [1 pancake (5"dia)]	40	1.4	76	30%	3	11	0.8
3417	Rice paste (Include Japanese Mochi) [2 oz]	56	2.0	132	2%	3	29	1.4
3418	**Waffle, plain [1 waffle (4"square)]**	37	1.3	98	28%	2	15	0.9
3419	Waffle, plain, fat free [1 waffle (4"square)]	30	1.1	74	1%	3	15	0.4
3420	Waffle, cornmeal [1 waffle (4"square)]	37	1.3	102	31%	3	14	0.8
3421	Waffle, fruit (Include blueberry waffle) [1 waffle (4"square)]	37	1.3	88	27%	2	14	0.9
3422	Waffle, multi-bran [1 waffle (4"square)]	38	1.3	103	38%	3	14	1.0
3423	Waffle, nut and honey [1 waffle (4"square)]	46	1.6	142	37%	4	19	0.0
3424	Waffle, oat bran (Include Eggo waffle) [1 waffle (4"square)]	38	1.3	97	32%	3	13	1.4
3425	Waffle, wheat, bran, or mixed grain (Include Roman Meal waffle, Nutri-Grain Raisin and Bran waffle) [1 waffle (4"square)]	37	1.3	111	34%	3	17	1.8
3426	Waffle, 100% whole wheat or 100% whole grain [1 waffle (4"square)]	37	1.3	99	38%	3	12	0.9
	Cooked Cereals (About 1/3 to 1/2 cup dry makes about 1 cup cooked; cooking in salted water can add several hundred mg sodium per cup of cereal.)							
3450	Barley, cooked without salt [1 cup]	162	5.7	199	3%	4	46	6.2
3451	Buckwheat groats, cooked without salt (Include kasha) [1 cup]	168	5.9	155	6%	6	33	4.5
3452	Bulgur, cooked without salt (Include wheat pilaf) [1 cup]	135	4.8	112	3%	4	25	6.1
3453	Cornmeal dumplings (Include boiled cornbread) [1 cup]	240	8.5	405	25%	14	60	4.8
3454	**Cornmeal mush, made with unsalted water (Include polenta) [1 cup]**	240	8.5	223	4%	5	47	4.5
3455	Cornmeal mush, made with whole milk [1 cup]	240	8.5	330	20%	15	51	3.4
3456	Cornmeal mush, cooked without salt, fried [1 slice]	51	1.8	80	21%	2	14	1.3
3457	Cornmeal, lime-treated, cooked without salt (Include masa harina, Fu Fu) [1 cup]	240	8.5	235	9%	6	49	6.2
3458	Cornmeal, made with milk, sugar, Puerto Rican style (Include Harina de maiz con leche) [1 cup]	227	8.0	297	21%	8	51	1.8
3459	Cornmeal sticks (cornmeal, coconut milk, molasses, anise seed), boiled (Include guanimes) [1 cup]	211	7.4	380	30%	5	63	4.6
3460	Couscous, cooked without salt [1 cup]	146	5.1	164	1%	6	34	2.0
3461	Couscous, cooked with margarine [1 cup]	162	5.7	237	29%	6	36	2.1
3462	Cream of rice, cooked without salt [1 cup]	244	8.6	127	2%	2	28	0.2
3463	Cream of rice, made with evaporated milk, sugar, Puerto Rican style [1 cup]	245	8.6	304	25%	9	48	0.3
3464	**Cream of wheat, instant, various flavors, cooked without salt (Include farina) [1 cup]**	241	8.5	134	3%	4	28	1.2
3465	Cream of wheat, quick, cooked (Include farina) [1 cup]	239	8.4	105	3%	3	22	0.8
3466	Cream of wheat, regular, cooked without salt (Include farina) [1 cup]	251	8.9	110	4%	3	23	1.1
3467	Cream of wheat, cooked with milk, sugar, Puerto Rican style [1 cup]	245	8.6	307	26%	10	47	1.0
3468	Cream of wheat, cooked with milk [1 cup]	243	8.6	213	24%	11	29	0.8
3469	**Grits, corn or hominy (regular, quick, or instant), cooked in unsalted water [1 cup]**	242	8.5	111	3%	3	24	0.5
3470	Grits, corn or hominy (regular, quick, or instant), cooked with whole milk [1 cup]	242	8.5	237	21%	11	35	0.5
3471	Grits, corn or hominy, flavored, instant, includes salt, cooked (Include Quaker Instant Grits) [1 cup]	242	8.5	168	14%	4	34	1.9
3472	Grits, corn or hominy, cooked with cheese [1 cup]	247	8.7	194	35%	8	23	0.4
3473	Millet, cooked without salt [1 cup]	131	4.6	156	8%	5	31	1.7
3474	Multi-grain cereal, cooked without salt (Include seven-grain cereals) [1 cup]	246	8.7	202	10%	7	40	3.9
3475	Muesli, prepared, instant, includes salt [1 cup]	254	9.0	232	14%	15	42	7.2

Food #	fat gm	sat fat gm	choles mg	sodium mg	potass mg	vit A	vit E	vit C	thia-min	ribo-flavin	nia-cin	vit B-6	fol-ate	vit B-12	cal-cium	phos-phorus	magne-sium	iron	zinc
3408	2	1	16	99	40	3	1	0	6	5	4	2	5	1	5	4	2	4	1
3409	1	0	0	1	162	0	1	0	7	2	5	7	6	0	1	7	6	3	4
3410	2	1	1	46	89	0	1	3	5	3	4	3	3	0	1	2	2	3	1
3411	1	0	4	204	29	1	1	0	10	11	8	1	5	1	2	15	1	8	2
3412	1	0	9	206	59	1	1	0	5	5	3	1	3	2	9	12	2	3	2
3413	4	1	15	111	184	1	2	0	5	5	3	4	3	1	4	5	7	6	2
3414	3	1	16	100	32	1	2	0	8	7	5	1	7	1	1	3	1	5	1
3415	4	1	24	128	96	2	3	0	4	5	4	3	2	2	8	9	5	4	3
3416	3	1	24	169	73	2	1	2	5	6	2	2	3	2	7	11	2	2	2
3417	0	0	0	7	14	0	0	0	2	1	2	2	0	0	0	1	2	1	4
3418	3	1	9	291	47	13	1	0	9	10	8	17	4	15	9	16	2	9	1
3419	0	0	0	130	38	0	0	0	5	7	3	0	3	0	3	5	1	3	1
3420	4	1	35	78	61	3	2	0	7	8	4	2	6	2	6	6	2	5	2
3421	3	0	8	250	47	12	1	2	8	9	7	14	4	13	7	13	2	8	1
3422	4	1	0	165	61	0	3	0	7	7	6	2	4	0	4	9	4	6	2
3423	6	1	15	283	255	18	3	0	12	12	12	12	6	12	2	12	7	12	3
3424	3	1	0	171	153	15	2	0	10	10	10	10	5	10	2	10	6	10	2
3425	4	1	25	133	112	6	2	4	9	10	7	5	7	6	11	11	7	8	5
3426	4	1	35	125	86	3	2	0	5	7	4	2	3	2	10	9	4	4	3
3450	1	0	0	5	151	0	0	0	9	6	17	9	6	0	2	9	9	12	9
3451	1	0	0	7	148	0	1	0	4	4	8	6	6	0	1	12	21	7	7
3452	0	0	0	7	92	0	0	0	5	2	7	6	6	0	1	5	11	7	5
3453	11	3	189	352	249	16	5	1	31	34	18	11	28	9	21	24	10	22	8
3454	1	0	0	14	99	2	1	0	23	13	14	7	20	0	1	5	7	14	4
3455	7	4	27	163	577	17	1	4	25	40	12	11	18	16	39	35	15	11	11
3456	2	0	0	4	29	1	1	0	6	4	4	2	5	0	0	2	2	4	1
3457	2	0	0	19	192	0	1	0	49	26	29	11	21	0	10	14	19	26	9
3458	7	4	26	99	307	6	1	2	11	22	6	4	9	1	23	20	8	7	6
3459	13	11	0	22	712	2	2	2	20	10	14	18	17	0	8	10	30	25	5
3460	0	0	0	7	85	0	0	0	6	2	7	4	5	0	1	3	3	3	3
3461	8	1	0	94	92	7	4	0	6	3	8	4	6	0	1	4	3	3	3
3462	0	0	0	2	49	0	0	0	0	0	5	3	2	0	1	4	2	3	3
3463	8	5	32	119	357	6	1	3	11	21	7	5	13	2	29	25	8	7	8
3464	1	0	0	12	42	0	0	0	11	4	7	2	33	0	6	4	4	58	3
3465	0	0	0	121	36	0	0	0	8	3	5	1	6	0	5	8	3	44	2
3466	0	0	0	10	34	0	0	0	8	3	6	2	6	0	5	3	3	45	2
3467	9	5	33	123	367	6	1	3	10	23	6	4	7	2	33	25	9	39	7
3468	6	3	22	133	436	13	1	4	12	27	5	6	7	13	35	28	10	33	8
3469	0	0	0	8	39	0	0	0	10	6	7	2	10	0	1	2	3	6	1
3470	6	3	21	128	435	12	1	3	16	30	8	7	12	12	31	26	10	7	7
3471	3	1	1	868	79	0	0	0	16	17	17	4	18	2	3	6	5	74	3
3472	8	5	19	352	109	6	1	0	10	12	6	4	9	5	17	16	4	7	7
3473	1	0	0	3	81	0	1	0	9	6	9	7	6	0	0	13	14	5	8
3474	2	0	0	2	138	0	11	0	26	27	22	23	4	0	7	18	17	30	6
3475	4	1	4	349	671	47	23	28	28	30	30	31	31	31	38	34	32	31	32

Grains, Beans, Nuts, Seeds

Food #	Food Description & Amount	wt gm	wt oz	calo-ries	%cal fat	prot gm	carbo gm	fiber gm
3476	Nestum, Puerto Rican cereal, without salt [1 cup]	245	8.6	42	6%	1	8	1.5
3477	Oat bran cereal, cooked without salt (Include Mother's Oat Bran) [1 cup]	242	8.5	81	26%	6	22	5.1
3478	Oat bran cereal, cooked with milk [1 cup]	242	8.5	206	32%	14	33	4.9
3479	Oatmeal, dry, regular or quick (sliced thinner), uncooked [1 cup]	81	2.9	311	15%	13	54	8.6
3480	Oatmeal, regular or quick, cooked without salt [1 cup]	234	8.3	146	15%	6	25	4.0
3481	Oatmeal with raisins, cooked without salt [1 cup]	234	8.3	190	11%	6	38	4.5
3482	Oatmeal with maple flavor, cooked without salt (Include Maypo) [1 cup]	240	8.5	170	13%	6	32	5.8
3483	**Oatmeal, instant, fortified**, includes salt (Include with spice, fruit) [1 cup]	**234**	**8.3**	**226**	**15%**	**9**	**39**	**6.7**
3484	Oatmeal, made with milk, sugar, Puerto Rican style (Avena con leche) [1 cup]	210	7.4	263	30%	10	37	1.8
3485	Oatmeal, with additional oat bran, instant, fortified, includes salt [1 packet]	152	5.4	142	15%	4	26	2.9
3486	Rye, cream of, cooked without salt (rye flour, water) [1 cup]	251	8.9	109	3%	2	24	4.3
3487	Wheat cereal, chocolate flavored, cooked without salt (Include cocoa wheat cereal, Chocolate Malt-O-Meal) [1 cup]	246	8.7	123	9%	4	27	4.3
3488	Wheat hearts, cooked without salt [1 cup]	245	8.6	114	5%	4	25	3.2
3489	Wheat, rolled, cooked without salt [1 cup]	242	8.5	114	5%	4	25	3.2
3490	Whole wheat cereal, cooked without salt (Include Wheatena, Ralston, Zoom, Roman Meal, Branola, home ground cereal, Roman Meal with oats) [1 cup, cooked]	246	8.7	114	5%	4	25	3.2
3491	Whole wheat cereal, wheat and barley, cooked without salt (Include Maltex, Malt-O-Meal) [1 cup]	249	8.8	171	5%	5	37	2.0
Ready to Eat Cereals (check product websites or labels for updates)								
3550	All-Bran, Kellogg's [1 cup]	62	2.2	160	11%	8	46	19.7
3551	All-Bran Bran Buds, Kellogg's [1 cup]	90	3.2	210	13%	6	72	39.0
3552	All-Bran Extra Fiber, Kellogg's [1 cup]	52	1.8	100	18%	6	40	26.0
3553	Alpha-Bits, Post [1 cup]	32	1.1	136	10%	3	27	1.1
3554	Alpha-Bits with marshmallows, Post [1 cup]	30	1.1	120	8%	2	26	1.0
3555	Apple Cinnamon Cheerios, General Mills [1 cup]	40	1.4	160	12%	2	33	2.0
3556	**Apple Jacks**, Kellogg's [1 cup]	**33**	**1.2**	**130**	**3%**	**1**	**30**	**0.9**
3557	Banana Nut Crunch Cereal, Post [1 cup]	72	2.5	305	22%	6	54	4.9
3558	Basic 4, General Mills [1 cup]	55	1.9	200	13%	4	42	3.0
3559	Berry Berry Kix, General Mills [1 cup]	40	1.4	160	9%	2	35	0.2
3560	Blueberry Morning, Post [1 cup]	55	1.9	220	12%	4	42	2.0
3561	Boo Berry, General Mills [1 cup]	30	1.1	120	4%	1	27	0.4
3562	Bran Flakes, Post [1 cup]	40	1.4	128	6%	4	32	7.0
3563	**Cap'n Crunch**, Quaker [1 cup]	**37**	**1.3**	**147**	**11%**	**2**	**32**	**1.2**
3564	Cap'n Crunch's Crunch Berries, Quaker [1 cup]	35	1.2	140	11%	2	30	0.8
3565	Cap'n Crunch's Peanut Butter Crunch, Quaker [1 cup]	35	1.2	146	19%	3	28	1.0
3566	**Cheerios**, General Mills [1 cup]	**30**	**1.1**	**110**	**15%**	**3**	**22**	**2.5**
3567	Cinnamon Crunch Crispix, Kellogg's [1 cup]	40	1.4	160	8%	2	35	0.2
3568	Cinnamon Grahams, General Mills [1 cup]	40	1.4	160	9%	2	35	1.4
3569	Cinnamon Toast Crunch, General Mills [1 cup]	40	1.4	173	22%	2	32	1.9
3570	Cocoa Blasts, Quaker [1 cup]	33	1.2	129	8%	1	29	0.8
3571	Cocoa Rice Krispies, Kellogg's [1 cup]	41	1.5	160	6%	2	36	0.5
3572	**Cocoa Pebbles**, Post [1 cup]	**29**	**1.0**	**120**	**7%**	**1**	**25**	**0.0**
3573	Cocoa Puffs, General Mills [1 cup]	30	1.1	120	7%	1	26	0.2
3574	Complete Oat Bran Flakes, Kellogg's [1 cup]	40	1.4	147	9%	4	31	5.2
3575	Complete Wheat Bran Flakes, Kellogg's [1 cup]	39	1.4	120	6%	4	31	6.2
3576	Cookie Crisp, General Mills [1 cup]	30	1.1	120	8%	1	26	0.4
3577	Corn Chex, General Mills [1 cup]	30	1.1	110	1%	2	26	0.5
3578	**Corn flakes**, Kellogg's [1 cup]	**28**	**1.0**	**100**	**2%**	**2**	**24**	**0.8**
3579	Corn Pops, Kellogg's [1 cup]	31	1.1	118	1%	1	28	0.7

% of Daily Value

Food #	fat gm	sat fat gm	choles mg	sodium mg	potass mg	vit A	vit E	vit C	thia-min	ribo-flavin	nia-cin	vit B-6	fol-ate	vit B-12	cal-cium	phos-phorus	magne-sium	iron	zinc
3476	0	0	0	8	31	0	0	6	3	5	2	4	1	0	4	5	4	2	2
3477	2	0	0	9	177	0	2	0	20	4	1	2	3	0	2	23	20	10	7
3478	7	4	21	127	566	12	2	3	26	27	2	7	6	12	33	47	27	10	13
3479	5	1	0	3	284	1	2	0	39	7	3	5	6	0	4	38	30	19	17
3480	2	0	0	8	126	0	1	0	15	3	1	2	2	0	2	17	15	9	8
3481	2	0	0	10	253	0	1	1	16	4	2	4	2	0	3	18	15	10	8
3482	2	0	0	10	211	70	6	48	48	42	47	48	2	48	12	25	13	47	10
3483	4	1	0	624	217	98	1	0	68	35	56	80	44	0	36	29	23	76	13
3484	9	5	30	113	370	6	1	3	9	21	2	3	3	2	28	29	13	5	9
3485	2	0	0	146	120	147	132	96	98	98	98	98	98	98	20	11	9	98	98
3486	0	0	0	7	66	0	1	0	5	1	1	3	1	0	1	5	6	3	4
3487	1	0	0	9	219	0	2	0	7	6	8	6	5	0	2	15	15	9	8
3488	1	0	0	8	123	0	2	0	7	5	7	6	5	0	2	12	11	6	6
3489	1	0	0	8	123	0	1	0	7	5	7	6	5	0	2	12	11	6	6
3490	1	0	0	8	124	0	2	0	7	5	7	6	5	0	2	12	11	6	6
3491	1	0	0	15	240	0	3	0	13	5	10	3	5	0	2	16	14	9	12
3550	2	0	0	160	700	20	4	20	50	50	50	200	200	200	20	70	50	50	20
3551	3	0	0	600	900	30	4	30	75	75	75	300	300	300	0	45	45	75	30
3552	2	0	0	240	540	20	4	20	50	50	50	200	200	200	20	40	40	50	20
3553	1	0	0	210	60	15	0	0	25	25	25	25	25	25	10	6	6	15	10
3554	1	0	0	230	50	15	1	0	25	25	25	25	25	25	10	4	4	15	10
3555	2	0	0	160	80	13	1	13	33	33	33	33	67	47	13	8	5	33	40
3556	0	0	0	150	35	10	0	25	25	25	25	25	25	25	0	2	2	25	10
3557	8	1	0	293	207	18	3	0	31	30	31	30	60	30	0	18	12	110	12
3558	3	0	0	320	150	10	2	0	25	25	25	25	25	25	25	20	8	25	25
3559	2	0	0	240	33	13	1	13	33	33	33	33	33	33	5	5	1	33	33
3560	3	0	0	250	95	15	8	0	25	25	25	25	25	25	2	9	6	10	6
3561	1	0	0	210	15	0	0	10	25	25	25	25	25	25	2	2	0	25	25
3562	1	0	0	293	246	20	0	0	33	33	33	33	33	33	2	20	20	60	13
3563	2	1	0	286	47	0	1	0	34	34	34	34	144	0	1	4	3	34	34
3564	2	0	0	256	49	1	1	0	34	34	34	34	136	0	1	4	3	34	36
3565	3	1	0	264	81	0	1	0	32	34	32	32	136	0	0	7	6	32	34
3566	2	0	0	280	95	10	1	10	25	25	25	25	50	25	10	10	10	45	25
3567	1	0	0	240	47	13	0	13	33	33	33	33	67	33	1	27	2	40	13
3568	2	0	0	320	60	13	1	13	33	33	33	33	33	33	13	3	3	33	33
3569	4	1	0	280	60	13	1	13	33	33	33	33	33	33	13	5	3	33	33
3570	1	0	0	133	71	33	1	22	28	27	27	27	105	0	1	6	5	28	28
3571	1	1	0	253	67	13	1	33	33	33	33	33	33	33	5	3	3	33	13
3572	1	1	0	180	50	15	0	0	25	25	25	25	25	25	10	2	0	10	10
3573	1	0	0	170	50	0	0	10	25	25	25	25	25	25	10	2	2	25	25
3574	1	0	0	280	160	20	133	133	133	133	133	133	133	133	2	13	13	133	133
3575	1	0	0	280	227	20	133	133	133	133	133	133	133	133	0	20	13	133	133
3576	1	0	0	180	40	10	0	10	25	25	25	25	25	25	10	4	0	25	25
3577	0	0	0	280	25	10	0	10	25	25	25	25	50	25	10	1	1	50	25
3578	0	0	0	200	25	10	0	10	25	25	25	25	25	25	0	1	1	45	1
3579	0	0	0	123	23	10	0	10	25	25	25	25	25	25	0	1	1	10	10

Grains, Beans, Nuts, Seeds

Food #	Food Description & Amount	wt gm	wt oz	calo-ries	%cal fat	prot gm	carbo gm	fiber gm
3580	Count Chocula, General Mills [1 cup]	30	1.1	120	7%	1	26	0.5
3581	Country Corn Flakes, General Mills [1 cup]	30	1.1	110	3%	2	26	0.5
3582	Cracklin' Oat Bran, Kellogg's [1 cup]	65	2.3	267	33%	5	47	6.7
3583	Crispix, Kellogg's [1 cup]	29	1.0	110	2%	2	25	0.7
3584	Crunchy Corn Bran, Quaker [1 cup]	36	1.3	120	9%	2	30	6.4
3585	Fiber One, General Mills [1 cup]	0	2.1	120	12%	4	48	28.5
3586	Franken Berry, General Mills [1 cup]	30	1.1	120	4%	1	27	0.2
3587	French Toast Crunch, General Mills [1 cup]	40	1.4	160	9%	1	35	0.9
3588	Froot Loops, Kellogg's [1 cup]	32	1.1	120	7%	1	28	0.6
3589	Froot Loops, Marshmallow, Kellogg's [1 cup]	30	1.1	120	4%	1	27	0.7
3590	Frosted Cheerios, General Mills [1 cup]	30	1.1	120	7%	2	25	0.9
3591	Frosted Flakes, Kellogg's [1 cup]	41	1.4	160	1%	1	37	0.9
3592	Frosted Shredded Wheat, bite size, Post [1 cup]	57	2.0	208	5%	5	48	5.5
3593	Fruit & Fibre Dates Raisins Walnuts, Post [1 cup]	55	1.9	190	13%	4	42	6.0
3594	Fruit & Fibre Peaches Raisins Almonds, Post [1 cup]	55	1.9	190	13%	4	42	6.0
3595	Fruity Pebbles, Post [1 cup]	27	1.0	110	8%	1	24	0.0
3596	Golden Crisp, Post [1 cup]	36	1.3	146	0%	1	33	0.0
3597	Golden Grahams, General Mills [1 cup]	40	1.4	160	8%	2	33	1.2
3598	Granola, homemade [1 cup]	122	4.3	570	47%	18	65	12.8
3599	Granola Oats and Honey, 100% Natural, Quaker [1 cup]	107	3.8	458	30%	10	75	7.7
3600	Granola with Raisins, 100% Natural, Quaker [1 cup]	110	3.9	496	37%	11	72	7.3
3601	Granola, Low Fat, with fruit, Nature Valley, General Mills [1 cup]	82	2.9	315	12%	6	64	4.1
3602	Granola, Low Fat, with raisins, 100% Natural, Quaker [1 cup]	87	3.1	338	12%	7	70	5.2
3603	Granola, Low Fat, with raisins, Kellogg's [1 cup]	90	3.2	330	12%	8	72	5.4
3604	Granola, Low Fat, without raisins, Kellogg's [1 cup]	98	3.5	380	14%	8	79	5.8
3605	Grape-Nuts Flakes, Post [1 cup]	29	1.0	110	9%	3	24	3.0
3606	Grape-Nuts, Post [1 cup]	109	3.8	383	4%	11	90	9.4
3607	Great Grains Crunchy Pecans Whole Grain Cereal, Post [1 cup]	93	3.3	386	25%	9	68	7.0
3608	Great Grains, Raisins, Dates, and Pecans Whole Grain Cereal, Post [1 cup]	97	3.4	377	23%	7	74	7.2
3609	Harmony, General Mills [1 cup]	44	1.6	160	5%	4	35	1.8
3610	Heartland Natural Cereal, plain [1 cup]	115	4.1	499	32%	12	79	7.0
3611	Heartland Natural Cereal, with coconut [1 cup]	105	3.7	463	33%	11	71	7.5
3612	Heartland Natural Cereal, with raisins [1 cup]	110	3.9	468	30%	11	76	6.1
3613	Honey Bunches of Oats, Post [1 cup]	40	1.4	160	11%	3	33	1.3
3614	Honey Bunches of Oats with Almonds, Post [1 cup]	43	1.5	173	20%	4	32	1.4
3615	Honey Crunch Corn Flakes, Kellogg's [1 cup]	40	1.4	160	7%	3	35	0.9
3616	Honey Nut Cheerios, General Mills [1 cup]	30	1.1	120	10%	3	24	1.7
3617	Honey Nut Chex, General Mills [1 cup]	40	1.4	155	5%	2	35	0.6
3618	Honey Nut Clusters, General Mills [1 cup]	55	1.9	210	15%	4	46	3.0
3619	Honey-Comb, Post [1 cup]	29	1.0	110	4%	2	26	1.0
3620	Honey-Comb, Strawberry Blasted, Post [1 cup]	30	1.1	120	4%	2	26	1.0
3621	Just Right Fruit and Nut, Kellogg's [1 cup]	60	2.1	220	7%	4	49	3.1
3622	Kaboom, General Mills [1 cup]	24	0.8	96	9%	1	21	1.2
3623	Kashi, Puffed [1 cup]	24	0.8	83	6%	3	18	2.4
3624	King Vitaman, Quaker [1 cup]	21	0.7	81	8%	2	18	0.8
3625	Kix, General Mills [1 cup]	23	0.8	96	5%	1	20	0.6
3626	Life, Quaker [1 cup]	44	1.6	167	11%	4	34	2.9
3627	Life, Cinnamon, Quaker [1 cup]	44	1.6	167	10%	4	35	2.7
3628	Lucky Charms, General Mills [1 cup]	30	1.1	120	8%	2	25	1.2
3629	Malt-O-Meal Corn Bursts [1 cup]	31	1.1	118	1%	1	29	0.4

Food #	fat gm	sat fat gm	choles mg	sodium mg	potass mg	vit A	vit E	vit C	thia-min	ribo-flavin	nia-cin	vit B-6	fol-ate	vit B-12	cal-cium	phos-phorus	magne-sium	iron	zinc
						% of Daily Value													
3580	1	0	0	180	69	0	0	10	25	25	25	25	25	25	2	4	3	25	25
3581	0	0	0	270	30	10	0	10	25	25	25	25	50	25	25	2	0	45	25
3582	9	3	0	187	293	20	1	33	33	33	33	33	33	33	3	20	20	13	13
3583	0	0	0	210	35	10	0	10	35	35	35	35	70	35	0	2	2	45	10
3584	1	0	0	338	75	1	1	0	7	33	33	33	133	0	3	5	5	56	33
3585	2	0	0	260	460	0	2	20	50	50	50	50	50	50	20	30	30	50	50
3586	1	0	0	210	15	0	0	10	25	25	25	25	25	25	2	2	0	25	25
3587	2	0	0	240	26	13	1	13	33	33	33	33	33	33	11	8	1	33	33
3588	1	0	0	150	35	10	0	25	25	25	25	25	25	25	0	2	2	25	10
3589	1	0	0	105	25	10	0	25	25	25	25	25	25	25	0	1	1	25	10
3590	1	0	0	210	55	10	0	10	25	25	25	25	25	25	10	6	4	25	25
3591	0	0	0	200	27	13	0	13	33	33	33	33	33	33	0	1	1	33	1
3592	1	0	0	11	186	0	1	0	27	27	27	27	27	27	0	17	11	11	11
3593	3	0	0	250	270	15	4	0	25	25	25	25	25	25	0	15	15	30	10
3594	2	0	0	260	280	15	4	0	25	25	25	25	25	25	0	20	15	30	10
3595	1	0	0	160	30	15	2	0	25	25	25	25	25	25	0	2	0	10	10
3596	0	0	0	33	60	20	0	0	33	33	33	33	33	33	0	4	5	13	13
3597	1	0	0	360	67	13	1	13	33	33	33	33	33	33	47	27	3	33	33
3598	30	6	0	29	656	0	52	3	60	20	13	20	26	0	10	56	54	28	33
3599	15	7	1	24	448	0	4	1	20	11	8	8	6	2	8	31	25	19	15
3600	20	14	0	47	538	1	3	0	21	38	10	8	11	2	16	35	31	17	14
3601	4	0	0	315	225	0	6	0	9	3	4	0	3	0	3	22	9	9	6
3602	5	1	1	224	294	0	2	1	17	6	8	6	5	0	5	21	17	12	11
3603	5	2	0	225	270	22	38	9	38	38	38	150	150	150	3	15	15	15	38
3604	6	1	0	240	240	30	0	8	50	50	50	200	200	200	4	20	20	20	50
3605	1	0	0	125	105	15	2	0	25	25	25	25	25	25	0	8	8	45	8
3606	2	0	0	657	301	42	3	0	47	47	47	47	47	47	4	40	28	85	15
3607	11	1	0	333	263	26	2	0	44	44	44	44	44	44	0	18	17	88	14
3608	9	1	0	287	215	27	2	0	45	45	45	45	45	45	0	19	18	90	14
3609	1	0	0	280	72	8	80	40	80	40	40	40	80	56	48	8	5	40	40
3610	18	5	0	293	385	1	3	2	24	9	8	10	16	0	7	42	37	24	20
3611	17	6	0	213	384	1	2	2	23	9	9	8	14	0	7	38	34	30	18
3612	16	4	0	226	415	1	3	2	21	8	8	10	11	0	7	38	35	22	19
3613	2	0	0	253	67	20	0	0	33	33	33	33	33	33	0	5	5	60	3
3614	4	0	0	253	80	20	2	0	33	33	33	33	33	33	0	5	5	60	3
3615	1	0	0	280	40	13	3	13	33	33	33	33	33	33	0	2	2	13	2
3616	1	0	0	270	90	10	1	10	25	25	25	25	50	25	10	10	8	25	25
3617	1	0	0	298	36	0	1	13	33	34	33	34	33	33	14	0	0	67	0
3618	3	0	0	270	135	0	10	10	25	25	25	25	25	25	2	10	8	25	25
3619	0	0	0	220	35	15	0	0	25	25	25	25	25	25	0	2	2	15	10
3620	0	0	0	150	40	15	0	0	25	25	25	25	25	25	0	4	2	15	10
3621	2	0	0	280	170	10	10	0	25	25	25	100	100	100	2	10	6	90	4
3622	1	0	0	168	16	8	0	8	20	20	20	20	40	20	8	3	3	36	20
3623	1	0	0	2	66	0	0	0	3	2	4	1	2	0	1	6	9	4	5
3624	1	0	0	178	58	21	5	14	18	18	18	18	70	18	0	5	4	33	18
3625	0	0	0	202	26	8	0	8	19	19	19	19	38	19	11	3	1	34	19
3626	2	0	0	226	125	0	1	0	37	37	37	37	140	0	15	18	11	68	37
3627	2	0	0	210	113	0	1	0	37	37	37	37	140	0	14	16	9	50	37
3628	1	0	0	210	60	10	0	10	25	25	25	25	50	25	10	8	5	25	25
3629	0	0	0	122	16	23	0	25	25	25	25	25	25	25	1	1	0	10	10

Grains, Beans, Nuts, Seeds

Food #	Food Description & Amount	wt gm	wt oz	calories	%cal fat	prot gm	carbo gm	fiber gm
3630	Malt-O-Meal Crispy Rice [1 cup]	28	1.0	106	3%	2	24	0.3
3631	Malt-O-Meal Marshmallow Mateys [1 cup]	30	1.1	115	8%	2	25	1.4
3632	**Malt-O-Meal Toasty O's [1 cup]**	28	1.0	109	15%	4	19	2.0
3633	Malt-O-Meal Tootie Fruities [1 cup]	28	1.0	109	8%	1	25	0.6
3634	Millet, puffed [1 cup]	21	0.7	74	10%	2	14	0.6
3635	Mini-Wheats, Frosted (Include all flavors), Kellogg's [1 cup]	60	2.1	203	4%	6	50	6.4
3636	Mini-Wheats, Raisin, Kellogg's [1 cup]	71	2.5	240	6%	7	56	6.7
3637	Mini-Wheats, Strawberry, Kellogg's [1 cup]	67	2.4	230	6%	5	54	6.7
3638	Mueslix with raisins, dates, and almonds, Kellogg's [1 cup]	85	3.0	289	13%	8	66	6.2
3639	Multi-Bran Chex, General Mills [1 cup]	58	2.0	200	4%	4	49	8.2
3640	Multi-Grain Cheerios, General Mills [1 cup]	30	1.1	110	9%	3	24	2.8
3641	Nesquik Chocolatey Rice and Corn Puffs, General Mills [1 cup]	40	1.4	160	12%	2	33	0.0
3642	**Oat bran**, plain, uncooked [1 cup]	98	3.5	241	26%	17	65	15.1
3643	Oatmeal Crisp Almond, General Mills [1 cup]	55	1.9	220	19%	5	42	4.3
3644	Oatmeal Crisp Apple Cinnamon, General Mills [1 cup]	55	1.9	210	9%	5	45	3.9
3645	Oatmeal Crisp Raisin, General Mills [1 cup]	55	1.9	210	10%	5	44	3.6
3646	Oh!s, Honey Graham, Quaker [1 cup]	36	1.3	149	15%	2	30	0.9
3647	Oreo O's, Post [1 cup]	36	1.3	147	14%	1	29	1.8
3648	Para Su Familia, Cinnamon Stars, General Mills [1 cup]	30	1.1	120	7%	1	26	0.3
3649	Para Su Familia, Fruitis, General Mills [1 cup]	30	1.1	120	7%	1	26	0.3
3650	Para Su Familia, Raisin Bran, General Mills [1 cup]	55	1.9	170	7%	5	41	6.6
3651	Product 19, Kellogg's [1 cup]	30	1.1	100	3%	2	25	1.3
3652	**Puffed Rice**, plain (Include Quaker, Malt-O-Meal) [1 cup]	14	0.5	54	2%	1	12	0.2
3653	Puffed Wheat, plain, (Include Quaker, Malt-O-Meal) [1 cup]	12	0.4	44	5%	2	9	1.1
3654	Quaker Oat Bran Cereal [1 cup]	46	1.6	172	12%	7	33	4.8
3655	Quaker Oatmeal Squares [1 cup]	57	2.0	220	11%	7	44	4.3
3656	Quisp, Quaker [1 cup]	30	1.1	121	12%	1	26	0.8
3657	Raisin Bran, Kellogg's [1 cup]	59	2.1	190	7%	5	45	7.5
3658	Raisin Bran Crunch, Kellogg's [1 cup]	53	1.9	190	5%	3	45	4.0
3659	**Raisin Bran**, Post [1 cup]	59	2.1	190	5%	4	46	8.0
3660	Raisin Nut Bran, General Mills [1 cup]	73	2.6	367	18%	5	55	5.3
3661	Reese's Puffs, General Mills [1 cup]	40	1.4	173	22%	3	31	0.5
3662	Rice Chex, General Mills [1 cup]	25	0.9	96	1%	1	22	0.5
3663	**Rice Krispies**, Kellogg's [1 cup]	26	0.9	96	3%	2	23	0.3
3664	Rice Krispies Treats, Kellogg's [1 cup]	40	1.4	160	12%	1	35	0.4
3665	Shredded Wheat with Oat Bran [1 cup spoon size biscuits]	51	1.8	180	9%	5	40	7.2
3666	Shredded Wheat, 100% [1 cup spoon-size biscuits]	50	1.8	172	3%	5	41	5.3
3667	Smacks (sweetened puffed wheat), Kellogg's [1 cup]	38	1.3	150	2%	2	34	1.0
3668	Smart Start, Kellogg's [1 cup]	50	1.8	180	3%	3	43	2.3
3669	**Special K**, Kellogg's [1 cup]	31	1.1	110	2%	7	22	0.7
3670	Special K, Red Berries, Kellogg's [1 cup]	31	1.1	110	2%	3	25	1.0
3671	Sweet Crunch, Quaker [1 cup]	27	1.0	108	12%	1	23	0.7
3672	Sweet Puffs, Quaker [1 cup]	34	1.2	133	4%	2	30	1.2
3673	Team Cheerios, General Mills [1 cup]	30	1.1	110	8%	2	25	2.0
3674	Toasties Corn Flakes, Post [1 cup]	28	1.0	100	0%	2	24	1.0
3675	**Total**, Whole Grain, General Mills [1 cup]	40	1.4	147	6%	3	31	3.5
3676	Total, Brown Sugar & Oat, General Mills [1 cup]	40	1.4	147	6%	3	31	1.6
3677	Total, Corn Flakes, General Mills [1 cup]	20	0.7	73	4%	1	16	0.5
3678	Total, Raisin Bran, General Mills [1 cup]	55	1.9	170	5%	4	41	4.7
3679	Trix, General Mills [1 cup]	30	1.1	120	8%	1	27	0.7

Food #	fat gm	sat fat gm	choles mg	sodium mg	potass mg	% of Daily Value													
						vit A	vit E	vit C	thia-min	ribo-flavin	nia-cin	vit B-6	fol-ate	vit B-12	cal-cium	phos-phorus	magne-sium	iron	zinc
3630	0	0	0	300	36	21	0	23	24	23	23	24	25	25	0	4	3	9	3
3631	1	0	0	211	62	15	0	10	25	25	25	25	50	25	10	8	5	32	28
3632	2	0	0	237	89	37	1	25	25	25	25	25	25	25	4	10	10	44	25
3633	1	0	0	118	30	25	0	25	25	25	25	25	25	25	10	2	2	25	25
3634	1	0	0	1	38	0	0	0	5	3	5	4	4	0	0	6	6	3	2
3635	1	0	0	2	200	0	2	0	28	28	29	27	30	29	2	17	15	98	12
3636	1	0	0	7	333	0	0	0	33	33	33	33	33	33	0	20	13	120	13
3637	1	0	0	20	228	0	0	0	33	33	33	33	33	33	3	20	20	120	13
3638	4	1	0	196	413	9	39	0	39	39	39	155	155	155	5	15	15	39	9
3639	1	0	0	380	220	10	2	10	25	25	25	25	100	25	10	20	15	90	25
3640	1	0	0	200	85	10	100	25	100	100	100	100	100	100	10	10	6	100	100
3641	2	1	0	253	87	13	0	13	33	33	33	33	33	33	13	5	3	33	33
3642	7	1	0	4	555	0	6	0	76	13	5	8	13	0	6	72	58	29	20
3643	5	1	0	240	180	0	10	10	25	25	25	25	25	25	2	15	15	25	25
3644	2	0	0	250	170	0	2	10	25	25	25	25	25	25	2	10	10	25	25
3645	2	0	0	220	200	0	5	0	25	25	25	25	25	25	2	10	10	25	25
3646	3	1	0	238	60	13	0	13	32	32	32	32	129	0	1	6	4	32	32
3647	2	0	0	120	93	20	2	0	33	33	33	33	33	33	0	5	3	13	13
3648	1	0	0	240	25	10	0	10	25	25	25	25	50	25	10	2	0	45	25
3649	1	0	0	210	20	10	0	10	25	25	25	25	50	25	10	4	2	45	25
3650	1	0	0	320	330	10	1	0	25	50	50	50	100	25	70	15	10	100	50
3651	0	0	0	210	50	15	100	100	100	100	100	100	100	100	0	4	4	100	100
3652	0	0	0	1	16	0	0	0	4	0	4	0	0	0	0	2	1	2	1
3653	0	0	0	1	44	0	0	0	3	2	7	1	1	1	0	4	4	3	2
3654	2	0	0	166	207	13	9	13	21	21	21	21	85	0	8	24	19	72	20
3655	3	0	0	268	232	10	10	10	25	25	25	25	100	0	10	20	15	90	25
3656	2	0	0	216	40	0	1	0	28	28	28	28	115	0	1	5	4	28	28
3657	1	0	0	350	360	10	2	0	25	25	25	25	25	25	2	20	20	25	10
3658	1	0	0	210	210	10	1	0	25	25	25	25	25	25	0	10	10	25	10
3659	1	0	0	360	360	15	2	0	25	25	25	25	25	25	2	20	20	60	15
3660	5	1	0	333	307	0	7	0	25	25	25	25	25	25	2	15	10	25	25
3661	4	1	0	227	60	13	2	13	33	33	33	33	33	33	13	3	0	33	33
3662	0	0	0	232	28	8	0	8	20	20	20	20	40	20	8	3	2	40	20
3663	0	0	0	256	32	8	0	5	20	20	20	20	20	20	0	3	3	8	3
3664	2	0	0	253	33	13	0	13	33	33	33	33	33	33	0	3	2	13	2
3665	2	0	0	5	234	3	2	2	11	4	11	6	6	0	2	18	14	11	11
3666	1	0	0	0	211	0	1	0	8	1	13	8	4	0	2	20	16	8	8
3667	0	0	0	64	57	14	1	14	35	35	35	35	35	35	0	6	3	3	3
3668	1	0	0	280	100	15	30	25	100	100	100	100	100	100	2	10	8	100	100
3669	0	0	0	220	60	15	35	35	35	35	35	100	100	100	1	6	4	45	6
3670	0	0	0	220	65	15	35	35	35	35	35	35	35	35	2	50	12	45	3
3671	1	0	0	194	36	0	0	0	25	25	25	25	110	0	1	4	4	25	25
3672	1	0	0	80	50	0	2	0	3	2	7	1	2	1	0	5	5	4	3
3673	1	0	0	200	70	10	50	15	70	70	60	70	70	60	15	6	4	60	60
3674	0	0	0	260	30	15	0	0	25	25	25	25	25	25	0	6	0	30	0
3675	1	0	0	253	120	13	133	133	133	133	133	133	133	133	133	11	8	133	133
3676	1	0	0	267	107	13	133	133	133	133	133	133	133	133	133	8	5	133	133
3677	0	0	0	140	20	7	67	67	67	67	67	67	67	67	67	1	0	67	67
3678	1	0	0	240	360	10	100	0	100	100	100	100	100	100	100	10	10	100	100
3679	1	0	0	190	15	10	2	10	25	25	25	25	25	25	10	2	0	25	25

Grains, Beans, Nuts, Seeds

Food #	Food Description & Amount	wt gm	wt oz	calo-ries	%cal fat	prot gm	carbo gm	fiber gm
3680	Waffle Crisp, Post [1 cup]	30	1.1	130	19%	1	25	0.5
3681	Weetabix Whole Wheat Cereal [1 cup]	57	2.0	213	7%	7	44	6.5
3682	Wheat bran, unprocessed, dry [1 cup]	58	2.0	125	18%	9	37	24.8
3683	Wheat Chex, General Mills [1 cup]	50	1.8	180	6%	5	40	4.5
3684	Wheat germ, plain [1 cup]	113	4.0	432	25%	33	56	14.6
3685	Wheat Germ, Honey Crunch, Kretschmer/Quaker [1 cup]	113	4.0	420	19%	30	66	11.5
3686	**Wheaties**, General Mills [1 cup]	**30**	**1.1**	**110**	**8%**	**3**	**24**	**2.6**
3687	Wheaties, Frosted, General Mills [1 cup]	40	1.4	147	1%	1	36	0.9
3688	Wheaties, Raisin Bran, General Mills [1 cup]	55	1.9	183	5%	4	44	5.0
	Rice, Pasta, & Noodles (About 1/3 to 1/2 cup dry makes about 1 cup cooked; cooking in salted water can add several hundred mg sodium per cup.)							
3800	**Pasta/Noodles (all shapes)**, cooked without salt (Include spaghetti, macaroni, linguini, vermicelli, fides, lasagna noodles, orzo, ziti, rotini, shells, wagon wheels, cart wheels, manicotti, rigatoni, mostaccioli, cavatoni ricci bows, twirls, spirals) [1 cup]	140	4.9	197	4%	7	40	1.8
3801	Pasta/noodles, high protein type, cooked without salt [1 cup]	140	4.9	230	1%	11	44	2.4
3802	Pasta/noodles, spinach, cooked without salt [1 cup]	140	4.9	191	4%	7	38	5.4
3803	Pasta/noodles, vegetable, cooked without salt [1 cup]	91	3.2	116	1%	4	24	3.9
3804	Pasta/noodles, whole wheat, cooked without salt [1 cup]	160	5.6	198	4%	9	42	4.5
3805	Noodles, chow mein, deep fried (including canned) [1 cup]	45	1.6	237	53%	4	26	1.8
3806	Noodles/pasta, egg, cooked without salt (Include pastina, egg noodles) [1 cup]	160	5.6	213	10%	8	40	1.8
3807	Noodles/pasta, egg, cooked, with margarine (Include pastina, egg noodles) [1 cup]	165	5.8	247	22%	8	40	1.8
3808	Noodles/pasta, spinach, cooked without salt [1 cup]	160	5.6	193	4%	7	39	5.5
3809	Noodles/pasta, corn-based, cooked without salt [1 cup]	119	4.2	148	5%	3	33	4.5
3810	Noodles, rice noodles (made from rice flour), cooked [1 cup]	152	5.4	163	3%	3	36	1.1
3811	Noodles made from mung beans, cooked without salt (Include transparent noodles, cellophane noodles) [1 cup]	190	6.7	160	0%	0	39	0.2
3812	Noodles made from soybeans, cooked without salt [1 cup]	140	4.9	500	0%	0	123	5.5
3813	**Rice, brown**, cooked without salt [1 cup]	**195**	**6.9**	**216**	**7%**	**5**	**45**	**3.5**
3814	Rice, brown, instant, cooked without salt [1 cup]	212	7.5	235	7%	5	49	3.8
3815	Rice, brown and wild, cooked [1 cup]	151	5.3	149	6%	4	31	1.6
3816	**Rice, white**, enriched (check label; most white rice is enriched), cooked without salt [1 cup]	**205**	**7.2**	**267**	**2%**	**6**	**58**	**0.8**
3817	Rice, white, not enriched (check label; most white rice is enriched), cooked without salt [1 cup]	204	7.2	267	2%	6	58	0.8
3818	Rice, white, instant, cooked without salt (Include Minute Rice, yellow rice) [1 cup]	165	5.8	162	1%	3	35	1.0
3819	Rice, white, converted, cooked without salt (Include Uncle Ben's rice) [1 cup]	175	6.2	200	2%	4	43	0.7
3820	Rice, white, glutinous, cooked without salt (Include sticky rice, Japanese-style plain rice) [1 cup]	174	6.1	169	2%	4	37	1.7
3821	Rice, white and wild, cooked without salt [1 cup]	151	5.3	147	2%	3	32	0.8
3822	**Rice, wild**, cooked without salt [1 cup]	**130**	**4.6**	**131**	**3%**	**5**	**28**	**2.3**
3823	Rice, sweet, cooked without salt (Include Japanese mochi rice) [1 cup]	175	6.2	246	2%	4	55	0.7
3824	Rice bran, uncooked (Include Ener-G Pure Rice Bran) [1 cup]	118	4.2	373	59%	16	59	24.8
3825	Rice polishings [1 cup]	105	3.7	278	43%	13	61	7.4
3826	Rice, cooked with oil, Puerto Rican style (Include Arroz blanco) [1 cup]	155	5.5	337	24%	5	57	0.9
3827	Rice, cooked, with whole milk [1 cup]	200	7.1	287	14%	10	50	0.7
	Beans & Peas/Legumes (About 1/3 to 1/2 cup dry makes about 1 cup cooked; cooking in salted water can add several hundred mg sodium per cup. For canned beans, see label for sodium content.)							
3850	Bean cake, made with flour, lima beans, oil, sugar [1 cake]	32	1.1	130	47%	2	16	0.9
3851	Black, brown, or Bayo beans, cooked with salt pork [1 cup]	177	6.2	294	37%	13	34	8.4
3852	Chickpeas, cooked without salt (Include garbanzo beans) [1 cup]	164	5.8	297	15%	16	49	14.2

Food #	fat gm	sat fat gm	choles mg	sodium mg	potass mg	vit A	vit E	vit C	thia-min	ribo-flavin	nia-cin	vit B-6	fol-ate	vit B-12	cal-cium	phos-phorus	magne-sium	iron	zinc
						|← % of Daily Value →|													
3680	3	0	0	110	25	15	0	0	25	25	25	25	25	25	0	2	2	10	10
3681	2	0	0	221	311	0	3	0	41	33	16	13	7	0	6	10	13	16	7
3682	2	0	0	1	686	0	4	0	20	20	39	38	11	0	4	59	89	34	28
3683	1	0	0	420	190	10	1	10	25	25	25	25	100	25	10	15	10	80	25
3684	12	2	0	5	1070	0	68	11	126	55	32	55	99	0	5	129	90	57	126
3685	9	2	0	12	1089	1	83	0	101	46	27	28	94	0	6	114	77	51	105
3686	1	0	0	220	105	10	1	10	50	50	50	50	50	50	2	10	8	45	50
3687	0	0	0	267	47	13	0	13	67	67	67	67	133	67	13	3	0	60	67
3688	1	0	0	250	230	10	3	0	50	50	50	50	50	50	2	10	10	45	50
3800	1	0	0	1	43	0	0	0	19	8	12	2	25	0	1	8	6	11	5
3801	0	0	0	7	59	0	0	0	28	13	13	4	29	0	1	7	11	6	5
3802	1	0	0	12	58	2	0	0	8	4	8	7	4	0	3	14	19	5	10
3803	0	0	0	5	28	0	0	0	7	3	5	1	15	0	1	5	4	2	3
3804	1	0	0	5	70	0	1	0	12	4	6	6	2	0	2	14	12	9	9
3805	14	2	0	198	54	0	0	0	17	11	13	2	10	0	1	7	6	12	4
3806	2	0	53	11	45	1	0	0	20	8	12	3	26	2	2	11	8	14	7
3807	6	1	53	56	47	5	2	0	20	8	12	3	26	2	2	11	8	14	7
3808	1	0	0	13	59	2	0	0	8	5	8	7	4	0	3	15	19	5	10
3809	1	0	0	4	121	1	1	0	6	2	5	4	3	0	0	10	12	2	5
3810	1	0	0	91	29	0	0	0	3	1	5	9	0	0	1	4	4	1	2
3811	0	0	0	8	3	0	0	0	3	0	0	1	0	0	1	1	1	5	1
3812	0	0	0	6	4	0	0	0	0	0	0	0	0	0	8	3	1	14	40
3813	2	0	0	10	84	0	5	0	12	3	15	14	2	0	2	16	21	5	8
3814	2	0	0	11	91	0	5	0	14	3	16	15	2	0	2	18	23	5	9
3815	1	0	0	7	98	0	1	0	8	3	11	9	2	0	1	13	15	3	7
3816	1	0	0	2	72	0	0	0	22	2	15	10	30	0	2	9	6	14	7
3817	1	0	0	2	72	0	0	0	3	2	4	10	2	0	2	9	6	2	7
3818	0	0	0	5	7	0	0	0	8	4	7	1	17	0	1	2	2	6	3
3819	0	0	0	5	65	0	0	0	29	2	12	2	22	0	3	7	5	11	4
3820	0	0	0	9	17	0	0	0	2	1	3	2	0	0	0	1	2	1	5
3821	0	0	0	7	63	0	0	0	11	2	9	4	15	0	1	6	5	8	5
3822	0	0	0	4	131	0	1	0	5	7	8	9	8	0	0	11	10	4	12
3823	0	0	0	2	63	0	0	0	18	2	12	8	24	0	2	7	5	11	6
3824	25	5	0	6	1752	0	24	0	217	20	201	240	19	0	7	198	230	122	48
3825	13	2	0	0	750	0	21	0	129	11	148	22	29	0	7	116	158	63	57
3826	9	1	0	7	78	0	6	0	22	2	15	6	29	0	2	8	5	16	5
3827	4	3	17	103	368	10	1	2	19	20	12	7	23	7	26	25	10	12	9
3850	7	1	0	1	58	0	4	0	5	3	3	1	4	0	0	2	2	4	1
3851	12	4	12	207	622	0	1	0	23	5	5	6	31	1	6	18	19	13	13
3852	5	1	0	21	500	1	2	4	12	8	4	12	40	0	8	25	18	23	17

% of Daily Value

Grains, Beans, Nuts, Seeds

Grains, Beans, Nuts, Seeds

Food #	Food Description & Amount	wt gm	wt oz	calories	%cal fat	prot gm	carbo gm	fiber gm
3853	Cowpeas, cooked without salt (Include blackeye peas, field peas) [1 cup]	169	6.0	196	4%	13	35	11.0
3854	Curd cheese (soybean product) [1 cup]	225	7.9	304	54%	28	14	0.0
3855	Fava beans, cooked without salt [1 cup]	170	6.0	187	3%	13	33	9.2
3856	Lentil loaf (lentils, onion, sunflower seeds, breadcrumbs, oil, soy sauce, vinegar) [1 slice]	47	1.7	83	38%	4	10	3.0
3857	Lentils, cooked without salt [1 cup]	191	6.7	222	3%	17	38	15.1
3858	**Lima beans**, cooked without salt (Include butter beans) [1 cup]	**184**	**6.5**	**212**	**3%**	**14**	**38**	**12.9**
3859	Mongo beans without salt [1 cup]	180	6.3	189	5%	14	33	11.5
3860	Mung beans, cooked without salt [1 cup]	200	7.1	225	3%	15	41	10.6
3861	Pink beans, cooked without salt [1 cup]	169	6.0	252	3%	15	47	9.0
3862	Pinto, calico, and red Mexican beans, cooked without salt (Include October beans, Shellie beans) [1 cup]	173	6.1	196	3%	12	36	14.0
3863	Red kidney beans, cooked without salt [1 cup]	172	6.1	218	4%	15	39	12.7
3864	Soy nuts (roasted soybean kernels) (Include pernuts) [1 package]	135	4.8	636	49%	48	45	23.9
3865	Soybean flour (Include soybean meal) [1 cup]	122	4.3	532	43%	42	43	11.7
3866	Soybeans, cooked without salt [1 cup]	180	6.3	311	47%	30	18	10.8
3867	Split peas, green or yellow, cooked with salt [1 cup]	196	6.9	230	3%	16	41	16.2
3868	**Tofu (soybean curd)** [1 cup (½" cubes)]	**184**	**6.5**	**140**	**57%**	**15**	**3**	**2.2**
3869	Tofu (soybean curd), breaded, fried [1 slice (2¾"x1"x½")]	29	1.0	47	58%	3	3	0.4
3870	Tofu (soybean curd), deep fried (Include aburage) [1 oz]	28	1.0	76	67%	5	3	1.1
3871	White beans, cooked without salt (Include Navy peas, Great Northern beans) [1 cup]	175	6.2	243	2%	17	44	11.0
	Nuts & Seeds							
3900	Almond butter [2Tbs]	32	1.1	203	84%	5	7	1.2
3901	Almond paste (Marzipan paste) [1 cup]	227	8.0	1040	54%	20	109	10.9
3902	Almonds, dry roasted, salted [about 22 almonds]	28	1.0	164	79%	5	7	3.8
3903	Almonds, dry roasted, unsalted [about 22 almonds]	28	1.0	164	79%	5	7	3.8
3904	Almonds, honey-roasted [about 20 almonds]	28	1.0	163	79%	5	7	2.8
3905	**Almonds**, roasted, salted [about 22 almonds]	**28**	**1.0**	**173**	**84%**	**6**	**4**	**3.1**
3906	Almonds, unroasted, unsalted [1 cup, whole almonds]	145	5.1	854	80%	29	30	15.8
3907	Brazil nuts [1 cup, shelled (about 32 kernels)]	140	4.9	918	91%	20	18	7.6
3908	Breadnuts [1 cup]	160	5.6	587	4%	14	127	23.8
3909	Butter nuts [1 cup]	120	4.2	734	84%	30	14	5.6
3910	Carob powder or flour [1 cup]	140	4.9	311	3%	6	124	55.7
3911	Cashew butter [2Tbs]	32	1.1	188	76%	6	9	0.6
3912	Cashew nuts, dry roasted, salted [1 cup]	137	4.8	786	73%	21	45	4.1
3913	Cashew nuts, honey-roasted, salted [about 10 whole cashews]	16	0.6	86	69%	2	6	0.5
3914	**Cashew nuts**, roasted, salted [about 18 whole cashews]	**28**	**1.0**	**161**	**75%**	**5**	**8**	**1.1**
3915	Cashew nuts, roasted, unsalted [about 18 whole cashews]	28	1.0	161	75%	5	8	1.1
3916	Chestnuts, roasted, unsalted [about 10 chestnuts]	84	3.0	206	8%	3	44	4.3
3917	Coconut cream (liquid expressed from grated coconut meat), canned, sweetened (Include Coco Lopez) [1 cup]	296	10.4	568	83%	8	25	6.5
3918	Coconut meat, dried, sweetened (Include flaked or shredded) [1 cup, shredded]	93	3.3	441	61%	3	44	4.0
3919	Coconut meat, fresh [1 piece (2"x2"x½")]	45	1.6	159	85%	1	7	4.1
3920	Coconut milk (liquid expressed from grated coconut meat, water added) [1 cup]	240	8.5	552	93%	5	13	5.3
3921	Coconut water (liquid from coconuts) [1 cup]	240	8.5	46	9%	2	9	2.6
3922	Filberts, hazelnuts [1 cup, whole]	135	4.8	853	89%	18	21	8.2
3923	Flax seeds [1 cup]	145	5.1	722	61%	26	54	24.5
3924	Ginkgo nuts [1 cup (about 78 kernels)]	155	5.5	172	13%	4	34	14.4
3925	Hickory nuts, unsalted [1 cup]	120	4.2	788	88%	15	22	7.7
3926	**Macadamia nuts**, roasted, salted [1 cup]	**134**	**4.7**	**962**	**96%**	**10**	**17**	**12.5**
3927	Macadamia nuts, unroasted, unsalted [1 cup, whole or halves]	134	4.7	941	95%	11	18	12.5

Food #	fat gm	sat fat gm	choles mg	sodium mg	potass mg	% of Daily Value													
						vit A	vit E	vit C	thia-min	ribo-flavin	nia-cin	vit B-6	fol-ate	vit B-12	cal-cium	phos-phorus	magne-sium	iron	zinc
3853	1	0	0	7	470	0	2	1	23	5	4	8	88	0	4	26	22	24	15
3854	18	3	0	45	448	1	5	0	0	19	6	8	12	0	42	50	128	70	26
3855	1	0	0	9	456	0	1	1	11	9	6	6	44	0	6	21	18	14	11
3856	4	0	0	44	156	0	7	1	10	3	3	4	16	0	2	9	7	8	4
3857	1	0	0	4	705	0	1	5	22	8	10	17	86	0	4	34	17	35	16
3858	1	0	0	4	935	0	1	0	20	6	4	15	38	0	3	20	20	24	12
3859	1	0	0	13	416	1	1	3	18	8	14	5	42	0	10	28	28	18	10
3860	1	0	0	13	567	1	1	3	16	6	5	8	46	0	8	20	23	20	10
3861	1	0	0	3	859	0	2	0	29	6	5	15	71	0	9	28	27	22	11
3862	1	0	0	9	573	0	0	5	14	6	3	9	36	0	6	22	19	16	9
3863	1	0	0	3	693	0	0	3	18	6	5	10	56	0	5	24	19	28	12
3864	34	5	0	220	1985	3	9	5	9	12	10	14	71	0	19	49	49	29	28
3865	25	4	0	16	3068	1	8	0	47	83	26	28	105	0	25	60	131	43	32
3866	16	2	0	2	927	0	12	5	19	30	4	21	24	0	18	44	39	51	14
3867	1	0	0	457	705	0	3	1	25	6	9	5	32	0	3	19	18	14	13
3868	9	1	0	13	223	2	0	0	10	6	2	4	7	0	19	18	47	55	10
3869	3	1	6	30	39	1	1	0	3	2	1	1	2	0	3	3	7	9	2
3870	6	1	0	4	41	0	0	0	3	1	0	1	2	0	10	8	4	8	4
3871	1	0	0	11	982	0	1	0	14	5	1	8	35	0	16	20	28	36	16
3900	19	2	0	144	243	0	22	0	3	12	5	1	5	0	9	17	24	7	7
3901	63	6	0	20	713	0	153	2	12	55	16	5	41	0	39	59	74	20	22
3902	14	1	0	218	216	0	5	0	2	10	4	1	4	0	8	15	21	6	9
3903	14	1	0	3	216	0	5	0	2	10	4	1	4	0	8	15	21	6	9
3904	14	1	0	192	170	0	5	0	2	14	4	1	4	0	6	14	19	5	8
3905	16	2	0	218	191	0	5	0	2	16	5	1	4	0	7	15	21	6	9
3906	76	7	0	16	1061	0	116	1	20	66	24	8	21	0	39	75	107	29	28
3907	93	23	0	3	840	0	35	2	93	10	11	18	1	0	25	84	79	26	43
3908	3	1	0	85	3218	4	19	124	3	13	17	55	45	0	15	28	46	41	20
3909	68	2	0	1	505	1	14	6	31	10	6	34	20	0	6	54	71	27	25
3910	1	0	0	49	1158	0	3	0	5	38	13	26	10	0	49	11	19	23	9
3911	16	3	0	196	175	0	2	0	7	4	3	4	5	0	1	15	21	9	11
3912	63	13	0	877	774	0	3	0	18	16	10	18	24	0	6	67	89	46	51
3913	7	1	0	86	74	0	1	0	4	1	1	2	2	0	1	6	9	3	4
3914	13	3	0	175	148	0	1	0	8	3	3	4	5	0	1	12	18	6	9
3915	13	3	0	5	148	0	1	0	8	3	3	4	5	0	1	12	18	6	9
3916	2	0	0	2	497	0	3	36	14	9	6	21	15	0	2	9	7	4	3
3917	52	47	0	148	299	0	7	9	4	7	1	4	11	0	0	7	13	8	12
3918	30	27	0	238	294	0	2	0	2	1	1	12	2	0	1	9	11	9	11
3919	15	13	0	9	160	0	1	2	2	1	1	1	3	0	1	5	4	6	3
3920	57	51	0	36	631	0	6	11	4	0	9	4	10	0	4	24	22	22	11
3921	0	0	0	252	600	0	0	10	5	8	1	4	2	0	6	5	15	4	2
3922	85	6	0	4	601	1	108	2	45	9	8	41	24	0	25	42	96	25	22
3923	49	5	0	96	1901	0	24	3	16	14	10	55	109	0	39	67	183	91	74
3924	3	0	0	476	279	5	18	24	14	5	28	15	13	0	1	8	6	2	2
3925	77	8	0	1	523	2	21	4	69	9	5	12	12	0	7	40	52	14	34
3926	103	15	0	348	441	0	2	0	19	9	14	13	5	0	6	27	39	13	10
3927	99	15	0	7	493	0	2	0	31	9	14	13	5	0	9	18	39	18	15

Grains, Beans, Nuts, Seeds

Food #	Food Description & Amount	wt gm	wt oz	calories	%cal fat	prot gm	carbo gm	fiber gm
3928	Mixed nuts, dry roasted, salted [1 cup]	137	4.8	814	78%	24	35	12.3
3929	Mixed nuts, in shell, unsalted [1 cup, in shell, edible yield]	26	0.9	167	88%	4	4	1.5
3930	Mixed nuts, roasted, without peanuts, salted [1 cup]	144	5.1	886	82%	22	32	7.9
3931	Mixed nuts, roasted, with peanuts, salted [1 cup]	142	5.0	876	82%	24	30	12.8
3932	Mixed nuts, honey-roasted, with peanuts [1 cup]	145	5.1	836	77%	21	43	11.4
3933	**Peanut butter** [2Tbs]	32	1.1	190	77%	8	6	1.9
3934	Peanut butter, unsalted [2Tbs]	32	1.1	190	77%	8	6	1.9
3935	Peanut butter, reduced fat [2Tbs]	36	1.3	187	59%	9	13	1.9
3936	Peanut spread (Include imitation peanut butter) [2Tbs]	32	1.1	192	78%	6	7	2.2
3937	Peanuts, boiled, salted [1 cup, shelled]	180	6.3	572	62%	24	38	15.8
3938	Peanuts, dry roasted, salted [1 cup]	144	5.1	842	76%	34	31	11.5
3939	Peanuts, dry roasted, unsalted [1 cup]	144	5.1	842	76%	34	31	11.5
3940	Peanuts, in shell (shell not eaten), salted [1 cup, in shell, edible portion]	51	1.8	296	76%	13	10	4.7
3941	**Peanuts**, roasted, salted [1 cup, halves and whole]	146	5.1	848	76%	38	28	13.4
3942	Peanuts, roasted, unsalted [1 cup, halves and whole]	146	5.1	848	76%	38	28	10.1
3943	Peanuts, honey-roasted, salted (Include **beer nuts**) [1 cup]	136	4.8	742	71%	31	37	10.9
3944	Pecans, unsalted [1 cup]	108	3.8	720	91%	8	20	8.2
3945	Pine nuts, unsalted (Include pignolias) [1 cup]	171	6.0	968	81%	41	24	7.7
3946	**Pistachio nuts**, roasted, salted [1 cup, in shell, edible yield]	58	2.0	351	78%	9	16	6.3
3947	Pistachio nuts, roasted, unsalted [1 cup, in shell, edible yield]	58	2.0	351	78%	9	16	6.3
3948	Pistachio nuts, unroasted, unsalted [1 cup, shelled]	128	4.5	739	75%	26	32	13.8
3949	Psyllium seed, husks [1 cup, ground]	134	4.7	67	9%	4	108	96.5
3950	**Pumpkin or squash seeds**, hulled, roasted, salted [1 cup]	227	8.0	1185	73%	75	30	8.9
3951	Pumpkin or squash seeds, hulled, unroasted, unsalted [about 142 seeds]	28	1.0	151	76%	7	5	1.1
3952	Sesame butter (made from kernels) (Include tahini) [2Tbs]	30	1.1	178	81%	5	6	1.4
3953	Sesame paste (sesame butter made from whole seeds) [2Tbs]	32	1.1	190	77%	6	8	1.8
3954	Sesame sauce (sesame seeds, water, lemon juice, garlic, salt) [1 cup]	192	6.8	384	74%	12	21	7.8
3955	Sesame seeds, toasted, salted [1 cup]	150	5.3	851	76%	25	39	25.4
3956	Sesame seeds, whole seed, unsalted [1 cup]	144	5.1	825	78%	26	34	17.0
3957	Sunflower seeds, hulled, dry roasted, salted [¼ cup without hulls; ¾ cup with hulls, edible portion]	30	1.1	175	77%	6	7	2.7
3958	**Sunflower seeds**, hulled, roasted, salted [¼ cup without hulls; ¾ cup with hulls, edible portion]	30	1.1	185	84%	6	4	2.0
3959	Sunflower seeds, hulled, roasted, unsalted [¼ cup without hulls; ¾ cup with hulls, edible portion]	30	1.1	185	84%	6	4	2.0
3960	Sunflower seeds, hulled, unroasted, unsalted [¼ cup without hulls; ¾ cup with hulls, edible portion]	30	1.1	171	78%	7	6	3.2
3961	Trail mix (peanuts, raisins, sunflower seeds, cashews, walnuts, almonds) (Include gorp) [1 cup]	140	4.9	702	64%	22	55	9.5
3962	Walnuts, unsalted [1 cup, chopped]	120	4.2	770	87%	17	22	5.8
3963	Walnuts, honey-roasted [1 cup]	114	4.0	676	81%	14	31	4.7
Your Additions								

Food #	fat gm	sat fat gm	choles mg	sodium mg	potass mg	% of Daily Value													
						vit A	vit E	vit C	thia-min	ribo-flavin	nia-cin	vit B-6	fol-ate	vit B-12	cal-cium	phos-phorus	magne-sium	iron	zinc
3928	70	9	0	917	818	0	27	1	18	16	32	20	17	0	10	60	77	28	35
3929	16	2	0	2	138	0	7	1	11	3	2	5	3	0	4	11	13	4	6
3930	81	13	0	1008	783	0	29	1	48	41	14	13	20	0	15	65	90	21	45
3931	80	12	0	926	825	0	28	1	47	19	36	17	29	0	15	66	83	25	48
3932	71	11	0	823	743	0	25	1	42	17	32	15	26	0	14	59	74	23	43
3933	16	3	0	149	214	0	11	0	2	2	21	7	6	0	1	12	13	3	6
3934	16	3	0	5	214	0	11	0	2	2	21	7	6	0	1	12	13	3	6
3935	12	3	0	194	241	0	8	0	6	1	26	6	5	0	1	13	15	4	7
3936	17	2	0	191	170	0	9	0	2	2	20	5	6	0	2	10	14	4	6
3937	40	5	0	1352	324	0	19	0	31	7	47	14	34	0	10	36	46	10	22
3938	72	10	0	1171	948	0	36	0	42	8	97	18	52	0	8	52	63	18	32
3939	72	10	0	9	948	0	37	0	42	8	97	18	52	0	8	52	63	18	32
3940	25	3	0	221	348	0	13	0	9	3	36	7	16	0	4	26	24	5	23
3941	72	10	0	632	996	0	36	0	25	9	104	19	46	0	13	75	68	15	65
3942	72	10	0	9	996	0	36	0	25	9	104	19	46	0	13	75	68	15	65
3943	58	8	0	514	818	0	29	0	20	8	85	15	37	0	11	61	55	12	53
3944	73	6	0	1	423	1	11	4	61	8	5	10	11	0	4	31	35	13	39
3945	87	13	0	7	1024	1	20	5	92	19	31	9	24	0	4	87	100	87	48
3946	31	4	0	452	563	1	12	7	16	8	4	7	9	0	4	28	19	10	5
3947	31	4	0	3	563	1	10	7	16	8	4	7	9	0	4	28	19	10	5
3948	62	8	0	8	1399	3	22	15	70	13	7	16	19	0	17	64	51	48	11
3949	1	0	0	47	240	3	3	1	63	6	9	16	23	0	27	18	12	26	24
3950	96	18	0	1305	1830	9	8	7	32	43	20	10	33	0	10	266	303	188	113
3951	13	2	0	5	226	1	1	1	4	5	2	3	4	0	1	33	37	23	14
3952	16	2	0	11	138	0	2	2	32	2	8	2	7	0	4	24	7	7	9
3953	16	2	0	4	186	0	2	0	5	4	11	13	8	0	31	21	29	34	16
3954	32	4	0	11	377	0	5	41	30	9	14	27	14	0	63	41	57	52	34
3955	72	10	0	59	609	1	11	0	121	41	41	11	36	0	20	116	130	65	102
3956	72	10	0	16	674	0	11	0	76	21	33	57	35	0	140	91	126	116	74
3957	15	2	0	234	255	0	50	1	2	4	11	12	18	0	2	35	10	6	11
3958	17	2	0	181	145	0	40	1	6	5	6	12	18	0	2	34	10	11	10
3959	17	2	0	1	145	0	50	1	6	5	6	12	18	0	2	34	10	11	10
3960	15	2	0	1	207	0	50	1	46	4	7	12	17	0	3	21	27	11	10
3961	50	6	0	12	998	0	52	4	18	14	43	25	32	0	12	67	51	21	37
3962	74	7	0	12	602	1	10	6	31	10	6	33	20	0	11	38	51	16	22
3963	61	6	0	36	484	3	9	5	20	8	5	25	13	0	9	30	40	14	17

We're advised to eat more whole grains, e.g., oats, whole wheat, brown rice. For people who aren't used to eating any, oatmeal is a good place to start. You can also gradually make switches from white to whole wheat bread, and from white to brown rice, either by combining the white and brown, or by choosing brown some of the time.

You can buy packets of instant oatmeal, but by making your own, you can customize them to your taste. The first time you make this, experiment a bit, to find out how sweet or thick you like your oatmeal.

Microwave time will vary, depending on the shape of your mug and the microwave you use. Your mug may overflow the 1st time you try this, so put a plate underneath. If it overflows, mix the oatmeal half-way through the microwaving—or use a wider or bigger mug.

Do what's tastiest and convenient for you. You can cool down the oatmeal at the end by mixing in some cold milk. Or leave out the dry milk, and start with milk in your mug instead of water.

If you dash off to work without breakfast, keep these packets in your office drawer. Most workplaces have microwaves, and many have a pot of hot water available all day. If you start the day with the oatmeal, it's easier to resist the pastries and other office treats that so many of us face daily in the workplace.

Mug-of-Oatmeal Packet

½ cup dry quick oatmeal (*quick* is sliced thinner than *regular*)
¼ cup dry nonfat milk
2 Tbs brown sugar, more or less, to taste
Optional: salt, raisins, nuts, cinnamon, dried chopped apricots

Put all the ingredients in a seal-top sandwich bag. (Make many packets at once; they don't need to be refrigerated.) Put about ¾ cup hot water (amount depends on how thick you like your oatmeal) into a wide-mouth mug (if the water is cold, microwave it in the mug). Mix in an oatmeal packet. Microwave for about a minute, and it's ready to eat.

*   *   *   *   *   *   *   *   *   *   *   *

Bread-Machine Packet

1 cup white bread flour	2 Tbs dry nonfat milk	¾ tsp salt
1 cup whole wheat flour	1 Tbs butter	1 cup water
¼ cup dry oatmeal	1 Tbs sugar	1 tsp dry yeast

Even if you normally only eat white bread, you'll like this half-way-to-whole-grain bread. Put all but the water and yeast into a sandwich bag (make many packets at once). Empty a packet into the bread pan and add water and yeast. Use the 3-hour rapid-bake setting on your breadmaker, or whatever works best in your machine. If you aren't going to eat all the bread by the next day, put it in the freezer. All bread keeps better in the freezer than in the refrigerator or at room temperature. It's easy to pull off frozen bread slices in the freezer.

Meat, Poultry, and Fish

Beef and Veal *4000*

Pork *4150*

Lamb *4250*

Chicken *4300*

Turkey and Other Poultry *4450*

Other Meats and Sausages *4550*

Fish and Shellfish *4750*

Your Additions

End-of-Section Recipes
Scallops Bordelaise
Halibut with Mango Salsa

Meat, Poultry, Fish

Food #	Food Description & Amount	wt gm	wt oz	calo-ries	%cal fat	prot gm	carbo gm	fiber gm
	Beef & Veal (weight columns are for cooked, boneless part)							
4000	Beef brisket, cooked, lean and fat eaten [1 slice (4½"x2½"x¼")]	42	1.5	144	69%	10	0	0.0
4001	Beef brisket, cooked, lean only eaten [1 slice (4½"x2½"x¼")]	42	1.5	97	45%	12	0	0.0
4002	Beef, cow head, cooked [2 oz, boneless, cooked]	57	2.0	163	60%	15	0	0.0
4003	**Beef jerky** [1 cup, pieces]	90	3.2	369	56%	30	10	1.6
4004	Beef liver, battered, fried [2 oz, cooked]	56	2.0	132	33%	14	8	0.1
4005	Beef liver, braised [2 oz, cooked]	56	2.0	120	24%	17	5	0.0
4006	Beef liver, breaded, fried (Include floured, fried) [2 oz, cooked]	56	2.0	130	30%	14	7	0.1
4007	Beef liver, fried or broiled, no coating [2 oz, cooked]	56	2.0	122	33%	15	4	0.0
4008	Beef steak, battered, fried, lean and fat eaten [1 medium steak]	243	8.6	765	58%	57	19	0.8
4009	Beef steak, battered, fried, lean only eaten [1 medium steak]	186	6.6	487	45%	49	15	0.6
4010	Beef steak, braised, lean and fat eaten [1 medium steak]	187	6.6	547	56%	56	0	0.0
4011	Beef steak, braised, lean only eaten [1 medium steak]	146	5.1	328	36%	49	0	0.0
4012	Beef steak, breaded or floured, baked or fried, lean and fat eaten [1 medium steak]	243	8.6	805	55%	59	27	0.9
4013	Beef steak, breaded or floured, baked or fried, lean only eaten [1 medium steak]	186	6.6	518	43%	50	21	0.7
4014	**Beef steak**, broiled, grilled, or baked, lean and fat eaten [1 medium steak]	204	7.2	521	53%	57	0	0.0
4015	Beef steak, broiled, grilled, or baked, lean only eaten [1 medium steak]	156	5.5	310	36%	46	0	0.0
4016	Beef steak, fried, lean and fat eaten [1 medium steak]	204	7.2	592	54%	63	0	0.0
4017	Beef steak, fried, lean only eaten [1 medium steak]	156	5.5	362	37%	53	0	0.0
4018	Beef, bacon, cooked [2 slices]	13	0.5	58	69%	4	0	0.0
4019	Beef, bacon, cooked, lean only eaten [2 slices]	12	0.4	21	20%	3	1	0.0
4020	Beef, bacon, formed, lean meat added, cooked (Include Sizzlean) [1 strip]	11	0.4	49	69%	3	0	0.0
4021	Beef, dried, chipped, cooked in fat [1 oz, cooked]	28	1.0	71	61%	7	0	0.0
4022	Beef, dried, chipped, uncooked [1 oz]	28	1.0	46	21%	8	0	0.0
4023	Beef, neck bones, cooked [5 oz, with bone, cooked]	55	1.9	183	65%	15	0	0.0
4024	Beef, oxtails, cooked [3 oz, with bone, cooked]	48	1.7	126	49%	15	0	0.0
4025	Beef, pastrami (beef, smoked, spiced) [2 slices]	56	2.0	195	75%	10	2	0.0
4026	Beef, pickled [2 oz, boneless]	56	2.0	141	68%	10	0	0.0
4027	**Beef, pot roast (Include chuck roast, arm roast, blade roast, shoulder roast)**, braised or boiled, lean and fat eaten [1 slice (4½"x2½"x¼")]	42	1.5	129	61%	12	0	0.0
4028	Beef, pot roast, braised or boiled, lean only eaten [1 slice (4½"x2½"x¼")]	42	1.5	99	43%	13	0	0.0
4029	Beef, roast, canned (Include beef, steak, canned) [2 oz, boneless]	56	2.0	125	52%	14	0	0.0
4030	**Beef, roast (Include prime ribs, rib roast)**, roasted, lean and fat eaten [1 slice (4½"x2½"x¼")]	42	1.5	112	59%	11	0	0.0
4031	Beef, roast, roasted, lean only eaten [1 slice (4½"x2½"x¼")]	42	1.5	83	39%	12	0	0.0
4032	Beef, sandwich steak (flaked, formed, thinly sliced) (Include Steak-umms) [1 steak]	41	1.4	105	58%	10	0	0.0
4033	Beef, short ribs, barbecued, with sauce, lean and fat eaten [1 medium rib]	66	2.3	251	77%	11	2	0.2
4034	Beef, short ribs, barbecued, with sauce, lean only eaten [1 medium rib]	51	1.8	108	50%	10	3	0.3
4035	Beef, short ribs, cooked, lean and fat eaten (Include beef rib tips) [1 medium rib]	66	2.3	311	80%	14	0	0.0
4036	Beef, short ribs, cooked, lean only eaten (Include beef rib tips) [1 medium rib]	51	1.8	150	55%	16	0	0.0
4037	Beef, stew meat, cooked, lean and fat eaten [2 oz, boneless, cooked]	56	2.0	172	61%	16	0	0.0
4038	Beef, stew meat, cooked, lean only eaten [2 oz, boneless, cooked]	56	2.0	132	43%	18	0	0.0
4039	Calves liver, braised [2 oz, cooked]	56	2.0	92	38%	12	2	0.0
4040	Calves liver, breaded, fried (Include floured, fried) [2 oz, cooked]	56	2.0	144	38%	16	5	0.1
4041	Calves liver, fried or broiled, no coating [2 oz, cooked]	56	2.0	137	42%	17	2	0.0
4042	**Corned beef**, canned, ready-to-eat [1 slice]	40	1.4	100	54%	11	0	0.0
4043	Corned beef, cooked, lean and fat eaten [1 slice (4½"x2½"x¼")]	42	1.5	105	68%	8	0	0.0
4044	Corned beef, cooked, lean only eaten [1 slice (4½"x2½"x¼")]	42	1.5	105	54%	11	0	0.0

Food #	fat gm	sat fat gm	choles mg	sodium mg	potass mg	vit A	vit E	vit C	thia-min	ribo-flavin	nia-cin	vit B-6	fol-ate	vit B-12	cal-cium	phos-phorus	magne-sium	iron	zinc
													% of Daily Value						
4000	11	4	39	26	102	0	0	0	2	5	7	5	1	16	0	8	2	6	15
4001	5	2	39	29	120	0	0	0	2	5	8	6	1	18	0	10	2	7	19
4002	11	4	50	35	181	0	0	0	3	7	10	9	1	23	1	12	3	8	23
4003	23	10	43	1992	537	0	1	0	9	8	8	8	30	15	2	37	11	27	49
4004	5	1	239	42	186	513	2	19	10	97	35	19	36	600	1	20	3	25	17
4005	3	1	296	27	121	658	2	23	9	75	24	18	34	578	0	19	2	19	20
4006	4	1	247	95	197	550	1	20	9	126	38	37	29	956	2	24	3	19	19
4007	4	1	270	59	204	601	1	21	8	136	40	40	31	1043	1	26	3	20	20
4008	49	17	190	361	810	1	6	0	26	45	46	43	9	107	5	61	15	45	73
4009	24	8	146	285	698	1	5	0	22	38	38	37	7	90	4	51	13	38	63
4010	34	13	183	105	507	0	1	0	9	27	29	25	3	80	2	40	10	33	83
4011	13	5	144	88	431	0	1	0	7	23	24	22	3	67	1	35	9	29	76
4012	49	16	182	455	861	1	8	0	29	41	47	43	11	105	12	50	18	48	73
4013	25	7	141	356	736	1	6	0	25	35	39	37	9	88	9	43	15	40	63
4014	31	12	170	124	744	0	1	0	13	26	47	40	4	83	2	43	13	30	70
4015	13	5	126	102	642	0	1	0	11	22	41	36	4	66	1	36	11	24	61
4016	36	13	199	142	905	0	1	0	15	33	46	52	5	112	2	52	16	36	66
4017	15	5	153	115	767	0	1	0	13	28	39	44	5	92	1	44	13	30	56
4018	4	2	15	293	54	0	0	0	1	2	4	2	0	7	0	3	1	2	6
4019	0	0	5	173	51	0	0	0	1	1	3	2	0	5	0	2	1	2	3
4020	4	2	13	248	45	0	0	0	1	2	4	2	0	6	0	3	1	2	5
4021	5	2	22	15	94	0	0	0	2	4	4	4	1	13	0	6	2	4	8
4022	1	0	12	972	124	0	0	0	2	3	8	5	1	12	0	5	2	7	10
4023	13	5	54	33	135	0	0	0	3	8	9	8	1	27	1	12	3	10	25
4024	7	3	51	34	126	0	0	0	3	8	6	7	1	20	1	11	3	10	33
4025	16	6	52	687	128	0	0	0	4	6	14	5	1	16	1	8	3	6	16
4026	11	4	55	635	81	0	0	0	1	6	8	6	1	15	0	7	2	6	17
4027	9	3	42	26	106	0	0	0	2	6	6	6	1	17	0	9	2	7	21
4028	5	2	43	28	116	0	0	0	2	7	7	6	1	18	0	10	2	8	25
4029	7	3	45	34	145	0	0	0	1	8	12	4	1	22	1	6	3	8	23
4030	7	3	33	26	143	0	0	0	2	5	8	7	1	17	0	9	2	5	16
4031	4	1	32	28	159	0	0	0	3	5	8	7	1	18	0	9	3	6	18
4032	7	3	33	29	128	0	0	0	2	6	10	6	1	14	0	7	2	5	15
4033	22	9	47	172	144	2	1	2	2	5	7	6	1	22	1	9	3	7	17
4034	6	2	29	203	136	2	1	3	2	4	6	5	1	18	1	8	3	7	16
4035	28	12	62	33	148	0	1	0	2	6	8	7	1	29	1	11	2	8	21
4036	9	4	47	30	160	0	0	0	2	6	8	7	1	29	1	12	3	10	27
4037	12	5	56	35	141	0	0	0	3	8	8	8	1	23	1	12	3	10	28
4038	6	2	57	37	155	0	0	0	3	9	9	9	1	25	1	14	3	11	33
4039	4	1	314	30	115	451	1	29	5	64	24	14	106	341	0	18	3	8	36
4040	6	2	169	108	235	289	1	19	10	102	45	22	42	547	2	23	4	17	27
4041	6	2	185	74	245	315	1	21	9	111	47	24	45	597	1	25	4	16	29
4042	6	2	34	402	54	0	0	0	1	3	5	3	1	11	0	4	1	5	10
4043	8	3	41	476	61	0	0	0	1	4	6	5	1	11	0	5	1	4	13
4044	6	3	36	423	57	0	0	0	1	4	5	3	1	11	1	5	1	5	10

Meat, Poultry, Fish

Food #	Food Description & Amount	wt gm	wt oz	calo-ries	%cal fat	prot gm	carbo gm	fiber gm
4045	**Ground beef** (hamburger patty), regular, cooked [1 medium patty (4 oz, raw)]	**85**	**3.0**	**246**	**64%**	**20**	**0**	**0.0**
4046	Ground beef, breaded, cooked [1 medium patty (4 oz, raw)]	101	3.6	350	62%	17	15	0.5
4047	Ground beef with textured vegetable protein, cooked [1 medium patty]	84	3.0	219	58%	20	1	0.8
4048	Ground beef, extra lean, cooked (Include ground sirloin, ground round) [1 medium patty (4 oz, raw)]	96	3.4	246	57%	24	0	0.0
4049	Ground beef, lean, cooked (Include ground chuck) [1 medium patty (4 oz, raw)]	88	3.1	239	61%	22	0	0.0
4050	Ground beef, meatballs, meat only [2 medium]	56	2.0	158	57%	16	0	0.0
4051	Ground beef, raw [2 oz]	56	2.0	155	73%	10	0	0.0
4052	Veal chop, broiled, lean and fat eaten [1 medium (6.5 oz, with bone, raw)]	107	3.8	232	51%	27	0	0.0
4053	Veal chop, broiled, lean only eaten [1 medium (6.5 oz, with bone, raw)]	85	3.0	135	32%	22	0	0.0
4054	Veal chop, fried, lean and fat eaten (Include breaded) [1 medium (6.5 oz, with bone, raw)]	107	3.8	244	36%	29	11	0.3
4055	Veal chop, fried, lean only eaten (Include breaded) [1 medium (6.5 oz, with bone, raw)]	85	3.0	203	36%	25	7	0.2
4056	Veal cutlet or steak, broiled, lean and fat eaten [2 oz, boneless, cooked]	56	2.0	90	26%	16	0	0.0
4057	Veal cutlet or steak, broiled, lean only eaten [2 oz, boneless, cooked]	56	2.0	102	23%	19	0	0.0
4058	Veal cutlet or steak, fried, lean and fat eaten (Include breaded or floured) [2 oz, boneless, cooked]	56	2.0	128	36%	15	6	0.2
4059	Veal cutlet or steak, fried, lean only eaten (Include breaded or floured) [2 oz, boneless, cooked, lean only]	56	2.0	102	23%	19	0	0.0
4060	Veal loaf [2 slices]	56	2.0	172	77%	8	2	0.0
4061	Veal patty, breaded, cooked [1 medium patty (4 oz, raw)]	79	2.8	212	54%	16	7	0.2
4062	Veal, ground or patty, cooked [1 medium patty (4 oz, raw)]	67	2.4	115	40%	16	0	0.0
4063	Veal, roasted, lean and fat eaten [1 slice (4½"x2½"x¼")]	42	1.5	97	44%	13	0	0.0
4064	Veal, roasted, lean only eaten [1 slice (4½"x2½"x¼")]	42	1.5	67	32%	11	0	0.0
	Pork (weight columns are for cooked, boneless part)							
4150	**Bacon** (pork), smoked or cured, cooked [2 slices]	16	0.6	92	77%	5	0	0.0
4151	Bacon (pork), smoked or cured, cooked, lean only eaten [2 slices]	12	0.4	22	41%	3	0	0.0
4152	Bacon (pork), formed, lean meat added, cooked (Include breakfast strips; Sizzlean) [2 strips]	22	0.8	101	72%	6	0	0.0
4153	Bacon or side pork, fresh, cooked [1 slice (¼" thick)]	26	0.9	150	77%	8	0	0.0
4154	Canadian bacon, cooked [1 slice]	23	0.8	43	41%	6	0	0.0
4155	Fat back, cooked [1 oz, raw (yield after cooking)]	20	0.7	162	98%	1	0	0.0
4156	Pork, fried chunks, Puerto Rican style (Carne de cerdo frita, masitas fritas) [1 piece (2½"x2"x1")]	38	1.3	104	53%	11	0	0.0
4157	Pork jerky [1 cup, pieces]	126	4.4	519	45%	67	0	0.0
4158	Ham, breaded, fried, lean and fat eaten (Include smoked, cured, canned; chicken fried ham) [1 slice (4½"x2½"x¼")]	42	1.5	97	53%	8	3	0.1
4159	Ham, breaded, fried, lean only eaten (Include smoked, cured, canned; chicken fried ham) [1 slice (4½"x2½"x¼")]	42	1.5	87	42%	9	3	0.1
4160	**Ham**, fresh, cooked, lean and fat eaten [1 slice (4½"x2½"x¼")]	**42**	**1.5**	**115**	**58%**	**11**	**0**	**0.0**
4161	Ham, fresh, cooked, lean only eaten [1 slice (4½"x2½"x¼")]	42	1.5	89	40%	12	0	0.0
4162	Ham, fried, lean and fat eaten (Include smoked, cured, canned) [1 slice (4½"x2½"x¼")]	42	1.5	94	60%	9	0	0.0
4163	Ham, fried, lean only eaten (Include smoked, cured, canned) [1 slice (4½"x2½"x¼")]	42	1.5	81	48%	10	0	0.0
4164	Ham, luncheon meat, chopped, minced, pressed, spiced, not canned [1 slice (4¼"x4¼"x1/8")]	42	1.5	102	70%	7	0	0.0
4165	Ham, luncheon meat, chopped, minced, pressed, spiced, lowfat, not canned [1 slice (4¼"x4¼"x1/8")]	42	1.5	55	34%	8	0	0.0
4166	Ham and pork, luncheon meat, chopped, minced, pressed, spiced, canned (Include Spam, Treet) [1 slice (½" thick)]	57	2.0	188	80%	8	1	0.0
4167	Ham, pork and chicken, luncheon meat, chopped, minced, pressed, spiced, canned (Include Spam Lite) [1 slice (½" thick)]	57	2.0	117	63%	9	1	0.0

Food #	fat gm	sat fat gm	choles mg	sodium mg	potass mg	% of Daily Value													
						vit A	vit E	vit C	thia-min	ribo-flavin	nia-cin	vit B-6	fol-ate	vit B-12	cal-cium	phos-phorus	magne-sium	iron	zinc
4045	18	7	77	71	248	0	1	0	2	10	25	11	2	42	1	14	4	12	29
4046	24	6	54	231	236	1	8	0	10	12	24	9	5	30	7	14	6	15	22
4047	14	5	59	145	232	0	1	0	12	14	26	19	5	35	1	17	4	11	26
4048	16	6	81	67	300	0	1	0	4	15	24	13	2	35	1	15	5	13	35
4049	16	6	77	68	265	0	1	0	3	11	23	11	2	34	1	14	5	10	31
4050	10	4	56	50	193	0	0	0	2	8	17	9	1	27	1	10	3	8	23
4051	12	5	44	38	142	0	0	0	2	6	13	7	1	22	0	8	2	6	14
4052	13	6	110	100	348	0	2	0	4	18	47	18	4	22	2	23	7	5	22
4053	5	2	115	92	264	0	1	0	4	16	34	11	3	27	2	18	5	5	26
4054	10	3	120	486	397	1	2	0	11	22	55	21	7	22	4	27	8	10	20
4055	8	2	93	220	274	0	3	0	7	17	42	14	5	17	3	20	6	7	18
4056	3	1	58	38	218	0	1	0	2	11	28	9	2	11	0	13	4	3	11
4057	3	1	60	43	248	0	1	0	3	12	35	14	2	14	0	16	4	3	13
4058	5	2	63	254	208	1	1	0	6	12	29	11	4	12	2	14	4	5	10
4059	3	1	60	43	248	0	1	0	3	12	35	14	2	14	0	16	4	3	13
4060	15	6	36	744	116	0	0	0	4	7	10	5	1	36	1	7	2	7	9
4061	13	4	80	142	227	1	3	0	6	13	29	14	4	12	4	15	5	6	13
4062	5	2	69	56	226	0	0	0	3	11	27	13	2	14	1	15	4	4	17
4063	5	2	48	37	137	0	1	0	2	8	17	7	2	11	1	10	3	3	13
4064	2	1	57	45	131	0	1	0	2	8	17	5	1	13	1	9	3	2	13
4150	8	3	14	255	78	0	0	0	7	3	6	2	0	5	0	5	1	1	3
4151	1	0	7	186	47	0	0	0	7	1	4	3	0	2	0	4	1	1	1
4152	8	3	23	462	103	0	0	0	11	5	8	4	0	6	0	6	1	2	5
4153	13	5	22	415	126	0	0	0	12	4	10	4	0	8	0	9	2	2	6
4154	2	1	13	356	90	0	0	0	13	3	8	5	0	3	0	7	1	1	3
4155	18	6	10	2	12	0	0	0	1	1	1	0	0	0	0	1	0	0	1
4156	6	2	34	30	162	0	0	1	28	7	10	9	1	5	1	10	3	2	6
4157	26	9	113	3623	879	1	2	1	108	48	58	53	7	28	2	35	8	15	51
4158	6	2	27	464	127	0	2	0	19	7	10	7	1	4	1	9	2	4	6
4159	4	1	27	495	120	0	2	0	17	7	10	8	1	4	1	9	2	3	6
4160	7	3	39	25	148	0	0	0	18	8	10	8	1	5	1	11	2	2	8
4161	4	1	39	27	157	0	0	0	19	9	10	9	1	5	0	12	3	3	9
4162	6	2	22	504	135	0	2	0	20	6	10	7	0	5	0	9	2	3	7
4163	4	1	22	529	126	0	2	0	18	6	10	9	0	5	0	9	2	2	7
4164	8	3	24	557	128	0	0	0	18	5	8	7	0	6	0	6	2	2	5
4165	2	1	20	600	147	0	0	0	26	6	10	10	0	5	0	9	2	2	5
4166	17	6	40	758	233	0	1	0	12	6	10	6	0	4	0	9	2	2	6
4167	8	3	43	539	352	0	0	30	7	7	10	8	1	6	0	6	2	4	7

Meat, Poultry, Fish

Food #	Food Description & Amount	wt gm	wt oz	calo-ries	%cal fat	prot gm	carbo gm	fiber gm
4168	Ham, pork, and chicken, luncheon meat, chopped, minced, pressed, spiced, canned, reduced sodium (Include Spam 25% Less Salt) [1 slice (½" thick)]	57	2.0	172	80%	7	1	0.0
4169	Ham, prosciutto [2 oz, boneless]	56	2.0	109	38%	16	0	0.0
4170	Ham, sliced, extra lean, prepackaged or deli-sliced (including 95% or more fat-free) [1 slice (6¼"x4"x1/16")]	56	2.0	73	34%	11	1	0.0
4171	Ham, sliced, low salt, prepackaged or deli-sliced (including low salt boiled ham) [2 slices (6¼"x 4"x1/16")]	56	2.0	92	42%	12	0	0.0
4172	Ham, sliced, prepackaged or deli-sliced (Include boiled ham) [2 slices (6¼"x4"x1/16")]	56	2.0	91	47%	10	1	0.0
4173	**Ham, smoked or cured, canned, lean and fat eaten [1 slice (4½"x2½"x¼")]**	**42**	**1.5**	**80**	**62%**	**7**	**0**	**0.0**
4174	Ham, smoked or cured, canned, lean only eaten [1 slice (4½"x2½"x¼")]	42	1.5	50	34%	8	0	0.0
4175	Ham, smoked or cured, cooked, lean and fat eaten (Include country ham, cottage ham, picnic ham) [1 slice (4½"x2½"x¼")]	42	1.5	72	44%	9	0	0.0
4176	Ham, smoked or cured, cooked, lean only eaten (Include country ham, cottage ham, picnic ham) [1 slice (4½"x2½"x¼")]	42	1.5	66	32%	11	0	0.0
4177	Ham, smoked or cured, ground patty [2 oz, cooked]	56	2.0	192	81%	7	1	0.0
4178	Ham, smoked or cured, low sodium, cooked, lean and fat eaten (Include canned ham) [1 slice (4½"x2½"x¼")]	42	1.5	72	43%	9	0	0.0
4179	Ham, smoked or cured, low sodium, cooked, lean only eaten (Include canned) [1 slice (4½"x2½"x¼")]	42	1.5	61	34%	9	1	0.0
4180	Pork chop, battered, fried, lean and fat eaten [1 medium (5.5 oz, with bone, raw)]	110	3.9	297	53%	26	7	0.2
4181	Pork chop, battered, fried, lean only eaten [1 medium (5.5 oz, with bone, raw)]	84	3.0	212	49%	21	5	0.2
4182	Pork chop, breaded, broiled or baked, lean and fat eaten (Include Shake-n-Bake pork chop) [1 medium (5.5 oz, with bone, raw)]	100	3.5	256	45%	25	8	0.3
4183	Pork chop, breaded, broiled or baked, lean only eaten (Include Shake-n-Bake pork chop) [1 medium (5.5 oz, with bone, raw)]	80	2.8	182	36%	21	7	0.2
4184	Pork chop, breaded, fried, lean and fat eaten [1 medium (5.5 oz, with bone, raw)]	110	3.9	345	53%	24	15	0.5
4185	Pork chop, breaded, fried, lean only eaten [1 medium (5.5 oz, with bone, raw)]	84	3.0	241	46%	19	12	0.4
4186	Pork chop, broiled, grilled, or baked, lean and fat eaten (Include floured pork chop) [1 medium (5.5 oz, with bone, raw)]	85	3.0	206	52%	23	0	0.0
4187	Pork chop, broiled, grilled, or baked, lean only eaten (Include floured pork chop) [1 medium (5.5 oz, with bone, raw)]	67	2.4	141	42%	19	0	0.0
4188	**Pork chop, fried, lean and fat eaten (Include floured pork chop) [1 medium (5.5 oz, with bone, raw)]**	**92**	**3.2**	**249**	**57%**	**25**	**0**	**0.0**
4189	Pork chop, fried, lean only eaten (Include floured) [1 medium (5.5 oz, with bone, raw)]	70	2.5	159	46%	20	0	0.0
4190	Pork chop, smoked or cured, cooked, lean and fat eaten [1 medium (5.5 oz, with bone, raw)]	84	3.0	235	69%	17	0	0.0
4191	Pork chop, smoked or cured, cooked, lean only eaten [1 medium (5.5 oz, with bone, raw)]	67	2.4	114	37%	17	0	0.0
4192	Pork chop, stewed, lean and fat eaten [1 medium (5.5 oz, with bone, raw)]	77	2.7	184	51%	21	0	0.0
4193	Pork chop, stewed, lean only eaten [1 medium (5.5 oz, with bone, raw)]	66	2.3	139	43%	19	0	0.0
4194	Pork ears, tail, head, snout, miscellaneous parts, cooked [1 ear]	111	3.9	327	73%	20	0	0.0
4195	Pork liver, braised [2 oz, cooked]	56	2.0	92	24%	15	2	0.0
4196	Pork liver, breaded or floured, fried [2 oz, cooked]	56	2.0	143	33%	17	6	0.1
4197	**Pork roast, loin, cooked, lean and fat eaten [1 slice (4½"x2½"x¼")]**	**42**	**1.5**	**104**	**53%**	**11**	**0**	**0.0**
4198	Pork roast, loin, cooked, lean only eaten [1 slice (4½"x2½"x¼")]	42	1.5	88	41%	12	0	0.0
4199	Pork roast, shoulder, cooked, lean and fat eaten [1 slice (3"dia x ½")]	56	2.0	164	66%	13	0	0.0
4200	Pork roast, shoulder, cooked, lean only eaten [1 slice (3"dia x ½")]	56	2.0	129	53%	14	0	0.0
4201	Pork roast, smoked or cured, cooked, lean and fat eaten [1 slice (4½"x2½"x¼")]	42	1.5	69	42%	9	0	0.0
4202	Pork roast, smoked or cured, cooked, lean only eaten [1 slice (4½"x2½"x¼")]	42	1.5	66	32%	11	0	0.0
4203	Pork roll, cured, fried [2 slices]	56	2.0	199	82%	7	1	0.0
4204	Pork skin, boiled [1 slice]	33	1.2	208	91%	4	0	0.0

Food #	fat gm	sat fat gm	choles mg	sodium mg	potass mg	vit A	vit E	vit C	thia-min	ribo-flavin	nia-cin	vit B-6	fol-ate	vit B-12	cal-cium	phos-phorus	magne-sium	iron	zinc
						% of Daily Value													

Food #	fat gm	sat fat gm	choles mg	sodium mg	potass mg	vit A	vit E	vit C	thia-min	ribo-flavin	nia-cin	vit B-6	fol-ate	vit B-12	cal-cium	phos-phorus	magne-sium	iron	zinc
4168	15	5	43	539	321	0	0	30	10	6	9	8	1	6	0	6	2	2	8
4169	5	2	39	1509	286	0	0	0	21	8	11	12	1	8	1	18	4	3	10
4170	3	1	26	800	196	0	1	0	35	7	14	13	1	7	0	12	2	2	7
4171	4	1	32	543	203	0	0	0	28	9	15	10	0	6	0	14	3	4	10
4172	5	2	30	716	166	0	0	0	33	8	14	11	0	7	0	13	3	3	8
4173	5	2	16	521	133	0	0	0	27	6	7	10	1	5	0	7	1	2	5
4174	2	1	16	527	153	0	0	0	23	6	11	9	1	6	0	9	2	2	5
4175	4	1	24	606	162	0	0	0	21	8	12	7	0	5	0	11	2	3	7
4176	2	1	23	557	133	0	0	0	19	6	11	10	0	5	0	10	2	2	7
4177	17	6	40	595	137	0	0	0	13	6	9	4	0	7	1	6	1	5	7
4178	3	1	24	407	162	0	0	0	20	8	12	7	0	5	0	11	2	3	7
4179	2	1	22	407	121	0	0	0	21	5	8	8	0	5	0	8	1	3	8
4180	18	6	78	82	412	1	3	1	55	20	26	18	4	10	4	24	7	6	13
4181	11	3	58	63	324	1	2	1	44	16	20	15	3	8	3	19	5	5	10
4182	13	5	72	345	398	2	1	1	55	19	24	22	3	10	2	23	7	6	15
4183	7	3	57	278	329	2	1	1	46	16	20	18	2	9	1	19	6	5	12
4184	20	6	100	240	371	2	5	1	50	21	26	16	6	10	7	23	7	11	14
4185	12	3	76	190	293	2	4	1	40	17	20	13	4	8	5	18	6	9	11
4186	12	4	68	53	360	0	1	1	50	16	21	20	1	10	2	21	6	4	14
4187	7	2	53	43	293	0	1	1	41	13	18	16	1	8	1	17	5	3	11
4188	16	6	73	57	390	0	1	1	52	17	24	18	1	11	2	22	6	4	14
4189	8	3	55	46	312	0	1	1	43	14	19	15	1	9	1	17	5	3	12
4190	18	6	49	900	217	0	1	0	34	9	17	12	1	13	1	19	3	4	14
4191	5	2	32	825	196	0	1	0	32	9	16	12	1	12	1	16	3	4	13
4192	10	4	62	37	288	0	1	1	32	12	17	14	1	7	2	14	4	5	12
4193	7	2	53	37	242	0	1	1	30	10	15	12	1	6	1	11	3	4	12
4194	27	10	112	91	185	0	1	0	14	8	10	11	1	8	2	9	3	7	13
4195	2	1	199	27	84	302	1	22	10	72	24	16	23	174	1	13	2	56	25
4196	5	1	234	101	191	379	2	26	12	125	49	16	36	269	2	21	4	97	30
4197	6	2	34	25	171	0	0	0	28	8	12	11	1	5	1	10	3	2	6
4198	4	1	34	24	179	0	0	0	28	8	12	12	1	5	1	10	3	3	7
4199	12	4	50	38	184	0	0	0	22	11	11	8	1	7	1	12	3	4	14
4200	8	3	50	42	194	0	0	0	24	12	12	9	1	8	1	12	3	5	16
4201	3	1	24	582	152	0	0	0	21	7	11	7	0	5	0	10	2	3	7
4202	2	1	23	557	133	0	0	0	19	6	11	10	0	5	0	10	2	2	7
4203	18	6	39	581	133	0	1	0	13	6	9	4	0	6	0	6	1	5	7
4204	21	8	31	11	78	0	1	0	7	2	4	2	0	2	2	5	1	1	3

Meat, Poultry, Fish

Food #	Food Description & Amount	wt gm	wt oz	calo-ries	%cal fat	prot gm	carbo gm	fiber gm
4205	Pork skin, rinds, deep-fried (Include snack type) [10 rinds]	10	0.4	54	52%	6	0	0.0
4206	Pork steak or cutlet, battered, fried, lean and fat eaten [3 oz]	75	2.6	210	55%	17	5	0.1
4207	Pork steak or cutlet, battered, fried, lean only eaten [3 oz]	63	2.2	152	47%	15	4	0.1
4208	Pork steak or cutlet, breaded, broiled or baked, lean and fat eaten [3 oz]	75	2.6	203	50%	18	6	0.2
4209	Pork steak or cutlet, breaded, broiled or baked, lean only eaten [3 oz]	63	2.2	149	40%	16	5	0.2
4210	Pork steak or cutlet, breaded, fried, lean and fat eaten [3 oz]	75	2.6	210	51%	17	7	0.2
4211	Pork steak or cutlet, breaded, fried, lean only eaten [3 oz]	87	3.1	228	46%	21	9	0.3
4212	Pork steak or cutlet, broiled or baked, lean and fat eaten (Include floured) [3 oz]	75	2.6	177	51%	20	0	0.0
4213	Pork steak or cutlet, broiled or baked, lean only eaten (Include floured) [3 oz]	72	2.5	153	44%	20	0	0.0
4214	**Pork steak or cutlet, fried, lean and fat eaten (Include floured) [3 oz]**	**75**	**2.6**	**204**	**57%**	**21**	**0**	**0.0**
4215	Pork steak or cutlet, fried, lean only eaten (Include floured) [3 oz]	63	2.2	144	47%	18	0	0.0
4216	Pork, cracklings, cooked [1 cup]	91	3.2	524	77%	28	1	0.0
4217	Pork, dehydrated, oriental style [1 cup]	22	0.8	135	91%	3	0	0.0
4218	Pork, ground or patty, breaded, cooked [2 oz, cooked]	56	2.0	196	61%	10	9	0.3
4219	Pork, ground or patty, cooked [2 oz, cooked]	56	2.0	166	63%	14	0	0.0
4220	Pork, neck bones, cooked (Include pork backbone) [1 neck bone]	47	1.7	98	41%	13	0	0.0
4221	Pork, pickled [2 boneless pieces (1 cubic inch]	36	1.3	73	72%	5	0	0.0
4222	Pork, pig's feet, cooked [1 foot]	87	3.1	169	58%	17	0	0.0
4223	Pork, pig's feet, pickled [1 foot]	87	3.1	177	72%	12	0	0.0
4224	Pork, pig's hocks, cooked (Include ham hocks) [1 ham hock]	51	1.8	168	64%	14	0	0.0
4225	Pork, spareribs, cooked, lean and fat eaten (Include flank end) [1 medium rib]	35	1.2	139	69%	10	0	0.0
4226	Pork, spareribs, cooked, lean only eaten (Include flank end) [1 medium rib]	26	0.9	54	41%	7	0	0.0
4227	**Pork, spareribs, barbecued, with sauce, lean and fat eaten [2 oz, with bone, cooked]**	**42**	**1.5**	**130**	**65%**	**9**	**2**	**0.2**
4228	Pork, spareribs, barbecued, with sauce, lean only eaten [2 oz, with bone, cooked]	32	1.1	71	48%	7	1	0.1
4229	Pork, tenderloin, baked [2 oz, boneless, cooked]	56	2.0	97	31%	16	0	0.0
4230	Pork, tenderloin, battered, fried [2 oz, boneless, cooked]	56	2.0	117	36%	14	4	0.1
4231	Pork, tenderloin, braised [2 oz, boneless, cooked]	56	2.0	114	40%	16	0	0.0
4232	Pork, tenderloin, breaded, fried (Include floured) [2 oz, boneless, cooked]	56	2.0	110	42%	11	4	0.1
4233	Salt pork or fat back, cooked (Include hog jowl) [1 slice (4"x1¾"x½")]	47	1.7	337	96%	3	0	0.0
	Lamb (weight columns are for cooked, boneless part)							
4250	Lamb hocks, cooked (Include mutton hocks) [2 oz]	38	1.3	92	50%	11	0	0.0
4251	Lamb liver, cooked (Include mutton) [2 oz, cooked]	56	2.0	123	36%	17	1	0.0
4252	Lamb, ground or patty, cooked (Include mutton, ground or patty) [1 patty (4 oz, raw)]	77	2.7	218	62%	19	0	0.0
4253	Lamb, loin chop, cooked, lean and fat eaten (Include lamb steak, mutton loin chop, mutton steak) [1 medium (5 oz, with bone, raw)]	89	3.1	281	66%	22	0	0.0
4254	Lamb, loin chop, cooked, lean only eaten (Include lamb steak, mutton loin chop, mutton steak) [1 medium (5 oz, with bone, raw)]	62	2.2	134	41%	19	0	0.0
4255	Lamb, ribs, cooked, lean and fat eaten (Include mutton ribs) [1 rib]	46	1.6	166	74%	10	0	0.0
4256	Lamb, ribs, cooked, lean only eaten (Include mutton ribs) [2 ribs]	50	1.8	118	50%	14	0	0.0
4257	**Lamb, roast, cooked, lean and fat eaten (Include mutton roast; lamb leg; mutton leg) [1 slice (3"dia x ½")]**	**56**	**2.0**	**150**	**61%**	**13**	**0**	**0.0**
4258	Lamb, roast, cooked, lean only eaten (Include mutton roast; lamb leg; mutton leg) [1 slice (3"dia x ½")]	56	2.0	110	42%	15	0	0.0
4259	Lamb, shoulder chop, cooked, lean and fat eaten (Include mutton shoulder chop) [1 chop (7 oz, with bone, raw)]	127	4.5	351	65%	29	0	0.0
4260	Lamb, shoulder chop, cooked, lean only eaten (Include mutton shoulder chop) [1 chop (7 oz, with bone, raw)]	91	3.2	186	48%	23	0	0.0
4261	Lamb, shoulder, cooked, lean and fat eaten (Include mutton shoulder) [1 slice (3"dia x ½")]	56	2.0	155	65%	13	0	0.0
4262	Lamb, shoulder, cooked, lean only eaten (Include mutton shoulder) [1 slice (3"dia x ½")]	56	2.0	114	48%	14	0	0.0

Food #	fat gm	sat fat gm	choles mg	sodium mg	potass mg	% of Daily Value													
						vit A	vit E	vit C	thia-min	ribo-flavin	nia-cin	vit B-6	fol-ate	vit B-12	cal-cium	phos-phorus	magne-sium	iron	zinc
4205	3	1	9	184	13	0	0	0	1	2	1	0	0	1	0	1	0	0	0
4206	13	4	61	64	241	1	2	1	38	15	16	11	2	9	4	16	4	5	14
4207	8	2	49	51	205	1	2	0	31	13	14	9	2	8	3	13	4	5	13
4208	11	4	61	79	251	0	1	1	40	17	17	14	3	10	3	16	5	7	16
4209	7	2	51	69	221	0	1	1	36	15	15	13	2	9	2	14	4	6	15
4210	12	4	73	131	238	1	2	1	36	17	16	13	3	10	4	16	5	8	15
4211	12	3	83	157	281	1	3	1	44	20	19	16	3	12	4	19	6	9	19
4212	10	4	67	47	269	0	1	1	40	17	17	14	1	11	2	17	4	5	17
4213	8	3	64	49	279	0	1	1	45	17	17	16	1	12	2	17	5	6	17
4214	13	5	60	46	325	0	1	1	41	14	19	15	1	9	2	18	5	3	12
4215	8	3	49	41	280	0	1	1	36	13	17	13	1	8	1	16	4	3	11
4216	45	16	77	1452	442	0	2	0	42	15	33	12	1	27	1	31	5	8	20
4217	14	5	15	151	31	0	0	0	7	2	2	2	0	1	0	3	1	1	2
4218	13	3	31	125	154	0	4	0	20	7	10	7	3	3	4	10	3	6	8
4219	12	4	53	41	203	0	0	1	26	7	12	11	1	5	1	13	3	4	12
4220	5	2	38	313	164	0	0	0	21	8	13	9	1	7	0	11	2	4	12
4221	6	2	33	332	85	0	0	0	0	1	1	7	0	4	1	1	0	1	3
4222	11	4	87	26	127	0	1	0	1	3	2	4	0	3	4	4	1	2	6
4223	14	5	80	803	204	0	1	0	0	2	2	17	1	9	3	3	1	3	7
4224	12	4	56	45	188	0	0	0	18	9	13	9	1	6	1	11	2	5	14
4225	11	4	42	33	112	0	0	0	10	8	10	6	0	6	2	9	2	4	11
4226	2	1	18	11	105	0	0	0	11	4	7	4	0	2	1	5	1	1	4
4227	9	3	36	140	120	1	1	2	8	7	9	6	0	5	2	8	2	4	9
4228	4	1	27	103	113	1	1	1	11	5	5	4	0	4	1	4	2	3	9
4229	3	1	44	31	242	0	0	0	35	13	13	12	1	5	0	14	4	5	10
4230	5	1	42	42	218	1	1	0	31	13	12	10	2	5	2	13	4	5	9
4231	5	2	44	28	217	0	0	1	25	9	13	11	1	5	1	10	3	4	9
4232	5	1	42	74	165	1	3	1	24	10	10	9	2	6	2	11	4	5	7
4233	36	13	40	601	30	0	0	0	3	2	4	1	0	2	0	2	1	1	4
4250	5	2	40	27	98	0	0	0	1	4	10	2	2	14	1	6	2	5	19
4251	5	2	281	31	124	419	1	4	9	133	34	14	10	714	0	24	3	26	29
4252	15	6	75	62	261	0	1	0	5	11	26	5	4	33	2	15	5	8	24
4253	21	9	92	62	254	0	0	0	6	15	33	6	3	37	2	18	5	9	19
4254	6	2	59	52	233	0	0	0	5	10	21	5	4	26	1	14	4	7	17
4255	14	6	46	35	124	0	0	0	3	6	16	3	2	19	1	8	3	5	12
4256	6	2	46	43	157	0	0	0	3	7	16	4	3	22	1	11	4	6	18
4257	10	4	52	37	158	0	0	0	4	8	18	4	3	24	1	10	3	6	18
4258	5	2	49	38	169	0	0	0	4	9	17	4	3	25	1	11	4	7	20
4259	25	11	117	84	319	0	1	0	8	18	39	8	7	56	3	23	7	14	44
4260	10	4	79	62	241	0	1	0	5	14	26	7	6	41	2	18	6	11	37
4261	11	5	52	37	140	0	0	0	3	8	17	4	3	25	1	10	3	6	20
4262	6	2	49	38	148	0	0	0	3	9	16	4	4	25	1	11	4	7	23

Meat, Poultry, Fish

Food #	Food Description & Amount	wt gm	wt oz	calo-ries	%cal fat	prot gm	carbo gm	fiber gm
	Chicken (weight columns are for cooked, boneless part)							
4300	Chicken, back, battered, fried, skin eaten (Include extra-crispy fried chicken) [1 back]	212	7.5	703	60%	47	22	0.7
4301	Chicken, back, battered or breaded, fried or baked with added fat, skin and coating not eaten [1 back]	119	4.2	344	48%	36	7	0.2
4302	Chicken, back, breaded, fried or baked with added fat, skin eaten (Include regular fried chicken, Shake-n-Bake chicken) [1 back]	212	7.5	698	57%	58	14	0.4
4303	Chicken, back, broiled or grilled, skin eaten [1 back]	134	4.7	402	63%	35	0	0.0
4304	Chicken, back, broiled or grilled, skin not eaten [1 back]	112	4.0	268	50%	32	0	0.0
4305	Chicken, back, floured, seasoned, fried or baked with added fat, skin eaten [1 back]	128	4.5	424	56%	36	8	0.3
4306	Chicken, back, floured, seasoned, fried or baked with added fat, skin not eaten [1 back]	103	3.6	300	48%	31	6	0.2
4307	Chicken, back, fried, no coating, skin eaten [1 back]	128	4.5	416	62%	37	0	0.0
4308	Chicken, back, fried, no coating, skin not eaten [1 back]	103	3.6	289	52%	32	0	0.0
4309	Chicken, back, roasted, skin eaten [1 back]	94	3.3	282	63%	24	0	0.0
4310	Chicken, back, roasted, skin not eaten [1 back]	72	2.5	172	50%	20	0	0.0
4311	Chicken, back, stewed, skin eaten [1 back]	106	3.7	273	63%	24	0	0.0
4312	Chicken, back, stewed, skin not eaten [1 back]	75	2.6	157	48%	19	0	0.0
4313	**Chicken, breast, battered, fried,** skin eaten (Include extra crispy fried chicken) [½ breast]	140	4.9	364	46%	35	13	0.4
4314	Chicken, breast, battered or breaded, fried or baked with added fat, skin and coating not eaten [½ breast]	88	3.1	165	23%	29	0	0.0
4315	Chicken, breast, breaded, fried or baked with added fat, skin eaten (Include regular fried chicken, Shake-n-Bake chicken) [½ breast]	140	4.9	325	33%	42	9	0.3
4316	Chicken, breast, broiled or grilled, skin eaten [½ breast]	92	3.2	181	36%	27	0	0.0
4317	Chicken, breast, broiled or grilled, skin not eaten [½ breast]	81	2.9	134	19%	25	0	0.0
4318	Chicken, breast, floured, seasoned, fried or baked with added fat, skin eaten [½ breast]	98	3.5	218	36%	31	2	0.1
4319	Chicken, breast, floured, fried or baked with added fat, skin not eaten [½ breast]	86	3.0	161	23%	29	0	0.0
4320	Chicken, breast, fried, no coating, skin eaten (Include sauteed chicken) [½ breast]	98	3.5	214	37%	32	0	0.0
4321	Chicken, breast, fried, no coating, skin not eaten (Include sauteed chicken) [½ breast]	86	3.0	160	23%	29	0	0.0
4322	**Chicken, breast, roasted,** skin eaten [½ breast]	98	3.5	193	36%	29	0	0.0
4323	Chicken, breast, roasted, skin not eaten [½ breast]	86	3.0	142	19%	27	0	0.0
4324	Chicken, breast, skinless, battered, fried, coating eaten (Include Chicken Tenders) [4 tenders/pieces]	48	1.7	112	37%	12	5	0.1
4325	Chicken, breast, skinless, battered or breaded, fried or baked with fat, coating not eaten [½ breast]	98	3.5	183	23%	33	1	0.0
4326	Chicken, breast, skinless, breaded, cooked, breading eaten (Include Weaver Crispy Light Fried Chicken, Perdue Done It Chicken Breast Tenders) [½ breast]	124	4.4	277	25%	36	13	0.4
4327	Chicken, breast, stewed, skin eaten [½ breast]	110	3.9	202	36%	30	0	0.0
4328	Chicken, breast, stewed, skin not eaten [½ breast]	95	3.4	143	18%	28	0	0.0
4329	Chicken, canned, dark meat [1 can (5 oz), meat portion]	125	4.4	239	42%	32	0	0.0
4330	Chicken, canned, light and dark meat [1 can (5 oz), meat portion]	125	4.4	230	40%	32	1	0.0
4331	Chicken, canned, light meat [1 can (5 oz), meat portion]	125	4.4	198	23%	36	0	0.0
4332	Chicken, crackling, Puerto Rican style (Include Chicharron de pollo) [2 pieces (1½"x1"boneless)]	50	1.8	196	56%	11	10	0.4
4333	**Chicken, drumstick, battered, fried,** skin eaten (Include extra crispy fried chicken) [1 drumstick]	72	2.5	193	53%	16	6	0.2
4334	Chicken, drumstick, battered or breaded, fried or baked with added fat, skin and coating not eaten [1 drumstick]	46	1.6	90	37%	13	0	0.0
4335	Chicken, drumstick, breaded, fried or baked with added fat, skin eaten (Include regular fried chicken, Shake-n-Bake chicken) [1 drumstick]	72	2.5	182	47%	18	5	0.2
4336	Chicken, drumstick, floured, baked or fried, prepared skinless, coating eaten [1 drumstick]	42	1.5	91	43%	12	1	0.0

Food #	fat gm	sat fat gm	choles mg	sodium mg	potass mg	% of Daily Value													
						vit A	vit E	vit C	thia-min	ribo-flavin	nia-cin	vit B-6	fol-ate	vit B-12	cal-cium	phos-phorus	magne-sium	iron	zinc
4300	47	12	186	671	381	8	9	0	17	27	62	25	10	9	6	29	10	18	28
4301	18	5	111	118	299	3	2	0	9	18	46	21	4	6	3	21	7	11	22
4302	44	12	187	695	493	11	5	1	14	29	75	33	6	10	5	35	12	19	35
4303	28	8	118	117	281	13	1	0	5	15	45	18	2	6	3	21	7	11	20
4304	15	4	101	108	265	3	1	0	5	14	40	19	2	6	3	18	6	9	20
4305	27	7	114	116	290	5	3	0	9	18	47	19	5	6	3	21	7	12	21
4306	16	4	95	102	258	3	2	0	8	15	39	18	4	5	3	18	6	9	19
4307	29	7	123	125	304	5	3	0	6	17	48	20	2	7	3	22	7	11	22
4308	17	4	103	110	271	3	2	0	5	15	40	19	2	6	3	19	6	9	20
4309	20	5	83	82	197	9	1	0	4	11	32	13	1	4	2	14	5	7	14
4310	9	3	65	69	171	2	1	0	3	9	25	12	1	4	2	12	4	6	13
4311	19	5	83	68	154	9	1	0	3	9	23	8	1	3	2	13	4	7	14
4312	8	2	64	50	119	2	1	0	2	8	17	8	1	3	2	10	3	5	12
4313	18	5	120	385	282	3	5	0	11	12	74	30	5	7	3	26	9	10	9
4314	4	1	80	69	243	1	1	0	5	6	65	28	1	5	1	22	7	6	6
4315	12	3	117	433	357	4	2	0	10	11	91	39	3	7	2	31	10	10	10
4316	7	2	77	65	225	2	1	0	4	6	58	26	1	5	1	20	6	5	6
4317	3	1	69	60	207	0	1	0	4	5	56	24	1	5	1	18	6	5	5
4318	9	2	88	74	253	1	1	0	5	7	67	28	1	6	2	23	7	7	7
4319	4	1	79	68	237	1	1	0	5	6	64	27	1	5	1	21	7	5	6
4320	9	2	90	76	257	1	1	0	5	7	68	29	1	6	1	23	7	6	7
4321	4	1	79	68	238	1	1	0	5	6	64	28	1	5	1	21	7	5	6
4322	8	2	82	70	240	3	1	0	4	7	62	27	1	5	1	21	7	6	7
4323	3	1	73	64	220	1	1	0	4	6	59	26	1	5	1	20	6	5	6
4324	5	1	41	144	100	1	2	0	4	4	26	11	2	2	1	9	3	3	3
4325	5	1	90	77	270	1	1	0	5	7	72	31	1	6	2	24	8	6	7
4326	8	2	97	546	321	3	3	1	10	10	81	35	3	6	2	28	9	9	8
4327	8	2	83	68	196	3	1	0	3	7	43	16	1	4	1	17	6	6	7
4328	3	1	73	60	178	1	1	0	3	7	40	16	1	4	1	16	6	5	6
4329	11	3	110	238	226	3	1	0	5	15	30	13	2	5	2	18	6	9	22
4330	10	3	63	169	191	4	1	0	0	7	15	12	1	21	2	19	6	9	21
4331	5	1	96	226	224	1	1	0	4	9	49	21	1	5	2	20	7	6	10
4332	12	3	39	115	106	2	4	6	6	7	18	8	4	2	1	8	3	6	5
4333	11	3	62	194	134	2	3	0	5	9	18	10	3	3	1	11	4	5	11
4334	4	1	43	44	115	1	1	0	2	6	14	9	1	3	1	9	3	3	10
4335	9	2	61	232	163	3	2	0	5	10	21	12	2	4	1	12	4	6	13
4336	4	1	38	39	100	1	1	0	2	6	13	8	1	2	0	8	3	3	9

Meat, Poultry, Fish

Food #	Food Description & Amount	wt gm	wt oz	calo-ries	%cal fat	prot gm	carbo gm	fiber gm
4337	Chicken, drumstick, broiled or grilled, skin eaten [1 drumstick]	52	1.8	112	46%	14	0	0.0
4338	Chicken, drumstick, broiled or grilled, skin not eaten [1 drumstick]	45	1.6	77	30%	13	0	0.0
4339	Chicken, drumstick, floured, fried or baked with added fat, skin eaten [1 drumstick]	49	1.7	120	50%	13	1	0.0
4340	Chicken, drumstick, floured, fried or baked with added fat, skin not eaten [1 drumstick]	42	1.5	82	37%	12	0	0.0
4341	Chicken, drumstick, fried, no coating, skin eaten [1 drumstick]	49	1.7	119	52%	13	0	0.0
4342	Chicken, drumstick, fried, no coating, skin not eaten [1 drumstick]	42	1.5	82	37%	12	0	0.0
4343	**Chicken, drumstick, roasted, skin eaten [1 drumstick]**	52	1.8	112	46%	14	0	0.0
4344	Chicken, drumstick, roasted, skin not eaten [1 drumstick]	44	1.6	76	30%	12	0	0.0
4345	Chicken, drumstick, skinless, breaded, baked or fried, breading eaten (Include Kentucky Fried Lite 'N Crispy) [1 drumstick]	64	2.3	148	35%	16	7	0.2
4346	Chicken, drumstick, skinless, breaded, baked or fried, breading not eaten [1 drumstick]	55	1.9	127	35%	14	6	0.2
4347	Chicken, drumstick, stewed, skin eaten [1 drumstick]	57	2.0	116	47%	14	0	0.0
4348	Chicken, drumstick, stewed, skin not eaten [1 drumstick]	46	1.6	78	30%	13	0	0.0
4349	Chicken, feet, roasted [1 foot]	34	1.2	73	61%	7	0	0.0
4350	Chicken, ground [1 cup, cooked, or 2 medium patties]	127	4.5	304	51%	35	0	0.0
4351	**Chicken, leg (drumstick+thigh), battered, fried, skin eaten (Include extra crispy fried chicken) [1 leg]**	158	5.6	430	53%	34	14	0.4
4352	Chicken, leg, battered or breaded, fried or baked with added fat, skin and coating not eaten [1 leg]	102	3.6	212	40%	29	1	0.0
4353	Chicken, leg, breaded, fried or baked with added fat, skin eaten (Include regular fried chicken, Shake-n-Bake chicken) [1 leg]	158	5.6	412	48%	40	11	0.3
4354	Chicken, leg, broiled or grilled, skin eaten [1 leg]	109	3.8	253	52%	28	0	0.0
4355	Chicken, leg, broiled or grilled, skin not eaten [1 leg]	97	3.4	185	40%	26	0	0.0
4356	Chicken, leg, floured, fried or baked with added fat, skin eaten [1 leg]	112	4.0	285	51%	30	3	0.1
4357	Chicken, leg, floured, fried or baked with added fat, skin not eaten [1 leg]	94	3.3	195	40%	27	1	0.0
4358	Chicken, leg, fried, no coating, skin eaten [1 leg]	112	4.0	280	53%	31	0	0.0
4359	Chicken, leg, fried, no coating, skin not eaten [1 leg]	94	3.3	194	41%	27	0	0.0
4360	**Chicken, leg (drumstick+thigh), roasted, skin eaten [1 leg]**	114	4.0	264	52%	30	0	0.0
4361	Chicken, leg, roasted, skin not eaten [1 leg]	95	3.4	181	40%	26	0	0.0
4362	Chicken, leg, stewed, skin eaten [1 leg]	125	4.4	275	53%	30	0	0.0
4363	Chicken, leg, stewed, skin not eaten [1 leg]	101	3.6	187	39%	27	0	0.0
4364	Chicken, liver paste or pate [1 slice (1 oz)]	28	1.0	56	59%	4	2	0.0
4365	Chicken, liver, battered, fried [1 oz, cooked]	28	1.0	60	36%	6	3	0.1
4366	Chicken, liver, braised [1 oz, cooked]	28	1.0	44	31%	7	0	0.0
4367	Chicken, liver, breaded or floured, fried [1 oz, cooked]	28	1.0	78	35%	8	4	0.1
4368	**Chicken, liver, fried or sauteed, no coating [1 oz, cooked]**	28	1.0	71	40%	9	2	0.0
4369	Chicken, neck, breaded, baked or fried, skin eaten (Include Shake-n-Bake) [1 neck]	52	1.8	172	63%	12	3	0.1
4370	Chicken, neck, breaded, baked or fried, skin not eaten [1 neck]	25	0.9	57	47%	7	0	0.0
4371	Chicken, neck, floured, salted, fried or baked with added fat, skin eaten [1 neck]	36	1.3	119	64%	9	2	0.1
4372	Chicken, neck, floured, fried or baked with added fat, skin not eaten [1 neck]	22	0.8	50	47%	6	0	0.0
4373	Chicken, neck, fried, no coating, skin eaten [1 neck]	36	1.3	118	68%	9	0	0.0
4374	Chicken, neck, fried, no coating, skin not eaten [1 neck]	22	0.8	49	49%	6	0	0.0
4375	Chicken, neck, roasted, skin eaten [1 neck]	36	1.3	108	69%	8	0	0.0
4376	Chicken, neck, roasted, skin not eaten [1 neck]	24	0.8	56	56%	6	0	0.0
4377	Chicken, neck, stewed, skin eaten [1 neck]	38	1.3	94	66%	7	0	0.0
4378	Chicken, neck, stewed, skin not eaten [1 neck]	18	0.6	32	41%	4	0	0.0
4379	**Chicken nuggets, breaded, fried (Include Weaver mini drums; Tyson chicken sticks) [4 nuggets]**	72	2.5	204	55%	12	11	0.3
4380	Chicken nuggets, lowfat (includes soy), breaded, baked [4 nuggets]	72	2.5	140	29%	14	10	0.5

Food #	fat gm	sat fat gm	choles mg	sodium mg	potass mg	% of Daily Value													
						vit A	vit E	vit C	thia-min	ribo-flavin	nia-cin	vit B-6	fol-ate	vit B-12	cal-cium	phos-phorus	magne-sium	iron	zinc
4337	6	2	47	47	119	2	0	0	2	7	16	9	1	3	1	9	3	4	10
4338	3	1	42	43	111	1	0	0	2	6	14	9	1	3	1	8	3	3	10
4339	7	2	44	44	112	1	1	0	3	6	15	9	1	3	1	9	3	4	9
4340	3	1	40	41	105	1	1	0	2	6	13	8	1	2	0	8	3	3	9
4341	7	2	45	44	113	1	1	0	2	6	15	9	1	3	1	9	3	4	10
4342	3	1	40	41	105	1	1	0	2	6	13	8	1	2	0	8	3	3	9
4343	6	2	47	47	119	2	0	0	2	7	16	9	1	3	1	9	3	4	10
4344	2	1	41	42	108	1	0	0	2	6	13	9	1	2	1	8	3	3	9
4345	6	1	51	300	150	2	1	0	5	9	18	11	3	3	1	11	4	5	12
4346	5	1	44	257	129	2	1	0	4	8	16	10	2	3	1	9	3	5	10
4347	6	2	47	43	105	2	1	0	2	6	12	5	1	2	1	8	3	4	10
4348	3	1	40	37	92	1	0	0	2	6	10	5	1	2	1	7	2	4	9
4349	5	1	29	23	11	1	0	0	1	4	1	0	7	3	3	3	0	2	2
4350	17	5	112	104	283	6	2	0	5	13	54	25	2	6	2	23	7	9	16
4351	25	6	142	441	300	4	6	0	12	21	43	21	7	7	3	24	8	12	23
4352	10	2	101	97	259	2	1	0	6	15	34	20	2	6	1	20	6	8	20
4353	22	6	141	509	368	6	3	1	11	22	50	26	5	8	2	28	9	13	27
4354	15	4	100	95	245	4	1	0	5	14	34	18	2	5	1	19	6	8	19
4355	8	2	91	88	235	2	1	0	5	13	31	18	2	5	1	18	6	7	18
4356	16	4	106	99	261	3	2	0	7	16	37	19	3	6	1	20	7	9	20
4357	9	2	93	90	239	2	1	0	5	14	31	18	2	5	1	18	6	7	19
4358	17	4	109	102	266	3	2	0	5	15	37	19	2	6	1	21	7	9	20
4359	9	2	94	90	240	2	1	0	5	14	31	18	2	5	1	18	6	7	19
4360	15	4	105	99	257	4	1	0	5	14	35	19	2	6	1	20	7	8	20
4361	8	2	89	86	230	2	1	0	5	13	30	18	2	5	1	17	6	7	18
4362	16	4	105	91	220	5	1	0	5	14	29	11	2	4	1	17	6	9	20
4363	8	2	90	79	192	2	1	0	4	13	24	11	2	4	1	15	5	8	19
4364	4	1	109	108	27	6	1	5	1	23	11	4	22	38	0	5	1	14	4
4365	2	1	147	22	67	151	2	15	3	35	13	8	52	100	1	8	2	15	7
4366	2	1	177	14	39	138	1	7	3	29	6	8	54	90	0	9	1	13	8
4367	3	1	198	30	90	208	3	20	4	48	17	10	71	138	1	11	2	21	9
4368	3	1	210	32	93	221	3	22	3	50	18	11	75	147	1	12	2	22	10
4369	12	3	47	165	96	4	2	0	3	8	13	7	1	2	2	7	2	7	10
4370	3	1	26	25	53	1	1	0	1	5	6	4	1	1	1	3	1	4	7
4371	9	2	34	29	65	2	1	0	2	6	10	5	1	2	1	5	2	5	7
4372	3	1	23	22	47	1	1	0	1	4	6	4	1	1	1	3	1	4	6
4373	9	2	35	31	67	2	1	0	1	5	10	5	0	2	1	5	2	5	8
4374	3	1	24	22	48	1	1	0	1	4	6	4	0	1	1	3	1	4	6
4375	8	2	48	27	59	3	0	0	1	6	8	4	0	2	1	5	1	5	7
4376	4	1	26	22	45	1	0	0	1	4	5	4	0	1	1	3	1	4	6
4377	7	2	27	20	41	2	0	0	1	6	6	2	0	1	1	5	1	5	7
4378	1	0	14	12	25	1	0	0	1	3	4	1	0	1	1	2	1	3	5
4379	12	4	43	383	177	2	5	0	4	6	24	11	5	4	1	14	4	5	5
4380	5	1	35	342	116	1	1	0	3	3	27	11	1	2	1	11	4	4	4

Meat, Poultry, Fish

Food #	Food Description & Amount	wt gm	wt oz	calo-ries	%cal fat	prot gm	carbo gm	fiber gm
4381	Chicken, patty with cheese, breaded, cooked (Include Cheese Recipe Chicken Rondelets) [1 patty]	85	3.0	237	54%	13	14	0.5
4382	Chicken, patty, breaded, cooked (Include Chicken Rondelets) [1 patty]	75	2.6	213	55%	12	11	0.3
4383	Chicken roll, roasted, dark meat [2 slices]	56	2.0	114	43%	15	0	0.0
4384	Chicken roll, roasted, light and dark meat [2 slices]	56	2.0	106	35%	16	0	0.0
4385	Chicken roll, roasted, light meat [2 slices]	56	2.0	89	42%	11	1	0.0
4386	Chicken, skin, roasted [skin from ½ chicken]	56	2.0	254	81%	11	0	0.0
4387	Chicken, tail, roasted [1 tail]	7	0.2	27	76%	2	0	0.0
4388	**Chicken, thigh, battered, fried**, skin eaten (Include extra crispy fried chicken) [1 thigh]	**86**	**3.0**	**237**	**54%**	**19**	**8**	**0.2**
4389	Chicken, thigh, battered or breaded, fried or baked with added fat, skin not eaten [1 thigh]	54	1.9	118	43%	15	1	0.0
4390	Chicken, thigh, breaded, fried or baked with added fat, skin eaten (Include regular fried chicken, Shake-n-Bake chicken) [1 thigh]	86	3.0	229	49%	22	6	0.2
4391	Chicken, thigh, broiled or grilled, skin eaten [1 thigh]	58	2.0	143	56%	15	0	0.0
4392	Chicken, thigh, broiled or grilled, skin not eaten [1 thigh]	52	1.8	109	47%	13	0	0.0
4393	Chicken, thigh, floured, fried or baked with added fat, skin eaten [1 thigh]	62	2.2	162	51%	17	2	0.1
4394	Chicken, thigh, floured, fried or baked with added fat, skin not eaten [1 thigh]	52	1.8	113	43%	15	1	0.0
4395	Chicken, thigh, fried, no coating, skin eaten [1 thigh]	62	2.2	159	55%	17	0	0.0
4396	Chicken, thigh, fried, no coating, skin not eaten [1 thigh]	52	1.8	112	44%	15	0	0.0
4397	**Chicken, thigh, roasted**, skin eaten [1 thigh]	**62**	**2.2**	**153**	**56%**	**16**	**0**	**0.0**
4398	Chicken, thigh, roasted, skin not eaten [1 thigh]	52	1.8	109	47%	13	0	0.0
4399	Chicken, thigh, skinless, battered, fried, coating eaten [1 thigh]	63	2.2	160	48%	14	6	0.2
4400	Chicken, thigh, skinless, battered, fried, coating not eaten [1 thigh]	52	1.8	113	43%	15	1	0.0
4401	Chicken, thigh, skinless, breaded, baked or fried, breading eaten (Include Weaver Crispy Light Fried Chicken) [1 thigh]	78	2.8	202	47%	19	8	0.3
4402	Chicken, thigh, skinless, breaded, baked or fried, breading not eaten [1 thigh]	70	2.5	182	47%	17	7	0.2
4403	Chicken, thigh, smoked, skin eaten [1 thigh]	84	3.0	162	56%	16	0	0.0
4404	Chicken, thigh, smoked, skin not eaten [1 thigh]	70	2.5	95	47%	12	0	0.0
4405	Chicken, thigh, stewed, skin eaten [1 thigh]	68	2.4	158	57%	16	0	0.0
4406	Chicken, thigh, stewed, skin not eaten [1 thigh]	55	1.9	107	45%	14	0	0.0
4407	**Chicken, wing, battered, fried**, skin eaten (Include extra crispy fried chicken) [1 wing]	**49**	**1.7**	**159**	**61%**	**10**	**5**	**0.2**
4408	Chicken, wing, battered or breaded, fried or baked with added fat, skin and coating not eaten [1 wing]	22	0.8	46	39%	7	0	0.0
4409	Chicken, wing, breaded, fried or baked with added fat, skin eaten (Include regular fried chicken, Shake-n-Bake chicken) [1 wing]	49	1.7	158	59%	12	3	0.1
4410	Chicken, wing, broiled or grilled, skin eaten [1 wing]	35	1.2	102	60%	9	0	0.0
4411	Chicken, wing, broiled or grilled, skin not eaten [1 wing]	20	0.7	41	36%	6	0	0.0
4412	Chicken, wing, floured, fried or baked with added fat, skin eaten [1 wing]	32	1.1	103	62%	8	1	0.0
4413	Chicken, wing, floured, fried or baked with added fat, skin not eaten [1 wing]	20	0.7	42	39%	6	0	0.0
4414	Chicken, wing, fried, no coating, skin eaten [1 wing]	32	1.1	102	65%	8	0	0.0
4415	Chicken, wing, fried, no coating, skin not eaten [1 wing]	20	0.7	42	39%	6	0	0.0
4416	Chicken, wing, roasted, skin eaten [1 wing]	34	1.2	99	60%	9	0	0.0
4417	Chicken, wing, roasted, skin not eaten [1 wing]	21	0.7	43	36%	6	0	0.0
4418	Chicken, wing, stewed, skin eaten [1 wing]	40	1.4	100	61%	9	0	0.0
4419	Chicken, wing, stewed, skin not eaten [1 wing]	24	0.8	43	36%	7	0	0.0
	Turkey & Other Poultry (weight columns are for cooked, boneless part)							
4450	Cornish game hen, roasted, skin eaten [1 hen (1¼ lb, raw)]	306	10.8	796	63%	68	0	0.0
4451	Cornish game hen, roasted, skin not eaten [1 hen (1¼ lb, raw)]	249	8.8	334	26%	58	0	0.0
4452	Dove, roasted (Include squab, pigeon) [1 dove]	111	3.9	243	53%	27	0	0.0
4453	Dove, floured, fried (Include squab, pigeon) [1 dove]	111	3.9	258	54%	26	2	0.1
4454	Duck, battered, fried [1 leg (drumstick+thigh)]	70	2.5	156	45%	16	5	0.2

Food #	fat gm	sat fat gm	choles mg	sodium mg	potass mg	% of Daily Value														
						vit A	vit E	vit C	thia-min	ribo-flavin	nia-cin	vit B-6	fol-ate	vit B-12	cal-cium	phos-phorus	magne-sium	iron	zinc
4381	14	4	33	588	122	4	5	0	9	9	17	7	4	2	12	17	4	9	8
4382	13	4	45	399	185	2	5	1	5	6	25	12	5	4	1	15	4	5	5
4383	5	1	52	141	134	1	0	0	3	7	18	10	1	3	1	10	3	4	10
4384	4	1	50	135	136	1	0	0	3	6	26	13	1	3	1	11	3	4	8
4385	4	1	28	327	128	1	0	0	2	4	15	6	0	1	2	9	3	3	3
4386	23	6	46	36	76	4	1	0	1	4	16	3	0	2	1	7	2	5	5
4387	2	1	6	5	12	1	0	0	0	1	2	1	0	0	0	1	0	0	1
4388	14	4	80	248	165	2	3	0	7	12	25	11	4	4	2	13	4	7	12
4389	6	2	55	51	140	1	1	0	3	8	19	10	1	3	1	11	3	4	10
4390	12	3	80	277	204	4	1	0	6	12	29	14	3	4	1	16	5	8	14
4391	9	3	54	49	129	3	1	0	3	7	18	9	1	3	1	10	3	4	9
4392	6	2	49	46	124	1	0	0	3	7	17	9	1	3	1	10	3	4	9
4393	9	3	61	54	147	2	1	0	4	9	22	10	2	3	1	12	4	5	10
4394	5	1	53	49	135	1	1	0	3	8	19	10	1	3	1	10	3	4	10
4395	10	3	63	56	151	2	1	0	3	9	22	11	1	3	1	12	4	5	11
4396	5	1	54	50	136	1	1	0	3	8	19	10	1	3	1	10	3	4	10
4397	10	3	58	52	138	3	1	0	3	8	20	10	1	3	1	11	3	5	10
4398	6	2	49	46	124	1	0	0	3	7	17	9	1	3	1	10	3	4	9
4399	9	2	59	197	124	1	2	0	5	9	18	9	3	3	1	10	3	5	9
4400	5	1	53	49	135	1	1	0	3	8	19	10	1	3	1	10	3	4	10
4401	11	2	67	354	186	3	1	0	6	12	25	13	3	4	1	14	5	7	12
4402	9	2	60	318	167	3	1	0	6	10	22	12	3	3	1	12	4	6	11
4403	10	3	61	539	146	3	1	0	3	8	21	10	1	3	1	11	4	5	10
4404	5	1	43	393	108	1	0	0	2	6	15	8	1	2	1	8	3	3	8
4405	10	3	57	48	116	3	1	0	3	8	17	6	1	2	1	9	3	5	10
4406	5	1	50	41	101	1	0	0	2	7	14	6	1	2	1	8	3	4	9
4407	11	3	39	157	68	2	2	0	3	4	13	7	2	2	1	6	2	4	5
4408	2	1	18	20	46	0	0	0	1	2	8	7	0	1	0	4	1	1	3
4409	10	3	37	153	88	2	1	0	2	4	16	10	1	2	1	7	2	4	6
4410	7	2	29	29	64	2	0	0	1	3	12	7	0	2	1	5	2	2	4
4411	2	0	17	18	42	0	0	0	1	2	7	6	0	1	0	3	1	1	3
4412	7	2	26	25	57	1	1	0	1	3	11	7	1	1	0	5	2	2	4
4413	2	0	17	18	42	0	0	0	1	2	7	6	0	1	0	3	1	1	3
4414	7	2	26	25	58	1	1	0	1	2	11	7	0	2	0	5	2	2	4
4415	2	0	17	18	42	0	0	0	1	2	7	6	0	1	0	3	1	1	3
4416	7	2	29	28	63	2	0	0	1	3	11	7	0	2	1	5	2	2	4
4417	2	0	18	19	44	0	0	0	1	2	8	6	0	1	0	3	1	1	3
4418	7	2	28	27	56	2	0	0	1	2	9	4	0	1	0	5	2	3	4
4419	2	0	18	18	37	0	0	0	1	2	6	4	0	1	0	3	1	1	3
4450	56	15	401	196	750	10	3	3	14	36	90	47	2	14	4	45	14	15	30
4451	10	2	264	157	623	5	2	2	12	33	78	45	1	12	3	37	12	11	25
4452	14	4	129	63	284	3	0	5	21	23	42	32	2	8	2	37	7	36	28
4453	16	4	124	61	276	3	1	5	21	23	41	31	2	7	2	36	7	36	27
4454	8	2	74	50	186	2	3	6	16	21	19	11	5	4	1	14	3	12	11

Meat, Poultry, Fish

Food #	Food Description & Amount	wt gm	wt oz	calories	%cal fat	prot gm	carbo gm	fiber gm
4455	Duck, pressed, Chinese [2 oz, cooked]	56	2.0	107	47%	4	11	0.5
4456	**Duck, roasted,** skin eaten [½ duck]	**382**	**13.5**	**1287**	**76%**	**73**	**0**	**0.0**
4457	Duck, roasted, skin not eaten [½ duck]	221	7.8	444	50%	52	0	0.0
4458	Goose, wild, roasted [3 oz, with bone, cooked]	57	2.0	174	65%	14	0	0.0
4459	Pheasant, cooked (Include grouse) [½ pheasant breast]	127	4.5	314	44%	41	0	0.0
4460	Quail, cooked (Include partridge) [1 quail]	76	2.7	178	54%	19	0	0.0
4461	Turkey, back, roasted [1 back]	524	18.5	1273	53%	139	0	0.0
4462	Turkey, bacon, cooked [2 slices]	22	0.8	84	66%	7	1	0.0
4463	Turkey, canned [1 can (5 oz)]	125	4.4	204	38%	30	0	0.0
4464	**Turkey, dark meat, roasted,** skin eaten [1 slice (3"x2"x½")]	**56**	**2.0**	**124**	**47%**	**15**	**0**	**0.0**
4465	Turkey, dark meat, roasted, skin not eaten [1 slice (3"x2"x½")]	56	2.0	105	35%	16	0	0.0
4466	Turkey, drumstick, roasted, skin eaten [1 drumstick (14-18 lb bird)]	204	7.2	424	42%	57	0	0.0
4467	Turkey, drumstick, roasted, skin not eaten [1 drumstick (14-18 lb bird)]	188	6.6	352	35%	54	0	0.0
4468	Turkey, drumstick, smoked, salted, skin eaten [1 drumstick (14-18 lb bird)]	204	7.2	424	42%	57	0	0.0
4469	Turkey, gizzard, cooked [1 gizzard]	67	2.4	103	22%	18	1	0.0
4470	Turkey, ground, cooked [1 patty (4 oz, raw)]	60	2.1	141	50%	16	0	0.0
4471	Turkey ham roll [2 slices]	56	2.0	72	36%	11	0	0.0
4472	**Turkey, light and dark meat, roasted,** skin eaten [1 slice (3"x2"x½")]	**56**	**2.0**	**116**	**42%**	**16**	**0**	**0.0**
4473	Turkey, light and dark meat, roasted, skin not eaten [1 slice (3"x2"x½")]	56	2.0	95	26%	16	0	0.0
4474	Turkey, light meat, breaded, fried or baked with added fat, skin eaten [1 slice (3"x2"x½")]	56	2.0	124	37%	15	4	0.1
4475	Turkey, light meat, breaded, fried or baked with added fat, skin not eaten [1 slice (3"x2"x½")]	56	2.0	93	23%	16	0	0.0
4476	**Turkey, light meat, roasted,** skin eaten [1 slice (3"x2"x½")]	**56**	**2.0**	**110**	**38%**	**16**	**0**	**0.0**
4477	Turkey, light meat, roasted, skin not eaten [1 slice (3"x2"x½")]	56	2.0	88	18%	17	0	0.0
4478	Turkey, light or dark meat, battered, fried, skin eaten [1 slice (3"x2"x½")]	56	2.0	158	57%	8	9	0.3
4479	Turkey, light or dark meat, battered, fried, skin not eaten [1 slice (3"x2"x½")]	56	2.0	104	30%	16	1	0.0
4480	Turkey, light or dark meat, smoked, cooked, skin eaten [1 slice (3"x2"x½")]	56	2.0	116	42%	16	0	0.0
4481	Turkey, light or dark meat, smoked, cooked, skin not eaten [1 slice (3"x2"x½")]	56	2.0	95	26%	16	0	0.0
4482	Turkey, light or dark meat, stewed, skin eaten [1 slice (3"x2"x½")]	56	2.0	97	33%	15	0	0.0
4483	Turkey, light or dark meat, stewed, skin not eaten [1 slice (3"x2"x½")]	56	2.0	98	34%	15	0	0.0
4484	Turkey, liver, cooked [2 oz]	56	2.0	95	32%	13	2	0.0
4485	Turkey, neck, cooked [1 neck]	152	5.4	274	36%	41	0	0.0
4486	Turkey, nuggets (breaded, fried) [4 nuggets]	72	2.5	181	33%	16	13	0.4
4487	Turkey, pastrami [2 slices]	56	2.0	79	40%	10	1	0.0
4488	Turkey, roll, light or dark meat, roasted, [2 slices]	56	2.0	87	34%	12	2	0.0
4489	Turkey, salami [2 slices]	56	2.0	110	63%	9	0	0.0
4490	Turkey, tail, cooked [1 tail]	58	2.0	199	72%	13	0	0.0
4491	**Turkey, thigh, roasted,** skin eaten [1 thigh (14-18 lb bird)]	**297**	**10.5**	**618**	**42%**	**83**	**0**	**0.0**
4492	Turkey, thigh, roasted, skin not eaten [1 thigh (14-18 lb bird)]	274	9.7	512	35%	78	0	0.0
4493	Turkey, wing, roasted, skin eaten [1 wing]	174	6.1	398	49%	48	0	0.0
4494	Turkey, wing, roasted, skin not eaten [1 wing]	146	5.1	238	19%	45	0	0.0
4495	Turkey, wing, smoked, salted, skin eaten [1 wing]	174	6.1	398	49%	48	0	0.0
	Other Meats & Sausages (weight columns are for cooked, boneless part)							
4550	Armadillo, cooked [2 oz, boneless, cooked]	56	2.0	90	25%	16	0	0.0
4551	Bear, cooked [2 oz, boneless, cooked]	56	2.0	145	47%	18	0	0.0
4552	Beaver, cooked [2 oz, boneless, cooked]	56	2.0	119	30%	20	0	0.0
4553	Bison, cooked [1 cup]	134	4.7	192	15%	38	0	0.0
4554	Caribou, cooked [2 oz, boneless, cooked]	56	2.0	94	24%	17	0	0.0
4555	Frog legs, battered, fried [2 oz, boneless, cooked]	56	2.0	144	42%	10	11	0.4
4556	Frog legs, steamed [2 oz, boneless, cooked]	56	2.0	59	4%	13	0	0.0

Food #	fat gm	sat fat gm	choles mg	sodium mg	potass mg	vit A	vit E	vit C	thia-min	ribo-flavin	nia-cin	vit B-6	fol-ate	vit B-12	cal-cium	phos-phorus	magne-sium	iron	zinc
														% of Daily Value					
4455	6	2	18	51	104	2	2	5	5	5	6	3	2	1	1	4	2	5	3
4456	108	37	321	225	779	24	9	0	44	60	92	34	6	19	4	60	15	57	47
4457	25	9	197	144	557	5	5	0	38	61	56	28	6	15	3	45	11	33	38
4458	12	4	52	40	188	1	3	0	3	11	12	11	0	4	1	15	3	9	10
4459	15	4	113	55	344	7	1	5	6	13	48	48	2	15	2	31	7	10	12
4460	11	3	65	40	164	5	2	3	11	13	30	24	1	5	1	21	4	19	16
4461	75	22	477	383	1362	0	10	0	19	69	90	79	10	30	17	99	29	64	137
4462	6	2	22	503	87	0	0	0	1	3	4	4	0	1	0	10	2	3	4
4463	9	3	83	584	280	0	1	4	1	13	41	21	2	6	2	20	6	13	20
4464	6	2	50	43	153	0	1	0	2	8	10	9	1	3	2	11	3	7	16
4465	4	1	48	44	162	0	1	0	2	8	10	10	1	3	2	11	3	7	17
4466	20	6	173	157	571	0	4	0	8	29	36	34	5	12	7	41	12	26	58
4467	14	5	160	149	545	0	4	0	8	27	34	34	4	12	6	38	11	24	56
4468	20	6	173	2032	571	0	4	0	8	29	36	34	5	12	7	41	12	26	58
4469	2	1	130	45	120	4	3	2	1	10	13	4	9	22	1	10	3	15	20
4470	8	2	61	64	162	0	1	0	2	6	14	12	1	3	2	12	4	6	11
4471	3	1	31	558	182	0	1	0	2	8	10	7	1	2	1	11	2	9	11
4472	5	2	46	38	157	0	1	0	2	6	14	11	1	3	1	11	4	6	11
4473	3	1	43	39	167	0	1	0	2	6	15	13	1	3	1	12	4	6	12
4474	5	1	38	165	152	1	1	0	3	5	17	12	1	3	1	11	4	5	7
4475	2	1	38	35	168	0	0	0	2	4	19	15	1	3	1	12	4	4	8
4476	5	1	43	35	160	0	0	0	2	4	18	13	1	3	1	12	4	4	8
4477	2	1	39	36	171	0	0	0	2	4	19	15	1	3	1	12	4	4	8
4478	10	3	35	448	154	1	4	0	4	6	6	6	4	2	1	15	2	7	5
4479	3	1	41	38	162	0	1	0	3	6	15	12	1	3	1	12	4	6	11
4480	5	2	46	558	157	0	1	0	2	6	14	11	1	3	1	11	4	6	11
4481	3	1	43	558	167	0	1	0	2	6	15	13	1	3	1	12	4	6	12
4482	4	1	48	34	108	0	1	0	2	6	9	8	1	2	1	9	3	6	11
4483	4	1	47	34	114	0	1	0	2	7	10	8	1	3	1	10	3	5	11
4484	3	1	351	36	109	209	5	2	2	47	17	15	93	443	1	15	2	24	12
4485	11	4	185	85	226	0	3	0	4	17	13	16	3	6	6	19	6	19	72
4486	7	2	40	499	184	3	2	1	7	9	17	14	3	3	2	13	4	8	11
4487	3	1	30	585	146	0	0	0	2	8	10	8	1	2	1	11	2	5	8
4488	3	1	30	381	167	0	1	0	2	5	18	8	1	14	0	14	3	5	9
4489	8	2	46	562	137	0	1	0	2	6	10	7	1	2	1	6	2	5	7
4490	16	5	54	36	128	0	2	0	2	6	8	7	1	3	2	9	3	6	13
4491	29	9	252	229	832	0	6	0	12	42	53	49	7	18	10	59	17	38	85
4492	20	7	233	216	795	0	6	0	12	40	50	49	6	17	9	56	16	35	81
4493	22	6	141	106	463	0	1	0	6	14	50	37	3	10	4	34	11	14	24
4494	5	2	149	114	298	0	0	0	3	14	30	43	3	10	4	25	8	14	37
4495	22	6	141	1733	463	0	1	0	6	13	50	37	3	10	4	34	11	14	24
4550	2	1	43	34	222	0	0	0	12	5	12	12	1	7	1	8	4	3	11
4551	7	2	55	40	147	0	0	0	4	27	9	8	1	23	0	10	3	33	38
4552	4	1	66	33	226	0	1	3	2	10	6	13	2	77	1	16	4	31	8
4553	3	1	110	76	484	0	1	0	9	21	25	27	3	64	1	28	9	25	33
4554	2	1	61	34	174	0	0	3	9	30	16	9	1	62	1	13	4	19	20
4555	7	2	74	159	162	3	4	3	9	12	7	4	5	4	5	10	4	9	5
4556	0	0	41	47	208	1	3	0	7	11	4	4	2	5	1	9	4	6	5

Meat, Poultry, Fish

Food #	Food Description & Amount	wt gm	wt oz	calo-ries	%cal fat	prot gm	carbo gm	fiber gm
4557	Goat, head, cooked [2 oz, boneless, cooked]	56	2.0	80	34%	12	0	0.0
4558	Goat, liver, fried or broiled, no coating [2 oz, cooked]	56	2.0	133	48%	14	2	0.0
4559	Goat, ribs, cooked [1 rib]	46	1.6	66	19%	12	0	0.0
4560	Goat, baked or boiled [2 oz, boneless, cooked]	56	2.0	80	19%	15	0	0.0
4561	Goat, fried [2 oz, boneless, cooked]	56	2.0	87	27%	15	0	0.0
4562	Ground hog, cooked [3 oz, with bone, cooked]	69	2.4	174	53%	19	0	0.0
4563	Mock chicken leg (veal, pork, flour, egg), cooked (Include city chicken, pork and veal on a stick) [2 oz, cooked]	56	2.0	131	53%	12	3	0.1
4564	Moose, cooked [2 oz, boneless, cooked]	56	2.0	75	7%	16	0	0.0
4565	Opossum, cooked [3 oz, with bone, cooked]	69	2.4	152	42%	21	0	0.0
4566	**Rabbit, stewed [1 piece]**	**105**	**3.7**	**216**	**37%**	**32**	**0**	**0.0**
4567	Rabbit, domestic, breaded, fried [2 oz, boneless, cooked]	56	2.0	137	42%	16	3	0.1
4568	Rabbit, wild, cooked [3 oz, with bone, cooked]	69	2.4	119	18%	23	0	0.0
4569	Raccoon, cooked [2 oz, boneless, cooked]	56	2.0	143	51%	16	0	0.0
4570	Snails, steamed or poached [5 snails]	25	0.9	69	3%	12	4	0.0
4571	Squirrel, cooked [3 oz, with bone, cooked]	69	2.4	119	24%	21	0	0.0
4572	Turtle (terrapin) steamed or poached [1 cup, cooked]	140	4.9	158	5%	35	0	0.0
4573	Udder, cooked (Include milk ducts) [1 cup, pieces]	140	4.9	144	36%	21	0	0.0
4574	**Venison chop, fried (Include deer, antelope, caribou) [1 chop]**	**89**	**3.1**	**186**	**41%**	**26**	**0**	**0.0**
4575	Venison, jerky [2 strips (4" long)]	28	1.0	96	41%	10	4	0.0
4576	Venison, ribs, fried [3 oz, with bone, cooked]	69	2.4	118	18%	23	0	0.0
4577	Venison, roasted [2 oz, boneless]	56	2.0	96	18%	18	0	0.0
4578	Venison, sausage or bologna [2 oz]	56	2.0	175	82%	7	0	0.0
4579	Venison, steak, battered, fried [1 steak]	101	3.6	210	33%	22	11	0.4
4580	Venison, steak, fried (Include cured or ground venison) [2 oz, boneless, cooked]	56	2.0	97	19%	18	0	0.0
4581	Venison, stewed [2 oz, boneless, cooked]	56	2.0	96	18%	18	0	0.0
4582	Wild pig, smoked [2 oz, boneless]	56	2.0	90	25%	16	0	0.0
4583	Beef, pressed, luncheon meat (including smoked) [2 slices]	56	2.0	99	20%	16	3	0.0
4584	Bockwurst [1 sausage (7 per lb)]	65	2.3	184	72%	12	0	0.0
4585	Bologna ring (pork and beef), smoked (including Alderfers) [2 slices]	56	2.0	177	80%	7	2	0.0
4586	**Bologna, beef (Include veal bologna) [2 slices]**	**56**	**2.0**	**175**	**82%**	**7**	**0**	**0.0**
4587	Bologna, beef, lowfat [2 slices]	56	2.0	129	74%	7	2	0.0
4588	Bologna, beef and pork [2 slices]	56	2.0	172	81%	7	1	0.0
4589	Bologna, beef and pork, lowfat [2 slices]	56	2.0	129	76%	6	1	0.0
4590	Bologna, beef, chicken, and pork [2 slices]	56	2.0	155	78%	7	1	0.0
4591	Bologna, Lebanon [2 slices]	56	2.0	119	56%	11	2	0.0
4592	**Bologna, pork [2 slices]**	**56**	**2.0**	**138**	**72%**	**9**	**0**	**0.0**
4593	Bologna, turkey (Include chicken bologna) [2 slices]	56	2.0	111	69%	8	1	0.0
4594	Bologna, with cheese [2 slices]	56	2.0	178	79%	7	2	0.0
4595	Brains and scrambled eggs, cooked [1 cup]	243	8.6	355	74%	17	6	1.0
4596	Brains, cooked [1 cup]	140	4.9	226	66%	18	0	0.0
4597	Bratwurst, [1 stick]	85	3.0	256	77%	12	2	0.0
4598	Bratwurst, with cheese [1 stick]	85	3.0	260	76%	13	2	0.0
4599	Capicola [2 slices (4¼"x4¼"x1/16")]	42	1.5	55	34%	8	0	0.0
4600	Cervalat, soft [2 slices (4-1/8"dia x 1/8")]	46	1.6	154	79%	7	0	0.0
4601	Chicken or turkey loaf or roll, luncheon meat (including pressed, smoked) [2 slices]	56	2.0	85	43%	11	1	0.0
4602	Chicken salad spread [1 can (7.5 oz)]	213	7.5	426	61%	25	16	0.0
4603	Chitterlings, cooked [1 cup]	125	4.4	379	85%	13	0	0.0
4604	Chorizos (Include Spanish sausage, lenguica, Portuguese sausage) [1 link (4" long)]	60	2.1	273	76%	14	1	0.0
4605	Corned beef spread [1 can (5.5 oz)]	156	5.5	390	54%	42	0	0.0

Food #	fat gm	sat fat gm	choles mg	sodium mg	potass mg	% of Daily Value													
						vit A	vit E	vit C	thia-min	ribo-flavin	nia-cin	vit B-6	fol-ate	vit B-12	cal-cium	phos-phorus	magne-sium	iron	zinc
4557	3	1	406	57	190	0	1	4	4	16	10	1	1	36	1	14	1	10	15
4558	7	3	276	69	197	437	1	12	13	151	47	27	56	800	1	24	3	32	21
4559	1	0	35	40	186	0	0	0	3	17	9	0	1	9	1	9	0	10	16
4560	2	1	42	48	227	0	0	0	3	20	11	0	1	11	1	11	0	12	20
4561	3	1	41	47	223	0	1	0	3	20	11	0	1	11	1	11	0	11	19
4562	10	4	59	39	250	0	1	0	39	13	17	14	1	9	2	16	4	4	12
4563	8	2	49	40	160	0	2	0	10	10	14	8	2	10	1	11	3	3	13
4564	1	0	44	39	187	0	0	5	2	11	15	10	1	59	0	10	3	13	14
4565	7	1	89	40	302	0	2	0	5	15	29	16	2	95	1	19	6	18	10
4566	9	3	90	39	315	0	3	0	4	11	38	18	2	114	2	24	5	14	17
4567	6	2	48	58	163	0	3	0	4	5	18	9	2	53	2	12	3	10	8
4568	2	1	85	31	237	0	2	0	1	3	22	12	1	75	1	17	5	19	11
4569	8	2	54	44	223	0	1	0	22	17	13	13	2	77	1	15	4	22	8
4570	0	0	33	88	121	1	0	3	1	2	2	7	1	45	3	5	9	13	5
4571	3	1	83	82	243	0	2	0	3	12	16	13	2	75	0	15	5	26	8
4572	1	0	89	108	326	5	3	0	12	13	8	9	5	24	21	26	8	13	12
4573	6	3	140	68	398	0	0	7	1	14	0	2	1	28	1	12	3	16	24
4574	8	2	96	49	305	0	3	0	12	29	29	13	1	95	1	21	6	20	16
4575	4	2	38	820	106	0	0	0	3	11	10	4	0	30	0	7	2	8	6
4576	2	1	83	43	250	0	1	0	8	26	23	9	1	72	0	17	5	19	14
4577	2	1	68	35	203	0	1	0	6	21	19	7	1	59	0	14	4	15	11
4578	16	7	32	549	88	0	0	0	2	4	7	4	1	13	1	5	2	5	8
4579	8	2	103	181	274	1	4	0	15	27	27	11	4	73	4	19	6	21	14
4580	2	1	68	34	202	0	1	0	6	21	19	7	1	59	0	14	4	15	11
4581	2	1	68	22	139	0	1	0	5	19	14	5	1	50	0	10	3	15	11
4582	2	1	43	34	222	0	0	0	12	5	12	12	1	7	1	8	4	3	11
4583	2	1	23	806	240	0	0	0	3	6	15	10	2	24	1	9	3	8	15
4584	15	5	43	728	202	0	0	0	16	7	14	6	0	8	1	10	3	2	7
4585	16	6	31	571	101	0	0	0	6	5	7	5	1	12	1	5	2	5	7
4586	16	7	32	549	88	0	0	0	2	4	7	4	1	13	1	5	2	5	8
4587	11	4	21	632	82	0	0	1	2	3	7	4	1	13	1	10	2	3	7
4588	16	6	32	566	111	0	1	0	13	5	8	5	0	11	1	5	2	3	6
4589	11	4	22	620	87	0	0	0	6	4	7	5	1	12	1	10	2	2	6
4590	13	5	39	545	104	0	1	0	5	5	8	5	1	9	2	6	2	5	7
4591	7	3	39	749	168	0	0	0	2	6	12	7	0	24	1	8	2	8	15
4592	11	4	33	663	157	0	0	0	20	5	11	8	1	9	1	8	2	2	8
4593	9	3	55	492	111	0	1	0	2	5	10	6	1	3	5	7	2	5	6
4594	16	6	32	582	105	1	0	0	6	5	7	5	1	12	4	7	2	4	8
4595	29	6	2351	280	511	20	16	30	10	24	14	18	7	151	4	47	7	19	12
4596	17	4	3001	83	259	0	7	37	12	16	18	11	1	196	1	32	4	13	13
4597	22	8	51	473	180	0	1	1	29	9	14	9	0	13	4	13	3	6	13
4598	22	9	52	547	186	3	1	1	25	11	12	9	1	14	10	17	4	6	14
4599	2	1	20	600	147	0	0	0	26	6	10	10	0	5	0	9	2	2	5
4600	14	6	35	571	125	0	0	0	5	9	10	6	0	42	1	5	2	6	8
4601	4	1	28	310	140	0	0	0	3	7	16	7	1	2	2	9	2	4	5
4602	29	7	64	803	390	9	16	4	3	9	18	12	3	13	2	7	5	7	15
4603	36	13	179	49	10	0	1	0	0	6	1	1	1	21	3	6	3	26	42
4604	23	9	53	741	239	0	0	0	25	11	15	16	0	20	0	9	3	5	14
4605	23	10	134	1569	212	0	1	0	2	13	19	10	4	42	2	17	5	18	37

Meat, Poultry, Fish

Food #	Food Description & Amount	wt gm	wt oz	calories	%cal fat	prot gm	carbo gm	fiber gm
4606	Corned beef, pressed [2 slices]	56	2.0	140	54%	15	0	0.0
4607	Giblets, excluding liver, cooked [2 giblets]	46	1.6	70	22%	12	1	0.0
4608	Ham and cheese loaf [2 slices]	56	2.0	145	70%	9	1	0.0
4609	Ham loaf, luncheon meat (Include ham sausage, hamettes) [2 slices (4¼"x4¼"x1/16")]	42	1.5	140	82%	5	1	0.0
4610	Ham salad spread [1 can (7.5 oz)]	213	7.5	460	65%	18	23	0.0
4611	**Ham, deviled** or potted [1 can (3 oz)]	**85**	**3.0**	**284**	**82%**	**11**	**2**	**0.0**
4612	Head cheese (Include jellied pork) [2 slices (4"x4"x3/32")]	56	2.0	119	67%	9	0	0.0
4613	Heart (all animals), boiled, simmered, or braised [2 oz, cooked]	56	2.0	98	29%	16	0	0.0
4614	Heart (all animals), fried [2 oz, cooked]	56	2.0	139	44%	14	5	0.2
4615	Hog lights, cooked (Include hog lungs, pork lungs, pig lungs) [1 cup]	140	4.9	139	28%	23	0	0.0
4616	Hog maws, cooked (Include hog stomach, pork stomach, pig stomach) [1 cup]	140	4.9	349	55%	37	0	0.0
4617	Honey loaf, beef and pork [2 slices]	56	2.0	72	31%	9	3	0.0
4618	Kidney (all animals), braised, broiled, or simmered [1 kidney, cooked, beef]	227	8.0	327	22%	58	2	0.0
4619	Kidney (all animals), breaded or floured, fried [1 kidney, cooked, beef]	414	14.6	1127	38%	126	42	1.2
4620	Knockwurst (Include Knoblauch) [1 link (4"x1")]	68	2.4	209	81%	8	1	0.0
4621	Liver, raw (all types) [2 oz]	56	2.0	77	25%	11	3	0.0
4622	**Liverwurst** (Include liver cheese, Braunschweiger, liver sausage, liver loaf, liver pudding, liver bacon, goose bacon, goose liver sausage) [1 slice (3"dia x ½")]	**56**	**2.0**	**201**	**80%**	**8**	**2**	**0.0**
4623	Luncheon loaf (olive, pickle, or pimiento) [2 slices (1 oz) (4"x4"x3/32")]	56	2.0	139	68%	7	4	0.0
4624	Luncheon meat (Include tavern loaf, breakfast loaf, macaroni loaf, luxury loaf) [2 slices (4¼"x4¼"x1/16")]	42	1.5	148	82%	5	1	0.0
4625	Luncheon meat, ham and chicken, chopped, minced, pressed, spiced, canned [1 slice (½" thick)]	57	2.0	117	63%	9	1	0.0
4626	Luncheon meat, turkey ham, sliced, extra lean, prepackaged or deli [1 slice (4"x4"x1/8")]	42	1.5	50	29%	8	1	0.0
4627	Luncheon meat, turkey or chicken breast (including pressed, smoked) [2 slices]	56	2.0	62	13%	13	0	0.0
4628	Meat spread or potted meat [1 can (5.5 oz)]	156	5.5	521	82%	20	3	0.0
4629	Mettwurst [2 oz]	56	2.0	174	79%	7	1	0.0
4630	Mortadella [4 slices (15 per 8 oz pkg)]	60	2.1	187	73%	10	2	0.0
4631	Pepperoni [10 slices (1¼"dia x 1/8")]	60	2.1	298	80%	13	2	0.0
4632	Roast beef spread [1 can (5.5 oz)]	156	5.5	367	66%	12	19	0.3
4633	Salami, beef (Include kosher salami) [2 slices (4"dia x 1/8") (10 per 8 oz pkg)]	46	1.6	121	71%	7	1	0.0
4634	**Salami, dry** or hard (Include Italian salami, Goteborg) [2 slices (1¾"dia x 1/8")]	**40**	**1.4**	**167**	**74%**	**9**	**1**	**0.0**
4635	Salami, soft, cooked (Include cotto salami, beer bologna, beer sausage, beerwurst) [2 slices (4"dia x 1/8")]	46	1.6	115	72%	6	1	0.0
4636	Sandwich loaf, luncheon meat (Include old fashioned loaf, Dutch loaf, pepper loaf, praski) [2 slices]	56	2.0	109	56%	9	3	0.0
4637	Sausage, beef [1 patty (raw dimensions: 4"dia x ¼")]	27	1.0	85	81%	3	0	0.0
4638	Sausage, beef, brown and serve, links, cooked [2 links (2 oz, raw)]	26	0.9	85	81%	3	0	0.0
4639	Sausage, beef, fresh, bulk, patty or link, cooked [2 links]	26	0.9	87	71%	6	0	0.0
4640	Sausage, beef, smoked (Include Eckrich, Hillshire Farms) [2 links (2"x¾")]	32	1.1	100	81%	4	1	0.0
4641	Sausage, beef, smoked, stick (Include beef jerky) [2 sticks]	20	0.7	108	82%	4	1	0.0
4642	Sausage, beef, with cheese, smoked (Include Hillshire Farms) [1 link]	86	3.0	275	81%	11	1	0.0
4643	Sausage, blood (Include blutwurst, blood pudding) [4 slices (2¼"dia x 1/8")]	32	1.1	121	82%	5	0	0.0
4644	Sausage, chicken and beef, smoked [1 sausage (5"x¾")]	57	2.0	169	73%	11	0	0.0
4645	Sausage, Italian (Include hot links) [1 link (5" long)]	68	2.4	220	72%	14	1	0.0
4646	Sausage, pickled (Include Penrose hot or firecracker sausage) [2 sausages]	28	1.0	81	72%	4	1	0.0
4647	Sausage, Polish [1 sausage (10"x1¼")]	227	8.0	704	79%	30	5	0.0
4648	Sausage, pork and beef (Include brown and serve sausage) [1 patty, cooked]	27	1.0	107	82%	4	1	0.0
4649	**Sausage, pork**, fresh, bulk, patty or link, cooked (Include brown and serve sausage, country style sausage, breakfast sausage) [1 patty (raw dimensions: 4"dia x ¼")]	**27**	**1.0**	**100**	**76%**	**5**	**0**	**0.0**

Food #	fat gm	sat fat gm	choles mg	sodium mg	potass mg	vit A	vit E	vit C	thia-min	ribo-flavin	nia-cin	vit B-6	fol-ate	vit B-12	cal-cium	phos-phorus	magne-sium	iron	zinc
						% of Daily Value													
4606	8	3	48	563	76	0	0	0	1	5	7	4	1	15	1	6	2	6	13
4607	2	0	89	31	82	3	2	1	1	7	9	3	6	15	0	7	2	11	13
4608	11	4	32	752	165	1	1	0	22	6	10	7	0	8	3	14	2	3	7
4609	13	5	26	541	90	0	0	1	10	5	7	4	1	6	0	3	1	2	4
4610	33	11	79	1943	320	0	12	0	62	15	22	16	1	27	2	26	5	7	16
4611	26	9	53	1096	183	0	1	1	21	10	13	9	1	13	1	7	2	3	8
4612	9	3	45	704	17	0	0	0	1	6	3	5	0	10	1	3	1	4	5
4613	3	1	108	35	130	0	1	1	5	51	11	6	0	133	0	14	4	23	12
4614	7	1	88	29	113	0	4	1	7	43	11	5	2	109	0	12	3	21	10
4615	4	2	542	113	211	0	1	18	7	27	10	6	1	47	1	26	4	128	23
4616	21	8	429	52	201	0	2	0	8	8	22	2	1	22	2	24	3	16	27
4617	3	1	19	739	192	0	0	0	18	8	9	9	1	10	1	8	2	4	9
4618	8	2	878	304	406	85	1	3	29	542	68	59	56	1941	4	69	10	92	64
4619	47	12	2761	1569	1861	52	14	51	132	774	227	86	42	2852	19	172	31	151	104
4620	19	7	39	687	135	0	1	0	16	6	9	6	0	13	1	7	2	3	8
4621	2	1	211	42	167	523	2	24	8	84	33	25	53	529	0	17	3	23	14
4622	18	6	87	640	111	236	1	0	9	50	23	9	6	188	1	9	2	29	10
4623	11	4	21	804	178	1	0	0	11	8	5	6	0	11	6	7	3	2	5
4624	14	5	23	543	85	0	0	0	9	4	6	4	1	9	0	4	1	2	5
4625	8	3	43	539	352	0	0	30	7	7	10	8	1	6	0	6	2	4	7
4626	2	1	28	436	126	0	1	0	1	6	7	5	1	2	0	13	2	3	7
4627	1	0	23	801	156	0	0	0	1	4	23	10	1	19	0	13	3	1	4
4628	47	17	97	2011	335	0	1	3	38	18	24	16	2	23	1	13	4	6	15
4629	15	6	38	603	152	0	0	0	9	7	8	5	1	15	2	8	2	5	8
4630	15	6	34	748	98	0	0	0	5	5	8	4	0	15	1	6	2	5	8
4631	26	10	47	1224	208	0	0	0	13	9	15	8	1	25	1	7	2	5	10
4632	27	9	59	1580	172	1	9	0	18	12	13	9	1	29	2	9	3	7	11
4633	10	4	30	541	103	0	0	0	3	5	7	4	0	23	0	5	2	6	7
4634	14	5	32	744	151	0	0	0	16	7	10	10	0	13	0	6	2	3	9
4635	9	4	30	490	91	0	0	0	7	10	8	5	0	28	1	5	2	7	7
4636	7	2	26	776	216	0	0	0	13	9	8	7	0	15	4	9	3	4	9
4637	8	3	16	275	45	0	0	0	1	2	3	2	0	7	0	2	0	2	4
4638	8	3	17	270	44	0	0	0	1	2	3	1	0	6	1	2	0	2	4
4639	7	3	20	247	79	0	0	0	1	3	4	3	0	12	0	4	1	3	9
4640	9	4	19	326	53	0	0	0	1	2	4	2	0	8	1	3	0	3	5
4641	10	4	20	338	57	0	0	0	2	2	6	3	0	11	0	3	1	3	5
4642	25	11	54	900	139	2	1	0	3	7	9	6	1	20	7	13	2	7	13
4643	11	4	38	218	12	0	0	0	2	2	2	1	0	5	0	1	1	11	3
4644	14	4	40	581	79	2	1	0	2	4	12	5	1	4	1	6	2	3	7
4645	17	6	53	627	207	0	1	2	28	9	14	11	1	15	2	12	3	6	11
4646	6	3	21	444	64	0	0	0	5	7	6	3	0	20	0	4	1	5	5
4647	62	22	152	2443	615	0	2	0	35	29	33	20	3	61	10	34	9	18	31
4648	10	3	19	217	51	0	0	0	6	2	5	1	0	2	0	3	1	2	3
4649	8	3	22	349	97	0	0	1	13	4	6	4	0	8	1	5	1	2	5

Meat, Poultry, Fish

Food #	Food Description & Amount	wt gm	wt oz	calo-ries	%cal fat	prot gm	carbo gm	fiber gm
4650	Sausage, pork with rice links, brown and serve, cooked (Include Jones Dairy Farm Light Links) [2 links, cooked]	50	1.8	120	71%	7	1	0.0
4651	Sausage, smoked link, pork and beef [1 link (4"long x 1"dia)]	68	2.4	228	81%	9	1	0.0
4652	Sausage, smoked, pork [1 link (4"x1")]	68	2.4	265	73%	15	1	0.0
4653	Sausage, turkey breakfast, bulk [1 patty]	42	1.5	86	42%	12	0	0.0
4654	Sausage, turkey, smoked (Include chicken sausage) [2 slices]	56	2.0	111	69%	8	1	0.0
4655	Sausage, turkey and pork, fresh, bulk, patty or link, cooked [2 oz, cooked]	56	2.0	172	67%	13	0	0.0
4656	Sausage, turkey, pork, and beef, reduced fat, smoked [1 sausage (2"x1½")]	39	1.4	94	63%	7	1	0.0
4657	**Sausage, Vienna**, canned [2 sausages (2"x¾")]	**32**	**1.1**	**89**	**81%**	**3**	**1**	**0.0**
4658	Sausage, Vienna, chicken, canned [2 sausages]	32	1.1	82	68%	4	2	0.0
4659	Scrapple, cooked [2 slices (2¾"x2"x¼")]	50	1.8	114	57%	5	8	0.4
4660	Souse [2 slices (4"square x 1/8")]	56	2.0	97	67%	7	0	0.0
4661	Sweetbreads (thymus), cooked [2 oz, cooked]	56	2.0	97	22%	18	0	0.0
4662	Thuringer (Include summer sausage) [2 slices (4¼"dia x 1/8") (10 per 8 oz pkg)]	46	1.6	154	79%	7	0	0.0
4663	Tongue (all animals), braised [2 oz, cooked]	56	2.0	158	66%	12	0	0.0
4664	Tongue (all animals), deviled [½ cup]	113	4.0	326	71%	21	1	0.0
4665	Tongue, pot roast, Puerto Rican style (Include Lengua al caldero) [1 slice (5"x2"x1")]	110	3.9	352	66%	27	1	0.1
4666	Tongue, smoked, cured, or pickled, cooked [2 slices (3"x2"x1/8")]	40	1.4	110	66%	9	0	0.0
4667	Tripe, battered, fried [4 pieces (1 cubic inch, raw)]	44	1.6	71	49%	6	3	0.1
4668	Tripe, cooked [2 oz, cooked]	56	2.0	58	36%	9	0	0.0
	Fish & Shellfish (weight columns are for cooked, edible part)							
4750	Anchovy, canned [1 can (2 oz) drained]	45	1.6	95	42%	13	0	0.0
4751	Barracuda, baked or broiled (or sauteed or fried with no coating) [2 oz, boneless, cooked]	56	2.0	119	52%	13	0	0.0
4752	Barracuda, floured or breaded, fried [2 oz, boneless, cooked]	56	2.0	139	53%	13	2	0.1
4753	Barracuda, steamed or poached [2 oz, boneless, cooked]	56	2.0	112	45%	14	0	0.0
4754	**Carp**, baked or broiled (or sauteed or fried with no coating) (Include **bream, buffalo fish, chub, sucker**) [2 oz, boneless, cooked]	**56**	**2.0**	**115**	**52%**	**13**	**0**	**0.0**
4755	Carp, floured or breaded, fried [2 oz, boneless, cooked]	56	2.0	157	51%	12	7	0.2
4756	Carp, smoked [2 oz]	56	2.0	111	40%	16	0	0.0
4757	Carp, steamed or poached [2 oz, boneless, cooked]	56	2.0	90	40%	13	0	0.0
4758	**Catfish**, battered, fried (Include **bullhead**) [1 filet]	**81**	**2.9**	**236**	**66%**	**12**	**8**	**0.3**
4759	Catfish, breaded or battered, baked [2 oz, boneless, cooked]	56	2.0	171	58%	10	7	0.2
4760	Catfish, broiled or baked (or sauteed or fried with no coating) [1 medium catfish]	272	9.6	591	60%	55	2	0.1
4761	Catfish, floured or breaded, fried [1 medium]	332	11.7	968	56%	62	42	1.4
4762	Catfish, steamed or poached [2 oz, boneless, cooked]	56	2.0	95	51%	11	0	0.0
4763	**Cod**, battered, fried [2 oz, boneless, cooked]	**56**	**2.0**	**97**	**41%**	**10**	**4**	**0.1**
4764	Cod, breaded or battered, baked with added margarine[1 filet]	56	2.0	112	41%	11	5	0.2
4765	Cod, broiled or baked (or sauteed or fried with no coating) [2 oz, boneless, cooked]	56	2.0	69	27%	12	0	0.0
4766	Cod, dried, salted [1 piece (5½"x1½"x½")]	80	2.8	232	7%	50	0	0.0
4767	Cod, dried, salted, salt removed in water [2 oz, dried, soaked in water]	68	2.4	56	7%	12	0	0.0
4768	Cod, floured or breaded, fried [1 filet]	87	3.1	185	46%	17	7	0.2
4769	Cod, smoked [2 oz, boneless]	56	2.0	46	7%	10	0	0.0
4770	Cod, steamed or poached [2 oz, boneless, cooked]	56	2.0	57	7%	13	0	0.0
4771	**Croaker**, baked or broiled (or sauteed or fried with no coating) (Include **angelfish, butterfly fish, drumfish, goatfish, kingfish, sea trout, freshwater sheepshead, spadefish, spot, surgeonfish, weakfish, weke**) [1 filet]	**62**	**2.2**	**120**	**47%**	**15**	**0**	**0.0**
4772	Croaker, breaded or battered, baked with added margarine [1 filet]	81	2.9	179	47%	16	7	0.2
4773	Croaker, floured or breaded, fried [2 oz, boneless, cooked]	56	2.0	160	48%	12	8	0.3
4774	Croaker, steamed or poached [2 oz, boneless, cooked]	56	2.0	74	27%	13	0	0.0

Food #	fat gm	sat fat gm	choles mg	sodium mg	potass mg	% of Daily Value													
						vit A	vit E	vit C	thia-min	ribo-flavin	nia-cin	vit B-6	fol-ate	vit B-12	cal-cium	phos-phorus	magne-sium	iron	zinc
4650	9	3	35	325	105	0	0	1	21	5	7	5	1	11	1	5	2	3	6
4651	21	7	48	643	129	0	0	0	12	7	11	6	0	17	1	7	2	5	10
4652	22	8	46	1020	228	0	1	2	32	10	15	12	1	18	2	11	3	4	13
4653	4	1	34	289	116	0	0	0	2	4	11	8	1	2	1	8	3	4	8
4654	9	3	55	492	111	0	1	0	2	5	10	6	1	3	5	7	2	5	6
4655	13	4	47	492	189	0	1	1	19	8	12	10	1	12	2	11	3	5	12
4656	7	2	25	373	80	0	0	0	5	3	6	5	0	3	1	6	2	2	6
4657	8	3	17	305	32	0	0	0	2	2	3	2	0	5	0	2	1	2	3
4658	6	2	32	438	27	1	0	0	1	2	5	5	0	1	3	3	1	4	2
4659	7	3	23	382	122	0	0	0	4	2	4	2	0	2	0	3	1	2	5
4660	7	2	37	578	14	0	0	0	1	5	3	4	0	8	1	3	1	3	4
4661	2	1	263	37	192	0	1	69	2	5	6	3	0	20	0	38	2	6	12
4662	14	6	35	571	125	0	0	0	5	9	10	6	0	42	1	5	2	6	8
4663	12	5	60	34	101	0	1	0	1	12	6	4	1	55	0	8	2	11	18
4664	26	11	124	1609	185	0	1	0	3	7	7	8	1	94	2	13	4	17	28
4665	26	11	130	77	226	0	2	1	2	25	12	6	1	89	2	17	6	24	39
4666	8	3	42	416	70	0	0	0	1	8	4	3	0	38	0	6	2	7	12
4667	4	1	36	48	91	0	1	2	2	5	1	1	1	8	1	5	1	5	6
4668	2	1	56	27	159	0	0	3	0	6	0	1	0	11	1	5	1	6	10
4750	4	1	38	1651	245	1	8	0	2	10	45	5	1	7	10	11	8	12	7
4751	7	2	31	76	271	2	3	3	5	16	27	10	0	41	2	8	5	4	3
4752	8	2	29	213	256	1	3	2	6	16	27	9	1	39	1	8	5	5	3
4753	6	2	33	55	245	1	2	2	4	16	25	9	0	44	2	8	4	5	3
4754	7	1	47	66	244	3	3	4	5	2	6	6	3	16	3	30	5	5	7
4755	9	2	55	115	212	1	4	1	7	5	7	5	4	13	5	25	5	7	7
4756	5	1	58	382	291	1	2	2	6	3	7	7	3	19	4	36	6	6	9
4757	4	1	47	31	201	1	1	1	4	2	5	5	2	15	3	26	5	5	7
4758	17	4	49	66	224	1	8	1	17	7	10	6	4	21	3	16	5	5	4
4759	11	2	44	186	193	8	5	0	15	6	9	5	3	17	3	13	4	5	4
4760	39	9	164	336	1072	17	20	15	80	16	40	30	8	122	4	71	20	10	17
4761	60	13	267	705	1150	10	28	3	90	36	55	32	20	105	18	80	26	31	23
4762	5	1	33	33	178	1	3	1	13	3	7	5	1	24	1	13	4	2	3
4763	4	1	28	51	215	0	2	2	3	3	6	9	2	7	2	10	3	2	2
4764	5	1	33	147	241	5	3	2	4	4	7	10	2	8	2	11	4	3	2
4765	2	0	24	66	269	2	1	4	1	2	6	12	1	9	1	12	4	1	2
4766	2	0	122	5622	1166	3	2	5	14	11	30	35	5	133	13	76	27	11	8
4767	0	0	29	1227	240	1	0	1	3	2	6	7	1	27	3	17	6	3	2
4768	9	2	50	151	364	2	4	3	5	6	12	16	3	12	3	17	6	5	3
4769	0	0	24	30	231	1	0	1	3	2	5	6	1	8	1	11	4	1	2
4770	0	0	26	45	240	0	1	3	1	2	6	11	1	9	0	11	4	1	2
4771	6	2	51	89	295	5	5	4	4	5	17	11	3	31	1	18	8	2	2
4772	9	2	67	201	303	8	6	0	8	8	19	11	5	30	4	19	9	5	3
4773	9	2	56	135	223	2	5	0	7	7	15	8	4	21	4	14	7	5	3
4774	2	1	43	36	208	1	2	0	3	4	13	9	2	25	1	13	6	1	2

Meat, Poultry, Fish

Food #	Food Description & Amount	wt gm	wt oz	calo-ries	%cal fat	prot gm	carbo gm	fiber gm
4775	Eel, smoked [2 oz, boneless]	56	2.0	162	57%	16	0	0.0
4776	Eel, steamed or poached [2 oz, boneless, cooked]	56	2.0	130	57%	13	0	0.0
4777	**Fish sticks, battered or breaded, frozen, baked from frozen [2 sticks]**	**48**	**1.7**	**131**	**40%**	**8**	**11**	**0.0**
4778	Fish sticks, battered, fried [2 sticks]	48	1.7	99	50%	9	3	0.1
4779	Fish sticks, breaded or floured, fried [2 sticks]	48	1.7	106	45%	10	4	0.1
4780	**Flounder**, baked or broiled (or sauteed or fried with no coating) (Include **dab, fluke, halibut, sole, turbot**) [1 filet (6"x2½"x¼")]	**57**	**2.0**	**76**	**29%**	**13**	**0**	**0.0**
4781	Flounder, battered, fried [2 oz, boneless, cooked]	56	2.0	115	51%	10	4	0.1
4782	Flounder, breaded or battered, baked [1 filet]	56	2.0	117	42%	12	5	0.2
4783	Flounder, floured or breaded, fried [1 filet]	81	2.9	179	46%	16	7	0.2
4784	Flounder, raw [2 oz, boneless, raw]	56	2.0	51	12%	11	0	0.0
4785	Flounder, smoked [2 oz, boneless]	56	2.0	123	12%	25	0	0.0
4786	Flounder, steamed or poached [2 oz, boneless, cooked]	56	2.0	64	12%	13	0	0.0
4787	**Haddock**, baked or broiled (or sauteed or fried with no coating) (Include **burbot, cusk, hake, ling, monkfish, pollock, scrod**) [2 oz, boneless, cooked]	**56**	**2.0**	**73**	**26%**	**12**	**0**	**0.0**
4788	Haddock, battered, fried [1 filet]	178	6.3	316	41%	33	12	0.4
4789	Haddock, breaded or battered, broiled [2 oz, boneless, cooked]	56	2.0	115	41%	12	5	0.2
4790	Haddock, floured or breaded, fried [1 filet]	81	2.9	176	45%	16	7	0.2
4791	Haddock, smoked [2 oz, boneless]	56	2.0	65	7%	14	0	0.0
4792	Haddock, steamed or poached [2 oz, boneless, cooked]	56	2.0	62	7%	13	0	0.0
4793	**Herring**, baked or broiled (or sauteed or fried with no coating) (Include **alewife, milkfish, shad**) [2 oz, boneless, cooked]	**56**	**2.0**	**137**	**59%**	**13**	**0**	**0.0**
4794	Herring, dried, salted [2 oz, boneless]	56	2.0	225	51%	25	0	0.0
4795	Herring, floured or breaded, fried [2 oz, boneless, cooked]	56	2.0	176	56%	12	7	0.2
4796	Herring, pickled (Include herring in wine sauce) [2 oz, boneless]	56	2.0	147	62%	8	5	0.0
4797	Herring, pickled, in cream sauce [2 oz, boneless]	56	2.0	141	66%	7	5	0.0
4798	Herring, raw [2 oz, boneless, raw]	56	2.0	88	51%	10	0	0.0
4799	Herring, smoked, kippered [2 oz, boneless]	56	2.0	122	51%	14	0	0.0
4800	Jellyfish, pickled [1 cup]	58	2.0	21	35%	3	0	0.0
4801	**Mackerel**, baked or broiled (or sauteed or fried with no coating) (Include **enenui, garfish, ono, needlefish, wahoo**) [2 oz, boneless, cooked]	**56**	**2.0**	**125**	**56%**	**13**	**0**	**0.0**
4802	Mackerel, canned [2 oz, boneless]	56	2.0	87	36%	13	0	0.0
4803	Mackerel, dried [2 oz, boneless]	56	2.0	171	74%	10	0	0.0
4804	Mackerel, floured or breaded, fried [2 oz, boneless, cooked]	56	2.0	164	59%	12	5	0.2
4805	Mackerel, pickled [2 oz, boneless]	56	2.0	144	61%	13	0	0.0
4806	Mackerel, raw [2 oz, boneless, raw]	56	2.0	94	50%	11	0	0.0
4807	Mackerel, salted [2 oz, dried, soaked, drained, and cooked]	44	1.6	134	74%	8	0	0.0
4808	Mackerel, smoked [2 oz, boneless]	56	2.0	112	45%	14	0	0.0
4809	Mullet, baked or broiled (Include sauteed; fried with no coating) [1 filet (6"x2½"x¼")]	57	2.0	111	45%	14	0	0.0
4810	Mullet, floured or breaded, fried (Include fried) [2 oz, boneless, cooked]	56	2.0	154	47%	12	7	0.2
4811	Mullet, raw [2 oz, raw]	56	2.0	66	29%	11	0	0.0
4812	Mullet, steamed or poached [2 oz, boneless, cooked]	56	2.0	83	29%	14	0	0.0
4813	**Ocean Perch**, baked, broiled (or sauteed or fried with no coating) (Include **bocaccio, menpachi, orange roughy, redfish, rockfish**) [2 oz, boneless, cooked]	**56**	**2.0**	**77**	**32%**	**12**	**0**	**0.0**
4814	Ocean Perch, battered, fried [2 oz, boneless, cooked]	56	2.0	116	52%	10	4	0.1
4815	Ocean Perch, breaded or battered, baked [2 oz, boneless, cooked]	56	2.0	104	32%	12	5	0.2
4816	Ocean Perch, floured or breaded, fried [2 oz, boneless, cooked]	56	2.0	125	48%	11	5	0.2
4817	Ocean Perch, raw [2 oz, boneless, raw]	56	2.0	53	16%	10	0	0.0
4818	Ocean Perch, steamed or poached [2 oz, boneless, cooked]	56	2.0	66	16%	13	0	0.0
4819	Octopus, cooked [2 oz, cooked]	56	2.0	106	39%	9	6	0.2

Food #	fat gm	sat fat gm	choles mg	sodium mg	potass mg	% of Daily Value													
						vit A	vit E	vit C	thia-min	ribo-flavin	nia-cin	vit B-6	fol-ate	vit B-12	cal-cium	phos-phorus	magne-sium	iron	zinc
4775	10	2	111	45	239	83	12	2	9	2	15	3	3	35	2	19	4	2	9
4776	8	2	89	33	164	63	9	2	6	2	11	2	2	30	1	14	3	2	8
4777	6	2	54	279	125	1	2	0	4	5	5	1	2	14	1	9	3	2	2
4778	5	1	37	48	158	1	3	0	3	6	8	6	1	20	4	10	7	2	2
4779	5	1	43	90	179	1	2	0	3	7	9	6	2	22	4	11	8	3	2
4780	2	1	32	74	245	2	5	3	4	3	9	6	1	15	1	12	5	1	2
4781	6	1	32	54	187	1	6	1	4	4	8	5	2	12	2	10	4	2	2
4782	5	1	39	152	218	5	6	1	6	5	10	6	3	14	3	12	5	4	2
4783	9	2	55	148	307	2	8	2	8	7	14	8	3	18	4	16	7	5	3
4784	1	0	27	45	202	1	4	2	3	3	8	6	1	14	1	10	4	1	2
4785	2	0	65	110	488	1	9	3	7	6	19	13	2	31	2	25	10	3	4
4786	1	0	34	51	215	1	4	1	3	3	9	6	1	15	1	12	5	1	2
4787	2	0	37	64	210	3	2	2	1	1	12	9	2	12	2	12	6	4	2
4788	14	3	120	158	537	3	9	0	10	10	34	22	9	30	9	35	17	14	6
4789	5	1	44	145	191	6	3	0	4	4	12	8	3	10	4	12	6	6	2
4790	9	2	62	138	268	2	4	0	5	5	18	11	4	15	5	17	9	8	3
4791	1	0	43	427	232	1	1	0	2	2	14	11	2	15	3	14	8	4	2
4792	1	0	40	43	187	1	1	0	1	1	11	9	2	12	2	12	4	4	2
4793	9	2	44	93	243	4	4	3	4	10	12	10	2	124	4	17	6	4	5
4794	13	3	85	952	464	3	3	1	7	19	23	19	3	242	9	34	12	9	9
4795	11	2	52	140	209	2	4	1	7	11	12	8	3	114	6	15	6	7	5
4796	10	1	7	487	39	14	2	0	1	5	9	5	0	40	4	5	1	4	2
4797	10	3	11	395	47	14	2	0	1	5	7	4	1	32	5	5	1	3	2
4798	5	1	34	50	183	2	2	1	3	8	9	8	1	128	3	13	4	3	4
4799	7	2	46	514	250	2	2	1	5	11	12	12	2	175	5	18	6	5	5
4800	1	0	3	5620	2	0	0	0	0	0	1	0	0	0	0	1	0	7	2
4801	8	2	42	71	259	3	3	3	6	12	22	11	0	43	1	12	8	4	3
4802	4	1	44	212	109	7	3	1	1	7	17	6	1	65	13	17	5	6	4
4803	14	4	53	2492	291	3	5	0	1	6	9	11	2	112	4	14	8	4	4
4804	11	3	47	101	227	2	4	1	7	12	20	10	2	35	3	11	7	6	3
4805	10	2	49	63	220	4	4	0	8	13	32	14	0	102	1	15	13	6	3
4806	5	1	36	44	218	2	2	1	5	10	18	11	0	48	1	10	6	3	2
4807	11	3	42	1958	229	2	4	0	1	5	7	9	2	88	3	11	7	3	3
4808	6	2	33	223	290	1	2	2	5	18	30	11	0	39	2	9	5	5	3
4809	6	1	36	80	267	5	4	4	4	3	18	14	1	2	3	16	5	4	3
4810	8	2	46	126	226	3	4	1	7	6	17	11	3	3	5	15	5	7	3
4811	2	1	27	36	200	2	2	1	3	3	15	12	1	2	2	12	4	3	2
4812	3	1	35	41	215	2	2	1	3	3	16	12	1	2	3	14	5	4	2
4813	3	0	28	69	183	2	4	2	4	4	6	7	1	10	7	14	5	3	2
4814	7	1	29	51	145	1	5	1	5	5	6	5	2	8	6	12	4	4	2
4815	4	1	37	130	176	3	4	1	7	6	8	7	3	9	8	14	5	5	3
4816	7	1	35	99	165	1	5	1	6	6	7	6	2	8	7	13	5	5	2
4817	1	0	24	42	153	1	2	1	4	4	6	6	1	9	6	12	4	3	2
4818	1	0	29	47	162	1	3	1	4	4	6	6	1	10	7	14	5	4	2
4819	5	1	40	188	213	3	4	4	4	4	8	9	3	166	5	12	5	19	7

Meat, Poultry, Fish

Food #	Food Description & Amount	wt gm	wt oz	calo-ries	%cal fat	prot gm	carbo gm	fiber gm
4820	Octopus, dried [2 oz]	56	2.0	175	11%	32	5	0.0
4821	Octopus, dried, boiled [1 cup, cooked]	106	3.7	174	11%	32	5	0.0
4822	Octopus, smoked [2 oz, boneless, cooked]	56	2.0	78	11%	14	2	0.0
4823	Octopus, steamed [2 oz, cooked]	56	2.0	92	11%	17	2	0.0
4824	**Perch, freshwater, baked or broiled (or sauteed or fried with no coating) (Include freshwater bass, bluegill, crappie, sunfish, walleye) [2 oz, boneless, cooked]**	56	2.0	75	27%	13	0	0.0
4825	Perch, freshwater, battered, fried [2 oz, boneless, cooked]	56	2.0	102	41%	11	4	0.1
4826	Perch, freshwater, breaded or battered, baked [2 oz, boneless, cooked]	56	2.0	102	29%	12	5	0.2
4827	Perch, freshwater, floured or breaded, fried [2 oz, boneless, cooked]	56	2.0	148	43%	13	8	0.3
4828	Perch, freshwater, steamed or poached [2 oz, boneless, cooked]	56	2.0	64	9%	14	0	0.0
4829	**Pike, baked or broiled (or sauteed or fried with no coating) (Include muskellunge, pickerel) [2 oz, boneless, cooked]**	56	2.0	73	26%	13	0	0.0
4830	Pike, battered, fried [2 oz, boneless, cooked]	56	2.0	114	50%	10	4	0.1
4831	Pike, floured or breaded, fried [2 oz, boneless, cooked]	56	2.0	122	45%	11	5	0.2
4832	Pike, steamed or poached [2 oz, boneless, cooked]	56	2.0	62	7%	14	0	0.0
4833	**Pompano, baked or broiled (or sauteed or fried with no coating) (Include akule, blackfish, bluefish, butterfish, dolphin, jack, mahi-mahi, paplo, parrot fish, sablefish, scad, tilefish, ulva, yellowtail) [2 oz, boneless, cooked]**	56	2.0	143	60%	13	0	0.0
4834	Pompano, battered, fried [2 oz, boneless, cooked]	56	2.0	150	63%	10	4	0.1
4835	Pompano, floured or breaded, fried [2 oz, boneless, cooked]	56	2.0	179	56%	12	7	0.2
4836	Pompano, raw [2 oz, boneless, raw]	56	2.0	92	52%	10	0	0.0
4837	Pompano, smoked [2 oz, boneless, raw]	56	2.0	108	52%	12	0	0.0
4838	Pompano, steamed or poached [2 oz, boneless, cooked]	56	2.0	115	52%	13	0	0.0
4839	**Porgy, baked or broiled (or sauteed or fried with no coating) (Include scup, sea bream, marine sheepshead, snapper) [2 oz, boneless, cooked]**	56	2.0	109	44%	14	0	0.0
4840	Porgy, battered, fried [2 oz, boneless, cooked]	56	2.0	164	61%	10	6	0.2
4841	Porgy, breaded or battered, baked [2 oz, boneless, cooked]	56	2.0	149	50%	11	7	0.2
4842	Porgy, floured or breaded, fried [2 oz, boneless, cooked]	56	2.0	161	47%	12	8	0.3
4843	Porgy, raw [2 oz, boneless, raw]	56	2.0	59	23%	11	0	0.0
4844	Porgy, steamed or poached [2 oz, boneless, cooked]	56	2.0	74	23%	13	0	0.0
4845	**Ray, baked or broiled (or sauteed or fried with no coating) (Include skate) [2 oz, boneless, cooked]**	56	2.0	114	41%	16	0	0.0
4846	Ray, floured or breaded, fried [2 oz, boneless, cooked]	56	2.0	161	47%	13	7	0.2
4847	Ray, steamed or poached [2 oz, boneless, cooked]	56	2.0	92	31%	15	0	0.0
4848	Roe, cod and shad, cooked [2 oz]	56	2.0	110	51%	14	1	0.0
4849	Roe, herring [2Tbs]	28	1.0	39	41%	6	0	0.0
4850	Roe, sturgeon (Include caviar) [2Tbs]	32	1.1	81	64%	8	1	0.0
4851	**Salmon, baked or broiled (or sauteed or fried with no coating) (Include saltwater trout) [2 oz, boneless, cooked]**	56	2.0	97	40%	14	0	0.0
4852	Salmon, battered, fried [2 oz, boneless, cooked]	56	2.0	127	54%	10	4	0.1
4853	Salmon, canned [2 oz]	56	2.0	79	40%	11	0	0.0
4854	Salmon, dried [2 oz, boneless]	56	2.0	81	27%	14	0	0.0
4855	Salmon, floured or breaded, fried [2 oz, boneless, cooked]	56	2.0	134	44%	12	6	0.2
4856	Salmon, raw [2 oz, boneless, raw]	56	2.0	82	37%	12	0	0.0
4857	Salmon, smoked (Include lox) [2 oz, boneless]	56	2.0	66	33%	10	0	0.0
4858	Salmon, steamed or poached [2 oz, boneless, cooked]	56	2.0	81	27%	14	0	0.0
4859	**Sardines, canned in oil [1 can (3.75 oz), drained]**	92	3.2	191	50%	23	0	0.0
4860	Sardines, cooked [2 oz, cooked]	56	2.0	116	50%	14	0	0.0
4861	Sardines, dried [4 sardines (5" long)]	28	1.0	57	51%	6	0	0.0
4862	Sardines, skinless, boneless, packed in water [1 can (4.375 oz, 4 sardines), drained]	84	3.0	182	51%	21	0	0.0

Food #	fat gm	sat fat gm	choles mg	sodium mg	potass mg	vit A	vit E	vit C	thia-min	ribo-flavin	nia-cin	vit B-6	fol-ate	vit B-12	cal-cium	phos-phorus	magne-sium	iron	zinc
														% of Daily Value					
4820	2	0	102	490	745	8	9	17	4	4	21	36	8	674	11	40	16	63	24
4821	2	0	102	488	668	9	4	14	4	5	20	34	6	636	11	30	16	56	24
4822	1	0	46	219	334	4	4	8	2	2	10	16	4	302	5	18	7	28	11
4823	1	0	54	258	353	5	4	7	2	3	11	18	3	336	6	16	8	30	13
4824	2	0	59	60	180	2	1	3	3	4	5	4	1	19	5	13	5	3	5
4825	5	1	54	47	148	1	2	1	4	5	5	3	2	15	5	11	4	4	4
4826	3	1	64	122	173	3	2	1	5	6	6	4	2	18	6	13	5	5	5
4827	7	1	71	133	180	1	3	1	6	7	7	4	3	16	7	14	6	7	5
4828	1	0	63	39	160	1	0	1	3	4	5	3	1	19	6	13	5	4	5
4829	2	0	26	45	174	3	1	5	2	2	7	4	2	20	4	15	5	2	3
4830	6	1	28	34	138	1	3	2	4	4	7	3	3	15	4	12	4	3	3
4831	6	1	33	80	157	2	3	3	4	4	8	3	3	17	5	13	5	4	3
4832	0	0	28	25	156	1	0	3	2	2	7	3	2	20	4	14	5	2	3
4833	10	3	36	79	281	5	2	3	26	5	11	7	3	12	2	14	5	2	3
4834	10	3	33	46	197	1	3	0	17	5	8	5	3	10	2	11	4	3	3
4835	11	3	47	126	239	2	3	0	21	8	11	6	4	10	4	13	5	6	4
4836	5	2	28	36	213	2	0	0	21	4	8	6	2	12	1	11	4	2	3
4837	6	2	33	43	251	2	0	0	23	5	10	6	2	12	1	13	4	2	3
4838	7	2	35	41	227	2	0	0	21	4	9	6	2	13	2	12	4	2	3
4839	5	1	39	70	223	5	3	3	5	4	15	10	3	16	3	14	4	2	2
4840	11	2	37	43	149	1	5	0	6	6	11	6	4	10	4	11	3	4	2
4841	8	2	44	180	167	8	4	0	7	6	12	7	4	11	5	11	4	5	3
4842	8	2	51	127	191	2	4	0	8	7	15	8	4	12	5	13	5	6	3
4843	2	0	29	24	161	2	1	0	4	3	11	8	2	13	2	10	3	2	2
4844	2	0	36	26	171	2	1	0	4	4	12	8	2	14	3	12	4	2	2
4845	5	1	38	81	123	7	3	2	2	3	10	13	1	17	3	16	9	3	2
4846	8	2	47	134	117	4	4	0	5	6	11	11	3	13	4	14	8	6	3
4847	3	1	36	50	96	4	2	0	2	2	9	11	0	15	2	13	8	3	2
4848	6	1	241	84	147	7	16	16	9	28	6	5	11	102	2	25	3	2	4
4849	2	0	105	25	62	2	7	6	4	12	3	2	5	37	1	11	1	1	2
4850	6	1	188	480	58	18	7	0	4	12	0	5	4	107	9	11	24	21	2
4851	4	1	35	68	223	4	3	2	7	2	24	6	1	25	1	16	4	3	2
4852	8	1	34	47	169	2	4	0	7	4	18	5	2	19	2	13	4	4	2
4853	4	1	29	307	188	1	3	0	1	6	18	9	2	33	12	18	5	3	4
4854	2	0	36	47	226	2	2	0	8	2	25	6	1	26	1	16	5	3	3
4855	7	1	44	108	201	2	4	0	8	5	22	6	2	21	3	15	5	5	3
4856	3	1	25	26	237	2	1	1	4	5	20	15	1	39	2	15	4	2	2
4857	2	1	13	439	98	1	3	0	1	3	13	8	0	30	1	9	3	3	1
4858	2	0	36	42	192	2	2	0	6	2	21	6	1	30	1	14	4	3	3
4859	11	1	131	465	365	6	1	0	5	12	24	8	3	137	35	45	9	15	8
4860	6	1	80	283	222	4	1	0	3	7	15	5	2	83	21	27	5	9	5
4861	3	1	22	32	117	1	1	0	2	5	6	5	1	61	2	8	3	2	2
4862	10	2	69	771	375	3	3	1	7	16	18	17	3	262	7	27	10	7	8

Meat, Poultry, Fish

Food #	Food Description & Amount	wt gm	wt oz	calo-ries	%cal fat	prot gm	carbo gm	fiber gm
4863	**Sea bass**, baked or broiled (or sauteed or fried with no coating) (Include **grouper, striped bass, wreakfish**) [2 oz, boneless, cooked]	56	2.0	84	36%	13	0	0.0
4864	Sea bass, breaded or battered, baked [2 oz, boneless, cooked]	56	2.0	106	34%	12	5	0.2
4865	Sea bass, floured or breaded, fried [2 oz, boneless, cooked]	56	2.0	124	42%	12	6	0.2
4866	Sea bass, pickled (Include Mero en escabeche) [2 oz, boneless]	56	2.0	154	80%	7	1	0.1
4867	Sea bass, steamed or poached [2 oz, boneless, cooked]	56	2.0	68	19%	13	0	0.0
4868	**Shark**, baked or broiled (or sauteed or fried with no coating) (Include **dogfish, grayfish**) [2 oz, boneless, cooked]	56	2.0	101	41%	14	0	0.0
4869	Shark, steamed or poached [2 oz, boneless, cooked]	56	2.0	92	31%	15	0	0.0
4870	**Smelt**, battered, fried (Include **capelin**) [2 oz, boneless, cooked]	56	2.0	146	59%	9	5	0.2
4871	Smelt, broiled or baked (or sauteed) [2 oz, boneless, cooked]	56	2.0	95	42%	13	0	0.0
4872	Smelt, floured or breaded, fried [2 oz, boneless, cooked]	56	2.0	143	46%	12	7	0.2
4873	Smelt, steamed or poached [2 oz, boneless, cooked]	56	2.0	69	22%	12	0	0.0
4874	**Squid**, baked, broiled (or sauteed) (Include **cuttlefish, calamari**) [1 squid]	272	9.6	377	31%	51	10	0.0
4875	Squid, breaded, fried [2 oz, cooked]	56	2.0	111	38%	10	7	0.2
4876	Squid, canned (Include calameres en su tinta, squid in its own ink) [1 cup]	187	6.6	199	13%	34	7	0.0
4877	Squid, dried [2 oz, boneless]	56	2.0	196	13%	33	7	0.0
4878	Squid, pickled [2 oz, boneless]	56	2.0	53	13%	9	2	0.0
4879	Squid, raw [2 oz, boneless, raw]	56	2.0	52	14%	9	2	0.0
4880	Squid, steamed or boiled [2 oz, boneless, cooked]	56	2.0	60	13%	10	2	0.0
4881	Sturgeon, baked or broiled (or sauteed or fried with no coating) [2 oz, boneless, cooked]	56	2.0	76	35%	12	0	0.0
4882	Sturgeon, floured or breaded, fried (Include fried) [2 oz, boneless, cooked]	56	2.0	131	54%	10	5	0.2
4883	Sturgeon, smoked [2 oz, boneless]	56	2.0	97	23%	17	0	0.0
4884	Sturgeon, steamed [2 oz, boneless, cooked]	56	2.0	74	35%	11	0	0.0
4885	**Swordfish**, baked or broiled (or sauteed or fried with no coating) (Include **marlin**) [2 oz, boneless, cooked]	56	2.0	100	42%	13	0	0.0
4886	Swordfish, floured or breaded, fried [2 oz, boneless, cooked]	56	2.0	140	51%	12	5	0.2
4887	Swordfish, steamed or poached [2 oz, boneless, cooked]	56	2.0	86	30%	14	0	0.0
4888	**Trout**, baked or broiled (or sauteed or fried with no coating) (Include **cisco, lake herring, steelhead, whitefish**) [2 oz, boneless, cooked]	56	2.0	106	44%	14	0	0.0
4889	Trout, battered, fried [2 oz, boneless, cooked]	56	2.0	130	52%	11	4	0.1
4890	Trout, breaded or battered, baked [2 oz, boneless, cooked]	56	2.0	120	35%	14	5	0.2
4891	Trout, floured or breaded, fried [2 oz, boneless, cooked]	56	2.0	152	49%	13	6	0.2
4892	Trout, smoked [2 oz, boneless]	56	2.0	149	40%	21	0	0.0
4893	Trout, steamed or poached [2 oz, boneless, cooked]	56	2.0	98	35%	15	0	0.0
4894	Tuna, canned, oil pack (Include low sodium) [2 oz]	56	2.0	111	37%	16	0	0.0
4895	Tuna, canned, water pack (Include low sodium) [2 oz]	56	2.0	65	6%	14	0	0.0
4896	**Tuna**, fresh, baked or broiled (or sauteed or fried with no coating) (Include **ahi, aku, bonito**) [2 oz, boneless, cooked]	56	2.0	86	24%	15	0	0.0
4897	Tuna, fresh, dried [1 cup]	42	1.5	76	31%	12	0	0.0
4898	Tuna, fresh, floured or breaded, fried [2 oz, boneless, cooked]	56	2.0	133	42%	14	5	0.2
4899	Tuna, fresh, raw [2 oz, boneless, raw]	56	2.0	60	8%	13	0	0.0
4900	Tuna, fresh, smoked [2 oz, boneless]	56	2.0	113	45%	14	0	0.0
4901	Tuna, fresh, steamed or poached [2 oz, boneless, cooked]	56	2.0	77	8%	17	0	0.0
4902	Whiting, baked or broiled (or sauteed or fried with no coating) [2 oz, boneless, cooked]	56	2.0	74	30%	12	0	0.0
4903	Whiting, battered, fried [2 oz, boneless, cooked]	56	2.0	101	43%	10	4	0.1
4904	Whiting, breaded or battered, baked [2 oz, boneless, cooked]	56	2.0	116	42%	11	5	0.2
4905	Whiting, floured or breaded, fried (Include fried) [2 oz, boneless, cooked]	56	2.0	123	47%	11	5	0.2
4906	Whiting, steamed or poached [2 oz, boneless, cooked]	56	2.0	64	13%	13	0	0.0

Food #	fat gm	sat fat gm	choles mg	sodium mg	potass mg	vit A	vit E	vit C	thia-min	ribo-flavin	nia-cin	vit B-6	fol-ate	vit B-12	cal-cium	phos-phorus	magne-sium	iron	zinc
% of Daily Value																			
4863	3	1	28	69	178	5	2	2	5	5	5	12	1	3	1	13	7	1	2
4864	4	1	37	126	166	6	2	0	7	6	6	11	2	3	2	13	7	3	2
4865	6	1	38	108	164	3	3	0	6	7	7	11	2	3	3	13	7	4	2
4866	14	2	16	44	111	2	6	0	3	3	3	7	1	2	1	8	4	1	1
4867	1	0	29	43	152	3	1	0	4	4	5	11	1	3	1	12	6	1	2
4868	5	1	34	71	109	6	3	2	2	2	10	12	1	12	2	14	8	3	2
4869	3	1	36	50	96	4	2	0	2	2	9	11	0	15	2	13	8	3	2
4870	10	2	44	49	151	1	5	0	3	6	5	3	2	24	4	12	4	4	6
4871	4	1	51	75	215	4	3	3	1	5	5	5	1	37	4	17	5	4	8
4872	7	2	58	124	189	2	3	0	4	7	7	4	3	29	6	15	5	6	7
4873	2	0	50	38	175	1	1	0	0	5	4	4	1	35	4	15	5	4	8
4874	13	3	768	242	815	11	17	25	4	64	34	9	4	68	11	73	27	12	34
4875	5	1	142	85	156	1	4	3	3	15	8	2	2	11	4	14	5	5	6
4876	3	1	504	86	425	2	9	12	2	42	19	5	2	35	7	38	16	8	22
4877	3	1	496	94	524	2	9	16	3	41	22	6	2	44	7	47	18	8	22
4878	1	0	129	25	138	0	2	3	1	13	6	1	1	11	2	12	5	2	6
4879	1	0	130	25	138	1	2	4	1	14	6	2	1	12	2	12	5	2	6
4880	1	0	151	26	127	1	3	4	1	13	6	1	1	11	2	11	5	2	7
4881	3	1	43	39	204	14	1	0	3	3	28	6	2	23	1	15	6	3	2
4882	8	2	45	88	171	10	3	0	5	4	24	5	3	18	2	13	6	4	2
4883	2	1	45	414	212	16	1	0	3	3	31	8	3	27	1	16	7	3	2
4884	3	1	42	30	159	13	1	0	3	3	28	6	2	24	1	12	5	2	2
4885	5	1	26	84	199	4	2	3	2	4	31	10	0	18	0	18	5	3	5
4886	8	2	33	107	173	2	3	1	4	5	28	8	2	15	2	16	4	5	5
4887	3	1	28	57	174	2	1	1	1	4	29	9	0	18	0	17	4	3	5
4888	5	1	39	42	300	6	1	4	9	3	27	18	2	35	4	19	5	1	2
4889	7	1	38	42	194	1	2	0	12	11	12	5	3	59	3	14	3	6	3
4890	5	1	48	95	233	2	1	0	14	13	15	6	3	69	4	16	4	8	3
4891	8	2	47	100	222	2	2	0	14	13	15	6	3	65	4	15	4	7	3
4892	7	1	58	52	362	2	1	1	21	19	21	9	3	117	4	25	6	8	4
4893	4	1	42	22	272	5	0	3	8	3	25	18	2	38	5	18	5	1	2
4894	5	1	10	198	116	1	2	0	1	4	35	3	1	21	1	17	4	4	3
4895	0	0	17	189	133	1	1	0	1	2	37	10	1	28	1	9	4	5	3
4896	2	0	30	44	296	3	2	3	17	2	31	27	0	5	1	13	8	3	2
4897	3	1	20	20	132	31	2	0	8	7	22	11	0	74	0	13	7	3	2
4898	6	1	37	79	256	1	3	1	16	4	28	22	2	5	3	12	8	5	3
4899	1	0	25	21	249	1	1	1	16	2	27	25	0	5	1	11	7	2	2
4900	6	2	34	62	292	1	2	2	5	18	30	11	0	39	2	9	5	5	3
4901	1	0	32	24	268	1	1	1	16	2	30	26	0	5	1	12	8	3	2
4902	3	0	44	67	167	3	1	2	2	2	4	5	2	23	3	15	4	1	4
4903	5	1	43	52	138	1	3	0	4	3	5	4	3	18	4	13	3	2	3
4904	5	1	49	147	157	6	3	0	4	4	5	4	3	19	5	14	4	3	4
4905	6	1	48	97	152	2	3	0	4	4	5	4	3	19	4	13	4	3	4
4906	1	0	47	46	150	2	1	0	2	2	4	4	2	23	3	14	3	1	4

Meat, Poultry, Fish

Food #	Food Description & Amount	wt gm	wt oz	calo-ries	%cal fat	prot gm	carbo gm	fiber gm
4907	Abalone, floured or breaded, fried [2 oz, cooked]	56	2.0	107	32%	11	6	0.1
4908	Abalone, steamed or poached [2 oz, cooked]	56	2.0	118	7%	19	7	0.0
4909	**Clams**, baked, broiled, or sauteed, with margarine [1 cup (8 large clams, 12 medium clams, 15 small clams)]	150	5.3	210	45%	23	5	0.0
4910	Clams, battered, fried [1 cup (5 large clams, 8 medium clams, 10 small clams), cooked]	102	3.6	223	48%	15	14	0.4
4911	Clams, canned [2 oz]	56	2.0	52	12%	9	2	0.0
4912	Clams, floured or breaded, fried (or baked with fat) [1 cup (8 large clams, 12 medium clams, 15 small clams)]	150	5.3	271	40%	22	17	0.4
4913	Clams, raw [4 clams]	64	2.3	47	12%	8	2	0.0
4914	Clams, smoked, in oil [2 oz]	56	2.0	98	59%	8	2	0.0
4915	Clams, steamed or boiled [1 cup (8 large clams, 12 medium clams, 15 small clams)]	150	5.3	139	12%	24	5	0.0
4916	Conch, battered, fried [2 oz, raw]	50	1.8	104	44%	10	4	0.1
4917	Conch, baked or broiled [2 oz, raw]	34	1.2	44	8%	9	1	0.0
4918	**Crab**, baked or broiled (or sauteed) [1 cup, flaked and pieces]	118	4.2	163	42%	23	0	0.0
4919	Crab, canned (Include white or king meat) [2 oz]	56	2.0	55	11%	11	0	0.0
4920	Crab, hard shell, steamed or boiled [1 cup, flaked and pieces]	118	4.2	120	16%	24	0	0.0
4921	Crab, soft shell, floured or breaded, fried [2 oz, cooked]	56	2.0	187	54%	11	10	0.3
4922	Crayfish, boiled or steamed [2 oz, without shell, cooked]	56	2.0	46	13%	9	0	0.0
4923	Crayfish, floured or breaded, fried [2 oz, without shell, cooked]	56	2.0	124	47%	10	6	0.2
4924	**Lobster**, baked or broiled (or sauteed) [1 cup, cooked, diced]	145	5.1	169	23%	29	2	0.0
4925	Lobster, battered, fried [1 cup]	145	5.1	306	47%	28	11	0.3
4926	Lobster, canned [2 oz]	56	2.0	55	5%	11	1	0.0
4927	Lobster, floured or breaded, fried [2 oz, without shell, cooked]	56	2.0	123	46%	11	5	0.2
4928	Lobster, steamed or boiled [1 cup, cooked, diced]	145	5.1	142	5%	30	2	0.0
4929	Mussels, raw [4 mussels]	64	2.3	55	23%	8	2	0.0
4930	Mussels, steamed or poached [4 mussels]	32	1.1	55	23%	8	2	0.0
4931	**Oysters**, baked or broiled (or sauteed) [4 eastern oysters]	48	1.7	51	60%	3	2	0.0
4932	Oysters, battered, fried [4 eastern oysters]	32	1.1	68	54%	3	5	0.1
4933	Oysters, canned [1 cup, drained]	162	5.7	122	32%	12	7	0.0
4934	Oysters, floured or breaded, fried [4 eastern oysters]	32	1.1	64	57%	3	4	0.1
4935	Oysters, raw [4 eastern oysters]	60	2.1	41	33%	4	2	0.0
4936	Oysters, smoked [6 oysters]	30	1.1	33	33%	3	2	0.0
4937	Oysters, steamed [4 eastern oyster]	48	1.7	41	33%	4	2	0.0
4938	**Scallops**, baked or broiled (or sauteed) [4 scallops]	100	3.5	134	27%	20	3	0.0
4939	Scallops, battered, fried [4 scallops]	32	1.1	74	45%	6	4	0.1
4940	Scallops, floured or breaded, fried [4 scallops]	100	3.5	218	45%	18	11	0.3
4941	Scallops, steamed or boiled [4 scallops]	100	3.5	107	27%	16	2	0.0
4942	Sea urchin (roe) [2Tbs]	24	0.8	35	52%	4	0	0.0
4943	**Shrimp**, baked or broiled (or sauteed) (Include **prawns**) [1 cup, cooked]	145	5.1	226	30%	36	2	0.0
4944	Shrimp, canned [1 cup]	128	4.5	154	15%	30	1	0.0
4945	Shrimp, dried [20 shrimp]	10	0.4	30	15%	6	0	0.0
4946	Shrimp, floured or breaded, fried [1 cup, cooked]	129	4.6	318	45%	27	15	0.5
4947	Shrimp, steamed or boiled [1 cup, cooked]	145	5.1	202	15%	39	2	0.0
	Your Additions							

Food #	fat gm	sat fat gm	choles mg	sodium mg	potass mg	vit A	vit E	vit C	thia-min	ribo-flavin	nia-cin	vit B-6	fol-ate	vit B-12	cal-cium	phos-phorus	magne-sium	iron	zinc
						% of Daily Value													
4907	4	1	53	189	160	0	10	2	8	4	5	4	2	6	2	12	8	12	4
4908	1	0	95	287	196	0	15	3	13	5	6	7	1	8	3	15	11	18	6
4909	11	2	60	202	559	22	10	36	9	18	15	5	7	1382	8	30	4	137	16
4910	12	2	85	126	316	10	8	15	10	18	12	4	7	618	6	19	4	74	10
4911	1	0	24	39	198	6	2	12	4	8	6	2	2	519	3	9	2	49	6
4912	12	2	85	246	518	14	9	26	14	24	18	5	9	1039	12	29	6	122	16
4913	1	0	22	36	201	6	2	14	3	8	6	2	3	527	3	11	1	50	6
4914	6	1	21	35	197	6	5	13	3	8	6	2	3	516	3	11	1	49	6
4915	2	0	64	105	530	15	6	33	10	22	15	5	6	1391	9	24	4	131	17
4916	5	1	31	69	72	0	10	0	3	3	3	1	18	33	5	9	23	4	5
4917	0	0	22	52	55	0	7	0	1	2	2	1	15	30	3	7	20	3	4
4918	8	1	111	375	363	6	6	6	7	3	18	10	14	135	12	23	9	6	31
4919	1	0	50	186	209	0	2	3	3	3	4	4	6	4	6	15	5	3	15
4920	2	0	118	329	382	0	4	6	8	3	19	11	15	144	12	24	10	6	33
4921	11	2	69	187	180	1	6	2	9	6	11	5	9	48	7	12	5	6	14
4922	1	0	74	53	166	1	3	1	2	3	6	2	6	20	3	15	5	3	7
4923	7	1	85	70	168	2	7	1	6	5	8	3	7	15	3	15	4	5	5
4924	4	2	111	571	496	7	5	0	1	6	8	5	4	73	9	26	12	3	27
4925	16	3	113	511	474	3	11	0	6	10	10	5	6	56	11	27	12	6	25
4926	0	0	40	213	197	1	2	0	0	2	3	2	2	29	3	10	5	1	11
4927	6	1	63	217	166	2	5	0	3	4	6	2	2	7	4	9	4	3	12
4928	1	0	104	551	510	4	5	0	1	6	8	6	4	75	9	27	13	3	28
4929	1	0	18	183	205	3	2	9	7	8	5	2	7	128	2	13	5	14	7
4930	1	0	18	156	143	3	2	6	6	6	4	1	5	77	2	9	5	13	7
4931	3	1	24	122	72	3	2	3	3	2	3	1	1	139	2	6	5	17	274
4932	4	1	32	82	55	2	2	1	4	4	3	1	2	77	2	5	4	12	168
4933	4	1	97	197	403	16	5	15	18	17	11	8	4	562	8	24	24	66	1068
4934	4	1	23	98	58	1	2	2	3	3	3	1	1	84	2	5	4	13	185
4935	1	0	32	127	94	2	2	4	4	3	4	2	2	195	3	8	7	22	363
4936	1	0	26	103	76	1	1	3	3	3	3	2	1	158	2	7	6	18	295
4937	1	0	32	127	84	2	2	3	4	3	4	2	1	175	3	6	7	20	363
4938	4	1	40	231	392	5	6	6	1	4	7	9	5	29	3	27	17	2	8
4939	4	1	26	68	101	1	2	1	2	3	3	2	2	7	1	7	4	2	2
4940	11	2	54	259	341	2	7	4	5	8	9	7	6	22	5	24	15	6	7
4941	3	1	32	185	282	4	4	4	1	4	5	7	3	22	2	16	14	1	6
4942	2	0	74	18	32	1	6	6	2	11	2	2	5	40	1	10	1	1	2
4943	7	1	267	312	327	12	7	6	3	3	21	9	1	32	9	36	16	24	13
4944	3	0	221	216	269	2	4	5	2	3	18	7	1	24	8	30	13	19	11
4945	0	0	44	43	53	0	1	1	0	1	3	1	0	5	1	6	3	4	2
4946	16	3	238	261	256	9	9	3	10	11	19	7	6	21	9	28	12	22	11
4947	3	1	290	240	247	9	5	5	3	3	18	9	1	22	10	27	15	23	14

These dishes are fancy enough for company, yet easy to make, and you get a vegetable or fruit portion with each serving.

Scallops Bordelaise (serves 4)

4 slices French bread, lightly buttered	½ lb fresh mushrooms, sliced
1 Tbs butter	1 lb scallops
1 small onion, minced	½ cup red wine
1 small carrot, minced	¼ cup brandy
1 piece of celery, minced	8-oz can diced tomatoes
2 Tbs minced parsley	Salt, black pepper, cayenne pepper

The French bread slices should be about an inch thick and lightly buttered on both sides. Lightly grill them on both sides in a frying pan, and set them aside.

In the same pan, melt the butter, and add the onion, carrot, celery, parsley, and mushrooms. Sauté and stir until onions turn yellow. Add the scallops, wine, and brandy. Set the alcohol fumes ablaze with a match. When the flames die out, add the tomatoes, cover the pan, and simmer for about 5 minutes. Add salt and peppers to taste, and serve over the French bread, allowing the bread to soak up the liquid.

You can make this dish surrounded by your guests. Prepare the ingredients ahead of time and present them attractively, e.g., the minced vegetables attractively arranged in a small bowl. (Mince the onion, carrot, celery, parsley sequentially. Put the onions in the bowl; push a hole into the center of the onions; put the carrot in the hole; push a hole in the center of the carrots; do the same with the celery and then the parsley. The vegetables are now in colorful concentric circles.) Dim the lights when you light the alcohol fumes.

* * * * * * * * * * * * *

Halibut with Mango Salsa (serves 6)

6 halibut filets (about 5 oz each)	salt and pepper, to taste
1½ cups chopped macadamia nuts	2 Tbs butter, melted

Mango Salsa:

2 sweet red peppers, cut in ¼" pieces	3 Tbs fresh lemon juice
2 mangos, cut in ¼" pieces	1 tsp minced fresh garlic
1 cup fresh cilantro, finely chopped	¼ tsp cayenne pepper
1 small red onion, finely chopped	salt, black pepper, to taste

Preheat oven to 350° Pat the halibut dry with paper towels. Rub in salt and pepper. Mix the filets with the melted butter. Lay the filets about 2" apart on a lightly buttered or oiled baking sheet. Press the macadamia nuts on the top and sides of the filets. Bake for about 20 minutes, until the filets are just opaque in the center. Serve surrounded by the salsa.

Soups, Sauces, Fats, and Miscellaneous

Soups *5000*

Sauces, Gravies, and Dips *5300*

Fats and Oils *5400*

Dressings *5500*

Condiments *5600*

Spices and Miscellaneous *5700*

End-of-Section Recipes
Harira (Moroccan Soup)
Caesar Salad Dressing

Soups, Sauces, Fats, & Misc.

Food #	Food Description & Amount	wt gm	wt oz	calo- ries	%cal fat	prot gm	carbo gm	fiber gm
	Soups, Sauces, Fats, Miscellaneous							
5000	Asparagus soup, cream of, made with milk [1 cup]	248	8.7	148	40%	6	17	0.5
5001	Asparagus soup, cream of, made with water [1 cup]	244	8.6	87	43%	2	11	0.5
5002	Bacon soup, cream of, made with water (Include Albertson brand) [1 cup]	244	8.6	520	71%	22	15	0.5
5003	Barley soup (Include beef barley, chicken barley, mushroom barley soup) [1 cup]	244	8.6	96	7%	5	18	3.6
5004	Barley soup, sweet, with or without nuts, oriental Style [1 cup]	244	8.6	217	13%	2	47	3.0
5005	Bean soup (Include Navy bean soup) [1 cup]	253	8.9	137	26%	7	19	8.6
5006	Bean soup, home recipe [1 cup]	247	8.7	141	3%	9	27	6.7
5007	Bean soup, mixed beans [1 cup]	238	8.4	129	10%	8	22	6.2
5008	Bean with bacon or pork soup [1 cup]	253	8.9	173	31%	8	23	7.9
5009	Bean soup with ham, chunky style [1 cup]	243	8.6	224	28%	11	29	4.9
5010	Bean and ham soup, canned, reduced sodium, prepared with water or ready-to-serve [1 cup]	249	8.8	184	13%	10	34	10.0
5011	Bean and ham soup, home recipe [1 cup]	247	8.7	226	39%	17	18	4.7
5012	Bean soup with macaroni (Include Pasta e Fagiole without meat; Pasta e Fagioli) [1 cup]	253	8.9	156	22%	8	22	3.7
5013	Bean soup with macaroni and meat (Include Pasta Fagiole) [1 cup]	253	8.9	205	50%	6	20	3.1
5014	Bean and rice soup [1 cup]	253	8.9	155	22%	8	23	3.5
5015	Bean soup with vegetables, rice, and pork [1 cup]	243	8.6	194	30%	9	25	3.4
5016	Bean soup with vegetables and rice, canned, reduced sodium, prepared with water or ready-to-serve [1 cup]	241	8.5	140	6%	5	27	5.5
5017	Beef broth, bouillon, or consomme [1 cup]	240	8.5	17	28%	3	0	0.0
5018	Beef broth, bouillon, or consomme, canned, low sodium [1 cup]	240	8.5	38	34%	5	1	0.0
5019	Beef broth, bouillon, or consomme, dry, not reconstituted [1 cube]	4	0.1	7	28%	1	1	0.0
5020	Beef broth, bouillon, or consomme, low sodium, dry, not reconstituted [1 cube]	4	0.1	10	47%	1	1	0.0
5021	Beef broth, home recipe [1 cup]	240	8.5	31	6%	5	3	0.0
5022	Beef dumpling soup [1 cup]	241	8.5	314	40%	24	21	0.7
5023	Beef and mushroom soup [1 cup]	256	9.0	553	61%	43	8	0.3
5024	Beef and mushroom soup, canned, low sodium, chunky style (Include beef soup, canned, low sodium or no salt added) [1 cup]	251	8.9	173	30%	11	19	0.5
5025	Beef noodle soup, canned, condensed [½ cup condensed or 1 cup diluted 1:1 with water]	244	8.6	84	33%	5	9	0.8
5026	Beef noodle soup, chunky style [1 cup]	240	8.5	152	24%	15	13	1.1
5027	Beef noodle soup, home recipe [1 cup]	244	8.6	167	33%	19	8	1.2
5028	Beef noodle soup, Puerto Rican style (Sopa de carne y fideos) [1 cup]	250	8.8	140	22%	15	12	1.6
5029	Beef rice soup [1 cup]	241	8.5	111	25%	8	12	0.5
5030	Beef and rice soup, Puerto Rican style [1 cup]	250	8.8	140	22%	15	12	1.5
5031	Beef and rice noodle soup, oriental style (Vietnamese Pho Bo) [1 cup]	244	8.6	174	20%	17	17	1.0
5032	Beef stroganoff soup, chunky style (Include creamed beef soup) [1 cup]	240	8.5	235	42%	12	22	1.4
5033	Beef vegetable soup with potato, stew type (Include chunky style) [1 cup]	240	8.5	170	27%	12	20	1.4
5034	Beef vegetable soup with noodles, stew type, chunky style [1 cup]	240	8.5	182	25%	12	23	1.5
5035	Beef vegetable soup with rice, stew type, chunky style [1 cup]	240	8.5	181	24%	11	23	1.4
5036	Beef vegetable soup, Mexican style (Sopa caldo de Res) [1 cup]	239	8.4	141	37%	12	11	1.6
5037	Beer soup, made with milk [1 cup]	245	8.6	109	29%	5	11	0.6
5038	Beet soup (borscht) [1 cup]	245	8.6	78	46%	3	8	1.7
5039	Bird's nest soup (chicken, ham, and noodles) [1 cup]	244	8.6	112	22%	14	6	0.0
5040	Black bean soup [1 cup]	247	8.7	116	12%	6	20	4.4
5041	Bouillabaisse [1 cup]	227	8.0	241	33%	34	5	0.6
5042	Broccoli cheese soup, made with milk [1 cup]	239	8.4	165	48%	6	15	2.2
5043	Broccoli soup (Include cream of broccoli soup) [1 cup]	237	8.4	205	53%	9	17	2.0
5044	Cabbage soup [1 cup]	245	8.6	67	45%	4	6	1.7

Food #	fat gm	sat fat gm	choles mg	sodium mg	potass mg	vit A	vit E	vit C	thia-min	ribo-flavin	nia-cin	vit B-6	fol-ate	vit B-12	cal-cium	phos-phorus	magne-sium	iron	zinc

Food #	fat gm	sat fat gm	choles mg	sodium mg	potass mg	vit A	vit E	vit C	thia-min	ribo-flavin	nia-cin	vit B-6	fol-ate	vit B-12	cal-cium	phos-phorus	magne-sium	iron	zinc
5000	7	3	15	1044	364	10	2	6	6	16	4	3	7	7	18	16	5	5	9
5001	4	1	5	985	173	5	2	4	4	5	4	1	6	1	3	4	1	5	6
5002	41	13	54	1155	564	18	8	3	31	25	29	13	10	20	14	31	8	8	15
5003	1	0	0	723	184	0	0	0	3	4	14	4	2	3	2	8	6	5	3
5004	3	0	0	8	104	0	0	0	3	3	5	4	2	0	1	6	6	3	5
5005	4	1	3	918	357	5	1	2	5	8	2	2	5	1	7	11	9	9	6
5006	0	0	0	39	602	66	1	8	9	4	2	9	18	0	10	11	15	19	9
5007	1	0	5	76	421	2	1	10	13	5	5	8	23	1	4	13	11	12	7
5008	6	2	3	956	403	9	1	3	6	2	3	2	8	1	8	13	11	11	7
5009	7	1	12	341	546	51	4	2	17	8	10	12	13	2	7	15	12	16	10
5010	3	1	5	466	393	24	2	5	9	4	4	6	8	1	9	3	12	14	9
5011	10	4	45	345	512	48	2	11	22	11	14	14	13	4	6	19	12	13	16
5012	4	1	0	445	490	3	2	18	9	7	14	8	14	2	6	12	9	13	6
5013	11	4	12	201	256	0	1	1	10	3	4	3	14	1	4	7	9	11	6
5014	4	1	0	440	487	3	2	18	9	5	14	8	14	2	6	12	9	13	6
5015	6	2	16	714	479	2	1	12	17	7	14	13	14	6	4	13	8	10	7
5016	1	0	2	472	352	3	1	4	9	3	4	4	9	0	7	9	8	9	4
5017	1	0	0	782	130	0	0	0	0	3	9	1	1	3	1	3	1	2	0
5018	1	0	0	72	206	0	0	0	0	4	16	1	1	4	1	7	1	3	2
5019	0	0	0	738	15	0	0	0	0	1	1	0	0	1	0	1	0	0	0
5020	1	0	0	38	11	1	0	0	0	1	0	0	0	0	1	1	1	0	0
5021	0	0	0	475	444	0	1	0	5	13	10	7	19	0	2	7	4	4	3
5022	14	5	117	1324	350	5	2	0	15	20	22	14	9	35	13	28	8	19	23
5023	38	14	156	854	570	0	5	2	6	23	53	23	5	85	5	33	9	26	63
5024	6	4	15	63	351	49	1	13	7	16	14	8	4	11	3	13	1	14	18
5025	3	1	5	956	99	6	0	1	4	3	5	2	4	3	2	5	2	6	11
5026	4	1	48	495	239	28	1	2	8	10	15	9	10	21	2	14	6	13	21
5027	6	2	66	92	419	56	1	4	10	13	13	12	5	44	3	20	7	15	38
5028	3	1	40	55	584	3	1	35	8	11	15	15	6	27	2	17	8	13	23
5029	3	1	15	573	210	17	0	1	6	5	13	8	7	12	2	9	4	7	7
5030	3	1	38	55	582	3	1	35	8	10	15	15	6	27	2	16	8	13	22
5031	4	1	42	522	334	2	0	7	6	10	15	14	4	31	2	17	10	12	25
5032	11	6	50	1044	336	20	5	0	6	13	1	7	4	10	5	12	1	12	18
5033	5	3	14	866	336	26	1	12	4	9	14	7	3	10	3	12	1	13	18
5034	5	2	19	801	315	24	1	11	6	9	14	6	6	10	3	12	2	14	17
5035	5	2	13	801	317	24	1	11	5	8	14	7	6	10	3	12	2	13	17
5036	6	2	24	462	676	30	2	17	10	15	16	15	19	11	4	15	8	9	14
5037	4	1	101	63	144	7	1	1	4	15	3	5	5	7	9	11	4	2	3
5038	4	2	7	496	288	4	1	15	3	5	7	5	12	2	5	6	5	4	2
5039	3	1	27	747	246	0	1	0	7	7	26	9	1	5	1	13	3	5	6
5040	2	0	0	1198	274	5	0	1	5	3	3	5	6	0	4	11	10	12	9
5041	9	2	90	416	733	9	7	20	16	11	25	19	7	173	8	34	18	22	12
5042	9	3	15	886	434	18	6	6	4	14	2	6	7	6	19	16	8	2	5
5043	12	4	15	204	481	26	8	80	8	23	4	8	11	6	26	22	10	5	7
5044	3	1	0	310	307	4	3	21	7	9	6	8	13	26	3	6	3	3	2

Soups, Sauces, Fats, & Misc.

Food #	Food Description & Amount	wt gm	wt oz	calo-ries	%cal fat	prot gm	carbo gm	fiber gm
5045	Cabbage with meat soup [1 cup]	245	8.6	121	35%	14	5	1.4
5046	Carrot soup with rice and milk [1 cup]	245	8.6	88	16%	5	13	1.3
5047	Cauliflower soup, cream of, made with milk [1 cup]	248	8.7	197	55%	8	15	1.5
5048	Carrot soup with milk [1 cup]	237	8.4	60	24%	5	6	1.3
5049	Celery soup, cream of, canned, condensed [½ cup condensed or 1 cup diluted 1:1 with water]	244	8.6	90	56%	2	9	0.8
5050	Celery soup, cream of, made with milk [1 cup]	248	8.7	152	48%	6	15	0.8
5051	Cheddar cheese soup, made with milk [1 cup]	251	8.9	217	54%	9	16	1.0
5052	Cheddar cheese soup, canned, condensed [1 cup condensed]	257	9.1	311	61%	11	21	2.1
5053	Chicken corn soup, home recipe [1 cup]	251	8.9	203	30%	14	25	1.5
5054	Chicken or turkey and mushroom soup, cream of, made with milk [1 cup]	248	8.7	199	53%	8	15	0.3
5055	Chicken, broth, bouillon, or consomme (Include chicken broth powder, reconstituted; Lipton's Trim Chicken Cup-a-Soup) [1 cup]	244	8.6	39	32%	5	1	0.0
5056	Chicken broth, bouillon, or consomme, dry, not reconstituted [1 cube]	4	0.1	11	47%	1	1	0.0
5057	Chicken broth, without tomato, home recipe [1 cup]	240	8.5	86	30%	6	8	0.0
5058	Chicken broth soup stock, Mexican style [1 cup]	242	8.5	130	16%	6	22	2.4
5059	Chicken broth, canned, reduced sodium [1 cup]	240	8.5	17	0%	3	1	0.0
5060	Chicken broth, canned, low sodium (Include Campbell's low sodium chicken broth) [1 cup]	240	8.5	17	13%	2	1	1.0
5061	Chicken gumbo soup [1 cup]	244	8.6	56	23%	3	8	2.0
5062	Chicken noodle soup, canned, condensed (Include chicken and stars soup) [½ cup condensed, or 1 cup diluted 1:1 with water]	241	8.5	75	27%	4	9	0.7
5063	Chicken noodle soup, canned, low sodium, ready-to-serve [1 cup]	246	8.7	76	29%	4	10	0.7
5064	Chicken noodle soup, canned, reduced sodium, ready-to-serve (Include Campbell's, Healthy Choice) [1 cup]	238	8.4	84	24%	8	7	1.0
5065	Chicken noodle soup, chunky style [1 cup]	240	8.5	175	31%	13	17	3.8
5066	Chicken noodle soup, with carrots [1 cup]	241	8.5	128	19%	18	7	1.0
5067	Chicken noodle soup, cream of [1 cup]	245	8.6	136	31%	8	15	0.7
5068	Chicken or turkey soup, cream of, made with milk [1 cup]	248	8.7	178	50%	7	15	0.3
5069	Chicken or turkey soup, cream of, canned, condensed [½ cup condensed or 1 cup diluted 1:1 with water]	244	8.6	117	57%	3	9	0.3
5070	Chicken or turkey soup, cream of, canned, made with water, reduced sodium (Include Campbell's Healthy Request Cream of Chicken Soup) [1 cup]	244	8.6	73	20%	2	12	0.5
5071	Chicken or turkey vegetable soup, stew type (Include chunky style; chicken or turkey vegetable soup with noodles) [1 cup]	240	8.5	170	33%	12	17	1.4
5072	Chicken soup with vegetables (broccoli, carrots, celery, potatoes and onions), oriental style [1 cup]	228	8.0	54	25%	6	4	0.8
5073	Chicken or turkey rice soup, home recipe [1 cup]	231	8.1	161	25%	15	14	0.7
5074	Chicken vegetable soup with noodles, stew type, chunky style [1 cup]	240	8.5	167	29%	11	20	2.8
5075	Chicken vegetable soup with rice, Mexican style (Sopa/Caldo de Pollo) [1 cup]	242	8.5	177	20%	13	22	2.1
5076	Chicken vegetable soup with rice, stew type, chunky style, made with milk [1 cup]	242	8.5	130	26%	9	15	0.8
5077	Chicken or turkey vegetable soup, home recipe [1 cup]	239	8.4	133	26%	14	11	1.4
5078	Chicken rice soup, canned, condensed [1 cup condensed or 1 cup diluted 1:1 with water]	241	8.5	60	29%	4	7	0.6
5079	Chicken rice soup, canned, reduced sodium, ready-to-serve (Include Campbell's) [1 cup]	241	8.5	59	29%	2	8	0.7
5080	Chicken rice soup, chunky style (Include turkey rice soup) [1 cup]	240	8.5	127	23%	12	13	1.0
5081	Chicken rice soup, Puerto Rican style (Sopa de pollo con arroz) [1 cup]	220	7.8	200	39%	16	14	1.0
5082	Chicken soup with dumplings and potatoes [1 cup]	251	8.9	113	41%	6	11	0.9
5083	Chicken soup with dumplings [1 cup]	241	8.5	97	51%	6	6	0.5
5084	Chicken soup with noodles and potatoes, Puerto Rican style [1 cup]	220	7.8	165	29%	14	14	1.1

						% of Daily Value													
Food #	fat gm	sat fat gm	choles mg	sodium mg	potass mg	vit A	vit E	vit C	thia-min	ribo-flavin	nia-cin	vit B-6	fol-ate	vit B-12	cal-cium	phos-phorus	magne-sium	iron	zinc
5045	5	1	31	282	430	3	3	18	30	17	14	15	11	26	3	16	6	6	9
5046	2	1	2	622	268	83	1	2	5	6	13	7	6	4	5	9	3	5	3
5047	12	4	15	193	365	17	5	39	7	20	3	7	9	6	23	20	8	3	6
5048	2	1	2	566	279	89	1	2	2	7	12	6	3	4	5	9	3	3	3
5049	6	1	14	954	123	3	1	0	2	3	2	1	1	1	4	4	2	4	1
5050	8	3	24	1012	313	9	1	2	5	14	2	3	2	7	19	15	6	4	4
5051	13	8	40	1022	345	17	1	2	4	19	3	4	2	7	29	25	5	4	7
5052	21	13	59	1920	308	22	1	0	2	16	4	3	2	0	29	27	2	8	9
5053	7	2	32	460	365	6	2	9	6	14	23	13	15	4	7	18	9	5	10
5054	12	4	20	1033	349	17	0	2	4	18	9	5	2	7	18	14	6	5	10
5055	1	0	0	776	210	0	0	0	1	4	17	1	1	4	1	7	1	3	2
5056	1	0	1	743	12	1	0	0	0	1	0	0	0	0	1	1	1	0	0
5057	3	1	7	343	252	0	0	1	6	12	19	7	13	0	1	6	2	3	2
5058	2	1	5	261	692	81	1	29	10	12	20	16	13	0	2	10	7	7	4
5059	0	0	0	554	204	0	0	2	0	2	8	1	1	2	2	4	1	3	1
5060	0	0	0	379	192	0	0	28	0	1	6	1	1	2	1	3	1	3	1
5061	1	0	5	954	76	1	0	8	2	3	3	3	1	0	2	2	1	5	3
5062	**2**	**1**	**6**	**931**	**55**	**6**	**0**	**0**	**4**	**4**	**8**	**1**	**5**	**3**	**2**	**4**	**2**	**4**	**2**
5063	2	1	7	74	57	7	0	0	3	4	7	1	10	2	2	4	1	4	3
5064	2	1	13	459	303	24	1	4	2	6	20	8	4	4	4	10	3	10	4
5065	6	1	19	850	108	12	3	0	5	10	22	2	10	5	2	7	2	8	6
5066	3	1	61	79	290	49	1	6	8	9	34	13	5	4	2	16	7	6	9
5067	5	2	16	990	245	12	0	2	7	15	8	4	6	9	16	15	5	5	5
5068	10	4	20	1049	278	12	1	2	5	15	5	3	2	7	18	15	5	4	7
5069	7	2	10	990	88	6	1	0	2	4	4	1	0	1	4	4	1	3	4
5070	2	1	8	452	341	15	0	0	0	2	4	1	0	1	2	3	1	1	1
5071	6	2	29	850	168	12	1	2	5	10	21	2	1	4	2	11	2	9	6
5072	1	0	16	567	142	18	1	11	2	4	7	6	3	1	2	5	4	3	4
5073	4	1	38	323	284	31	1	3	8	11	25	11	12	1	2	12	5	7	8
5074	**5**	**1**	**22**	**834**	**449**	**70**	**2**	**11**	**9**	**7**	**20**	**13**	**7**	**2**	**3**	**13**	**7**	**6**	**6**
5075	4	1	27	246	655	70	1	25	11	13	27	18	13	1	3	13	8	8	8
5076	4	1	11	885	259	47	1	5	4	10	12	4	2	6	10	11	4	8	6
5077	4	1	34	511	459	23	4	31	8	11	28	18	12	2	3	13	7	8	8
5078	2	0	6	819	100	7	0	0	1	1	6	1	0	3	2	2	0	4	2
5079	2	1	7	411	204	12	0	54	3	3	10	3	1	2	2	6	2	1	2
5080	3	1	12	888	108	59	0	6	2	6	21	2	1	5	3	7	2	10	6
5081	9	2	52	206	440	2	1	15	7	7	27	16	5	3	2	15	7	7	9
5082	5	1	31	800	210	5	0	6	3	4	10	6	1	3	1	7	3	4	3
5083	6	1	33	865	116	5	0	0	1	4	9	2	1	3	2	6	1	4	3
5084	5	1	48	211	441	1	1	16	9	9	21	14	5	3	2	14	7	7	11

Soups, Sauces, Fats, & Misc.

Food #	Food Description & Amount	wt gm	wt oz	calo-ries	%cal fat	prot gm	carbo gm	fiber gm
5085	Chicken soup [1 cup]	241	8.5	75	30%	4	9	0.7
5086	Chicken soup, canned, undiluted [1 cup]	246	8.7	150	27%	8	19	1.5
5087	Chicken soup with vegetables and fruit, Oriental Style [1 cup]	234	8.3	136	25%	16	9	1.2
5088	Chili beef soup [1 cup]	250	8.8	170	35%	7	21	9.5
5089	Chili beef soup, chunky style [1 cup]	240	8.5	192	34%	16	16	4.5
5090	Chunky pea and ham soup [1 cup]	240	8.5	185	19%	11	27	4.1
5091	Clam chowder, Manhattan (Include chunky style) [1 cup]	240	8.5	106	24%	5	15	2.2
5092	Clam chowder, New England, canned, reduced sodium, ready-to-serve [1 cup]	251	8.9	124	17%	6	20	1.1
5093	**Clam chowder, New England, made with milk [1 cup]**	248	8.7	150	30%	10	17	0.8
5094	Clam chowder, New England, made with water [1 cup]	244	8.6	95	27%	5	12	1.5
5095	Codfish soup with noodles, Puerto Rican style [1 cup]	245	8.6	174	24%	14	18	1.4
5096	Codfish, rice, and vegetable soup, Puerto Rican style [1 cup]	245	8.6	166	22%	13	19	1.0
5097	Corn soup, cream of, made with milk [1 cup]	248	8.7	224	47%	8	24	1.4
5098	Corn soup, cream of, made with water [1 cup]	244	8.6	167	50%	6	16	0.8
5099	Crab soup, made with milk (Include crab bisque, seafood bisque) [1 cup]	248	8.7	235	45%	20	12	0.3
5100	Crab soup, tomato-base [1 cup]	244	8.6	169	38%	14	12	1.1
5101	Cucumber soup, cream of, made with milk [1 cup]	248	8.7	197	56%	7	15	0.5
5102	Duck soup [1 cup]	244	8.6	410	81%	16	2	0.3
5103	**Egg drop soup [1 cup]**	244	8.6	73	47%	8	1	0.0
5104	Escarole soup [1 cup]	245	8.6	252	57%	9	18	1.0
5105	Fish and vegetable soup, Puerto Rican style (Sopa de pescado) [1 cup]	250	8.8	101	21%	16	3	0.6
5106	Fish broth [1 cup]	244	8.6	41	43%	6	0	0.0
5107	Fish chowder (Include fisherman's soup, seafood chowder) [1 cup]	244	8.6	193	25%	24	12	0.7
5108	Fish soup, with potatoes (Sopa de Pescado) [1 cup]	241	8.5	113	18%	16	6	0.6
5109	Fruit soup[1 cup]	242	8.5	176	1%	1	46	3.9
5110	Garbanzo or chickpea soup [1 cup]	253	8.9	208	14%	10	36	9.3
5111	Garlic egg soup, Puerto Rican style (Sopa de ajo) [1 cup]	202	7.1	180	53%	10	11	0.4
5112	**Gazpacho [1 cup]**	244	8.6	46	5%	7	4	0.5
5113	Gazpacho, canned, undiluted [1 can (10.5 oz), undiluted]	298	10.5	57	5%	9	5	0.6
5114	Ham, noodle, and vegetable soup, Puerto Rican style [1 cup]	250	8.8	154	24%	17	12	1.5
5115	Ham, pasta, and vegetable soup [1 cup]	244	8.6	62	14%	5	8	1.6
5116	Ham, rice, and potato soup, Puerto Rican style [1 cup]	240	8.5	157	33%	9	17	1.2
5117	Hot and sour soup (Include hot and spicy Chinese soup) [1 cup]	244	8.6	162	45%	15	5	0.5
5118	**Instant soup, chicken noodle [1 cup]**	240	8.5	55	22%	2	9	0.2
5119	Instant soup, noodle (Include meat and/or vegetable flavors) [1 cup]	240	8.5	47	20%	2	7	0.3
5120	Instant soup, noodle with egg, shrimp or chicken [1 cup]	240	8.5	184	23%	12	23	1.0
5121	Instant soup, rice (Include meat or chicken flavor) [1 cup]	240	8.5	58	21%	2	9	0.7
5122	Instant soup, cream of chicken and/or vegetable [1 cup]	254	9.0	104	46%	2	12	0.4
5123	Lamb, pasta, and vegetable soup, Puerto Rican style [1 cup]	250	8.8	168	39%	13	13	1.9
5124	Leek soup, cream of, made with milk [1 cup]	248	8.7	172	40%	7	19	0.5
5125	Leek soup, made from dry mix [1 cup]	254	9.0	71	26%	2	11	3.0
5126	**Lentil soup [1 cup]**	248	8.7	219	34%	12	26	13.1
5127	Lima bean soup [1 cup]	253	8.9	111	24%	5	17	5.1
5128	Liquid from stewed kidney beans, Puerto Rican style [1 cup]	228	8.0	75	87%	4	6	0.2
5129	Lobster bisque [1 cup]	248	8.7	251	47%	20	13	0.2
5130	Lobster gumbo [1 cup]	244	8.6	178	35%	10	20	3.0
5131	Macaroni and potato soup [1 cup]	244	8.6	211	14%	7	40	3.1
5132	Matzo ball soup [1 cup]	241	8.5	119	42%	7	10	0.4
5133	Meatball soup, Mexican style (Sopa de Albondigas) [1 cup]	237	8.4	195	61%	10	9	1.5
5134	Meat broth, Puerto Rican style (Caldo) [1 cup]	240	8.5	17	28%	3	0	0.0

Food #	fat gm	sat fat gm	choles mg	sodium mg	potass mg	vit A	vit E	vit C	thia-min	ribo-flavin	nia-cin	vit B-6	fol-ate	vit B-12	cal-cium	phos-phorus	magne-sium	iron	zinc
5085	2	1	7	1106	55	7	0	0	4	4	7	1	5	2	2	4	1	4	3
5086	5	1	12	1862	111	13	0	0	9	8	15	3	10	5	3	7	2	8	4
5087	4	1	46	172	261	2	1	11	6	7	19	12	3	2	2	10	6	6	8
5088	7	3	13	1035	525	15	1	7	4	4	5	8	4	5	4	15	8	12	9
5089	7	3	31	407	487	2	1	12	9	10	16	10	21	15	3	16	10	16	18
5090	4	2	7	965	305	49	0	12	8	6	13	11	1	4	3	18	10	12	21
5091	3	1	8	785	284	21	1	13	3	3	7	9	2	99	5	6	4	12	9
5092	2	1	14	558	289	4	2	11	4	6	5	5	2	315	4	9	3	31	5
5093	5	2	15	995	305	6	1	6	4	14	5	6	2	170	19	16	6	8	8
5094	3	0	5	915	146	0	0	3	1	3	5	4	1	133	4	5	2	8	5
5095	5	1	46	199	365	3	3	22	12	6	12	11	12	9	3	18	10	8	5
5096	4	1	27	200	376	3	3	23	10	4	11	13	11	8	3	16	9	7	4
5097	12	4	14	340	397	16	5	10	7	21	6	4	10	6	21	21	9	5	6
5098	9	3	12	649	238	11	3	5	4	12	5	3	5	4	12	12	5	4	5
5099	12	3	85	585	490	15	7	8	11	17	15	10	13	96	25	30	12	6	25
5100	7	1	60	475	527	10	7	33	9	5	15	13	13	73	8	16	9	8	19
5101	12	4	16	193	360	18	5	5	7	20	3	4	5	6	24	20	8	3	6
5102	37	13	89	93	351	6	2	6	15	19	28	10	4	4	2	20	6	19	14
5103	4	1	103	729	220	4	1	0	2	11	15	3	4	8	2	11	1	4	3
5104	16	5	19	780	459	14	6	5	10	27	4	5	10	12	31	25	10	4	8
5105	2	0	29	605	473	3	1	13	5	7	19	10	4	12	7	17	6	4	3
5106	2	0	2	381	351	0	10	0	5	11	14	5	12	28	1	14	4	0	1
5107	5	2	56	180	711	6	1	12	11	16	14	18	4	21	15	30	12	4	7
5108	2	0	29	622	523	1	1	4	5	6	20	12	4	13	7	21	7	4	4
5109	0	0	0	9	392	8	1	3	2	3	3	7	0	0	2	4	5	7	2
5110	3	0	0	18	345	0	1	4	9	6	3	8	26	0	6	17	12	16	11
5111	11	2	160	724	223	7	4	0	7	17	16	4	8	8	5	14	3	8	5
5112	0	0	0	739	224	26	2	12	3	1	5	7	2	0	2	4	2	5	2
5113	0	0	0	903	274	32	2	14	4	2	6	9	3	0	3	4	2	7	2
5114	4	1	38	1052	606	4	2	35	28	11	22	20	6	8	3	20	8	7	12
5115	1	0	8	267	223	21	1	17	10	5	8	6	5	1	3	6	5	5	5
5116	6	2	21	484	294	0	1	6	12	5	12	13	4	3	2	11	6	4	7
5117	8	3	34	1011	384	0	0	1	18	15	25	10	3	7	3	19	7	11	10
5118	1	0	10	550	31	0	0	0	13	4	5	1	4	1	0	3	2	3	1
5119	1	0	6	770	54	0	0	0	10	4	4	1	4	0	1	3	3	2	1
5120	5	1	110	562	218	4	1	1	12	13	20	5	17	9	3	16	6	12	7
5121	1	0	2	931	10	0	0	0	0	0	2	1	0	1	1	1	0	0	1
5122	5	2	1	1148	151	6	2	4	43	9	8	2	2	3	5	7	2	2	6
5123	7	3	42	53	525	5	1	66	8	10	23	13	8	21	3	15	8	10	20
5124	8	3	25	1016	313	9	3	4	6	16	3	4	3	7	18	15	6	4	4
5125	2	1	3	965	89	0	1	4	3	1	1	1	2	0	3	3	3	3	2
5126	8	3	5	48	330	20	2	6	7	5	4	8	17	0	3	17	10	17	10
5127	3	1	3	89	418	42	1	6	7	3	3	7	13	0	4	9	11	9	5
5128	7	3	9	5	930	0	0	0	15	12	4	3	19	1	3	20	21	25	7
5129	13	4	63	450	548	20	7	3	6	21	5	7	5	43	28	31	12	3	18
5130	7	1	23	441	607	18	7	45	14	7	11	10	21	17	11	13	14	9	10
5131	3	1	7	65	716	5	1	34	15	11	12	25	8	4	12	16	12	4	6
5132	5	1	63	757	190	2	2	0	5	10	15	2	5	5	3	9	2	7	3
5133	13	5	54	145	441	54	2	18	6	10	15	10	8	14	3	11	6	8	12
5134	1	0	0	782	130	0	0	0	0	3	9	1	1	3	1	3	1	2	0

% of Daily Value

Soups, Sauces, Fats, & Misc.

Food #	Food Description & Amount	wt gm	wt oz	calo-ries	%cal fat	prot gm	carbo gm	fiber gm
5135	Minestrone soup, canned, reduced sodium, ready-to-serve (Include Campbell's, Healthy Choice, Progresso) [1 cup]	239	8.4	120	14%	5	22	5.7
5136	Minestrone soup, home recipe [1 cup]	235	8.3	234	49%	9	22	3.8
5137	Meat and hominy soup, Mexican style (Pozole) [1 cup]	238	8.4	188	31%	16	15	1.5
5138	Mushroom soup, cream of, canned, condensed [½ cup condensed or 1 cup diluted 1:1 with water]	244	8.6	129	66%	2	9	0.4
5139	Mushroom soup, made from dry mix [1 cup]	253	8.9	96	45%	2	11	0.8
5140	Mushroom soup, with meat broth, made with water (Include Campbell's Beefy Mushroom) [1 cup]	244	8.6	85	42%	3	9	0.1
5141	Mushroom with chicken soup, cream of, made with milk [1 cup]	248	8.7	199	53%	8	15	0.3
5142	Noodle and potato soup, Puerto Rican style [1 cup]	245	8.6	72	5%	2	16	2.0
5143	Noodle soup with vegetables, made with milk [1 cup]	248	8.7	175	30%	10	21	0.9
5144	Noodle soup with vegetables, Oriental style (Include pai-cue-me Chinese soup) [1 cup]	228	8.0	112	25%	6	14	0.7
5145	Noodle soup with fish ball, shrimp, and dark green leafy vegetable [1 cup]	234	8.3	164	32%	11	16	1.2
5146	Onion soup, cream of, canned, condensed, undiluted [1 cup]	251	8.9	221	43%	6	26	1.0
5147	Onion soup, cream of, made with milk [1 cup]	248	8.7	172	40%	7	19	0.5
5148	Onion soup, dry mix, not reconstituted [1 pkg (1.5 oz)]	39	1.4	115	18%	5	21	4.1
5149	Onion soup, French [1 cup]	241	8.5	58	27%	4	8	1.0
5150	Onion soup, made from dry mix [1 cup]	246	8.7	27	19%	1	5	1.0
5151	Oxtail soup [1 cup]	244	8.6	68	32%	3	9	0.5
5152	Oyster stew [1 cup]	245	8.6	211	57%	12	11	0.0
5153	Pea soup, canned, low sodium, made with water [1 cup]	250	8.8	165	16%	9	27	0.8
5154	Pea soup, instant type [1 cup]	271	9.6	133	11%	8	23	3.0
5155	Pea soup, made with milk [1 cup]	254	9.0	226	22%	13	32	2.9
5156	Pea soup, made with lowfat milk [1 cup]	254	9.0	219	19%	13	32	2.9
5157	Pea soup, made with water [1 cup]	250	8.8	165	16%	9	27	2.8
5158	Pepperpot (tripe) soup (Include menudo; mondongo soup; pork, potatoes, yuca) [1 cup]	241	8.5	104	40%	6	9	0.5
5159	Pigeon pea asopao [1 cup]	250	8.8	245	26%	10	38	6.2
5160	Pinto bean soup [1 cup]	253	8.9	191	3%	11	36	12.6
5161	Plantain soup, Puerto Rican style (Sopa de platano) [1 cup]	245	8.6	97	11%	6	18	1.3
5162	Pork, rice, and vegetable soup [1 cup]	244	8.6	124	32%	12	8	0.7
5163	Pork, vegetable soup with potatoes, stew type [1 cup]	240	8.5	136	16%	13	17	4.2
5164	Pork with vegetable (no carrots, broccoli, or dark-green leafy) soup, asian style [1 cup]	228	8.0	77	35%	11	1	0.5
5165	Portuguese bean soup [1 cup]	253	8.9	145	10%	9	25	5.8
5166	Potato soup, instant, made from dry mix (Include Lipton's) [1 cup]	249	8.8	68	8%	2	15	1.5
5167	Potato soup, made with milk [1 cup]	248	8.7	136	32%	6	17	0.5
5168	Potato soup, made with water [1 cup]	244	8.6	74	29%	2	11	0.5
5169	Potato and cheese soup [1 cup]	248	8.7	187	39%	10	19	1.1
5170	Potato chowder (Include corn chowder) [1 cup]	248	8.7	220	55%	7	19	1.3
5171	Ramen noodle soup, instant (Include all flavors; spaghetti soup, Top Ramen, Oriental Noodle Soup, saimin soup) [1 cup]	244	8.6	165	38%	4	22	1.2
5172	Rice and potato soup, Puerto Rican style [1 cup]	245	8.6	185	23%	4	31	1.1
5173	Rice soup, made with tea [1 cup]	241	8.5	75	17%	2	14	0.7
5174	Salmon soup, cream style [1 cup]	248	8.7	261	44%	28	7	0.2
5175	Scotch broth (lamb, vegetables, and barley) [1 cup]	241	8.5	80	30%	5	9	1.2
5176	Seafood soup with potatoes and vegetables (no carrots, broccoli, or dark-green leafy) [1 cup]	244	8.6	160	14%	20	13	1.2
5177	Seafood soup with [above] vegetables without potatoes [1 cup]	244	8.6	154	15%	21	12	1.3
5178	Seafood soup with potatoes and vegetables (including carrots, broccoli, and/or dark-green leafy) [1 cup]	244	8.6	151	14%	21	11	1.3
5179	Seafood soup with [above] vegetables except potatoes [1 cup]	244	8.6	143	15%	20	9	1.6

Food #	fat gm	sat fat gm	choles mg	sodium mg	potass mg	vit A	vit E	vit C	thia-min	ribo-flavin	nia-cin	vit B-6	fol-ate	vit B-12	cal-cium	phos-phorus	magne-sium	iron	zinc
													% of Daily Value					
5135	2	0	0	514	445	20	1	23	10	6	8	7	13	0	5	8	8	10	5
5136	13	4	9	494	584	19	3	14	16	14	14	12	33	0	4	15	11	13	7
5137	6	2	42	408	318	1	1	2	11	15	25	12	11	2	2	14	6	8	14
5138	10	3	1	872	84	0	4	2	2	5	4	1	1	2	3	4	2	3	4
5139	5	1	0	1020	200	0	2	2	19	7	3	1	1	4	7	8	1	3	1
5140	4	2	8	974	158	13	0	2	2	6	6	2	2	0	1	4	2	5	9
5141	12	4	20	1032	349	17	0	2	4	18	9	5	2	7	18	14	6	5	10
5142	0	0	3	14	364	6	2	31	7	4	6	9	6	0	3	5	6	4	3
5143	6	3	28	122	354	32	2	3	10	21	4	7	9	10	25	23	9	5	7
5144	3	1	17	833	177	2	1	3	7	6	16	3	11	3	2	9	4	7	4
5145	6	1	46	638	327	3	2	7	9	8	18	7	11	7	3	15	6	9	5
5146	11	3	30	1908	246	6	6	4	7	9	5	3	4	2	7	8	3	7	2
5147	8	3	25	1016	313	9	3	4	6	16	3	4	3	7	18	15	6	4	4
5148	2	1	2	3493	260	0	1	1	7	14	10	2	2	0	5	13	6	3	2
5149	2	0	0	1053	67	0	1	2	2	1	3	2	4	0	3	1	1	4	4
5150	1	0	0	849	64	0	0	0	2	3	2	0	0	0	1	3	1	1	0
5151	2	1	2	1166	81	0	0	0	2	1	4	1	1	4	1	6	2	1	0
5152	13	8	80	341	394	18	3	6	9	20	6	6	3	255	24	26	15	32	516
5153	3	1	0	25	190	2	0	3	7	4	6	3	1	0	3	13	10	11	11
5154	2	0	3	1220	238	1	0	0	15	9	7	2	11	5	2	13	12	6	4
5155	5	3	10	979	381	8	1	4	10	15	6	5	2	6	18	24	14	11	15
5156	5	2	7	977	384	9	1	4	10	15	6	5	2	6	18	24	14	11	15
5157	3	1	0	918	190	2	0	3	7	4	6	3	0	0	3	13	10	11	11
5158	5	2	10	971	152	9	0	2	4	3	6	3	2	3	2	4	1	5	8
5159	7	2	8	226	855	9	3	68	27	13	14	11	36	1	5	17	22	12	9
5160	1	0	0	11	528	0	0	6	14	6	4	9	33	0	7	20	17	16	8
5161	1	1	0	1429	508	6	0	16	2	7	19	10	5	5	3	8	7	6	1
5162	4	2	41	55	206	30	1	2	17	8	13	10	4	4	2	10	4	6	13
5163	2	1	20	668	681	54	2	50	20	10	18	18	10	3	6	16	11	11	10
5164	3	1	30	34	318	0	1	2	20	8	12	11	1	4	1	12	3	3	9
5165	2	1	5	25	586	56	3	18	11	6	7	10	16	0	4	14	13	14	8
5166	1	0	2	129	249	0	0	5	1	3	4	2	2	0	4	6	4	3	2
5167	5	3	16	1063	327	9	1	2	5	14	3	4	2	7	17	16	4	3	7
5168	2	1	6	1004	137	3	0	0	2	2	3	2	1	2	5	5	1	3	4
5169	8	5	25	169	554	12	1	16	7	20	5	10	5	9	29	24	9	4	8
5170	13	5	20	232	484	8	1	15	7	15	6	10	5	7	16	17	8	3	6
5171	7	2	0	862	53	0	8	0	2	1	1	1	1	0	1	3	3	2	1
5172	5	2	7	188	176	1	1	10	13	2	9	7	13	1	2	6	5	8	4
5173	1	0	0	14	147	21	2	1	5	2	3	4	9	0	1	3	4	4	2
5174	13	3	75	1541	526	6	6	1	3	17	48	20	6	93	29	46	11	9	11
5175	3	1	5	1012	159	22	0	2	1	3	6	4	2	4	1	6	1	5	11
5176	3	1	42	248	645	1	1	11	11	12	23	18	12	13	3	21	10	5	5
5177	3	1	43	255	575	2	1	7	11	12	22	16	12	13	3	21	10	5	5
5178	2	1	42	257	707	15	2	16	10	13	22	20	18	13	5	21	13	8	5
5179	2	1	42	264	658	71	3	13	10	14	22	18	18	13	5	21	13	7	5

Soups, Sauces, Fats, & Misc.

Food #	Food Description & Amount	wt gm	wt oz	calo-ries	%cal fat	prot gm	carbo gm	fiber gm
5180	Seaweed soup [1 cup]	230	8.1	83	40%	8	6	0.6
5181	Shav soup [1 cup]	240	8.5	58	59%	2	4	0.9
5182	Shrimp gumbo [1 cup]	244	8.6	170	36%	10	19	2.7
5183	Shrimp soup, cream of, made with milk (Include shrimp bisque) [1 cup]	248	8.7	266	47%	22	13	0.2
5184	Shrimp soup, cream of, made with water [1 cup]	244	8.6	90	52%	3	8	0.2
5185	Sopa seca (dry soup) [1 cup]	218	7.7	340	42%	7	43	2.2
5186	Sopa seca de arroz (dry rice soup) [1 cup]	218	7.7	351	39%	6	47	2.0
5187	Sopa Seca de Fideo (dry pasta soup) [1 cup]	218	7.7	328	45%	8	38	2.4
5188	Sopa de Fideo Aguada, Mexican style noodle soup [1 cup]	242	8.5	194	39%	8	22	0.9
5189	Sopa de tortilla, Mexican style tortilla soup [1 cup]	240	8.5	238	52%	10	19	1.4
5190	Sour cherry soup [1 cup]	242	8.5	208	31%	3	35	1.3
5191	Soybean soup, made with milk [1 cup]	253	8.9	213	53%	14	13	3.7
5192	Soybean soup, miso broth [1 cup]	240	8.5	85	36%	6	8	2.0
5193	Spanish vegetable soup, Puerto Rican style (Caldo gallego) [1 cup]	250	8.8	289	57%	18	13	2.6
5194	Spinach soup, cream of [1 cup]	245	8.6	204	54%	9	16	1.7
5195	Split pea soup [1 cup]	250	8.8	165	16%	9	27	2.8
5196	Split pea soup, canned, reduced sodium, prepared with water or ready-to-serve (Include Progresso Healthy Classics Split Pea Soup) [1 cup]	250	8.8	178	12%	10	30	4.8
5197	Split pea and ham soup [1 cup]	253	8.9	195	19%	12	28	4.3
5198	Split pea and ham soup, canned, reduced sodium, prepared with water or ready-to-serve (Include Campbell's Health Request Split Pea with Ham Soup) [1 cup]	253	8.9	172	9%	10	29	4.8
5199	Sweet and sour soup [1 cup]	244	8.6	72	10%	3	14	1.6
5200	Tomato beef noodle soup, made with water [1 cup]	244	8.6	139	28%	4	21	1.5
5201	Tomato beef rice soup, made with water [1 cup]	244	8.6	126	21%	3	22	1.6
5202	Tomato beef soup, made with water [1 cup]	244	8.6	139	28%	4	21	1.5
5203	Tomato noodle soup, cream of (Include tomato macaroni made with milk) [1 cup]	248	8.7	185	28%	7	28	2.7
5204	Tomato noodle soup, made with water (Include tomato macaroni soup) [1 cup]	244	8.6	144	15%	4	27	1.0
5205	Tomato rice soup, canned, undiluted [1 can undiluted]	312	11.0	290	21%	5	53	4.1
5206	Tomato rice soup, made with water (Include Spanish rice soup) [1 cup]	247	8.7	119	21%	2	22	1.5
5207	Tomato soup, canned, low sodium, ready-to-serve (Include condensed made with water) [1 can ready-to-serve]	298	10.5	104	21%	2	20	0.6
5208	Tomato soup, canned, condensed, undiluted [1 cup]	251	8.9	171	20%	4	33	1.0
5209	Tomato soup, cream of (Include tomato bisque, canned tomato soup prepared with milk) [1 cup]	248	8.7	147	27%	6	22	0.5
5210	Tomato soup, instant type, made with water [1 cup]	265	9.3	103	21%	2	19	0.5
5211	Tomato soup, made with water [1 cup]	244	8.6	85	20%	2	17	0.5
5212	Tomato vegetable soup with noodles, made with water [1 cup]	241	8.5	72	24%	2	12	0.5
5213	Tomato vegetable soup, made with water [1 cup]	241	8.5	53	14%	2	10	0.5
5214	Turkey noodle soup [1 cup]	244	8.6	69	26%	4	9	0.8
5215	Turkey noodle soup, home recipe [1 cup]	244	8.6	149	18%	21	8	1.2
5216	Turkey noodle soup, chunky style [1 cup]	236	8.3	177	28%	15	16	1.3
5217	Turtle and vegetable soup (Include snapper soup) [1 cup]	244	8.6	118	32%	13	4	0.7
5218	Vegetable bean soup, made with water (Include minestrone) [1 cup]	241	8.5	83	27%	4	11	1.0
5219	Vegetable beef noodle soup, made with water [1 cup]	244	8.6	81	28%	5	10	0.6
5220	Vegetable beef soup, home recipe [1 cup]	241	8.5	231	47%	16	15	2.5
5221	Vegetable beef soup, made with lowfat milk [1 cup]	248	8.7	141	28%	10	16	2.0
5222	Vegetable beef soup with noodles or pasta, home recipe [1 cup]	241	8.5	245	42%	16	20	2.6
5223	Vegetable beef soup with rice, home recipe [1 cup]	244	8.6	242	43%	16	19	2.5
5224	Vegetable beef soup, chunky style [1 cup]	240	8.5	157	26%	11	18	2.8
5225	Vegetable beef soup, canned, undiluted [1 can]	305	10.8	192	22%	14	25	4.9

Food #	fat gm	sat fat gm	choles mg	sodium mg	potass mg	vit A	vit E	vit C	thia-min	ribo-flavin	nia-cin	vit B-6	fol-ate	vit B-12	cal-cium	phos-phorus	magne-sium	iron	zinc
5180	4	1	14	1149	223	2	3	4	3	12	14	4	21	12	10	11	16	12	10
5181	4	1	157	18	61	21	3	11	2	6	1	4	11	5	5	7	2	4	3
5182	7	1	51	343	516	16	6	42	13	6	13	10	19	5	10	13	13	13	6
5183	14	4	130	311	454	19	7	6	7	20	11	8	3	22	27	34	13	11	11
5184	5	3	17	976	59	1	3	0	1	2	2	2	1	10	2	3	2	3	5
5185	16	4	7	631	417	8	9	21	22	9	21	10	21	1	3	11	8	15	6
5186	15	4	7	614	402	8	9	20	19	5	19	11	23	1	3	10	7	16	6
5187	16	4	7	649	433	8	9	21	25	13	23	9	19	1	3	11	9	14	5
5188	8	1	7	322	365	3	5	15	15	16	24	10	19	0	1	9	5	7	4
5189	14	4	19	346	349	5	4	11	7	15	17	10	15	2	13	18	7	5	6
5190	7	4	80	20	125	13	1	2	4	7	1	4	3	4	5	6	3	4	2
5191	13	3	8	352	555	6	7	9	9	20	8	10	10	6	18	26	15	18	8
5192	3	1	0	988	361	45	2	7	4	9	13	8	14	3	6	10	9	10	6
5193	18	6	63	561	603	2	1	35	10	10	24	16	8	11	5	18	10	11	16
5194	12	4	14	636	596	60	6	13	11	29	4	12	26	9	32	22	21	15	8
5195	3	1	0	918	190	2	0	3	7	4	6	3	0	0	3	13	10	11	11
5196	2	1	5	415	458	18	1	0	12	4	6	9	13	0	4	14	9	11	7
5197	4	2	8	1017	321	51	1	12	8	6	13	11	1	4	4	19	10	13	22
5198	2	1	8	496	516	22	1	4	14	6	9	6	12	1	4	14	9	10	8
5199	1	0	5	1292	227	3	2	28	6	4	5	6	4	0	3	4	4	3	2
5200	4	2	5	917	220	5	3	0	6	5	9	4	5	3	2	6	2	6	5
5201	3	1	1	1185	388	7	3	24	4	4	10	4	4	1	3	5	2	5	3
5202	4	2	5	917	220	5	3	0	6	5	9	4	5	3	2	6	2	6	5
5203	6	3	26	642	396	10	8	97	12	14	9	8	10	7	14	15	6	12	3
5204	2	0	20	528	215	6	6	83	12	5	10	5	12	1	2	7	4	13	4
5205	7	1	3	1981	802	18	6	60	10	7	13	9	9	0	6	8	3	11	8
5206	3	1	2	815	331	8	3	25	4	3	5	4	3	0	2	3	1	4	3
5207	2	0	0	60	322	8	10	135	8	4	9	7	4	0	1	4	2	12	2
5208	4	1	0	1391	527	14	17	222	12	6	14	11	7	0	3	7	4	20	3
5209	4	2	10	757	454	13	9	113	9	14	8	8	5	6	16	15	6	10	5
5210	2	1	0	943	294	8	3	8	4	3	4	5	2	1	5	7	3	2	1
5211	2	0	0	699	264	7	8	111	6	3	7	6	3	0	2	3	2	10	2
5212	2	0	0	822	210	30	3	2	4	3	5	3	3	0	2	3	2	6	3
5213	1	0	0	1092	99	2	3	10	4	3	4	2	2	0	1	3	5	3	1
5214	2	1	5	819	75	3	0	0	5	4	7	2	5	3	1	5	2	5	4
5215	3	1	66	86	398	56	2	4	9	12	23	18	6	5	3	21	8	10	16
5216	5	1	59	531	229	30	1	2	8	9	18	11	9	4	3	14	6	10	10
5217	4	1	59	472	281	4	3	12	6	9	8	5	5	9	7	12	5	6	4
5218	3	1	1	915	313	23	2	2	3	3	5	5	8	0	4	6	2	5	5
5219	2	1	5	871	137	13	1	2	4	3	5	4	4	2	4	4	1	6	10
5220	12	5	47	255	621	20	1	21	10	16	15	16	14	16	3	17	9	14	29
5221	4	2	15	854	364	25	0	5	5	14	6	6	4	11	16	16	6	7	13
5222	11	4	52	234	573	18	1	19	13	15	16	15	17	15	3	18	10	15	27
5223	12	5	45	244	600	19	1	20	12	15	16	16	16	16	3	17	9	14	28
5224	4	2	22	893	384	53	2	16	10	10	14	13	8	9	3	13	7	11	17
5225	5	2	12	1925	421	46	0	10	6	7	13	9	6	13	4	10	4	15	25

Soups, Sauces, Fats, & Misc.

Food #	Food Description & Amount	wt gm	wt oz	calo-ries	%cal fat	prot gm	carbo gm	fiber gm
5226	Vegetable beef soup, made with water (Include vegetable with meat soups) [1 cup]	244	8.6	79	22%	6	10	2.0
5227	Vegetable beef soup with rice, made with water or ready-to-serve [1 cup]	244	8.6	96	17%	6	15	0.5
5228	**Vegetable broth, bouillon** (Include onion broth, pot liquor) [1 cup]	**240**	**8.5**	**17**	**1%**	**2**	**2**	**0.0**
5229	Vegetable chicken or turkey soup, canned, undiluted [1 cup]	246	8.7	149	36%	7	17	1.5
5230	Vegetable chicken or turkey soup, made with water or ready-to-serve [1 can ready-to-serve]	298	10.5	92	36%	4	11	0.9
5231	Vegetable chicken soup, canned, made with water, low sodium [1 cup]	241	8.5	166	26%	12	19	1.0
5232	Vegetable noodle soup, home recipe [1 cup]	241	8.5	121	37%	5	15	1.9
5233	Vegetable noodle soup, canned, reduced sodium, prepared with water or ready-to-serve [1 cup]	244	8.6	99	10%	4	18	3.4
5234	Vegetable chicken rice soup, made with water or ready-to-serve [1 cup]	241	8.5	67	32%	4	8	0.8
5235	Vegetable chicken noodle soup, made with water or ready-to-serve [1 cup]	241	8.5	75	31%	4	9	0.8
5236	Vegetable noodle soup, made with water (Include vegetable with dumplings, alphabet vegetable soup) [1 cup]	241	8.5	72	24%	2	12	0.6
5237	Vegetable rice soup, made with water [1 cup]	241	8.5	106	15%	3	20	0.7
5238	Vegetable soup, home recipe [1 cup]	234	8.3	100	40%	4	12	2.1
5239	Vegetable soup, canned, low sodium, made with water or ready-to-serve [1 cup]	241	8.5	78	12%	3	15	2.5
5240	Vegetable soup, canned, condensed [½ cup condensed or 1 cup diluted 1:1 with water]	241	8.5	81	21%	3	13	1.6
5241	**Vegetable soup, chunky style** [1 cup]	**240**	**8.5**	**122**	**27%**	**4**	**19**	**1.2**
5242	Vegetable soup, cream of, made with milk [1 cup]	248	8.7	211	42%	9	22	0.7
5243	Vegetable soup, dark leafy-greens, with meat, oriental style [1 cup]	228	8.0	52	30%	7	2	1.0
5244	Vegetable soup, cream of, made from dry mix, low sodium, made with water [1 cup]	260	9.2	168	3%	19	22	1.4
5245	Vegetable soup, dark leafy-greens, meatless, asian style [1 cup]	226	8.0	38	93%	0	1	0.5
5246	Vegetable soup, dry mix, not reconstituted [1Tbs]	1	0.0	4	14%	0	1	0.0
5247	Vegetable soup, made from dry mix [1 cup]	253	8.9	53	19%	3	8	0.5
5248	Vegetable soup, made from dry mix, low sodium (Include Hain brand) [1 cup]	253	8.9	56	12%	2	10	0.5
5249	Vegetable soup, Spanish style, stew type [1 cup]	227	8.0	192	33%	14	18	4.4
5250	Vegetable soup with chicken broth, Mexican style (Sopa Ranchera) [1 cup]	232	8.2	140	42%	6	16	1.7
5251	Vegetable soup with pasta, chunky style (Include Campbell's Chunky Mediterranean Vegetable) [1 cup]	240	8.5	127	20%	5	21	5.8
5252	Vegetarian bouillon, dry [1 cube]	4	0.1	13	14%	0	2	0.1
5253	Vegetarian vegetable soup, canned, condensed (½ cup condensed or 1 cup diluted 1:1 with water]	241	8.5	72	24%	2	12	0.6
5254	Vichyssoise soup [1 cup]	248	8.7	136	32%	6	17	0.5
5255	Watercress soup [1 cup]	245	8.6	26	14%	5	0	0.1
5256	White bean soup, Puerto Rican style (Sopon de habichuelas blancas) [1 cup]	275	9.7	242	26%	9	36	3.9
5257	Won-Ton soup [1 cup]	241	8.5	182	35%	14	14	0.9
5258	Zucchini soup, cream of [1 cup]	248	8.7	169	53%	6	14	1.3
	Sauces, Gravies, Dips							
5300	Alfredo sauce [½ cup]	122	4.3	126	61%	4	9	0.5
5301	Barbecue sauce (Include Szechwan sauce) [½ cup]	125	4.4	94	22%	2	16	1.5
5302	Black bean sauce [½ cup]	138	4.9	129	43%	3	14	2.0
5303	Cheese sauce, homemade with lowfat cheese [½ cup]	122	4.3	161	51%	11	8	0.1
5304	Cheese sauce, made by milk added to dehydrated cheese sauce [½ cup]	122	4.3	134	50%	7	10	0.4
5305	Clam sauce, white [½ cup]	120	4.2	301	64%	21	5	0.2
5306	Cranberry-raspberry sauce [½ cup]	140	4.9	219	1%	0	57	2.7
5307	**Cocktail sauce** [½ cup]	**137**	**4.8**	**119**	**7%**	**2**	**30**	**3.8**
5308	Duck sauce (Include hoisin sauce) [2Tbs]	30	1.1	70	52%	0	7	0.0
5309	Enchilada sauce, green [½ cup]	125	4.4	93	69%	2	7	1.9
5310	Enchilada sauce, red [½ cup]	125	4.4	161	88%	1	5	1.0

Food #	fat gm	sat fat gm	choles mg	sodium mg	potass mg	vit A	vit E	vit C	thia-min	ribo-flavin	nia-cin	vit B-6	fol-ate	vit B-12	cal-cium	phos-phorus	magne-sium	iron	zinc
						% of Daily Value													

Food #	fat gm	sat fat gm	choles mg	sodium mg	potass mg	vit A	vit E	vit C	thia-min	ribo-flavin	nia-cin	vit B-6	fol-ate	vit B-12	cal-cium	phos-phorus	magne-sium	iron	zinc
5226	2	1	5	795	173	19	0	4	2	3	5	4	3	5	2	4	2	6	11
5227	2	1	5	801	167	18	1	4	2	3	5	4	3	5	2	5	2	6	10
5228	0	0	0	3180	55	0	0	0	0	1	3	1	1	2	1	4	2	1	0
5229	6	2	10	1857	331	51	1	2	5	6	11	5	2	5	3	8	2	9	7
5230	4	1	6	1149	204	32	0	1	3	4	7	3	1	3	2	5	2	6	4
5231	5	1	17	84	369	60	0	9	3	10	17	5	3	4	3	11	2	8	14
5232	5	1	8	413	470	26	4	16	9	11	11	10	18	0	4	9	7	7	4
5233	1	0	3	465	301	22	1	4	14	7	9	5	11	0	5	8	8	7	3
5234	2	1	8	880	128	17	0	1	2	2	6	2	1	2	2	3	1	4	2
5235	3	1	7	940	105	17	0	1	3	4	7	2	3	2	2	4	2	5	2
5236	2	0	0	827	210	30	1	2	4	3	5	3	3	0	2	3	2	6	3
5237	2	0	0	840	192	26	1	2	4	3	5	4	2	0	2	4	3	6	4
5238	5	1	0	395	534	26	4	19	7	10	10	11	15	0	4	8	7	6	4
5239	1	0	0	468	522	30	6	2	9	7	9	10	4	0	3	5	8	4	3
5240	2	0	1	814	192	21	0	3	3	3	5	3	2	0	2	4	2	5	6
5241	4	1	0	1010	396	59	2	10	5	4	6	10	4	0	6	7	2	9	21
5242	10	4	19	1197	441	11	4	8	80	27	3	5	4	9	30	27	10	4	8
5243	2	1	17	476	234	15	2	34	12	6	9	9	15	3	4	7	7	4	4
5244	1	0	2	600	583	10	0	27	9	32	3	7	9	10	33	29	12	13	10
5245	4	1	0	20	96	11	4	6	1	2	1	2	6	0	2	1	4	3	1
5246	0	0	0	81	7	0	0	1	0	0	0	0	0	0	0	0	0	0	0
5247	1	1	0	1002	76	2	0	2	2	2	2	3	2	4	1	4	6	5	2
5248	1	1	0	51	104	2	3	10	3	3	4	3	3	0	1	3	5	4	1
5249	7	2	28	346	588	28	2	37	12	9	15	16	12	15	4	17	10	12	15
5250	7	2	10	235	430	7	4	33	9	11	17	11	13	0	2	9	7	5	3
5251	3	1	5	864	612	43	2	8	4	7	6	12	13	0	6	11	4	10	10
5252	0	0	0	269	24	0	0	2	1	1	1	1	1	0	0	1	1	1	0
5253	2	0	0	827	210	30	1	2	4	3	5	3	3	0	2	3	2	6	3.
5254	5	3	16	1063	327	9	1	2	5	14	3	4	2	8	17	16	4	3	7
5255	0	0	35	92	63	3	1	4	1	1	3	2	0	4	2	5	3	3	2
5256	7	2	9	184	504	1	1	19	15	4	10	10	20	1	6	11	11	17	9
5257	7	2	53	543	316	10	1	6	27	15	23	10	8	7	3	15	5	10	7
5258	10	3	13	159	453	16	4	8	7	18	4	6	6	5	20	19	10	3	5
5300	9	3	13	613	60	4	3	0	2	1	2	2	7	1	11	10	2	1	3
5301	2	0	0	1019	218	11	5	15	3	1	6	5	1	0	2	3	6	6	2
5302	6	1	0	861	187	1	3	4	5	3	2	3	9	0	3	5	5	5	3
5303	9	3	18	612	201	11	3	2	5	16	2	3	3	9	33	37	5	3	10
5304	7	4	23	682	241	5	0	2	4	14	1	3	1	8	25	19	5	1	3
5305	21	3	56	94	534	14	11	32	9	21	14	5	6	1372	8	28	4	131	15
5306	0	0	0	25	60	0	1	11	1	3	2	1	1	0	1	1	2	2	1
5307	1	0	0	1254	551	10	5	32	6	5	7	10	8	0	3	5	7	5	3
5308	4	1	4	1	36	0	0	11	1	0	0	0	1	0	0	0	0	0	0
5309	7	4	22	15	270	8	1	19	3	5	7	5	2	1	4	6	5	3	2
5310	16	8	46	18	168	17	3	17	3	4	2	4	2	1	3	4	3	2	1

Soups, Sauces, Fats, & Misc.

Food #	Food Description & Amount	wt gm	wt oz	calories	%cal fat	prot gm	carbo gm	fiber gm
5311	Fish sauce (Include bagoong) [½ cup]	136	4.8	48	0%	7	5	0.0
5312	Green tomato-chile sauce, cooked (Include Salsa verde) [½ cup]	123	4.3	91	69%	1	7	2.4
5313	Green tomato-chile sauce, raw (Include Salsa de tomate verde cruda) [½ cup]	120	4.2	31	24%	1	6	1.9
5314	Hoisin sauce [2Tbs]	36	1.3	79	14%	1	16	1.0
5315	Lobster sauce [½ cup]	117	4.1	193	57%	12	7	0.7
5316	Miso [2Tbs]	34	1.2	70	27%	4	10	1.8
5317	Miso sauce [½ cup]	120	4.2	188	16%	6	35	2.9
5318	**Mole poblano (sauce) [½ cup]**	133	4.7	157	66%	5	11	2.4
5319	Mole verde (sauce) [½ cup]	133	4.7	119	56%	7	8	1.9
5320	Natto [½ cup]	88	3.1	186	47%	16	13	4.7
5321	Oyster sauce (Include scalloped oysters) [½ cup]	128	4.5	163	58%	7	10	0.2
5322	Oyster-flavored sauce [½ cup]	117	4.1	62	0%	0	16	0.1
5323	Peanut sauce [2Tbs]	28	1.0	87	76%	4	3	0.9
5324	Plum sauce, asian-style [2Tbs]	39	1.4	78	2%	0	20	0.4
5325	Puerto Rican ground seasoning [½ cup]	120	4.2	94	71%	1	7	1.7
5326	Salsa, cruda (uncooked salsa, tomato, pepper, onion, coriander) [½ cup]	120	4.2	22	11%	1	5	1.3
5327	Salsa, cooked (Include salsa de chile rojo; taco or creole or picante sauce) (½ cup)	137	4.8	30	9%	2	7	2.6
5328	Salsa, red, cooked, homemade [½ cup]	117	4.1	105	80%	1	5	1.2
5329	Sofrito, Puerto Rican seasoning [½ cup]	120	4.2	307	78%	10	7	1.6
5330	**Soy sauce (Include shoyu) [2Tbs]**	36	1.3	19	1%	2	3	0.3
5331	Soy sauce, low sodium [2Tbs]	36	1.3	19	1%	2	3	0.3
5332	Spaghetti sauce (Include marinara sauce, cacciatore sauce, pizza sauce, spaghetti sauce with mushrooms) [1 cup]	250	8.8	143	33%	4	21	4.0
5333	Spaghetti sauce, fat free [1 cup]	250	8.8	103	16%	2	22	3.5
5334	Spaghetti sauce with meat, canned, no extra meat added [1 cup]	250	8.8	178	39%	7	19	3.8
5335	Spaghetti sauce, low sodium (Include marinara sauce, cacciatore sauce, pizza sauce, spaghetti sauce with mushrooms) [1 cup]	250	8.8	273	40%	5	40	7.5
5336	Steak sauce, tomato-base (Include A1 sauce) [2Tbs]	31	1.1	19	3%	0	5	0.5
5337	Sweet and sour sauce (Include Vietnamese sauce) [2Tbs]	30	1.1	28	0%	0	7	0.0
5338	**Tartar sauce [1Tbs]**	29	1.0	148	90%	0	4	0.1
5339	Tartar sauce, low calorie [1Tbs]	28	1.0	62	73%	0	5	0.1
5340	Teriyaki sauce [½ cup]	144	5.1	121	0%	9	23	0.1
5341	Teriyaki sauce, reduced sodium [1 cup]	255	9.0	214	0%	15	41	0.3
5342	Tomato and sofrito stewing sauce, Puerto Rican style [½ cup]	120	4.2	223	79%	6	7	1.5
5343	Tomato sauce, canned [½ cup]	122	4.3	37	5%	2	9	1.7
5344	Tomato sauce, canned, low sodium [½ cup]	122	4.3	37	6%	2	9	1.8
5345	White sauce, milk sauce [½ cup]	125	4.4	185	65%	5	11	0.2
5346	**Worcestershire sauce [2Tbs]**	34	1.2	23	0%	0	6	0.0
5347	Gravy, brown, nut, meatless (has almonds, soy sauce) [2Tbs]	30	1.1	37	77%	1	2	0.3
5348	Gravy, Chinese, or sauce (soy sauce, stock or bouillon, cornstarch) [½ cup]	117	4.1	48	5%	1	11	0.1
5349	Gravy, flour and water [½ cup]	120	4.2	96	2%	3	20	0.7
5350	Gravy, giblet (Include poultry gravy with pieces of meat) [½ cup]	119	4.2	89	48%	6	6	0.4
5351	**Gravy, meat or poultry, canned [½ cup]**	118	4.2	93	65%	2	6	0.5
5352	Gravy, meat or poultry, made with water, low sodium [½ cup]	118	4.2	63	41%	4	6	0.4
5353	Gravy, meat, with fruit (Include French sauce) [½ cup]	119	4.2	74	44%	3	8	0.5
5354	Gravy, meat, with wine [1 cup]	118	4.2	76	40%	2	5	0.3
5355	Gravy, meat-based, from Puerto-Rican style beef stew [½ cup]	104	3.7	86	92%	0	2	0.3
5356	Gravy, meat-based, from Puerto-Rican style stuffed pot roast [½ cup]	136	4.8	334	100%	0	0	0.0
5357	Gravy, milk quick gravy [½ cup]	125	4.4	177	65%	5	11	0.2
5358	Gravy, mushroom [½ cup]	119	4.2	32	11%	1	6	0.5

Food #	fat gm	sat fat gm	choles mg	sodium mg	potass mg	vit A	vit E	vit C	thia-min	ribo-flavin	nia-cin	vit B-6	fol-ate	vit B-12	cal-cium	phos-phorus	magne-sium	iron	zinc
						% of Daily Value													

Food #	fat gm	sat fat gm	choles mg	sodium mg	potass mg	vit A	vit E	vit C	thia-min	ribo-flavin	nia-cin	vit B-6	fol-ate	vit B-12	cal-cium	phos-phorus	magne-sium	iron	zinc
5311	0	0	0	10499	392	0	0	1	1	5	16	27	17	11	6	1	60	6	2
5312	7	2	3	2	313	2	3	24	3	3	10	6	2	0	1	5	6	4	2
5313	1	0	0	3	249	2	1	22	3	2	8	5	2	0	1	4	5	3	2
5314	1	0	1	581	43	0	0	0	0	5	2	1	2	0	1	1	2	2	1
5315	12	2	85	347	230	3	6	2	14	11	12	9	7	7	2	14	4	5	8
5316	2	0	0	1240	56	0	0	0	2	5	1	4	3	0	2	5	4	5	8
5317	3	0	0	1965	100	0	0	0	4	8	2	6	4	0	4	8	6	9	12
5318	12	3	1	223	284	2	6	7	5	5	9	5	4	1	4	14	15	9	7
5319	7	1	1	387	419	4	2	78	5	6	13	7	6	2	2	23	22	17	9
5320	10	1	0	6	638	0	0	19	9	10	0	6	2	0	19	15	25	42	18
5321	10	3	39	309	245	10	6	7	10	13	6	4	3	184	10	14	11	26	385
5322	0	0	0	2530	1	0	0	0	0	0	0	0	0	0	0	0	0	0	0
5323	7	1	0	68	105	0	5	5	1	1	10	3	3	0	1	5	6	1	3
5324	0	0	0	233	45	3	0	1	0	1	1	1	0	0	1	1	1	1	0
5325	7	1	0	7	241	6	6	79	4	3	3	8	5	0	2	3	3	3	1
5326	0	0	0	8	184	5	1	26	3	2	3	5	3	0	1	2	3	2	1
5327	0	0	0	354	253	9	3	46	4	3	5	8	5	0	6	3	4	5	3
5328	9	2	2	7	185	4	6	21	3	2	4	4	3	0	1	2	2	2	1
5329	27	9	41	1083	353	4	3	45	11	6	9	12	4	4	2	13	5	5	8
5330	0	0	0	2057	65	0	0	0	1	3	6	3	1	0	1	4	3	4	1
5331	0	0	0	1200	65	0	0	0	1	3	6	3	1	0	1	4	3	4	1
5332	5	1	0	1030	738	10	10	33	9	6	13	14	6	0	6	8	11	10	3
5333	2	0	0	1365	995	20	12	55	11	18	14	24	9	0	3	10	13	11	5
5334	8	2	15	982	742	9	10	31	9	7	17	16	6	8	5	10	11	12	8
5335	12	2	0	75	960	31	13	47	10	9	19	44	13	0	7	9	15	9	4
5336	0	0	0	454	126	3	2	8	1	1	2	2	0	0	1	1	2	2	1
5337	0	0	0	96	9	0	0	0	0	0	0	0	0	0	0	0	1	0	0
5338	15	2	11	205	11	3	7	0	0	0	0	4	1	1	1	1	0	1	0
5339	5	1	6	165	8	0	6	0	0	0	0	0	0	0	0	0	0	1	0
5340	0	0	0	5520	324	0	0	0	3	6	9	7	7	0	4	22	22	14	1
5341	0	0	0	4534	574	0	0	0	5	11	16	13	13	0	6	39	39	24	2
5342	20	7	26	524	256	5	3	66	10	5	8	11	4	2	1	7	4	4	5
5343	0	0	0	738	453	12	6	27	5	4	7	9	3	0	2	4	6	5	2
5344	0	0	0	13	453	12	6	27	6	4	7	10	3	0	2	4	6	5	2
5345	13	4	10	187	197	17	6	2	6	13	3	2	3	6	15	12	4	2	3
5346	0	0	0	333	272	0	0	7	2	3	1	0	0	0	4	2	1	10	0
5347	3	0	0	57	24	0	3	0	1	1	1	0	1	0	1	2	2	1	1
5348	0	0	0	767	22	0	0	0	0	1	1	1	0	1	0	2	1	1	0
5349	0	0	0	4	28	0	0	0	11	7	7	1	7	0	1	3	2	7	1
5350	5	1	50	625	138	30	1	1	2	10	7	3	11	36	1	6	1	8	9
5351	7	2	2	681	129	13	1	0	1	3	3	1	1	2	2	3	1	3	6
5352	3	1	4	21	96	0	0	0	2	3	4	1	1	2	1	4	1	5	8
5353	4	1	2	502	129	5	0	10	3	2	3	1	1	1	1	3	1	3	5
5354	3	1	2	472	110	5	0	0	1	2	2	1	1	1	1	3	1	3	5
5355	9	4	9	100	65	2	2	9	1	1	1	2	1	0	1	1	1	1	0
5356	37	15	30	3	0	0	6	0	0	0	0	0	0	0	0	0	0	0	0
5357	13	6	20	61	197	6	1	2	5	13	2	2	3	6	15	12	4	2	3
5358	0	0	0	646	26	0	0	1	2	2	2	1	0	1	2	2	1	1	1

Soups, Sauces, Fats, & Misc.

Food #	Food Description & Amount	wt gm	wt oz	calo-ries	%cal fat	prot gm	carbo gm	fiber gm
5359	Gravy, poultry-based from Puerto Rican-style chicken fricasse [½ cup]	120	4.2	254	91%	1	6	1.2
5360	Gravy, swiss steak [½ cup]	117	4.1	62	40%	4	6	0.5
5361	Chili con queso (tomato, pepper, and cheese dip) [½ cup]	120	4.2	251	64%	14	9	0.4
5362	Dip, bean, made with refried beans (Include garbanzo bean dip; jalapeno pepper bean dip; bean dip) [½ cup]	131	4.6	188	34%	8	24	9.0
5363	Dip, cheese base other than cream cheese [½ cup]	128	4.5	372	66%	21	11	0.0
5364	Dip, cream cheese base [½ cup]	120	4.2	391	87%	8	6	0.0
5365	Dip, eggplant (Include Baba Ghanoush) [½ cup]	117	4.1	190	72%	5	12	3.1
5366	Dip, shrimp, cream cheese base (Include clam dip) [½ cup]	118	4.2	290	77%	12	5	0.5
5367	**Dip, sour cream base (Include buttermilk type; onion dip) [½ cup]**	**122**	**4.3**	**268**	**81%**	**5**	**10**	**1.0**
5368	Dip, sour cream base, reduced calorie [½ cup]	120	4.2	176	71%	4	10	0.9
5369	Dip, spinach, sour cream base [½ cup]	120	4.2	215	73%	3	14	1.7
5370	Hummus [½ cup]	120	4.2	205	44%	6	24	6.1
	Fats & Oils							
5400	Almond oil (Include apricot oil) [1Tbs]	14	0.5	120	102%	0	0	0.0
5401	Bacon grease or meat drippings (Include ham, sausage, lamb, chicken) [1Tbs]	13	0.5	114	100%	0	0	0.0
5402	Butter replacement, fat-free powder (Include Butter Buds) [1Tbs]	5	0.2	19	2%	0	4	0.0
5403	**Butter, regular, salted (Include seasoned butter, garlic butter) [1Tbs]**	**14**	**0.5**	**102**	**100%**	**0**	**0**	**0.0**
5404	Butter, regular, unsalted [1Tbs]	14	0.5	102	100%	0	0	0.0
5405	Butter, whipped, salted [1Tbs]	9	0.3	67	100%	0	0	0.0
5406	Butter, whipped, unsalted [1Tbs]	9	0.3	67	100%	0	0	0.0
5407	Butter, light, stick, salted [1Tbs]	14	0.5	71	99%	0	0	0.0
5408	Butter, light, stick, unsalted [1Tbs]	14	0.5	71	99%	0	0	0.0
5409	Butter, light, whipped, tub, salted [1Tbs]	10	0.3	47	99%	0	0	0.0
5410	Butter and margarine or vegetable oil blend (Include Blue Bonnet Butter Spread, Land O Lakes Country Morning Blend) [1Tbs]	14	0.5	102	100%	0	0	0.0
5411	Butter and margarine or vegetable oil blend, unsalted (Include Land O Lakes Country Morning Blend) [1Tbs]	14	0.5	102	100%	0	0	0.0
5412	Margarine-butter spread, stick, salted (Include Kraft Touch of Butter Spread) [1Tbs]	14	0.5	77	100%	0	0	0.0
5413	Margarine-butter spread, stick, salted, reduced calorie (Include Land O Lakes Country Morning Blend Light [1Tbs]	13	0.5	60	100%	0	0	0.0
5414	Margarine-butter spread, tub, salted, reduced calorie (Include Land O Lakes Country Morning Blend Light [1Tbs]	13	0.5	59	100%	0	0	0.0
5415	Margarine, imitation (Include Shedd's Spread) [1Tbs]	15	0.5	50	100%	0	0	0.0
5416	Margarine, liquid, salted [1Tbs]	14	0.5	102	100%	0	0	0.0
5417	**Margarine, regular, salted [1Tbs]**	**14**	**0.5**	**102**	**100%**	**0**	**0**	**0.0**
5418	Margarine, regular, unsalted [1Tbs]	14	0.5	102	100%	0	0	0.0
5419	Margarine, whipped, salted [1Tbs]	9	0.3	68	100%	0	0	0.0
5420	Margarine, whipped, unsalted [1Tbs]	9	0.3	67	100%	0	0	0.0
5421	Margarine-like spread, liquid, salted (Include Parkay Squeeze Spread) [1Tbs]	14	0.5	88	100%	0	0	0.0
5422	Margarine-like spread, stick, unsalted (Include I Can't Believe It's Not Butter) [1Tbs]	14	0.5	77	100%	0	0	0.0
5423	**Margarine-like spread, tub, salted (Include Canola Sunrise Spread) [1Tbs]**	**14**	**0.5**	**77**	**100%**	**0**	**0**	**0.0**
5424	Margarine-like spread, tub, unsalted [1Tbs]	14	0.5	76	100%	0	0	0.0
5425	Margarine-like spread, tub, sweetened (Include Shedd's Country Crock Cinnamon or Honey Spread) [1Tbs]	14	0.5	76	88%	0	2	0.0
5426	Margarine-like spread, whipped, salted [1Tbs]	10	0.4	54	100%	0	0	0.0
5427	Margarine-like spread, reduced calorie, about 40% fat, stick, salted [1Tbs]	15	0.5	53	100%	0	0	0.0
5428	Margarine-like spread, tub, reduced calorie, about 20% fat, salted [1Tbs]	15	0.5	26	100%	0	0	0.0
5429	Margarine-like spread, tub, reduced calorie, about 20% fat, unsalted [1Tbs]	15	0.5	27	100%	0	0	0.0
5430	Margarine-like spread, tub, salted, "fat free" (Include Promise fat free)[1Tbs]	15	0.5	5	39%	0	0	0.0
5431	Margarine-like spread, liquid, salted, "fat free" (Include Fleischmann's fat free) [1Tbs]	14	0.5	6	63%	0	0	0.0

Food #	fat gm	sat fat gm	choles mg	sodium mg	potass mg	vit A	vit E	vit C	thia-min	ribo-flavin	nia-cin	vit B-6	fol-ate	vit B-12	cal-cium	phos-phorus	magne-sium	iron	zinc
						% of Daily Value													
5359	26	5	6	537	201	5	11	49	3	2	3	7	3	0	2	2	4	4	1
5360	3	1	3	652	94	0	0	0	2	2	4	1	1	2	1	3	1	5	8
5361	18	11	46	1178	292	18	2	11	4	22	2	6	2	5	48	60	7	3	15
5362	7	1	0	6	396	4	5	31	9	4	2	7	24	0	4	14	13	11	6
5363	27	17	71	1722	310	24	3	0	4	32	1	7	2	9	72	91	9	2	22
5364	38	22	110	400	153	38	5	1	2	12	1	3	3	8	9	11	2	7	4
5365	15	2	0	12	325	1	3	17	29	3	9	6	9	0	4	21	9	8	8
5366	25	14	123	300	169	25	4	3	2	8	5	4	3	10	7	14	5	9	5
5367	24	15	50	910	225	22	2	2	4	13	3	1	3	6	14	13	5	1	2
5368	14	8	43	846	203	12	2	2	4	13	3	1	3	6	13	13	4	1	4
5369	17	6	22	383	199	38	7	17	11	7	2	5	13	3	9	6	7	6	3
5370	10	2	0	293	209	0	4	16	7	4	2	24	18	0	6	13	9	10	9
5400	14	1	0	0	0	0	18	0	0	0	0	0	0	0	0	0	0	0	0
5401	13	6	13	70	0	0	1	0	0	0	0	0	0	0	0	0	0	0	0
5402	0	0	0	60	0	0	0	0	0	0	0	0	0	0	0	0	0	1	0
5403	12	7	31	117	4	11	1	0	0	0	0	0	0	0	0	0	0	0	0
5404	12	7	31	2	4	11	1	0	0	0	0	0	0	0	0	0	0	0	0
5405	8	5	21	78	2	7	0	0	0	0	0	0	0	0	0	0	0	0	0
5406	8	5	21	1	2	7	0	0	0	0	0	0	0	0	0	0	0	0	0
5407	8	5	15	64	10	10	1	0	0	1	0	0	0	0	1	0	0	1	0
5408	8	5	15	5	10	10	1	0	0	1	0	0	0	0	1	0	0	1	0
5409	5	3	10	43	7	6	0	0	0	0	0	0	0	0	0	0	0	1	0
5410	11	4	12	127	5	11	4	0	0	0	0	0	0	0	0	0	0	0	0
5411	11	4	10	4	5	14	4	0	0	0	0	0	0	0	0	0	0	0	0
5412	9	2	1	140	4	11	4	0	0	0	0	0	0	0	0	0	0	0	0
5413	7	2	7	76	1	12	4	0	0	0	0	0	0	0	0	0	0	0	0
5414	7	2	9	79	5	11	2	0	0	0	0	0	0	0	0	0	0	0	0
5415	6	1	0	139	4	12	1	0	0	0	0	0	0	0	0	0	0	0	0
5416	11	2	0	111	13	11	2	0	0	1	0	0	0	1	1	1	0	0	0
5417	11	2	0	134	6	11	6	0	0	0	0	0	0	0	0	0	0	0	0
5418	11	2	0	4	5	11	6	0	0	0	0	0	0	0	0	0	0	0	0
5419	8	1	0	89	4	8	4	0	0	0	0	0	0	0	0	0	0	0	0
5420	8	1	0	3	4	8	4	0	0	0	0	0	0	0	0	0	0	0	0
5421	10	2	0	141	4	15	4	0	0	0	0	0	0	0	0	0	0	0	0
5422	9	2	0	0	4	11	4	0	0	0	0	0	0	0	0	0	0	0	0
5423	9	1	0	142	4	11	4	0	0	0	0	0	0	0	0	0	0	0	0
5424	9	1	0	4	4	11	4	0	0	0	0	0	0	0	0	0	0	0	0
5425	7	1	0	77	4	15	6	0	0	0	0	0	0	0	0	0	0	0	0
5426	6	1	0	99	3	8	3	0	0	0	0	0	0	0	0	0	0	0	0
5427	6	1	0	149	5	16	2	0	0	0	0	0	0	0	0	0	0	0	0
5428	3	0	0	110	4	14	2	0	0	0	0	0	0	0	0	0	0	0	0
5429	3	0	0	4	5	16	1	0	0	0	0	0	0	0	0	0	0	0	0
5430	0	0	0	94	0	14	0	0	0	0	0	0	0	0	0	0	0	0	0
5431	0	0	0	118	7	11	0	0	0	0	0	0	0	0	1	0	0	0	0

Soups, Sauces, Fats, & Misc.

Food #	Food Description & Amount	wt gm	wt oz	calo- ries	%cal fat	prot gm	carbo gm	fiber gm
5432	Canola oil (Include rapeseed oil) [1Tbs]	14	0.5	120	100%	0	0	0.0
5433	Corn oil [1Tbs]	14	0.5	120	100%	0	0	0.0
5434	Corn and canola oil (Include Mazola Right Blend) [1Tbs]	14	0.5	124	100%	0	0	0.0
5435	Cottonseed oil [1Tbs]	14	0.5	120	100%	0	0	0.0
5436	Ghee, clarified butter (Include butter oil) [1Tbs]	13	0.5	112	100%	0	0	0.0
5437	Flaxseed oil [1Tbs]	14	0.5	120	100%	0	0	0.0
5438	Honey butter [1Tbs]	18	0.6	85	62%	0	9	0.0
5439	Lard with annatto, Puerto Rican (Manteca con achiote) [1Tbs]	15	0.5	135	100%	0	0	0.0
5440	Lard [1Tbs]	13	0.5	115	100%	0	0	0.0
5441	Lecithin [1Tbs]	8	0.3	61	100%	0	0	0.0
5442	**Olive oil** [1Tbs]	**14**	**0.5**	**119**	**100%**	**0**	**0**	**0.0**
5443	Peanut oil [1Tbs]	14	0.5	119	100%	0	0	0.0
5444	Safflower oil [1Tbs]	14	0.5	120	100%	0	0	0.0
5445	Sesame oil [1Tbs]	14	0.5	120	100%	0	0	0.0
5446	Shortening, animal (Include Spry) [1Tbs]	13	0.5	115	100%	0	0	0.0
5447	Shortening, vegetable (Include Crisco, Fluffo, Frymax) [1Tbs]	13	0.5	113	100%	0	0	0.0
5448	Soybean and sunflower oil [1Tbs]	14	0.5	120	100%	0	0	0.0
5449	Soybean oil (Include Crisco, Wesson) [1Tbs]	14	0.5	120	100%	0	0	0.0
5450	Sunflower oil (Include Wesson Sunlite) [1Tbs]	14	0.5	120	100%	0	0	0.0
5451	Walnut oil [1Tbs]	14	0.5	120	100%	0	0	0.0
5452	Wheat germ oil [1Tbs]	14	0.5	120	100%	0	0	0.0
	Dressings							
5500	Bacon and tomato dressing [2Tbs]	30	1.1	98	97%	1	1	0.1
5501	Bacon and tomato dressing, low calorie [2Tbs]	32	1.1	65	95%	1	1	0.1
5502	Bacon dressing (hot) [2Tbs]	29	1.0	103	96%	1	1	0.0
5503	**Blue or roquefort cheese dressing** [2Tbs]	**31**	**1.1**	**154**	**93%**	**1**	**2**	**0.0**
5504	Blue or roquefort cheese dressing, low-calorie [2Tbs]	31	1.1	30	65%	2	1	0.0
5505	Blue or roquefort cheese dressing, reduced calorie [2Tbs]	31	1.1	27	28%	1	4	0.0
5506	Blue or roquefort cheese dressing, reduced calorie, fat-free, cholesterol-free [2Tbs]	33	1.2	38	6%	1	8	1.1
5507	**Caesar dressing** [2Tbs]	**29**	**1.0**	**155**	**98%**	**0**	**1**	**0.0**
5508	Caesar dressing, low-calorie [2Tbs]	30	1.1	33	36%	0	6	0.0
5509	Celery seed dressing (Include celery seed and onion dressing) [2Tbs]	31	1.1	197	88%	0	7	0.3
5510	Coleslaw dressing [2Tbs]	31	1.1	122	77%	0	7	0.0
5511	Coleslaw dressing, reduced calorie [2Tbs]	34	1.2	69	88%	0	13	0.1
5512	Cream cheese dressing (Include Philadelphia brand) [2Tbs]	31	1.1	130	95%	1	2	0.0
5513	Creamy dressing, made with sour cream (or yogurt or buttermilk) and mayonnaise (or salad oil) (Include **Ranch Dressing**, French made with sour cream, Creamy Cucumber, Seven Seas Southern with Bacon, Wishbone Creamy Bacon, Creamy Italian) [2Tbs]	29	1.0	147	97%	0	2	0.0
5514	Creamy dressing, made with sour cream and/or buttermilk and oil, reduced calorie (Include Kraft Reduced Calorie Creamy Cucumber Dressing) [2Tbs]	30	1.1	48	79%	0	2	0.0
5515	Creamy dressing, made with sour cream and/or buttermilk and oil, reduced calorie, cholesterol-free [2Tbs]	30	1.1	42	51%	0	5	0.0
5516	Creamy dressing, made with sour cream and/or buttermilk and oil, reduced calorie, fat-free, cholesterol-free [2Tbs]	33	1.2	35	23%	0	7	0.0
5517	Feta cheese dressing (Include Marzetties') [2Tbs]	29	1.0	160	97%	1	1	0.0
5518	French dressing (Include Catalina, Sweet 'n Saucy, Holsum's 1867, Richelieu's Western dressing) [2Tbs]	31	1.1	134	86%	0	5	0.0
5519	French dressing, low-calorie [2Tbs]	32	1.1	43	39%	0	7	0.0
5520	French dressing, reduced calorie [2Tbs]	32	1.1	65	59%	0	9	0.0
5521	French dressing, reduced calorie, fat-free, cholesterol-free [2Tbs]	32	1.1	43	21%	0	7	0.1

Food #	fat gm	sat fat gm	choles mg	sodium mg	potass mg	vit A	vit E	vit C	thia-min	ribo-flavin	nia-cin	vit B-6	fol-ate	vit B-12	cal-cium	phos-phorus	magne-sium	iron	zinc
													% of Daily Value						
5432	14	1	0	0	0	0	9	0	0	0	0	0	0	0	0	0	0	0	0
5433	14	2	0	0	0	0	10	0	0	0	0	0	0	0	0	0	0	0	0
5434	14	1	0	0	0	0	10	0	0	0	0	0	0	0	0	0	0	0	0
5435	14	4	0	0	0	0	17	0	0	0	0	0	0	0	0	0	0	0	0
5436	13	8	33	0	1	12	1	0	0	0	0	0	0	0	0	0	0	0	0
5437	14	1	0	0	0	0	8	0	0	0	0	0	0	0	0	0	0	0	0
5438	6	4	16	60	7	5	0	0	0	0	0	0	0	0	0	0	0	0	0
5439	15	6	14	0	0	0	1	0	0	0	0	0	0	0	0	0	0	0	0
5440	13	5	12	0	0	0	1	0	0	0	0	0	0	0	0	0	0	0	0
5441	8	1	0	0	0	0	1	0	0	0	0	0	0	0	0	0	0	0	0
5442	14	2	0	0	0	0	6	0	0	0	0	0	0	0	0	0	0	0	0
5443	14	2	0	0	0	0	6	0	0	0	0	0	0	0	0	0	0	0	0
5444	14	1	0	0	0	0	20	0	0	0	0	0	0	0	0	0	0	0	0
5445	14	2	0	0	0	0	2	0	0	0	0	0	0	0	0	0	0	0	0
5446	13	5	12	0	0	0	1	0	0	0	0	0	0	0	0	0	0	0	0
5447	13	3	0	0	0	0	5	0	0	0	0	0	0	0	0	0	0	0	0
5448	14	2	0	0	0	0	19	0	0	0	0	0	0	0	0	0	0	0	0
5449	14	2	0	0	0	0	8	0	0	0	0	0	0	0	0	0	0	0	0
5450	14	1	0	0	0	0	23	0	0	0	0	0	0	0	0	0	0	0	0
5451	14	1	0	0	0	0	1	0	0	0	0	0	0	0	0	0	0	0	0
5452	14	3	0	0	0	0	87	0	0	0	0	0	0	0	0	0	0	0	0
5500	10	2	1	325	32	1	4	4	1	0	1	1	0	0	0	1	0	0	0
5501	7	1	1	351	35	1	4	5	1	0	1	1	0	0	0	1	0	0	0
5502	11	2	2	46	30	0	6	0	1	0	1	0	0	1	0	1	1	1	1
5503	16	3	5	335	11	2	9	1	0	2	0	1	1	1	2	2	0	0	1
5504	2	1	0	367	2	0	1	0	0	2	0	0	0	1	3	3	1	1	1
5505	1	0	3	502	16	0	1	0	0	1	0	0	0	1	2	1	0	0	1
5506	0	0	1	265	64	0	1	0	1	2	0	0	0	1	2	4	1	0	0
5507	17	3	1	317	9	0	5	0	0	0	0	0	0	0	0	1	1	0	0	0
5508	1	0	1	323	9	0	0	0	0	0	0	0	0	0	1	1	0	0	0
5509	19	2	0	1	47	2	13	3	1	1	0	2	1	0	1	1	1	2	0
5510	10	2	8	222	3	2	7	0	0	0	0	0	0	1	0	1	0	0	0
5511	7	1	8	538	17	0	5	0	0	0	0	0	0	1	1	1	0	0	0
5512	14	3	8	22	11	3	7	0	0	1	0	0	0	1	1	1	0	1	0
5513	16	2	1	2	8	1	10	0	0	0	0	0	0	0	0	0	0	0	0
5514	4	1	0	307	11	0	2	0	0	0	0	0	1	0	0	0	0	0	0
5515	2	0	0	280	15	0	5	0	0	1	0	0	0	1	1	3	0	0	0
5516	1	0	0	330	44	0	1	0	0	1	0	0	0	0	1	3	0	0	0
5517	17	3	7	91	13	1	6	0	1	4	0	2	1	2	4	3	1	1	2
5518	13	3	0	427	25	4	9	0	0	0	0	0	0	1	0	0	0	1	0
5519	2	0	0	255	26	4	1	0	0	0	0	0	0	0	0	0	0	1	0
5520	4	1	0	324	26	4	2	0	0	0	0	0	0	0	0	0	0	1	0
5521	1	0	0	252	25	4	2	0	0	0	0	0	0	0	0	0	0	1	0

Soups, Sauces, Fats, & Misc.

Food #	Food Description & Amount	wt gm	wt oz	calo-ries	%cal fat	prot gm	carbo gm	fiber gm
5522	Fruit dressing, made with fruit juice and cream [2Tbs]	30	1.1	62	56%	1	6	0.0
5523	Fruit dressing, made with honey, oil, and water (Include with herbs, lemon juice) [2Tbs]	29	1.0	149	85%	0	7	0.0
5524	Green Goddess dressing (Include Marie's Avocado Goddess Dressing) [2Tbs]	31	1.1	155	88%	1	5	0.0
5525	**Honey mustard dressing** (Include Naturally Fresh Honey Mustard dressing) [2Tbs]	31	1.1	102	49%	0	14	0.2
5526	Italian dressing, low-calorie (Include Wishbone Lite Dijon Vinegarette, McDonald's Lite Vinaigrette) [2Tbs]	30	1.1	32	84%	0	1	0.0
5527	**Italian dressing**, made with vinegar, oil, and garlic (Include Christie's Greek dressing, California Onion dressing, Green Onion dressing, Kraft Presto dressing, vinegarette dressing, Seven Seas Viva Italian dressing) [2Tbs]	29	1.0	137	93%	0	3	0.0
5528	Italian dressing, reduced calorie [2Tbs]	28	1.0	56	90%	0	2	0.1
5529	Italian dressing, reduced calorie, fat-free [2Tbs]	28	1.0	13	40%	0	2	0.1
5530	Korean dressing or marinade (Includes ginseng, garlic, onion, chili pepper, salt) [2Tbs]	30	1.1	10	3%	0	2	0.2
5531	Mayonnaise, imitation [2Tbs]	30	1.1	69	75%	0	5	0.0
5532	Mayonnaise, imitation, no cholesterol [2Tbs]	30	1.1	145	89%	0	5	0.0
5533	Mayonnaise, low-calorie or diet [2Tbs]	31	1.1	72	75%	0	5	0.0
5534	Mayonnaise, low-calorie or diet, low sodium [2Tbs]	28	1.0	65	75%	0	4	0.0
5535	Mayonnaise, made with tofu [2Tbs]	30	1.1	94	75%	3	3	0.2
5536	Mayonnaise, made with yogurt (Include Yogannaise) [2Tbs]	28	1.0	27	47%	1	3	0.0
5537	Mayonnaise, reduced calorie or diet, cholesterol-free [2Tbs]	29	1.0	97	90%	0	2	0.0
5538	**Mayonnaise, regular** (Include McDonald's House dressing) [2Tbs]	28	1.0	198	100%	0	1	0.0
5539	Mayonnaise-type dressing (Include Miracle Whip) [2Tbs]	29	1.0	115	77%	0	7	0.0
5540	Mayonnaise-type dressing, cholesterol free [2Tbs]	30	1.1	206	100%	0	0	0.0
5541	Mayonnaise-type dressing, fat-free [2Tbs]	32	1.1	24	31%	0	4	1.2
5542	Mayonnaise-type dressing, low-calorie or diet (Include Miracle Whip Light) [2Tbs]	28	1.0	73	66%	0	7	0.0
5543	Mayonnaise-type dressing, low-calorie or diet cholesterol-free (Include Miracle Whip Light (cholesterol-free)) [2Tbs]	30	1.1	96	80%	0	4	0.0
5544	Milk, vinegar, and artificial sweetener dressing [2Tbs]	31	1.1	24	44%	1	3	0.0
5545	Milk, vinegar, and sugar dressing [2Tbs]	33	1.2	42	23%	1	8	0.0
5546	Peppercorn dressing [2Tbs]	27	0.9	151	98%	0	1	0.0
5547	**Poppy seed dressing** (Include Naturally Fresh brand) [2Tbs]	29	1.0	131	83%	0	6	0.0
5548	Russian dressing [2Tbs]	31	1.1	151	93%	0	3	0.0
5549	Russian dressing, low-calorie [2Tbs]	32	1.1	46	25%	0	9	0.1
5550	Salad dressing, low-calorie (Include Nutri-System salad dressing) [2Tbs]	32	1.1	41	65%	0	4	0.1
5551	Sandwich spread [2Tbs]	31	1.1	119	79%	0	7	0.1
5552	Sesame dressing [2Tbs]	29	1.0	156	95%	0	3	0.2
5553	Sour cream dressing, filled, sour, non-dairy (Include King Sour, Zest) [2Tbs]	29	1.0	52	84%	1	1	0.0
5554	Sweet and sour dressing [2Tbs]	31	1.1	5	0%	0	1	0.0
5555	**Thousand Island dressing** (Include McDonald's Big Mac sauce) [2Tbs]	31	1.1	118	85%	0	5	0.0
5556	Thousand Island dressing, low-calorie [2Tbs]	31	1.1	49	61%	0	5	0.4
5557	Thousand Island dressing, reduced calorie, fat-free, cholesterol-free [2Tbs]	32	1.1	36	16%	0	10	0.1
5558	Vinegar, sugar, and water dressing [2Tbs]	32	1.1	17	0%	0	5	0.0
5559	Yogurt dressing [2Tbs]	31	1.1	23	46%	1	2	0.0
Condiments								
5600	Adobo fresco (Include adobo criollo, creole seasoning) [2Tbs]	36	1.3	81	83%	1	7	0.5
5601	Beans, string, green, pickled [½ cup]	68	2.4	19	3%	1	4	2.0
5602	Beets, pickled (Include pickled beets with onions, beet salad) [½ cup, sliced]	84	3.0	53	2%	1	13	1.5
5603	Cabbage, fresh, pickled, Japanese style [½ cup]	75	2.6	16	4%	1	3	2.3
5604	Cabbage, Kim Chee style [½ cup]	75	2.6	16	9%	1	3	0.9
5605	Cabbage, mustard, salted [½ cup]	64	2.3	13	4%	1	3	2.0
5606	Cabbage, red, pickled (Include sweet and sour red cabbage) [½ cup]	75	2.6	110	1%	0	29	0.6

Food #	fat gm	sat fat gm	choles mg	sodium mg	potass mg	vit A	vit E	vit C	thia-min	ribo-flavin	nia-cin	vit B-6	fol-ate	vit B-12	cal-cium	phos-phorus	magne-sium	iron	zinc
5522	4	2	36	11	33	5	0	7	1	2	0	1	2	1	1	2	1	1	1
5523	14	2	0	1	4	0	9	0	0	0	0	0	0	0	0	0	0	0	0
5524	15	2	12	331	18	0	8	0	0	1	0	0	0	1	1	1	1	1	1
5525	6	1	0	74	20	0	4	0	0	0	0	0	0	0	1	1	1	1	1
5526	3	0	2	236	5	0	2	0	0	0	0	0	0	0	0	0	0	0	0
5527	14	2	0	231	4	1	10	0	0	0	0	0	0	1	0	0	0	0	0
5528	6	1	0	398	9	0	1	0	0	0	0	0	1	0	0	0	0	0	0
5529	1	0	0	258	37	0	1	0	0	0	0	0	1	0	0	0	0	0	0
5530	0	0	0	83	32	0	0	17	0	0	1	1	1	0	1	1	1	1	0
5531	6	1	7	149	3	0	6	0	0	0	0	0	0	0	0	0	0	0	0
5532	14	2	0	106	3	0	9	0	0	0	0	0	0	0	0	0	0	0	0
5533	6	1	7	155	3	0	7	0	0	0	0	0	0	0	0	0	0	0	0
5534	5	1	7	31	3	0	4	0	0	0	0	0	0	0	0	0	0	0	0
5535	8	1	0	200	20	0	5	0	1	1	0	0	1	0	2	1	4	0	1
5536	1	1	12	139	27	0	1	0	0	2	0	0	1	2	2	0	1	0	
5537	10	1	0	214	20	0	6	0	0	0	0	0	0	0	0	0	0	0	0
5538	22	3	16	157	9	2	11	0	0	0	0	8	1	1	0	1	0	1	0
5539	10	1	8	209	3	2	4	0	0	0	0	0	0	1	0	1	0	0	0
5540	23	3	0	146	4	0	12	0	0	1	0	0	0	0	0	1	0	0	0
5541	1	0	0	380	30	0	2	0	0	0	0	0	0	0	0	0	0	0	0
5542	5	1	7	199	3	2	4	0	0	0	0	0	0	1	0	1	0	0	0
5543	9	1	0	204	0	0	4	0	0	0	0	0	0	0	0	0	0	0	0
5544	1	1	5	17	62	1	0	0	0	3	0	0	0	0	4	3	2	1	1
5545	1	1	4	15	56	1	0	0	0	3	0	0	0	0	4	3	2	1	1
5546	16	3	13	285	47	0	3	0	0	0	0	1	2	1	1	1	0	1	0
5547	12	2	0	127	5	0	7	0	0	0	0	0	0	0	0	0	1	0	0
5548	16	2	6	266	48	6	10	3	1	1	1	0	1	2	1	1	1	1	1
5549	1	0	2	281	51	1	1	3	0	0	0	0	0	1	1	1	0	1	0
5550	3	0	2	270	17	2	2	0	0	0	0	0	0	0	0	1	0	1	0
5551	10	2	23	306	11	3	7	0	0	0	0	0	0	1	0	1	0	0	2
5552	16	2	0	285	14	0	2	0	0	0	0	1	0	0	0	0	0	0	0
5553	5	4	2	14	47	0	0	0	1	3	0	0	1	2	3	3	1	0	1
5554	0	0	0	65	10	0	0	4	0	0	0	0	0	0	0	0	0	0	0
5555	11	2	8	218	35	3	1	0	0	0	0	0	0	1	0	1	0	1	0
5556	3	0	5	306	35	3	1	0	0	0	0	0	0	1	0	1	0	1	0
5557	1	0	1	273	52	0	1	0	1	1	0	1	0	1	1	1	1	1	0
5558	0	0	0	1	10	0	0	0	0	0	0	0	0	0	0	0	1	0	0
5559	1	1	3	12	45	1	0	1	1	2	0	0	1	2	3	2	1	0	1
5600	8	1	0	6175	67	1	3	3	1	1	1	0	0	0	4	1	2	6	1
5601	0	0	0	4	128	4	1	14	3	3	2	2	5	0	2	2	4	4	1
5602	0	0	0	53	205	0	1	3	1	2	1	2	10	0	1	3	4	3	2
5603	0	0	0	208	640	1	0	1	0	2	1	4	8	0	4	3	2	2	1
5604	0	0	0	498	188	21	0	66	2	3	2	8	11	0	7	3	3	4	1
5605	0	0	0	459	157	6	0	0	2	3	2	10	12	0	4	2	2	2	1
5606	0	0	0	14	159	0	0	26	1	1	1	3	2	0	4	2	5	4	1

Soups, Sauces, Fats, & Misc.

Food #	Food Description & Amount	wt gm	wt oz	calo-ries	%cal fat	prot gm	carbo gm	fiber gm
5607	Capers, canned, drained [1Tbs]	9	0.3	2	34%	0	0	0.3
5608	Catsup, tomato [2Tbs]	34	1.2	35	3%	1	9	0.4
5609	Catsup, tomato, low sodium [2Tbs]	34	1.2	35	3%	1	9	0.4
5610	Cauliflower, pickled [½ cup]	63	2.2	27	6%	1	6	1.2
5611	Celery, pickled [½ cup]	75	2.6	11	7%	0	3	1.1
5612	Chinese preserved sweet zucchini (or other vegetables) [5 slices]	60	2.1	222	0%	0	57	0.2
5613	Chutney [2Tbs]	34	1.2	52	3%	0	13	0.8
5614	Corn relish [2Tbs]	31	1.1	26	6%	1	6	0.5
5615	Cucumber, pickled, Kim Chee style [½ cup]	75	2.6	16	4%	1	4	1.1
5616	Eggplant, pickled [½ cup]	68	2.4	23	19%	1	5	1.7
5617	Horseradish [2Tbs]	30	1.1	16	33%	0	3	3.0
5618	Mushrooms, pickled [½ cup]	78	2.8	18	14%	1	4	0.8
5619	Mustard (Include horseradish mustard, Chinese mustard) [1Tbs]	15	0.5	11	53%	1	1	0.4
5620	Mustard sauce [2Tbs]	20	0.7	50	84%	0	2	0.2
5621	Okra, pickled [5 pods]	55	1.9	16	3%	1	4	1.5
5622	Olives, black [10 small]	34	1.2	36	82%	0	2	1.0
5623	Olives, green [½ cup]	67	2.3	77	99%	1	1	0.7
5624	Olives, green, stuffed [½ cup]	73	2.6	76	96%	1	1	0.8
5625	Pepper, hot, pickled (Include pickled jalapeno pepper) [½ cup]	56	2.0	27	3%	1	7	0.7
5626	Peppers, hot, sauce (Include Tabasco sauce) [1Tbs]	15	0.5	3	5%	0	1	0.3
5627	Peppers, pickled [½ cup]	68	2.4	27	4%	1	7	1.1
5628	Pickled green bananas (Include Guineos verdes en escabeche) [½ cup]	75	2.6	242	83%	1	12	1.3
5629	Pickles (cucumber), dill or sour [1 small]	37	1.3	7	10%	0	2	0.4
5630	Pickles, dill, reduced salt (Include Vlasic Half the Salt Kosher Crunchy Dill Spears; Vlasic Half the Salt Hamburger Dill Chips) [1 pickle (3¾" long)]	65	2.3	7	16%	0	1	0.8
5631	Pickles, fresh (Include bread and butter pickles) [½ cup]	85	3.0	62	2%	1	15	1.3
5632	Pickles, sweet (Include candied dill spears, semi-sweet) [1 Gherkin (2" long)]	6	0.2	7	2%	0	2	0.1
5633	Pickles, sweet, reduced salt (Include Vlasic Half the Salt Sweet Butter Chips) [5 slices]	30	1.1	35	2%	0	10	0.3
5634	Pickles, mixed [½ cup]	78	2.7	106	3%	0	29	0.9
5635	Pickles, relish, sweet (Include Indian sweet relish) [½ cup]	123	4.3	159	3%	0	43	1.3
5636	Pickle-mustard-onion relish (Include chow chow, hotdog relish) [2Tbs]	31	1.1	36	7%	0	8	0.5
5637	Radishes, pickled, Hawaiian style [½ cup]	75	2.6	17	12%	1	3	1.7
5638	Recaito (Puerto Rican little coriander) (Include Recaito congelado) [½ cup]	120	4.2	24	26%	3	3	2.8
5639	Seaweed, pickled [2Tbs]	19	0.7	28	1%	0	7	0.1
5640	Tomato chili sauce (catsup-type) [2Tbs]	34	1.2	35	3%	1	8	2.0
5641	Tomato relish (Include tomato preserves) [2Tbs]	40	1.4	58	2%	1	15	0.7
5642	Tsukemono, Japanese pickles (Include nara zuke, takuan zuke, wasabi zuke) [½ cup]	68	2.4	15	8%	1	3	1.8
5643	Turnip, pickled [½ cup]	78	2.7	32	3%	1	8	1.2
5644	Vegetable relish [½ cup]	70	2.5	25	5%	1	6	0.6
5645	Vegetables, pickled (Include giardiniera) [½ cup]	82	2.9	22	5%	1	5	1.7
5646	Vegetables, pickled, Hawaiian style [½ cup]	75	2.6	19	13%	1	4	2.0
5647	Vinegar [2Tbs]	30	1.1	4	0%	0	2	0.0
5648	Yeast extract spread (Include Vegemite, Marmite, Promite) [1 tsp]	6	0.2	10	0%	2	1	0.2
5649	Zucchini, pickled [½ cup]	85	3.0	30	6%	1	7	1.0
	Spices & Miscellaneous							
5700	Allspice, ground [1Tbs (3 tsp)]	6	0.2	15	30%	0	4	1.2
5701	Anise seed [1Tbs (3 tsp)]	6	0.2	21	42%	1	3	0.9
5702	Basil, fresh [½ cup (8Tbs)]	21	0.7	6	20%	1	1	0.8
5703	Basil, ground [1Tbs (3 tsp)]	4	0.1	11	14%	1	3	1.7
5704	Bay leaf, crumbled [1Tbs (3 tsp)]	2	0.1	6	24%	0	1	0.5

Food #	fat gm	sat fat gm	choles mg	sodium mg	potass mg	vit A	vit E	vit C	thia-min	ribo-flavin	nia-cin	vit B-6	fol-ate	vit B-12	cal-cium	phos-phorus	magne-sium	iron	zinc
5607	0	0	0	255	3	0	0	1	0	1	0	0	0	0	0	0	1	1	0
5608	0	0	0	405	164	3	2	9	2	1	2	3	1	0	1	1	2	1	1
5609	0	0	0	7	164	3	2	9	2	1	2	3	1	0	1	1	2	1	1
5610	0	0	0	11	129	2	0	34	2	2	1	5	4	0	1	2	2	2	1
5611	0	0	0	196	177	1	1	6	2	2	1	2	3	0	3	2	2	2	1
5612	0	0	0	1	49	1	0	2	1	1	0	1	1	0	0	1	1	1	0
5613	0	0	0	7	139	2	1	13	2	1	1	2	1	0	1	1	2	2	0
5614	0	0	0	4	60	2	0	13	1	1	1	2	2	0	0	1	1	1	1
5615	0	0	0	766	88	2	0	4	2	1	2	4	4	0	1	1	2	20	3
5616	0	0	0	1138	8	0	0	0	2	3	2	5	3	0	2	1	1	3	1
5617	1	0	0	94	74	0	0	2	0	0	1	1	4	0	2	1	2	1	2
5618	0	0	0	3	232	0	0	3	4	16	12	3	2	0	0	6	2	5	3
5619	1	0	0	188	20	0	1	0	1	0	0	1	0	0	1	1	1	2	1
5620	5	1	0	61	17	0	3	0	0	0	0	0	0	0	0	0	1	1	0
5621	0	0	0	4	135	3	1	13	5	2	2	4	7	0	4	3	7	2	2
5622	3	0	0	299	3	1	3	1	0	0	0	0	0	0	3	0	0	6	0
5623	8	1	0	1596	37	2	7	0	0	0	0	0	0	0	4	1	4	6	1
5624	8	1	0	1518	51	5	7	15	0	0	0	1	1	0	4	1	4	7	1
5625	0	0	0	469	150	23	1	163	3	2	2	6	3	0	1	2	3	3	1
5626	0	0	0	4	85	1	0	17	0	0	1	1	0	0	0	0	0	0	0
5627	0	0	0	1	105	16	1	117	2	1	1	7	3	0	1	1	2	1	1
5628	22	3	0	1	184	0	10	6	2	2	1	12	2	0	1	2	4	2	1
5629	0	0	0	474	43	1	0	1	0	1	0	0	0	0	0	1	1	1	0
5630	0	0	0	12	15	1	0	1	0	0	0	0	0	0	0	1	1	1	0
5631	0	0	0	572	170	1	0	13	0	2	0	0	1	0	3	2	0	2	0
5632	0	0	0	56	2	0	0	0	0	0	0	0	0	0	0	0	0	0	0
5633	0	0	0	5	10	0	0	1	0	1	0	0	0	0	0	0	0	1	0
5634	0	0	0	662	20	1	0	1	0	2	1	1	0	0	0	1	1	4	1
5635	1	0	0	993	31	2	0	2	0	2	1	1	0	0	0	2	2	6	1
5636	0	0	0	161	61	0	0	3	0	0	0	0	0	0	1	1	2	2	0
5637	0	0	0	592	250	0	0	0	1	1	1	4	2	0	2	2	2	1	1
5638	1	0	0	32	553	32	10	12	5	8	4	5	2	0	11	4	7	12	3
5639	0	0	0	27	36	1	0	1	0	1	0	0	2	0	1	1	2	2	0
5640	0	0	0	457	126	2	4	9	2	1	3	3	4	0	1	2	1	2	0
5641	0	0	0	947	157	6	1	39	2	1	1	3	1	0	2	2	3	3	0
5642	0	0	0	360	400	1	0	0	0	1	1	3	4	0	3	2	2	1	1
5643	0	0	0	33	115	3	0	24	2	1	1	3	2	0	2	2	2	1	1
5644	0	0	0	6	124	2	0	9	2	1	1	2	2	0	1	2	2	2	1
5645	0	0	0	166	174	56	1	47	3	2	2	6	3	0	2	2	2	2	1
5646	0	0	0	795	148	3	0	0	2	3	2	7	6	0	3	2	2	2	1
5647	0	0	0	0	30	0	0	0	0	0	0	0	0	0	0	0	2	1	0
5648	0	0	0	216	156	0	0	0	39	50	29	4	15	1	1	1	3	1	1
5649	0	0	0	3	170	5	0	22	3	1	1	4	3	0	1	3	4	2	1
5700	0	0	0	4	60	0	0	4	0	0	1	1	1	0	4	1	2	2	0
5701	1	0	0	1	91	0	0	2	1	1	1	1	0	0	4	3	3	13	2
5702	0	0	0	1	98	8	0	6	0	1	1	1	3	0	3	1	4	4	1
5703	0	0	0	1	144	4	0	4	0	1	1	3	3	0	9	2	4	10	2
5704	0	0	0	0	10	1	0	1	0	0	0	1	1	0	2	0	1	4	0

Soups, Sauces, Fats, & Misc.

Food #	Food Description & Amount	wt gm	wt oz	calo-ries	%cal fat	prot gm	carbo gm	fiber gm
5705	Caraway seed [1Tbs (3 tsp)]	6	0.2	21	39%	1	3	2.4
5706	Cardamon, ground [1Tbs (3 tsp)]	6	0.2	19	19%	1	4	1.7
5707	Cayenne or red pepper [1Tbs (3 tsp)]	5	0.2	17	49%	1	3	1.5
5708	Celery seed [1Tbs (3 tsp)]	6	0.2	24	58%	1	2	0.7
5709	Chervil, dried [1Tbs (3 tsp)]	2	0.1	4	15%	0	1	0.2
5710	Chili powder [1Tbs (3 tsp)]	8	0.3	24	48%	1	4	2.7
5711	Cinnamon, ground [1Tbs (3 tsp)]	7	0.2	18	11%	0	6	3.7
5712	Cloves, ground [1Tbs (3 tsp)]	6	0.2	20	56%	0	4	2.2
5713	Coriander leaf, dried [1Tbs (3 tsp)]	2	0.1	5	15%	0	1	0.2
5714	Coriander seed [1Tbs (3 tsp)]	5	0.2	16	54%	1	3	2.3
5715	Cumin seed [1Tbs (3 tsp)]	6	0.2	24	53%	1	3	0.7
5716	Curry powder [1Tbs (3 tsp)]	6	0.2	20	38%	1	3	2.0
5717	Dill seed [1Tbs (3 tsp)]	6	0.2	19	43%	1	3	1.3
5718	Dill weed, dried [1Tbs (3 tsp)]	3	0.1	8	16%	1	2	0.4
5719	Dill weed, fresh [½ cup (8Tbs)]	5	0.2	2	23%	0	0	0.1
5720	Fennel seed [1Tbs (3 tsp)]	6	0.2	21	39%	1	3	2.4
5721	Fenugreek seed [1Tbs (3 tsp)]	11	0.4	36	18%	3	6	2.7
5722	Garlic powder [1Tbs (3 tsp)]	8	0.3	28	2%	1	6	0.8
5723	Gelatin, plain, powder, dry [1 envelope (1Tbs)]	7	0.2	23	0%	6	0	0.0
5724	Ginger, ground [1Tbs (3 tsp)]	5	0.2	19	15%	0	4	0.7
5725	Mace, ground [1Tbs (3 tsp)]	5	0.2	24	61%	0	3	1.0
5726	Marjoram, dried [1Tbs (3 tsp)]	2	0.1	5	23%	0	1	0.7
5727	Mustard seed, yellow [1Tbs (3 tsp)]	10	0.3	46	55%	2	3	1.5
5728	Nutmeg, ground [1Tbs (3 tsp)]	7	0.2	35	62%	0	3	1.4
5729	Onion powder [1Tbs (3 tsp)]	6	0.2	22	3%	1	5	0.4
5730	Oregano, ground [1Tbs (3 tsp)]	5	0.2	14	30%	0	3	1.9
5731	Paprika [1Tbs (3 tsp)]	6	0.2	18	40%	1	4	1.3
5732	Parsley, dried [1Tbs (3 tsp)]	1	0.0	2	14%	0	0	0.3
5733	Pepper, black [1Tbs (3 tsp)]	6	0.2	16	12%	1	4	1.7
5734	Pepper, white [1Tbs (3 tsp)]	7	0.3	21	6%	1	5	1.9
5735	Peppermint, fresh [½ cup (8Tbs)]	13	0.5	9	12%	0	2	1.0
5736	Poppy seed [1Tbs (3 tsp)]	8	0.3	45	75%	2	2	0.8
5737	Poultry seasoning [1Tbs (3 tsp)]	5	0.2	14	22%	0	3	0.5
5738	Pumpkin pie spice [1Tbs (3 tsp)]	5	0.2	17	33%	0	4	0.8
5739	Rosemary, dried [1Tbs (3 tsp)]	4	0.1	12	41%	0	2	1.5
5740	Rosemary, fresh [½ cup (8Tbs)]	17	0.6	22	40%	1	3	2.4
5741	Saffron [1Tbs (3 tsp)]	2	0.1	7	17%	0	1	0.1
5742	Sage, ground [1Tbs (3 tsp)]	2	0.1	7	36%	0	1	0.8
5743	Salt, table (sodium chloride) [1 tsp]	6	0.2	0	0%	0	0	0.0
5744	Savory, ground [1Tbs (3 tsp)]	4	0.1	11	20%	0	3	1.9
5745	Spearmint, dried [1Tbs (3 tsp)]	2	0.1	4	19%	0	1	0.4
5746	Spearmint, fresh [½ cup (8Tbs)]	46	1.6	20	15%	2	4	3.1
5747	Tarragon, ground [1Tbs (3 tsp)]	5	0.2	14	22%	1	2	0.4
5748	Thyme, fresh [½ cup (8Tbs)]	19	0.7	19	15%	1	5	2.7
5749	Thyme, ground [1Tbs (3 tsp)]	4	0.1	12	24%	0	3	1.6
5750	Tumeric, ground [1Tbs (3 tsp)]	7	0.2	23	25%	1	4	1.4
5751	Vanilla extract [1Tbs (3 tsp)]	13	0.4	36	0%	0	2	0.0
5752	Vanilla extract, imitation [1Tbs (3 tsp)]	13	0.4	30	0%	0	0	0.0
5753	Vanilla extract, imitation, no alcohol [1Tbs (3 tsp)]	13	0.4	7	0%	0	2	0.0
5754	Yeast (Include brewers yeast) [1Tbs, dry]	8	0.3	24	14%	3	3	1.7

Food #	fat gm	sat fat gm	choles mg	sodium mg	potass mg	vit A	vit E	vit C	thia-min	ribo-flavin	nia-cin	vit B-6	fol-ate	vit B-12	cal-cium	phos-phorus	magne-sium	iron	zinc
5705	1	0	0	1	85	0	1	2	2	1	1	1	0	0	4	4	4	6	2
5706	0	0	0	1	67	0	0	2	1	1	0	0	0	0	2	1	3	5	3
5707	1	0	0	2	109	22	1	7	1	3	2	6	1	0	1	2	2	2	1
5708	2	0	0	10	84	0	0	2	1	1	1	1	0	0	11	3	7	15	3
5709	0	0	0	1	85	1	0	2	0	1	0	1	1	0	2	1	1	3	1
5710	1	0	0	79	149	27	0	8	2	4	3	7	2	0	2	2	3	6	1
5711	0	0	0	2	35	0	0	3	0	1	0	1	1	0	8	0	1	15	1
5712	1	0	0	15	69	0	0	8	0	1	0	4	1	0	4	1	4	3	0
5713	0	0	0	4	80	1	0	17	2	2	1	1	1	0	2	1	3	4	1
5714	1	0	0	2	68	0	0	2	1	1	1	0	0	0	4	2	4	5	2
5715	1	0	0	11	113	1	0	1	3	1	1	1	0	0	6	3	6	23	2
5716	1	0	0	3	93	1	0	1	1	1	1	2	2	0	3	2	4	10	2
5717	1	0	0	1	75	0	0	2	2	1	1	1	0	0	10	2	4	6	2
5718	0	0	0	6	99	2	0	3	1	1	0	2	0	0	5	2	3	8	1
5719	0	0	0	3	33	3	0	6	0	1	0	0	2	0	1	0	1	2	0
5720	1	0	0	5	102	0	0	2	2	1	2	0	0	0	7	3	6	6	1
5721	1	0	0	7	85	0	0	1	2	2	1	0	2	0	2	3	5	21	2
5722	0	0	0	2	92	0	0	3	3	1	0	11	0	0	1	4	1	1	1
5723	0	0	0	14	1	0	0	0	0	1	0	0	1	0	0	0	0	0	0
5724	0	0	0	2	73	0	0	1	0	1	1	3	1	0	1	1	2	3	2
5725	2	0	0	4	24	0	0	2	1	1	0	1	1	0	1	1	2	4	1
5726	0	0	0	1	27	1	0	2	0	0	0	1	1	0	4	1	2	8	0
5727	3	0	0	0	68	0	1	0	4	2	4	1	2	0	5	8	7	5	4
5728	2	2	0	1	23	0	1	0	2	0	0	1	1	0	1	1	3	1	1
5729	0	0	0	3	59	0	0	2	2	0	0	5	3	0	2	2	2	1	1
5730	0	0	0	1	75	3	0	4	1	1	1	3	3	0	7	1	3	11	1
5731	1	0	0	2	148	38	0	7	3	6	5	6	2	0	1	2	3	8	2
5732	0	0	0	4	34	2	0	2	0	1	0	0	0	0	1	0	1	5	0
5733	0	0	0	3	79	0	0	2	0	1	0	1	0	0	3	1	3	10	1
5734	0	0	0	0	5	0	1	3	0	1	0	1	0	0	2	1	2	6	1
5735	0	0	0	4	73	5	0	7	1	2	1	1	4	0	3	1	3	4	1
5736	4	0	0	2	59	0	1	0	5	1	0	2	1	0	12	7	7	4	6
5737	0	0	0	1	31	1	0	1	1	1	1	2	2	0	4	1	3	9	1
5738	1	0	0	3	34	0	0	2	0	0	1	1	1	0	3	1	2	6	1
5739	1	0	0	2	34	1	0	4	1	1	0	2	3	0	5	0	2	6	1
5740	1	0	0	4	112	5	0	6	0	2	1	3	5	0	5	1	4	6	1
5741	0	0	0	3	36	0	0	3	0	0	0	1	0	0	0	1	1	1	0
5742	0	0	0	0	22	1	0	1	1	0	1	1	1	0	3	0	2	3	1
5743	0	0	0	2325	0	0	0	0	0	0	0	0	0	0	0	0	0	0	0
5744	0	0	0	1	44	2	0	4	1	0	1	0	0	0	9	1	4	9	1
5745	0	0	0	5	29	2	0	0	0	1	0	2	2	0	2	0	2	7	0
5746	0	0	0	14	209	48	1	10	2	5	2	4	12	0	9	3	7	30	3
5747	0	0	0	3	145	2	0	4	1	4	2	3	3	0	5	2	4	9	1
5748	0	0	0	2	117	9	0	51	1	5	2	3	2	0	8	2	8	19	2
5749	0	0	0	2	34	2	0	4	1	1	1	3	3	0	8	1	2	29	2
5750	1	0	0	3	167	0	0	3	1	1	2	6	1	0	1	2	3	15	2
5751	0	0	0	1	19	0	0	0	0	1	0	0	0	0	0	0	0	0	0
5752	0	0	0	1	12	0	0	0	0	1	0	0	0	0	0	0	0	0	0
5753	0	0	0	0	0	0	0	0	0	0	0	0	0	0	0	0	0	0	0
5754	0	0	0	4	160	0	0	0	13	26	16	6	47	0	1	10	2	7	3

This soup is not only tasty and nutritious but easy and quick. You don't have to soak the lentils in advance, and you only have to simmer the soup for 45 minutes.

Harira (Moroccan Soup)

2 cloves garlic, minced	1 cup dry lentils
2 onions, chopped	2 Tbs uncooked rice
1 Tbs oil	6 cups water
1½ tsp salt	15-oz can of garbanzo beans, drained
1 tsp pepper	8-oz can of tomato sauce
2 Tbs ground coriander	½ cup chopped parsley
½ tsp cumin	Juice of 2 lemons

Sauté garlic and onions in oil in a pot until onions are limp. Mix in salt, pepper, spices, lentils, rice. Add water and bring to a boil. Simmer for about 30 minutes. Add garbanzo beans, tomato sauce, and parsley, and simmer 15 minutes. Add lemon juice and serve. Optional: top each bowl of soup with a dab of sour cream and a sprinkle of chopped parsley.

*   *   *   *   *   *   *   *   *   *   *   *

Salad dressings don't have to be fancy to taste good. A good olive oil combined with a good balsamic or red wine vinegar and a dash of salt and pepper tastes great. Those who like Big Macs will like a salad dressing of mayonaisse with some catsup mixed in.

The recipe below isn't a classic Caesar (it doesn't have anchovies or raw egg) but is a favorite of those who love garlic and hate anchovies.

Caesar Salad Dressing

2 cloves garlic, minced	1 tsp dry mustard
1½ tsp salt	½ tsp Worcheshire sauce
6 Tbs olive oil	¼ tsp black pepper
2 Tbs red wine vinegar	¼ cup grated parmesan cheese
2 Tbs fresh lemon juice	

Mash minced garlic and salt together (or process together in a food processor). Blend in the rest of the ingredients.

Mixed Dishes and Fast Foods

Beef and Veal Dishes *6000*

Pork Dishes *6200*

Lamb Dishes and Other Meat Dishes *6400*

Chicken and Turkey Dishes *6500*

Fish Dishes *6700*

Other Mixed Dishes *6900*

Sandwiches *7400*

Hamburgers and Hot Dogs *7600*

Pizza and Other Fast Foods *7700*

Your Additions

End-of-Section Recipes
Dump Chili
Toaster-Oven Tacos

Mixed Dishes & Fast Food

Food #	Food Description & Amount	wt gm	wt oz	calo-ries	%cal fat	prot gm	carbo gm	fiber gm
	Beef & Veal Dishes							
6000	Beef and barbecue sauce [1 cup]	263	9.3	457	41%	56	8	0.7
6001	Beef and cream or white sauce [1 cup]	256	9.0	367	55%	25	15	0.3
6002	Beef and macaroni with cheese sauce (mixture) [1 cup]	246	8.7	347	42%	21	27	0.8
6003	Beef and noodles with sauce made from cream of mushroom soup [1 cup]	249	8.8	373	36%	33	25	1.0
6004	Beef and noodles with cream or white sauce [1 cup]	249	8.8	389	45%	27	25	0.8
6005	Beef and noodles with gravy [1 cup]	249	8.8	302	28%	31	21	1.1
6006	Beef and noodles with tomato-based sauce (Include beef casserole, Hamburger Helper, Hamburger Helper Chili Tomato, Hamburger Helper Lasagna) [1 cup]	249	8.8	275	23%	29	24	2.1
6007	Beef and noodles, seasoned, no sauce (Include Hamburger Helper Beef Noodle) [1 cup]	156	5.5	262	29%	24	21	0.9
6008	Beef and potatoes with sauce made from cream of mushroom soup [1 cup]	252	8.9	324	35%	27	24	1.8
6009	Beef and potatoes with cheese sauce [1 cup]	249	8.8	510	55%	34	23	2.4
6010	Beef and potatoes with cream or white sauce (Include Hamburger Helper Potato Stroganoff) [1 cup]	252	8.9	303	35%	25	23	1.4
6011	Beef and potatoes with gravy in pie crust [1/6 of 8"square]	216	7.6	321	37%	18	32	2.5
6012	Beef and potatoes, seasoned, but no sauce [1 cup]	190	6.7	284	26%	30	21	1.9
6013	Beef and rice with sauce made from cream of mushroom soup [1 cup]	248	8.7	412	45%	21	34	0.7
6014	Beef and rice with cream sauce [1 cup]	248	8.7	417	44%	20	37	0.6
6015	Beef and rice with gravy [1 cup]	222	7.8	292	34%	18	30	0.7
6016	Beef and rice with tomato-based sauce, onions [1 cup]	244	8.6	307	29%	20	35	3.0
6017	Beef, sweet and sour (beef, pineapple, sweet and sour sauce [1 cup]	252	8.9	336	49%	16	28	1.7
6018	**Beef and vegetables (no carrots, broccoli, dark-green leafy, or potatoes), sauce made from cream of mushroom soup [1 cup]**	**252**	**8.9**	**360**	**57%**	**26**	**12**	**2.4**
6019	Beef and vegetables (as above), gravy [1 cup]	252	8.9	223	22%	27	15	3.9
6020	Beef and vegetables (as above), seasoned, but no sauce [1 cup]	162	5.7	238	47%	15	17	1.7
6021	Beef and vegetables (as above), soy-based sauce [1 cup]	217	7.7	247	42%	16	21	4.0
6022	Beef and vegetables (as above), tomato-based sauce [1 cup]	249	8.8	288	54%	22	12	2.2
6023	**Beef and vegetables (Including carrots, broccoli, and/or dark-green leafy, no potatoes), sauce made from cream of mushroom soup [1 cup]**	**252**	**8.9**	**369**	**54%**	**25**	**16**	**3.3**
6024	Beef and [above] vegetables, gravy [1 cup]	252	8.9	216	25%	28	11	2.1
6025	Beef and [above] vegetables, seasoned, but no sauce [1 cup]	162	5.7	244	48%	16	17	1.8
6026	Beef and [above] vegetables, soy-based sauce [1 cup]	217	7.7	196	47%	16	11	3.9
6027	Beef and [above] vegetables, tomato-based sauce [1 cup]	249	8.8	183	25%	24	9	2.3
6028	Beef and vegetables, Hawaiian style (including seaweed, bamboo shoots, taro, carrots, burdock root, soy sauce) [1 cup]	252	8.9	214	16%	10	37	4.9
6029	Beef in barbeque sauce on bun (Include Sloppy Joe) [1 beef with sauce on bun]	186	6.6	358	37%	18	36	2.4
6030	Beef bourguignon [1 cup]	244	8.6	200	38%	21	9	1.6
6031	Beef burgundy [1 cup]	244	8.6	291	36%	35	9	1.4
6032	Beef chow mein or chop suey with noodles [1 cup]	220	7.8	421	51%	22	31	3.7
6033	Beef chow mein or chop suey, no noodles [1 cup]	220	7.8	271	50%	22	12	2.7
6034	Beef curry [1 cup]	236	8.3	436	65%	27	13	2.7
6035	Beef goulash [1 cup]	249	8.8	270	39%	33	7	1.0
6036	Beef goulash with noodles [1 cup]	249	8.8	361	35%	30	27	1.7
6037	Beef goulash with potatoes [1 cup]	244	8.6	299	37%	27	19	1.9
6038	Beef hash, made from roast beef [1 cup]	190	6.7	312	46%	21	21	2.3
6039	Meat loaf, beef (including meatball or patty, with breading, no sauce) [1 slice]	108	3.8	231	54%	18	7	0.4
6040	Beef roll, stuffed with vegetables or meat mixture (Include roulades, paupiettes, bracciola) [1 beef roll]	134	4.7	279	46%	27	9	1.0
6041	Beef salad [1 cup]	182	6.4	495	70%	33	2	0.8
6042	Beef shishkabob [1 shishkabob]	202	7.1	178	27%	24	9	2.1

Food #	fat gm	sat fat gm	choles mg	sodium mg	potass mg	% of Daily Value														
						vit A	vit E	vit C	thia-min	ribo-flavin	nia-cin	vit B-6	fol-ate	vit B-12	cal-cium	phos-phorus	magne-sium	iron	zinc
6000	21	8	160	632	913	5	3	7	11	23	41	31	4	113	4	46	15	36	85
6001	22	6	68	301	586	22	8	2	12	30	18	13	6	43	20	35	11	17	29
6002	16	7	61	704	265	4	1	1	19	23	20	6	14	19	10	19	9	15	27
6003	15	5	100	651	518	2	3	1	15	21	27	20	11	51	7	35	12	22	35
6004	20	6	80	240	501	17	6	2	17	25	21	17	14	42	16	34	12	17	26
6005	9	3	91	606	453	0	1	0	16	16	26	19	13	47	2	29	10	22	35
6006	7	2	86	667	740	10	5	21	18	17	28	25	14	45	3	29	14	22	30
6007	8	2	82	74	320	2	1	0	15	13	21	16	15	38	1	24	9	18	25
6008	13	4	76	561	579	1	3	12	11	18	22	25	5	44	5	27	10	19	47
6009	31	14	115	885	761	13	3	12	10	26	33	28	6	51	31	43	14	16	43
6010	12	4	65	164	691	10	3	11	14	23	19	26	5	39	15	31	12	14	37
6011	13	3	38	462	563	3	5	12	17	15	22	23	5	23	3	19	9	14	25
6012	8	3	88	62	589	0	1	13	11	16	23	28	5	49	2	27	10	20	52
6013	21	7	61	803	346	3	5	2	12	16	28	13	11	34	10	22	8	17	29
6014	20	7	55	409	351	6	5	1	17	18	25	14	17	31	14	23	9	16	24
6015	11	4	47	878	247	0	1	0	13	8	24	11	15	25	2	15	6	16	26
6016	10	4	47	83	825	15	11	21	17	12	28	22	15	26	3	23	14	22	20
6017	18	6	54	930	336	3	4	36	8	11	13	16	3	27	3	15	8	15	26
6018	23	8	88	801	506	2	4	10	5	16	31	16	9	46	6	22	9	19	38
6019	5	2	71	853	416	4	1	18	16	17	20	17	12	38	4	26	10	22	45
6020	12	4	49	271	380	6	3	33	6	10	21	13	9	25	2	14	7	12	22
6021	11	2	39	464	458	7	7	27	10	15	14	13	10	27	5	17	11	17	20
6022	17	7	75	732	742	14	7	94	9	14	32	26	6	38	3	19	11	17	31
6023	22	8	86	638	653	190	5	14	9	16	33	20	7	45	6	23	9	17	36
6024	6	2	81	91	462	66	1	9	10	17	18	18	7	43	4	25	8	20	48
6025	13	4	51	283	403	35	3	34	7	11	22	13	9	26	3	15	8	12	22
6026	10	3	44	339	457	161	8	79	6	14	11	18	11	18	6	16	8	14	31
6027	5	2	70	116	473	93	1	16	8	14	16	18	5	37	4	22	8	17	42
6028	4	1	13	1747	811	79	8	11	11	13	17	20	21	10	11	20	22	15	13
6029	15	5	46	1008	368	7	6	10	19	16	29	11	18	26	9	15	9	20	21
6030	8	2	56	112	549	3	3	7	7	13	16	16	5	41	3	23	10	16	32
6031	12	3	94	114	844	1	4	7	13	29	34	22	6	68	3	38	13	27	53
6032	24	5	43	950	519	10	6	33	24	21	29	20	18	28	4	26	14	23	23
6033	15	4	50	924	556	12	7	39	12	15	21	21	12	33	4	24	10	16	23
6034	31	7	69	802	978	37	20	41	12	20	27	24	5	51	4	29	15	24	40
6035	12	3	84	225	698	3	6	15	10	18	29	23	6	54	2	34	11	20	35
6036	14	3	95	130	549	2	8	7	19	19	29	19	18	45	2	32	13	23	31
6037	12	3	65	179	912	2	8	29	11	16	27	26	7	42	2	29	13	19	29
6038	16	5	57	470	587	0	4	12	11	12	19	25	4	30	2	20	9	14	33
6039	14	5	90	133	295	2	0	1	5	16	20	7	4	28	4	16	6	11	24
6040	14	5	76	218	492	36	2	5	14	16	23	22	6	46	2	25	8	16	28
6041	39	9	130	291	418	3	13	5	7	19	15	26	5	45	4	27	7	23	73
6042	5	2	58	59	626	6	2	55	10	13	20	23	6	40	2	23	9	15	25

Mixed Dishes & Fast Food

Food #	Food Description & Amount	wt gm	wt oz	calo-ries	%cal fat	prot gm	carbo gm	fiber gm
6043	Beef steak with onions, Puerto Rican style (Include Biftec encebollado, Puerto Rican style stewed steak) [1 cup]	179	6.3	589	69%	38	7	1.4
6044	Beef stew, from dried beef, Puerto Rican style (Include Tasajo guisado, carne cecina guisada) [1 cup]	200	7.1	491	67%	34	6	1.0
6045	Beef stew, seasoned ground beef with potatoes, Mexican style (Include Picadillo de carne de rez con papas) [1 cup]	222	7.8	385	63%	24	10	1.4
6046	Beef stew, Mexican style, no potatoes, tomato-based sauce (Include Carne guisada sin papas) [1 cup]	244	8.6	455	35%	57	14	2.0
6047	Beef stew, Mexican style, no potatoes, tomato-based sauce with chili peppers (Include Carne guisada con chile) [1 cup]	244	8.6	386	31%	45	21	3.2
6048	Beef stew, Puerto Rican style, meat with gravy [1 cup]	235	8.3	437	68%	30	3	0.6
6049	Beef stew, Puerto-Rican style (Include Carne a la Judia) [1 cup]	195	6.9	422	59%	29	13	1.6
6050	**Beef stew with potatoes and vegetables (no carrots, broccoli, dark-green leafy), gravy [1 cup]**	**252**	**8.9**	**298**	**40%**	**25**	**18**	**2.4**
6051	Beef stew with potatoes & vegetables (as above), tomato-based sauce [1 cup]	252	8.9	292	40%	25	19	2.5
6052	**Beef stew with potatoes and vegetables (including carrots, broccoli, and/or dark-green leafy), gravy [1 cup]**	**252**	**8.9**	**176**	**18%**	**17**	**19**	**2.9**
6053	Beef stew with potatoes and [above] vegetables, tomato-based sauce [1 cup]	252	8.9	176	18%	17	20	3.1
6054	Beef stew with potatoes, gravy [1 cup]	252	8.9	221	21%	23	20	1.8
6055	Beef stew with potatoes, tomato-based sauce [1 cup]	252	8.9	230	20%	23	22	2.1
6056	Beef stroganoff with noodles (Include Hamburger Helper Beef Stroganoff) [1 cup]	256	9.0	344	50%	20	23	1.5
6057	Beef stroganoff [1 cup]	256	9.0	408	60%	26	16	1.4
6058	Beef wellington [1 slice]	116	4.1	355	57%	25	12	0.5
6059	Beef with tomato-based sauce (Include beef with tomatoes, meatballs with tomato sauce) [1 cup]	249	8.8	449	62%	32	10	2.1
6060	Beef and dumplings and vegetables (including carrots, broccoli, and/or dark-green leafy), gravy [1 cup]	249	8.8	230	43%	16	17	2.1
6061	**Beef and dumplings and vegetables (no carrots, broccoli, dark-green leafy), gravy [1 cup]**	**249**	**8.8**	**269**	**41%**	**19**	**21**	**2.6**
6062	Beef and noodles and vegetables (as above), sauce of cream of mushroom soup [1 cup]	249	8.8	342	52%	18	23	2.0
6063	Beef and noodles and vegetables (as above), gravy [1 cup]	249	8.8	276	36%	19	25	2.8
6064	Beef and noodles and vegetables (as above), seasoned, but no sauce [1 cup]	162	5.7	206	23%	19	20	2.3
6065	Beef and noodles and vegetables (as above), soy-based sauce [1 cup]	217	7.7	226	28%	12	28	2.0
6066	Beef and noodles and vegetables (as above), tomato-based sauce [1 cup]	249	8.8	231	18%	20	27	2.6
6067	**Beef and noodles and vegetables (including carrots, broccoli, and/or dark-green leafy), sauce made with cream of mushroom soup [1 cup]**	**249**	**8.8**	**342**	**52%**	**18**	**23**	**2.1**
6068	Beef and noodles and [above] vegetables, gravy [1 cup]	249	8.8	269	38%	18	24	2.4
6069	Beef and noodles and [above] vegetables, seasoned, but no sauce [1 cup]	162	5.7	205	23%	19	20	2.4
6070	Beef and noodles and [above] vegetables, soy-based sauce [1 cup]	217	7.7	222	28%	13	27	2.4
6071	Beef and noodles and [above] vegetables, tomato-based sauce [1 cup]	249	8.8	215	17%	18	26	2.9
6072	Beef and noodles and [above] vegetables, sauce of cream of mushroom soup [1 cup]	252	8.9	403	51%	27	22	2.4
6073	Beef & noodles and [above] vegetables, no sauce [1 cup]	162	5.7	182	24%	18	16	2.7
6074	**Beef and potatoes and vegetables (no carrots, broccoli, dark-green leafy), sauce made with cream of mushroom soup [1 cup]**	**252**	**8.9**	**402**	**52%**	**27**	**21**	**2.2**
6075	Beef and potatoes and vegetables (as above), seasoned, but no sauce [1 cup]	162	5.7	183	23%	19	16	2.6
6076	Beef and rice and vegetables (as above), sauce of cream of mushroom soup [1 cup]	249	8.8	363	43%	21	30	2.0
6077	Beef and rice and vegetables (as above), gravy [1 cup]	249	8.8	313	44%	21	22	2.1
6078	Beef and rice and vegetables (as above), but no sauce [1 cup]	162	5.7	204	20%	18	22	1.9
6079	Beef and rice and vegetables (as above), soy-based sauce [1 cup]	217	7.7	209	35%	13	21	1.4
6080	Beef and rice and vegetables (as above), tomato-based sauce [1 cup]	249	8.8	210	14%	16	28	2.9

Food #	fat gm	sat fat gm	choles mg	sodium mg	potass mg	vit A	vit E	vit C	thia-min	ribo-flavin	nia-cin	vit B-6	fol-ate	vit B-12	cal-cium	phos-phorus	magne-sium	iron	zinc

Food #	fat gm	sat fat gm	choles mg	sodium mg	potass mg	vit A	vit E	vit C	thia-min	ribo-flavin	nia-cin	vit B-6	fol-ate	vit B-12	cal-cium	phos-phorus	magne-sium	iron	zinc
6043	45	12	114	84	643	0	17	7	10	17	27	30	6	68	3	35	11	21	40
6044	37	7	56	4465	673	4	21	18	7	15	30	14	4	37	2	23	12	31	40
6045	27	11	97	95	625	3	2	47	7	18	30	17	5	38	2	21	9	16	35
6046	18	6	157	591	1301	6	6	18	20	36	49	36	8	113	4	57	21	41	86
6047	13	4	118	450	1363	13	7	409	21	33	42	41	12	84	5	48	23	38	67
6048	33	12	109	226	370	2	4	14	7	16	19	18	3	54	2	25	7	20	50
6049	28	9	86	291	868	3	8	24	10	15	28	25	4	45	2	30	12	19	30
6050	13	6	67	110	591	2	1	19	9	12	16	14	7	31	2	22	9	19	41
6051	13	5	65	138	620	3	1	24	9	12	17	14	7	30	3	22	9	19	40
6052	4	1	39	114	654	71	1	20	11	12	17	17	7	28	3	19	9	14	24
6053	4	1	38	140	686	71	1	24	12	12	18	17	8	28	3	19	10	15	24
6054	5	2	58	73	869	0	1	25	11	15	23	23	5	42	2	25	11	18	34
6055	5	2	58	188	794	2	2	26	12	14	24	26	6	42	2	25	12	17	34
6056	19	7	74	468	394	7	5	2	14	18	19	10	12	30	7	24	9	18	24
6057	27	11	85	677	556	10	8	3	12	23	23	14	7	43	9	31	10	20	33
6058	22	7	94	80	361	2	5	1	12	25	21	17	9	44	1	23	7	24	30
6059	31	12	114	403	808	10	6	36	8	19	44	24	5	55	5	26	12	23	46
6060	11	4	41	820	350	62	1	4	8	11	19	11	5	21	6	15	5	14	24
6061	12	5	44	908	353	2	1	8	13	13	22	10	8	23	8	18	6	17	26
6062	20	8	69	769	279	6	4	5	8	15	18	9	9	21	17	23	8	14	23
6063	11	5	58	795	331	2	1	8	13	11	22	10	11	22	3	18	7	18	27
6064	5	2	64	82	258	3	1	10	14	12	15	12	14	26	3	19	8	17	30
6065	7	1	45	592	275	2	4	32	13	10	15	12	16	15	2	15	8	13	12
6066	5	1	62	315	503	6	2	24	18	15	21	14	18	31	3	22	11	20	27
6067	20	8	68	775	286	43	4	5	8	14	18	10	9	21	17	23	8	13	22
6068	11	5	59	788	336	40	1	4	10	11	21	11	9	22	3	16	7	17	26
6069	5	2	64	80	264	41	1	8	14	12	15	13	14	26	3	19	8	17	30
6070	7	1	43	584	286	28	4	28	13	10	14	12	18	15	4	15	9	13	12
6071	4	1	55	288	516	60	3	24	17	14	19	14	16	27	4	21	11	18	24
6072	23	8	88	628	788	49	4	22	8	16	36	24	6	46	5	24	10	19	38
6073	5	2	50	85	424	44	1	14	10	11	15	19	6	28	3	18	8	14	31
6074	23	8	89	642	781	0	4	22	8	16	36	23	6	47	5	24	10	19	39
6075	5	2	50	88	418	3	1	16	11	11	15	18	7	28	2	18	8	14	31
6076	17	6	65	573	417	0	3	5	13	12	30	15	16	34	5	20	8	19	30
6077	15	6	65	359	448	3	3	61	10	11	29	20	13	36	3	18	8	17	27
6078	4	2	46	79	262	3	1	10	14	10	15	13	13	26	3	18	7	16	30
6079	8	2	32	437	307	0	2	11	10	12	16	12	13	13	3	15	7	13	15
6080	3	1	34	306	485	6	2	25	16	12	18	15	17	24	3	19	9	17	23

Mixed Dishes & Fast Food

Food #	Food Description & Amount	wt gm	wt oz	calo-ries	%cal fat	prot gm	carbo gm	fiber gm
6081	**Beef and rice and vegetables (including carrots, broccoli, and/or dark-green leafy), sauce made with mushroom soup [1 cup]**	**249**	**8.8**	**367**	**42%**	**21**	**31**	**2.3**
6082	Beef and rice and [above] vegetables, gravy [1 cup]	249	8.8	334	44%	22	23	2.2
6083	Beef and rice and [above] vegetables, seasoned, but no sauce [1 cup]	162	5.7	203	20%	18	22	2.0
6084	Beef and rice and [above] vegetables, soy-based sauce [1 cup]	217	7.7	200	34%	12	21	2.0
6085	Beef and rice and [above] vegetables, tomato-based sauce [1 cup]	249	8.8	213	15%	17	28	2.5
6086	Beef and tofu and [above] vegetables, soy-based sauce [1 cup]	217	7.7	272	47%	22	16	2.6
6087	Beef and tofu and vegetables (no carrots, broccoli, dark-green leafy, or potatoes), soy-based sauce [1 cup]	217	7.7	277	46%	23	17	3.1
6088	Brunswick stew [1 cup]	243	8.6	321	39%	29	19	2.8
6089	Bulgogi (Include Korean-style beef, teriyaki beef) [1 cup]	244	8.6	331	58%	24	8	0.3
6090	Chili con carne without beans [1 cup]	254	9.0	351	48%	25	21	3.7
6091	**Chili con carne with beans [1 cup]**	**254**	**9.0**	**322**	**40%**	**22**	**27**	**7.5**
6092	Chili con carne with beans and cheese [1 cup]	254	9.0	378	47%	26	25	6.9
6093	Chili con carne (pork) with beans [1 cup]	254	9.0	275	27%	24	27	7.5
6094	Corned beef hash [1 cup]	190	6.7	344	56%	17	20	1.0
6095	Corned beef with tomato sauce and onion, Puerto Rican style [1 cup]	235	8.3	472	55%	45	5	1.0
6096	Corned beef and potatoes and vegetables (no carrots, broccoli, and dark-green leafy), seasoned, but no sauce [1 cup]	162	5.7	180	42%	10	17	2.3
6097	Corned beef and potatoes and vegetables (including carrots, broccoli, and/or dark-green leafy), seasoned, but no sauce [1 cup]	162	5.7	169	40%	9	17	2.6
6098	Creamed chipped or dried beef [1 cup]	246	8.7	327	55%	18	18	0.3
6099	Ground beef patty (including onion) with gravy [1 patty with gravy]	115	4.1	138	30%	20	3	0.3
6100	Ground beef patty (including egg and onion) [1 patty]	85	3.0	218	59%	20	1	0.1
6101	Ground beef with tomato sauce and taco seasonings on a cornbread crust (Include Hamburger Helper Taco Bake) [1 cup]	179	6.3	364	39%	18	37	4.1
6102	Ground beef, stewed seasoned Mexican style (Include Picadillo de carne de rez) [1 cup]	222	7.8	462	69%	31	3	0.5
6103	Ground beef, stewed seasoned, Puerto Rican style (Include Picadillo guisado, picadillo de carne) [1 cup]	200	7.1	577	73%	32	5	1.1
6104	Ground beef, stewed seasoned, Puerto Rican style (Picadillo para relleno) [1 cup]	150	5.3	481	70%	30	5	1.1
6105	Liver (beef or calf) and onions, fried, seasoned [1 slice with onions]	143	5.0	215	30%	24	12	0.8
6106	Mexican style beef stew with potatoes, tomato-based sauce (Include Carne guisada con papas) [1 cup]	244	8.6	274	32%	32	13	1.6
6107	Pepper steak [1 cup]	217	7.7	320	58%	28	6	1.3
6108	**Salisbury steak with gravy [1 steak with gravy]**	**129**	**4.6**	**219**	**56%**	**16**	**7**	**0.4**
6109	Sloppy Joe (not including bun) [1 cup]	251	8.9	402	51%	28	23	2.4
6110	Soup meat, seasoned, shredded , Puerto Rican style (Include Ropa vieja, sopa de carne ripiada) [1 cup]	133	4.7	275	56%	24	5	1.2
6111	Steak tartare (raw ground beef seasoned with onion, egg yolk, anchovy) [1 cup]	224	7.9	511	65%	40	1	0.2
6112	Stuffed cabbage rolls with rice [1 roll]	103	3.6	126	45%	8	9	1.3
6113	Stuffed grape leaves with beef and rice [1 roll]	21	0.7	50	69%	2	2	0.7
6114	Stuffed green pepper, Puerto Rican style (Pimiento relleno) [1 pepper (3½"x3½"x2")]	250	8.8	433	40%	22	43	4.6
6115	Stuffed pot roast, Puerto Rican style, with gravy and stuffing [1 slice with gravy and stuffing]	134	4.7	379	70%	26	1	0.2
6116	Swedish meatballs with cream or white sauce [1 cup]	246	8.7	406	51%	31	17	0.6
6117	Swiss steak (floured, braised; cooked with tomato-vegetable sauce) [1 piece with sauce]	170	6.0	177	39%	20	7	1.1
6118	Swiss steak, with gravy [1 steak with gravy]	92	3.2	182	46%	15	8	3.4
6119	Tripe, stewed Puerto Rican style, with potatoes (Include Mondongo) [1 cup]	280	9.9	318	33%	27	27	5.2
6120	Variety meats, stewed Puerto Rican style (mostly liver) (Include Gandinga) [1 cup]	165	5.8	166	24%	23	8	1.4
6121	Veal and noodles with cream or white sauce [1 cup]	224	7.9	377	46%	27	22	0.7
6122	Veal cordon bleu [1 roll (with ham and sauce)]	229	8.1	476	67%	33	4	0.7

Food #	fat gm	sat fat gm	choles mg	sodium mg	potass mg	vit A	vit E	vit C	thia-min	ribo-flavin	nia-cin	vit B-6	fol-ate	vit B-12	cal-cium	phos-phorus	magne-sium	iron	zinc
														% of Daily Value					
6081	**17**	**6**	**65**	**558**	**428**	**61**	**3**	**6**	**14**	**12**	**31**	**15**	**15**	**34**	**5**	**20**	**8**	**19**	**30**
6082	16	6	69	393	488	74	2	8	11	12	31	17	13	38	4	20	8	17	29
6083	4	2	46	77	269	40	1	8	13	10	15	14	13	26	3	17	7	16	30
6084	7	2	29	410	334	45	3	25	10	9	14	13	14	12	3	14	7	12	14
6085	3	1	36	285	521	60	3	24	16	12	19	16	15	26	3	19	10	17	24
6086	14	3	36	1243	442	39	5	6	12	12	11	14	8	29	15	25	36	46	30
6087	14	3	36	1225	433	2	5	13	14	13	12	14	10	28	15	26	37	47	31
6088	14	4	77	393	634	9	4	16	33	18	32	22	7	8	5	26	14	12	20
6089	21	6	53	861	530	0	6	2	6	12	32	14	3	42	2	26	7	15	27
6090	19	7	81	911	830	16	8	47	13	18	35	23	7	44	6	23	13	22	34
6091	**14**	**5**	**60**	**912**	**765**	**12**	**6**	**35**	**13**	**16**	**27**	**18**	**11**	**32**	**6**	**23**	**14**	**21**	**27**
6092	20	9	76	965	724	17	6	33	13	19	25	17	11	33	20	32	14	20	29
6093	8	3	51	892	793	12	6	36	45	21	24	22	11	7	7	26	14	16	16
6094	21	7	63	1026	380	0	1	0	1	10	20	8	4	20	2	13	7	21	29
6095	29	11	142	1837	387	3	5	9	4	16	22	14	5	42	3	20	8	21	40
6096	8	3	42	493	344	0	1	22	7	6	12	17	5	12	2	9	6	6	15
6097	8	2	37	452	347	43	1	20	7	6	11	17	5	10	3	9	6	6	13
6098	20	6	32	1469	499	25	8	3	11	27	13	10	7	25	27	28	10	12	18
6099	5	2	54	62	364	0	0	1	6	12	16	11	2	39	1	19	6	13	30
6100	14	6	102	74	250	1	1	1	2	11	23	11	3	39	1	15	4	11	28
6101	16	5	76	975	414	9	4	16	14	18	24	14	12	25	9	36	9	16	21
6102	35	14	127	121	515	1	1	15	5	22	35	13	4	50	2	24	9	19	44
6103	47	16	126	1219	693	5	10	22	11	22	36	18	4	43	3	29	11	18	41
6104	38	12	105	1185	644	4	9	19	31	21	31	21	3	25	3	29	10	13	29
6105	7	2	424	415	410	943	2	38	14	215	64	66	50	1638	2	42	7	31	33
6106	10	3	87	329	862	4	3	16	12	21	29	24	5	62	2	33	13	24	48
6107	20	4	70	563	550	2	11	45	9	14	22	24	7	48	3	26	9	17	29
6108	**14**	**6**	**60**	**438**	**292**	**0**	**1**	**1**	**5**	**14**	**17**	**6**	**3**	**20**	**3**	**14**	**5**	**12**	**24**
6109	23	9	97	1100	935	11	7	30	9	17	38	25	7	53	5	24	13	22	40
6110	17	5	60	64	442	3	6	43	7	11	19	14	4	36	2	25	7	18	35
6111	37	15	240	268	617	5	3	1	9	33	49	29	7	74	4	33	11	24	58
6112	6	2	42	206	293	4	2	23	4	6	10	6	6	11	3	8	5	7	11
6113	4	1	5	15	47	13	1	3	1	2	2	2	2	2	2	2	2	2	2
6114	19	7	61	921	859	16	8	182	26	24	37	29	16	24	12	22	16	29	27
6115	29	10	93	381	260	0	3	1	7	13	16	14	2	42	1	21	5	16	41
6116	23	10	163	407	574	9	1	4	20	31	33	16	7	40	12	33	11	18	37
6117	8	2	49	142	496	21	3	14	8	12	19	14	4	32	3	20	8	13	21
6118	9	1	0	620	136	0	6	0	45	26	37	43	15	29	2	25	4	9	9
6119	12	3	118	571	1070	14	6	94	15	19	11	21	21	23	5	26	14	24	28
6120	4	1	281	92	465	429	3	80	24	165	66	25	34	278	2	30	7	115	37
6121	19	6	104	236	390	16	6	1	14	27	26	11	13	24	16	30	11	11	33
6122	35	19	172	599	503	20	3	8	14	24	49	23	6	27	18	37	11	8	28

Mixed Dishes & Fast Food

Food #	Food Description & Amount	wt gm	wt oz	calo-ries	%cal fat	prot gm	carbo gm	fiber gm
6123	Veal fricassee, Puerto Rican style (Include ternera en fricase) [1 cup]	230	8.1	391	42%	38	18	2.3
6124	Veal goulash with vegetables (no carrots, broccoli, dark-green leafy, or potatoes), tomato-base sauce (Include veal marengo, veal stew) [1 cup]	252	8.9	243	34%	32	7	1.0
6125	Veal goulash with vegetables (including carrots, broccoli, and/or dark-green leafy; no potatoes), tomato-base sauce (Include veal marengo, veal stew) [1 cup]	252	8.9	248	34%	33	7	1.1
6126	Veal Marsala [1 slice with sauce]	96	3.4	267	66%	12	6	0.2
6127	**Veal parmigiana** [1 piece with sauce and cheese]	182	6.4	359	53%	26	16	1.1
6128	Veal scaloppini [1 slice with sauce]	96	3.4	238	64%	18	1	0.4
6129	Veal stew with potatoes and vegetables (no carrots, broccoli, or dark-green leafy), tomato-based sauce) [1 cup]	252	8.9	198	30%	16	18	2.5
6130	Veal stew with potatoes and vegetables (including carrots, broccoli, and/or dark-green leafy), tomato-based sauce [1 cup]	252	8.9	190	31%	16	16	2.8
6131	Veal with butter sauce [1 piece with sauce]	99	3.5	156	54%	16	2	0.1
6132	Veal with cream sauce (Include veal paprikash) [1 cup]	246	8.7	281	39%	36	5	0.6
6133	Veal with gravy [1 slice with gravy]	65	2.3	100	44%	12	1	0.1
6134	Veal with vegetables (no carrots, broccoli, dark-green leafy, or potatoes), cream or white sauce [1 cup]	241	8.5	292	46%	30	9	1.2
6135	Veal with vegetables (including carrots, broccoli, and/or dark-green leafy; no potatoes), cream or white sauce [1 cup]	241	8.5	251	44%	26	9	1.8
Pork Dishes								
6200	Chitterlings, stewed Puerto Rican style (Include cuajo guisado) [1 cup]	240	8.5	618	83%	17	11	2.3
6201	Cabbage with ham hocks [1 cup]	200	7.1	191	55%	16	6	3.1
6202	Greens with ham or pork [1 cup]	144	5.1	78	41%	6	6	3.1
6203	Ham and noodles with cream or white sauce [1 cup]	244	8.6	381	39%	27	30	1.0
6204	Ham and noodles, no sauce [1 cup]	157	5.5	239	26%	19	24	1.1
6205	Ham and rice mixed with cream of mushroom soup [1 cup]	248	8.7	332	35%	17	35	0.7
6206	Ham and vegetables (no carrots, broccoli, dark-green leafy, or potatoes), seasoned, but no sauce [1 cup]	162	5.7	220	57%	19	5	2.2
6207	Ham and vegetables (including carrots, broccoli, and/or dark-green leafy; no potatoes), seasoned, but no sauce [1 cup]	162	5.7	226	55%	19	7	2.1
6208	Ham croquette [1 croquette (1½"x2")]	62	2.2	151	53%	9	8	0.2
6209	Ham loaf (not luncheon meat) (Include pork meatball with breading) [1 slice]	108	3.8	207	38%	25	6	0.3
6210	Ham or pork and potatoes with cheese sauce [1 cup]	249	8.8	385	52%	26	20	2.0
6211	**Ham or pork and potatoes with gravy** [1 cup]	252	8.9	255	34%	21	21	1.8
6212	Ham or pork and rice, no sauce [1 cup]	196	6.9	295	22%	21	34	0.5
6213	Ham or pork salad [1 cup]	182	6.4	396	69%	27	2	0.8
6214	Ham or pork with sauce made from cream of mushroom soup [1 slice with sauce]	65	2.3	97	48%	10	2	0.1
6215	Ham or pork with barbecue sauce [1 slice with sauce]	58	2.0	104	46%	12	2	0.1
6216	Ham or pork with gravy [1 slice with gravy]	65	2.3	77	38%	10	2	0.1
6217	Ham or pork with stuffing [1 stuffed pork chop]	155	5.5	287	28%	26	24	1.0
6218	Ham or pork with tomato-based sauce [1 slice with sauce]	65	2.3	85	49%	8	3	0.6
6219	Ham or pork, noodles and vegetables (no carrots, broccoli, or dark-green leafy), cheese sauce [1 cup]	241	8.5	443	43%	33	28	2.5
6220	Ham or pork, noodles, and vegetables (including carrots, broccoli, and/or dark-green leafy), tomato-based sauce [1 cup]	249	8.8	418	43%	31	29	2.9
6221	Ham, potatoes, and [above] vegetables, no sauce [1 cup]	162	5.7	228	50%	17	11	1.9
6222	Ham, potatoes, and vegetables (no carrots, broccoli, or dark-green leafy), no sauce [1 cup]	162	5.7	176	48%	13	10	2.3
6223	Ham pot pie [1 piece (1/6 of pie)]	105	3.7	251	54%	9	19	1.3
6224	Ham stroganoff (Include ham with cream or white sauce) [1 cup]	244	8.6	356	63%	21	11	1.4
6225	Pork and onions with soy-based sauce (mixture) [1 cup]	256	9.0	531	49%	34	35	2.0

Food #	fat gm	sat fat gm	choles mg	sodium mg	potass mg	% of Daily Value													
						vit A	vit E	vit C	thia-min	ribo-flavin	nia-cin	vit B-6	fol-ate	vit B-12	cal-cium	phos-phorus	magne-sium	iron	zinc
6123	18	4	129	760	963	4	12	43	12	23	57	31	8	19	3	31	14	13	29
6124	9	3	115	237	695	3	6	15	8	24	68	26	7	18	2	35	12	9	24
6125	9	3	119	251	736	50	7	15	9	25	71	27	7	18	2	36	12	10	24
6126	19	9	70	144	212	8	3	3	4	9	25	10	3	8	2	13	4	4	9
6127	21	8	145	648	538	13	8	12	11	25	43	21	7	15	20	34	11	12	20
6128	17	5	65	278	253	10	6	1	3	14	26	10	3	15	5	17	5	5	19
6129	7	3	55	160	614	3	1	24	9	13	34	21	8	9	3	19	9	8	14
6130	7	3	55	167	548	60	2	20	9	13	34	20	8	9	4	19	9	8	14
6131	9	5	73	218	197	8	1	0	3	10	24	8	3	9	1	12	3	4	11
6132	12	5	139	158	696	12	3	3	8	29	77	27	6	21	4	40	13	10	27
6133	5	2	43	190	142	0	1	0	2	7	16	6	2	10	1	10	3	3	14
6134	15	6	115	333	545	9	4	4	8	28	50	17	7	22	11	31	11	8	22
6135	12	5	95	309	689	58	5	42	10	29	42	22	25	18	15	28	20	16	21
6200	57	17	214	189	358	8	10	121	6	11	5	13	6	26	6	11	9	35	52
6201	12	4	41	802	320	2	1	45	32	13	17	20	7	7	5	16	6	4	11
6202	4	1	11	522	361	61	4	57	11	9	7	12	19	2	13	7	6	5	6
6203	17	5	70	1466	468	8	5	1	30	28	25	14	10	11	19	34	12	13	19
6204	7	2	63	788	208	3	2	0	38	13	22	15	16	8	2	20	8	12	14
6205	13	4	30	1405	317	3	5	2	31	16	22	15	10	8	10	22	8	12	15
6206	14	5	50	966	392	3	1	20	36	14	20	19	6	9	4	20	7	7	14
6207	14	5	50	998	416	129	2	29	35	14	20	23	3	9	5	20	7	7	14
6208	9	2	18	494	153	5	3	1	17	9	10	8	3	5	5	10	3	4	6
6209	9	3	104	986	355	3	3	6	29	18	24	16	3	10	3	25	6	8	17
6210	22	10	80	1266	688	10	3	11	35	25	26	25	4	13	26	42	12	8	22
6211	10	3	57	651	821	0	1	25	37	16	30	25	5	9	2	26	10	10	16
6212	7	2	39	984	270	3	2	0	46	12	27	22	18	8	2	22	8	12	16
6213	31	6	76	1618	474	3	14	5	49	17	27	36	5	14	3	26	7	7	19
6214	5	2	26	208	162	0	1	1	22	8	10	9	1	5	2	9	3	3	6
6215	5	2	33	430	187	1	1	2	24	8	12	9	1	5	1	11	3	4	8
6216	3	1	30	180	125	0	0	1	15	7	8	7	1	4	1	9	2	2	7
6217	9	3	62	1261	432	0	1	0	64	24	34	22	12	11	4	27	8	13	18
6218	5	1	22	465	273	3	2	8	14	6	11	8	1	3	1	9	4	4	6
6219	21	9	90	1143	539	19	5	8	49	33	27	21	15	14	29	45	13	15	25
6220	20	7	86	1114	622	124	6	17	51	28	30	28	13	12	21	38	13	17	24
6221	13	4	46	894	467	64	2	34	34	12	20	24	3	8	4	19	8	7	13
6222	9	3	34	652	334	1	1	29	27	10	15	19	5	6	3	14	6	4	9
6223	15	3	13	450	207	16	6	7	17	10	14	6	7	3	1	10	4	8	6
6224	25	11	65	1620	429	11	7	3	35	19	23	18	4	12	10	26	8	7	17
6225	29	5	87	758	797	3	13	18	56	25	38	28	10	12	8	35	13	15	20

Mixed Dishes & Fast Food

Food #	Food Description & Amount	wt gm	wt oz	calo-ries	%cal fat	prot gm	carbo gm	fiber gm
6226	Pork and rice with tomato-based sauce [1 cup]	244	8.6	349	29%	25	35	1.2
6227	**Pork and vegetables (including carrots, broccoli, and/or dark-green leafy; no potatoes), no sauce (Include chow yuk) [1 cup]**	162	5.7	223	40%	22	12	4.1
6228	Pork and [above] vegetables, tomato-based sauce [1 cup]	249	8.8	288	40%	33	9	2.3
6229	Pork and [above] vegetables, soy-based sauce [1 cup]	217	7.7	247	42%	14	22	3.2
6230	Pork and vegetables, Hawaiian style (includes bamboo shoots, onions, burdock root, carrots, mushrooms) [1 cup]	252	8.9	223	43%	14	20	4.9
6331	**Pork and vegetables (no carrots, broccoli, dark-green leafy, or potatoes), tomato-based sauce [1 cup]**	249	8.8	286	42%	33	7	1.7
6232	Pork and vegetables (described above), soy-based sauce [1 cup]	217	7.7	259	45%	16	21	4.0
6233	Pork and vegetables (described above), no sauce [1 cup]	162	5.7	211	42%	22	8	2.0
6234	Pork, potatoes, and vegetables (described above), gravy [1 cup]	252	8.9	227	28%	16	25	3.5
6235	Pork, potatoes, and vegetables (described above), no sauce [1 cup]	162	5.7	197	34%	14	18	2.3
6236	Pork, potatoes, and vegetables (described above), tomato-based sauce [1 cup]	252	8.9	230	26%	17	26	4.4
6237	**Pork, potatoes, and vegetables (including carrots, broccoli, and/or dark-green leafy), gravy [1 cup]**	252	8.9	218	29%	15	24	3.0
6238	Pork, potatoes, and [above] vegetables, no sauce [1 cup]	162	5.7	204	33%	14	20	3.3
6239	Pork, potatoes, and [above] vegetables, tomato-based sauce [1 cup]	252	8.9	220	27%	16	26	4.0
6240	Pork, rice, and [above] vegetables, soy-based sauce [1 cup]	217	7.7	247	29%	20	23	1.6
6241	Pork, rice, and [above] vegetables, tomato-based sauce [1 cup]	249	8.8	230	27%	16	27	2.7
6242	**Pork, rice, and vegetables (no carrots, broccoli, dark-green leafy, or potatoes), soy-based sauce (Include pork chop suey with rice) [1 cup]**	217	7.7	241	29%	19	23	1.5
6243	Pork, rice, and vegetables (described above), tomato-based sauce [1 cup]	249	8.8	254	26%	17	30	2.9
6244	Pork hash, Hawaiian style ground pork, vegetables (described above), soy-based sauce [1 cup]	190	6.7	347	62%	26	6	1.0
6245	Pork, tofu, and vegetables (described above), soy-based sauce [1 cup]	217	7.7	309	51%	23	17	3.1
6246	Pork, tofu, and vegetables (including carrots, broccoli, and/or dark-green leafy, no potatoes), soy-base sauce [1 cup]	217	7.7	303	52%	22	16	2.7
6247	Pork chop stewed with vegetables, Puerto Rican style (Chuletas a la jardinera) [1 cup]	235	8.3	224	28%	26	15	2.4
6248	**Pork chow mein or chop suey with noodles [1 cup]**	220	7.8	448	54%	22	31	3.7
6249	Pork chow mein or chop suey, no noodles [1 cup]	220	7.8	286	53%	22	12	2.7
6250	Pork or ham with soy-based sauce [1 cup]	244	8.6	337	50%	34	5	0.1
6251	Pork roast, stuffed, Puerto Rican style [1 slice (3"x¾") with stuffing]	120	4.2	237	48%	27	3	0.5
6252	Pork stew, Mexican style, no potatoes, tomato-based sauce (mixture) (Include cerdo guisado sin papas) [1 cup]	244	8.6	290	37%	35	9	1.2
6253	Pork stew, Mexican style, with potatoes, tomato-based sauce (mixture) (Include cerdo guisado con papas) [1 cup]	244	8.6	283	35%	32	13	1.6
6254	Pork and watercress with soy-based sauce [1 cup]	162	5.7	248	55%	20	8	0.7
6255	Pork with chili and tomatoes (Include Puerco con chile) [1 cup]	236	8.3	226	38%	28	6	1.5
6256	Sausage and vegetables (no carrots, broccoli, dark-green leafy, or potatoes), tomato-based sauce [1 cup]	249	8.8	443	71%	23	9	1.9
6257	**Sausage and vegetables (including carrots, broccoli, and/or dark-green leafy, no potatoes), tomato-based sauce [1 cup]**	249	8.8	408	69%	21	11	2.6
6258	Sausage, noodles, and [above] vegetables, tomato-based sauce [1 cup]	249	8.8	375	50%	20	27	2.5
6259	**Sausage, noodles, and vegetables (no carrots, broccoli, or dark-green leafy), tomato-based sauce [1 cup]**	249	8.8	379	50%	20	27	2.4
6260	Sausage, potatoes, and vegetables (described above), gravy [1 cup]	252	8.9	409	55%	18	28	3.4
6261	Sausage, potatoes, and vegetables (including carrots, broccoli, and/or dark-green leafy), gravy [1 cup]	252	8.9	403	57%	17	27	2.8
6262	Sausage and noodles with cream or white sauce [1 cup]	244	8.6	397	48%	17	34	2.7
6263	Sausage and peppers, no sauce [1 cup]	154	5.4	387	70%	24	4	0.4

Food #	fat gm	sat fat gm	choles mg	sodium mg	potass mg	% of Daily Value													
						vit A	vit E	vit C	thia-min	ribo-flavin	nia-cin	vit B-6	fol-ate	vit B-12	cal-cium	phos-phorus	magne-sium	iron	zinc
6226	11	4	63	803	562	6	4	13	58	16	31	27	18	8	3	24	11	14	17
6227	10	4	56	76	451	40	2	6	45	20	22	20	5	8	4	22	10	8	14
6228	13	4	94	205	885	102	4	26	60	24	39	31	5	12	5	35	13	11	21
6229	12	2	35	456	538	147	7	15	31	13	15	17	6	6	5	16	8	6	10
6230	11	3	35	45	807	69	6	18	32	15	16	25	10	4	6	19	11	9	14
6331	13	4	96	196	837	7	5	63	61	24	39	33	5	12	4	35	12	11	21
6232	13	2	39	465	468	7	7	28	35	18	17	15	10	7	6	17	11	10	11
6233	10	4	56	78	405	3	1	11	50	17	22	20	5	8	3	20	8	8	13
6234	7	2	36	583	501	5	2	17	29	11	18	20	7	5	3	16	9	7	11
6235	7	3	36	57	462	3	1	14	34	10	18	21	4	5	2	14	8	6	9
6236	7	2	36	682	814	13	6	34	31	13	21	26	8	4	4	17	12	10	12
6237	7	2	37	505	524	103	2	12	26	10	17	24	4	5	4	14	8	6	10
6238	7	3	35	58	485	21	2	12	31	12	18	21	4	5	3	15	9	6	10
6239	7	2	37	604	843	113	6	30	29	12	21	30	5	4	4	15	12	9	11
6240	8	3	49	509	554	39	2	17	38	14	28	20	12	6	5	22	9	12	12
6241	7	2	34	628	720	39	7	28	31	15	21	23	23	4	8	16	16	18	13
6242	8	3	48	495	533	5	2	37	37	14	27	20	12	6	5	21	9	12	12
6243	7	2	37	654	652	13	6	28	34	13	23	23	15	4	4	17	11	13	13
6244	24	8	112	284	598	1	2	9	40	25	29	19	4	14	4	29	9	11	26
6245	18	4	35	1214	450	3	6	14	34	15	17	16	10	4	15	26	37	42	15
6246	18	4	35	1220	464	46	6	7	32	15	16	16	8	4	15	25	37	41	14
6247	7	2	65	348	727	6	2	27	44	20	31	25	9	9	6	28	12	10	16
6248	27	5	48	848	489	2	9	34	52	25	31	21	18	7	4	25	13	18	17
6249	17	4	56	926	527	12	7	39	43	20	24	22	11	8	5	23	10	10	16
6250	19	6	100	2223	653	0	2	1	56	25	46	25	2	16	3	41	10	11	23
6251	13	4	93	289	422	2	3	15	35	18	26	20	2	10	1	20	6	10	27
6252	12	4	99	349	816	4	5	13	61	26	40	31	4	13	4	37	12	11	24
6253	11	4	89	315	873	4	4	17	56	24	38	31	4	12	4	34	12	11	22
6254	15	4	53	315	584	61	3	32	42	20	21	24	8	8	7	21	10	8	12
6255	10	3	75	383	736	7	3	54	48	21	32	27	4	10	3	29	11	9	16
6256	35	12	92	1925	671	7	2	72	56	19	29	26	5	30	7	23	9	11	20
6257	31	11	82	1754	729	105	2	27	52	18	27	23	4	27	8	23	9	11	18
6258	21	7	82	1044	550	20	5	38	42	17	25	20	16	16	4	21	11	17	16
6259	21	7	84	1063	545	7	5	34	42	17	25	21	16	16	5	21	11	17	17
6260	25	9	44	1215	797	9	4	42	30	17	21	22	8	14	15	24	11	11	17
6261	25	9	45	1205	846	75	5	39	28	17	20	23	5	14	16	23	11	10	16
6262	21	10	73	1116	332	14	2	18	32	21	16	11	15	13	21	27	10	15	15
6263	30	11	91	1021	399	2	2	43	47	17	23	21	2	24	3	19	6	11	19

Mixed Dishes & Fast Food

Food #	Food Description & Amount	wt gm	wt oz	calo-ries	%cal fat	prot gm	carbo gm	fiber gm
6264	Sausage and rice mixed with cream of mushroom soup [1 cup]	244	8.6	439	55%	16	32	0.6
6265	Sausage and rice with cheese sauce [1 cup]	244	8.6	461	51%	21	34	0.7
6266	Sausage and rice with tomato-based sauce [1 cup]	244	8.6	502	47%	20	45	3.3
6267	Sausage gravy [1 cup]	240	8.5	391	64%	17	17	0.3
6268	Sausage with tomato-based sauce [1 link with sauce]	42	1.5	55	65%	3	2	0.4
6269	Stewed pig's feet, Puerto Rican style (Patitas de cerdo guisadas) [1 cup with bones]	184	6.5	220	55%	16	8	0.8
6270	Stewed pork, Puerto Rican style [1 cup]	200	7.1	385	56%	37	5	1.0
6271	Stewed beans with pork, tomatoes, and chili peppers, Mexican style (Include Frijoles a la charra) [1 cup]	242	8.5	350	59%	13	24	4.7
6272	Sweet and sour pork with rice [1 cup]	244	8.6	270	21%	13	40	1.5
6273	Sweet and sour pork [1 cup]	226	8.0	231	32%	15	25	1.6
Lamb & Other Meat Dishes								
6400	Lamb curry [1 cup]	236	8.3	256	49%	28	3	1.0
6401	Lamb or mutton and noodles with gravy [1 cup]	249	8.8	367	43%	21	30	1.3
6402	Lamb or mutton and potatoes with gravy [1 cup]	252	8.9	256	36%	20	20	1.8
6403	Lamb or mutton and potatoes with tomato-based sauce [1 cup]	252	8.9	265	35%	21	22	2.3
6404	Lamb or mutton goulash [1 cup]	249	8.8	310	46%	33	8	1.1
6405	Lamb or mutton loaf [1 medium slice]	108	3.8	196	51%	15	9	0.4
6406	**Lamb or mutton stew with potatoes and vegetables (no carrots, broccoli, or dark-green leafy), tomato-based sauce [1 cup]**	252	8.9	241	19%	22	26	3.7
6407	Lamb or mutton stew with potatoes and vegetables (described above), gravy [1 cup]	252	8.9	253	22%	24	25	3.1
6408	**Lamb or mutton stew with potatoes and vegetables (including carrots, broccoli, and/or dark-green leafy), tomato-based sauce [1 cup]**	252	8.9	249	19%	22	29	5.1
6409	Lamb or mutton stew with potatoes and [above] vegetables, gravy [1 cup]	252	8.9	261	21%	24	28	4.6
6410	Lamb or mutton stew with [above] vegetables, gravy [1 cup]	252	8.9	299	32%	35	16	4.6
6411	**Lamb or mutton stew with vegetables (no carrots, broccoli, dark-green leafy, or potatoes), gravy [1 cup]**	252	8.9	285	34%	34	12	2.4
6412	Lamb or mutton, rice, and vegetables (described above), gravy [1 cup]	252	8.9	270	21%	18	35	4.4
6413	**Lamb or mutton, rice, and vegetables (including carrots, broccoli, and/or dark-green leafy), tomato-based sauce [1 cup]**	252	8.9	251	21%	16	34	3.8
6414	Lamb or mutton, rice, and [above] vegetables, gravy [1 cup]	252	8.9	255	35%	19	21	1.5
6415	Lamb or mutton with gravy [1 slice with gravy]	43	1.5	56	37%	8	1	0.1
6416	Lamb shishkabob [1 shishkabob]	202	7.1	245	41%	27	9	2.1
6417	Rabbit, stewed Puerto Rican style (Include Fricase de conejo) [1 cup, boneless]	219	7.7	470	53%	38	16	1.7
6418	Rabbit stew with potatoes and vegetables [1 cup]	252	8.9	160	26%	18	12	1.8
6419	Venison/Deer loaf (Include deer meatball with breading) [1 medium slice]	108	3.8	148	20%	22	6	0.4
6420	Venison and noodles with cream or white sauce [1 cup]	249	8.8	343	41%	27	23	0.7
6421	Venison stew with potatoes and vegetables (no carrots, broccoli, or dark-green leafy), tomato-based sauce [1 cup]	252	8.9	163	10%	19	18	3.2
6422	**Venison stew with potatoes and vegetables (including carrots, broccoli, and/or dark-green leafy), tomato-based sauce [1 cup]**	252	8.9	161	10%	18	18	3.3
6423	Venison, noodles, and [above] vegetables, tomato-based sauce [1 cup]	249	8.8	203	10%	16	29	3.2
6424	**Venison, noodles, and vegetables (no carrots, broccoli, or dark-green leafy), tomato-based sauce [1 cup]**	249	8.8	191	11%	16	26	2.9
6425	Venison, potatoes, and vegetables (described above), gravy [1 cup]	252	8.9	170	10%	19	18	2.8
6426	Venison, potatoes, and vegetables (including carrots, broccoli, and/or dark-green leafy), gravy [1 cup]	252	8.9	162	10%	18	19	3.2
6427	Venison with gravy [1 slice with gravy]	65	2.3	78	23%	13	1	0.1
6428	Venison with tomato-based sauce [1 cup]	249	8.8	227	17%	40	6	1.1
6429	Stewed goat, Puerto Rican style (Include Cabrito en fricase, chilindron de chivo, Puerto Rican stewed kid) [1 piece with gravy]	88	3.1	230	61%	20	2	0.4

Food #	fat gm	sat fat gm	choles mg	sodium mg	potass mg	vit A	vit E	vit C	thia- min	ribo- flavin	nia- cin	vit B-6	fol- ate	vit B-12	cal- cium	phos- phorus	magne- sium	iron	zinc
						\multicolumn{14}{}
6264	27	9	51	1499	341	1	4	4	40	15	23	14	13	20	8	20	7	12	16
6265	26	11	73	1465	489	5	1	4	42	24	20	16	13	25	28	34	10	10	15
6266	26	9	69	1081	518	3	6	16	56	15	31	23	22	24	5	23	8	15	18
6267	28	9	55	817	494	19	5	4	32	29	14	12	5	23	26	29	9	6	13
6268	4	1	10	340	155	3	1	7	7	3	4	4	1	4	1	3	2	2	3
6269	13	4	73	281	424	5	4	19	7	7	7	10	2	4	4	9	5	6	9
6270	24	6	108	453	822	5	8	17	61	26	41	32	3	14	4	38	12	12	25
6271	23	8	23	274	566	3	1	15	21	7	10	11	20	5	5	20	15	14	10
6272	6	2	28	618	311	2	3	24	36	10	19	19	13	4	3	14	9	11	10
6273	8	2	39	839	386	3	4	33	37	12	18	21	3	6	3	15	9	8	10
6400	14	4	89	323	496	0	4	2	6	17	40	10	7	48	4	28	10	17	44
6401	17	4	81	654	240	12	6	0	19	16	27	7	21	25	2	20	9	17	22
6402	10	4	65	73	761	0	1	24	9	13	32	17	8	33	3	22	11	13	32
6403	10	4	65	147	872	3	2	36	11	14	34	19	9	33	4	23	12	15	32
6404	16	5	107	272	613	3	7	16	17	23	47	18	14	75	4	32	12	18	53
6405	11	4	92	200	237	3	0	1	4	14	20	5	4	24	5	16	5	8	21
6406	5	2	60	575	687	7	3	28	16	13	28	21	9	25	3	18	13	15	28
6407	6	2	62	334	545	2	1	18	15	12	27	18	8	26	3	18	11	15	30
6408	5	2	60	572	716	30	4	24	13	15	27	21	8	25	4	19	14	15	29
6409	6	2	62	541	576	26	1	14	12	14	27	18	8	26	3	19	12	15	31
6410	11	4	98	464	459	46	2	5	10	21	32	9	10	42	5	25	12	20	46
6411	11	4	98	466	408	7	1	11	15	18	33	10	10	42	4	24	10	21	45
6412	6	2	38	548	464	4	2	54	19	11	23	20	23	16	3	18	11	15	23
6413	6	2	37	476	500	80	3	49	15	9	21	21	19	16	4	15	10	13	20
6414	10	3	57	239	330	40	2	5	13	13	25	10	14	29	4	17	8	13	29
6415	2	1	22	121	97	0	0	0	2	5	8	2	1	11	0	6	2	4	9
6416	11	4	88	79	572	6	2	55	11	19	33	15	11	45	3	24	10	15	42
6417	27	5	102	308	857	2	12	24	8	14	47	24	5	84	4	32	12	21	21
6418	5	1	45	42	447	42	2	11	8	11	25	15	6	57	3	17	6	11	11
6419	3	1	100	111	328	2	1	1	11	29	26	9	3	68	4	21	6	18	13
6420	15	4	99	218	421	16	6	2	19	38	27	11	12	70	15	30	11	23	17
6421	2	1	56	249	743	6	3	49	15	23	28	20	9	52	3	21	12	19	14
6422	2	1	55	245	771	74	3	44	15	23	27	20	8	51	3	20	11	19	13
6423	2	1	61	342	484	45	3	16	18	20	21	14	15	35	3	18	12	21	12
6424	2	1	62	351	493	6	3	17	17	19	20	13	15	36	3	18	12	20	12
6425	2	1	59	74	606	2	1	23	15	23	27	16	7	54	2	20	10	19	13
6426	2	1	54	77	610	70	1	23	15	22	26	16	7	50	3	19	10	18	12
6427	2	1	45	181	156	0	0	0	5	15	13	5	1	39	0	10	3	11	9
6428	4	2	144	529	592	7	5	17	14	43	34	17	2	107	2	25	10	35	25
6429	16	3	56	324	343	1	5	7	6	25	15	2	2	14	2	16	1	15	25

Mixed Dishes & Fast Food

Food #	Food Description & Amount	wt gm	wt oz	calo-ries	%cal fat	prot gm	carbo gm	fiber gm
	Chicken & Turkey Dishes							
6500	Almond chicken [1 cup]	242	8.5	280	47%	22	16	3.4
6501	Chicken cornbread [1 piece (2½"x2½"x1½")]	67	2.4	117	43%	10	6	0.5
6502	Chicken curry [1 cup]	236	8.3	294	49%	27	10	2.2
6503	Chicken fricassee, Puerto Rican style (Include Fricase de pollo, Pollo guisado) [1 cup, boneless]	223	7.9	430	64%	24	15	2.0
6504	Chicken kiev [1 serving (1 whole breast)]	258	9.1	643	46%	73	10	0.3
6505	Chicken livers, chopped, with eggs and onion [1 cup]	208	7.3	472	70%	27	6	1.0
6506	Chicken or turkey and noodles with soup-based (cream of mushroom) sauce [1 cup]	224	7.9	311	32%	22	30	1.2
6507	Chicken or turkey and noodles with cheese sauce [1 cup]	224	7.9	330	30%	25	32	1.4
6508	Chicken or turkey and noodles with cream or white sauce [1 cup]	224	7.9	319	31%	22	32	1.2
6509	**Chicken or turkey and noodles with gravy [1 cup]**	**224**	**7.9**	**304**	**36%**	**20**	**27**	**1.2**
6510	Chicken or turkey and noodles, no sauce [1 cup]	157	5.5	254	28%	20	24	1.1
6511	Chicken or turkey and noodles, tomato-based sauce [1 cup]	224	7.9	291	29%	20	31	2.4
6512	Chicken or turkey and potatoes with gravy (Include Chicken Helper Chicken with Potatoes and Gravy) [1 cup]	242	8.5	277	40%	19	22	1.7
6513	Chicken or turkey and rice, no sauce [1 cup]	196	6.9	314	24%	23	34	0.5
6514	Chicken or turkey and rice with soup-based (cream of mushroom) sauce [1 cup]	248	8.7	455	43%	28	35	0.9
6515	Chicken with rice, Puerto Rican style (Include Arroz con Pollo) [1 cup]	163	5.7	462	38%	18	51	1.1
6516	Chicken or turkey and rice with cream sauce (Include Chicken Helper Mushroom Chicken with Long Grain and Wild Rice) [1 cup]	248	8.7	357	38%	22	32	1.4
6517	Chicken or turkey and rice with soy-based sauce (Include Chicken Helper Chicken Teriyaki) [1 cup]	244	8.6	323	18%	42	22	0.2
6518	Chicken or turkey and rice with tomato-based sauce [1 cup]	244	8.6	229	10%	19	33	2.8
6519	**Chicken or turkey and vegetables (no carrots, broccoli, dark-green leafy, or potatoes), cheese sauce [1 cup]**	**249**	**8.8**	**309**	**37%**	**29**	**20**	**2.9**
6520	Chicken or turkey and vegetables (as above), gravy [1 cup]	252	8.9	289	43%	23	18	3.0
6521	Chicken or turkey and vegetables (as above), no sauce [1 cup]	162	5.7	153	23%	17	13	2.7
6522	Chicken or turkey and vegetables (as above), soy-based sauce [1 cup]	162	5.7	291	58%	22	8	0.9
6523	**Chicken or turkey and vegetables (including carrots, broccoli, and/or dark-green leafy, no potatoes), cheese sauce [1 cup]**	**249**	**8.8**	**321**	**42%**	**34**	**12**	**2.1**
6524	Chicken or turkey and [above] vegetables, gravy [1 cup]	252	8.9	281	45%	23	15	2.9
6525	Chicken or turkey and [above] vegetables, no sauce [1 cup]	162	5.7	148	24%	17	12	2.5
6526	Chicken or turkey and [above] vegetables, soy-based sauce (Include Szechwan chicken, Hunan chicken) [1 cup]	162	5.7	289	60%	22	6	0.8
6527	Chicken or turkey a la king with [above] vegetables, cream, white, or soup-based sauce [1 cup]	241	8.5	476	65%	25	17	1.5
6528	Chicken or turkey a la king with vegetables (no carrots, broccoli, dark-green leafy, or potatoes), cream, white, or soup-based sauce [1 cup]	241	8.5	468	66%	25	15	1.2
6529	Chicken or turkey cacciatore (including chicken or turkey with tomato-based sauce, chicken or turkey with tomatoes) [½ chicken breast with sauce]	128	4.5	241	50%	22	7	1.0
6530	Chicken or turkey cake, patty, or croquette [1 cake or patty]	85	3.0	218	53%	14	11	0.3
6531	**Chicken or turkey chow mein or chop suey with noodles [1 cup]**	**220**	**7.8**	**275**	**45%**	**19**	**20**	**2.3**
6532	Chicken or turkey chow mein or chop suey, no noodles [1 cup]	220	7.8	193	39%	20	10	2.1
6533	Chicken or turkey cordon bleu [1 roll (½ breast with ham and sauce)]	229	8.1	494	53%	44	11	0.5
6534	Chicken or turkey creole, without rice [1 cup]	246	8.7	192	19%	29	9	2.1
6535	Chicken or turkey divan [1 cup]	236	8.3	324	39%	41	8	3.0
6536	Chicken or turkey fricassee [1 cup]	244	8.6	323	51%	29	8	0.3
6537	Chicken or turkey fricassee, no potatoes, Puerto Rican style (with sauce) [1 cup]	223	7.9	457	68%	30	6	1.2
6538	Chicken or turkey fricassee, no sauce, no potatoes, Puerto Rican style [1 cup]	223	7.9	561	60%	52	0	0.0

Food #	fat gm	sat fat gm	choles mg	sodium mg	potass mg	vit A	vit E	vit C	thia-min	ribo-flavin	nia-cin	vit B-6	fol-ate	vit B-12	cal-cium	phos-phorus	magne-sium	iron	zinc
6500	15	2	40	526	549	4	13	11	6	12	47	22	7	5	7	25	15	11	11
6501	6	1	70	64	77	5	2	0	4	7	10	5	4	3	1	7	3	4	5
6502	16	3	84	629	626	20	10	31	9	13	51	25	5	5	4	25	13	12	14
6503	31	6	81	770	704	15	12	74	11	11	39	25	5	5	3	23	11	11	13
6504	33	16	283	454	623	22	5	0	17	21	160	69	6	15	6	56	18	18	17
6505	37	11	753	92	256	458	8	30	12	106	21	32	184	304	4	36	7	46	30
6506	11	3	81	550	220	3	3	1	15	15	27	10	16	5	7	20	9	14	14
6507	11	4	95	581	321	5	1	2	16	21	24	11	16	9	21	30	12	12	13
6508	11	3	81	139	276	10	3	1	17	20	25	10	18	6	13	24	11	13	13
6509	12	3	78	590	145	3	2	0	15	12	25	8	17	3	3	16	8	13	11
6510	8	2	82	47	130	1	1	0	14	10	25	9	16	4	2	15	8	12	12
6511	9	2	74	658	478	14	7	20	18	13	29	15	18	3	3	18	12	16	13
6512	12	4	54	1117	625	3	2	24	9	10	27	19	5	2	2	15	9	10	11
6513	8	2	62	513	171	1	1	0	16	8	31	15	19	3	2	16	7	13	13
6514	22	5	66	1170	395	16	9	2	14	10	63	21	12	5	6	27	10	15	11
6515	20	5	54	340	264	3	5	8	23	7	35	14	26	3	3	18	8	19	12
6516	15	4	56	415	326	14	6	6	17	15	37	16	16	7	12	23	9	13	13
6517	7	2	126	719	533	2	2	6	15	19	78	28	18	7	6	37	17	15	21
6518	3	1	49	94	698	15	11	22	16	10	42	22	14	3	4	20	14	16	11
6519	13	4	83	499	641	9	3	17	13	20	41	25	8	9	17	33	15	11	15
6520	14	4	76	94	449	5	2	30	10	12	40	19	8	3	3	21	11	10	11
6521	4	1	45	125	359	5	1	18	6	8	21	13	5	2	3	12	8	7	9
6522	19	5	83	627	379	4	3	5	6	10	39	17	3	4	2	19	7	7	11
6523	15	5	101	604	558	76	4	36	9	23	46	31	7	11	21	35	12	9	17
6524	14	4	79	104	467	57	2	31	10	11	39	18	7	4	3	20	10	11	11
6525	4	1	45	130	353	32	1	17	6	8	21	14	5	2	3	12	7	7	9
6526	19	5	85	642	346	5	3	13	5	10	40	16	3	4	2	20	7	8	11
6527	34	12	195	368	434	120	10	10	11	24	34	23	8	10	16	29	9	11	14
6528	34	12	194	493	400	35	10	9	12	23	36	20	8	10	15	30	9	11	15
6529	13	3	67	130	362	7	5	13	7	10	37	19	3	4	3	16	7	9	11
6530	13	3	39	176	180	7	5	2	7	11	22	10	4	4	7	13	5	7	7
6531	14	2	43	793	371	1	3	15	14	16	37	17	13	3	4	18	10	13	12
6532	8	2	50	651	415	1	3	17	8	13	35	19	13	4	4	19	9	10	11
6533	29	15	188	665	487	21	3	3	20	24	81	36	5	13	23	45	13	14	18
6534	4	1	70	436	710	10	7	55	10	10	70	31	5	5	5	27	14	10	8
6535	14	6	134	445	433	29	7	66	8	20	46	24	10	8	31	39	14	10	14
6536	18	5	86	504	295	1	2	0	8	14	40	13	5	6	2	19	6	10	14
6537	35	7	86	642	411	9	13	39	15	13	35	22	4	6	3	20	9	11	16
6538	38	9	165	142	352	9	6	0	7	18	59	23	3	7	3	29	10	14	25

Mixed Dishes & Fast Food

Food #	Food Description & Amount	wt gm	wt oz	calo-ries	%cal fat	prot gm	carbo gm	fiber gm
6539	Chicken or turkey fricassee, with sauce, no potatoes, Puerto Rican style (Include pollo en salsa, Puerto Rican style chicken or turkey in sauce) [1 cup]	223	7.9	470	61%	40	4	0.7
6540	Chicken or turkey garden salad (chicken and/or turkey, other vegetables but no tomato or carrots), no dressing [1 cup]	90	3.2	64	19%	11	2	0.8
6541	Chicken or turkey garden salad (chicken and/or turkey, tomato and/or carrots, other vegetables), no dressing (Include McDonald's Chicken Salad Oriental) [1 fast food order]	252	8.9	161	18%	27	6	2.5
6542	Chicken or turkey hash [1 cup]	190	6.7	212	36%	18	16	2.3
6543	Chicken or turkey loaf (including with breading, no sauce; chicken or turkey meatball, with breading, no sauce) [1 slice]	108	3.8	184	32%	22	8	0.6
6544	Chicken or turkey parmigiana [1 piece with sauce and cheese]	182	6.4	320	44%	28	16	1.1
6545	Chicken or turkey pate with vegetables, diet (Include Nu System Cuisine Chicken Pate with Vegetables) [1 container (3 oz)]	85	3.0	127	18%	24	0	0.0
6546	**Chicken or turkey pot pie [1 pie (8 oz, frozen)]**	**227**	**8.0**	**490**	**52%**	**20**	**38**	**3.1**
6547	Chicken or turkey salad with egg [1 cup]	182	6.4	385	68%	28	3	0.7
6548	Chicken or turkey salad [1 cup]	182	6.4	417	69%	30	2	0.8
6549	Chicken or turkey souffle [1 cup]	159	5.6	283	58%	20	9	0.2
6550	Chicken or turkey teriyaki (chicken or turkey with soy-based sauce) [½ chicken breast with sauce]	128	4.5	178	19%	27	7	0.4
6551	Chicken or turkey tetrazzini [1 cup]	246	8.7	366	48%	19	28	1.7
6552	Chicken or turkey with cream of mushroom soup-based sauce [½ chicken breast with sauce]	129	4.6	188	44%	21	4	0.1
6553	Chicken or turkey with barbecue sauce [½ chicken breast with sauce]	123	4.3	234	43%	28	3	0.3
6554	Chicken or turkey with cheese sauce [1 cup]	241	8.5	368	40%	44	9	0.3
6555	Chicken or turkey with cream sauce [½ chicken breast with sauce]	129	4.6	209	53%	16	8	0.1
6556	Chicken or turkey with dumplings (Include Chicken Helper Chicken and Dumplings) [1 cup]	244	8.6	372	46%	26	22	0.7
6557	Chicken or turkey with stuffing (Include Chicken Helper Chicken and Stuffing) [1 cup]	200	7.1	273	18%	35	19	0.8
6558	Chicken or turkey, dumplings, and vegetables (including carrots, broccoli, and/or dark-green leafy), gravy [1 cup]	249	8.8	264	30%	23	23	3.2
6559	**Chicken or turkey, dumplings, and vegetables (no carrots, broccoli, or dark-green leafy), gravy [1 cup]**	**249**	**8.8**	**273**	**34%**	**22**	**22**	**2.5**
6560	Chicken or turkey, noodles, and vegetables (as above), cheese sauce [1 cup]	244	8.6	388	38%	32	28	2.6
6561	Chicken or turkey, noodles, & vegetables (as above), cream or white sauce [1 cup]	244	8.6	340	34%	27	28	2.1
6562	Chicken or turkey, noodles, and vegetables (as above), gravy [1 cup]	224	7.9	257	35%	17	25	2.4
6563	Chicken or turkey, noodles, and vegetables (as above), no sauce [1 cup]	162	5.7	184	18%	15	22	2.7
6564	Chicken or turkey, noodles, & vegetables (as above), tomato-based sauce [1 cup]	224	7.9	285	35%	18	28	2.7
6565	Chicken or turkey, noodles, and vegetables (as above), cream, white, or cream of mushroom soup-based sauce [1 cup]	224	7.9	294	37%	19	28	2.4
6566	**Chicken or turkey, noodles, and vegetables (including carrots, broccoli, and/or dark-green leafy), cheese sauce [1 cup]**	**244**	**8.6**	**356**	**39%**	**30**	**24**	**2.1**
6567	Chicken or turkey, noodles, and [above] vegetables, cream or white sauce [1 cup]	224	7.9	306	35%	18	31	2.9
6568	Chicken or turkey, noodles, and [above] vegetables, gravy [1 cup]	224	7.9	267	35%	16	27	2.7
6569	Chicken or turkey, noodles, and [above] vegetables, no sauce [1 cup]	162	5.7	178	19%	15	21	2.4
6570	Chicken or turkey, noodles, and [above] vegetables, tomato-based sauce [1 cup]	224	7.9	293	34%	18	30	3.0
6571	Chicken or turkey, potatoes, and [above] vegetables, no sauce [1 cup]	162	5.7	195	26%	23	12	1.8
6572	**Chicken or turkey, potatoes, and vegetables (no carrots, broccoli, or dark-green leafy), no sauce [1 cup]**	**162**	**5.7**	**201**	**25%**	**24**	**12**	**2.0**
6573	Chicken or turkey, rice, and vegetables (as above), cream of mushroom soup-based sauce [1 cup]	252	8.9	372	38%	22	35	4.0
6574	Chicken or turkey, rice, and vegetables (as above), cheese sauce [1 cup]	249	8.8	347	30%	30	29	1.4
6575	Chicken or turkey, rice, and vegetables (as above), gravy [1 cup]	252	8.9	381	39%	23	34	2.7

Food #	fat gm	sat fat gm	choles mg	sodium mg	potass mg	% of Daily Value													
						vit A	vit E	vit C	thia-min	ribo-flavin	nia-cin	vit B-6	fol-ate	vit B-12	cal-cium	phos-phorus	magne-sium	iron	zinc
6539	32	7	122	441	394	9	9	23	12	16	46	23	3	6	3	25	10	13	20
6540	1	0	29	37	187	2	1	11	3	3	24	12	7	2	2	9	4	3	3
6541	3	1	69	91	536	23	3	37	10	9	58	30	18	5	4	22	10	9	7
6542	8	2	43	245	585	1	7	19	8	8	21	25	6	3	4	16	9	8	14
6543	7	2	93	139	240	4	1	6	7	13	33	17	5	5	5	18	6	8	11
6544	16	5	137	641	471	15	8	14	12	20	42	18	7	7	20	32	11	13	16
6545	3	1	64	70	157	3	1	0	2	6	35	14	1	3	1	14	5	4	5
6546	28	9	62	246	355	74	8	16	24	21	33	11	16	3	6	20	9	17	12
6547	29	6	214	448	311	9	12	6	5	18	27	22	8	10	5	20	6	9	14
6548	32	6	106	290	331	5	14	5	5	11	33	25	5	5	4	18	7	9	15
6549	18	5	221	234	266	22	7	1	7	25	20	13	7	10	11	23	6	8	11
6550	4	1	82	1683	309	2	1	5	5	11	44	23	3	5	3	20	9	10	13
6551	19	7	49	705	200	11	5	10	13	15	25	10	14	5	14	22	8	12	13
6552	9	3	63	411	217	2	2	1	4	10	33	17	1	5	4	16	5	6	11
6553	11	3	89	262	275	5	2	2	5	10	47	23	2	5	2	20	7	8	13
6554	16	6	136	739	535	7	2	1	10	27	60	33	3	15	25	43	13	9	21
6555	12	3	47	164	242	12	4	1	6	14	22	12	3	6	11	17	6	5	9
6556	19	5	89	244	297	5	3	3	15	18	47	15	9	5	13	26	9	14	13
6557	5	1	105	511	403	2	2	5	15	18	66	23	11	6	4	29	12	13	17
6558	9	2	57	421	417	59	2	9	15	16	36	21	11	5	13	23	9	13	14
6559	10	3	56	735	394	10	2	8	15	15	35	18	10	5	13	22	8	13	15
6560	16	6	102	378	456	15	4	9	17	26	39	17	15	8	24	39	15	15	21
6561	13	3	89	283	327	6	4	6	16	19	30	14	17	6	10	24	11	14	16
6562	10	3	40	712	190	2	2	0	13	10	23	6	11	1	2	15	8	12	11
6563	4	1	53	209	178	4	1	6	13	9	19	8	16	2	2	14	7	11	10
6564	11	3	66	437	332	7	5	7	14	11	26	9	12	2	3	17	10	15	12
6565	12	3	63	545	291	5	4	1	17	16	24	10	15	6	11	22	10	13	13
6566	16	6	97	370	429	21	6	26	12	24	35	16	14	8	24	36	13	13	18
6567	12	3	64	337	348	147	5	3	15	18	21	15	16	6	12	20	10	12	12
6568	10	3	61	494	238	131	2	2	13	11	21	13	14	3	4	14	8	12	10
6569	4	1	54	145	194	80	1	2	12	8	19	11	13	2	3	13	7	10	10
6570	11	3	66	307	367	92	5	8	13	12	24	12	12	2	4	16	10	15	11
6571	6	2	67	86	381	62	1	8	6	9	29	20	4	3	3	15	8	7	12
6572	6	2	67	132	368	3	1	11	8	10	29	18	6	3	2	16	8	8	13
6573	16	4	63	709	348	7	3	18	23	12	40	16	20	3	5	23	11	18	15
6574	12	4	84	596	400	6	2	3	14	18	34	17	14	8	18	30	11	12	17
6575	17	5	72	545	352	8	2	8	17	11	40	15	18	4	4	22	9	16	14

Mixed Dishes & Fast Food

Food #	Food Description & Amount	wt gm	wt oz	calories	%cal fat	prot gm	carbo gm	fiber gm
6576	**Chicken or turkey, rice, and vegetables (no carrots, broccoli, or dark-green leafy), no sauce [1 cup]**	**162**	**5.7**	**190**	**16%**	**16**	**23**	**2.2**
6577	Chicken or turkey, rice, and vegetables (as above), soy-based sauce [1 cup]	217	7.7	228	40%	15	19	1.7
6578	Chicken or turkey, rice, and vegetables (as above), tomato-based sauce [1 cup]	249	8.8	354	36%	22	34	3.4
6579	**Chicken or turkey, rice, and vegetables (including carrots, broccoli, and/or dark-green leafy), cream of mushroom soup-based sauce [1 cup]**	**252**	**8.9**	**338**	**42%**	**20**	**29**	**2.9**
6580	Chicken or turkey, rice, and [above} vegetables, cheese sauce [1 cup]	249	8.8	277	29%	24	25	3.2
6581	Chicken or turkey, rice, and [above} vegetables, gravy [1 cup]	252	8.9	345	40%	21	30	2.6
6582	Chicken or turkey, rice, and [above} vegetables, no sauce [1 cup]	162	5.7	191	18%	17	21	1.7
6583	Chicken or turkey, rice, and [above} vegetables, soy-based sauce [1 cup]	217	7.7	241	38%	15	22	2.3
6584	Chicken or turkey, rice, and [above} vegetables, tomato-based sauce [1 cup]	249	8.8	352	37%	21	33	2.7
6585	Chicken or turkey, stuffing, and [above} vegetables, gravy [1 cup]	244	8.6	359	36%	25	32	4.4
6586	Chicken or turkey, stuffing, and [above} vegetables, no sauce [1 cup]	162	5.7	232	35%	15	22	3.3
6587	**Chicken or turkey, stuffing, and vegetables (no carrots, broccoli, or dark-green leafy), gravy [1 cup]**	**244**	**8.6**	**324**	**44%**	**21**	**24**	**2.6**
6588	Chicken or turkey, stuffing, and vegetables (as above), no sauce [1 cup]	162	5.7	207	18%	21	20	1.7
6589	Chicken wing with hot pepper sauce (Include Hot Wings, Buffalo chicken wing drummette) [2 wings or drummettes]	48	1.7	148	64%	12	0	0.0
6590	Chicken with gravy [2 slices with gravy]	44	1.6	59	44%	7	1	0.1
6591	Gizzards, stewed, Puerto Rican style (Include Mollejitas guisadas) [1 cup]	260	9.2	501	50%	45	13	1.9
6592	General Tso chicken [1 cup]	146	5.1	293	52%	19	16	0.8
6593	Kung pao chicken (Include cashew chicken) [1 cup]	162	5.7	431	64%	29	11	2.2
6594	Lemon chicken or turkey, Chinese style (Include Orange chicken, Sesame chicken, sweet and sour chicken without vegetables) [1 cup]	252	8.9	659	50%	45	34	1.4
6595	Moo Goo Gai Pan [1 cup]	216	7.6	272	62%	15	12	2.7
6596	Sweet and Sour Chicken or turkey, includes pineapple and vegetables [1 cup]	252	8.9	226	25%	15	29	1.8
6597	Soupy rice with chicken, Puerto Rican style (Include Asopao de pollo) [1 cup, boneless]	263	9.3	346	39%	19	33	1.7
6598	Spaghetti sauce with poultry, home-made style [1 cup]	249	8.8	261	48%	16	21	4.2
6599	**Stew, chicken or turkey, with potatoes and vegetables (no carrots, broccoli, or dark-green leafy), tomato-based sauce [1 cup]**	**247**	**8.7**	**227**	**16%**	**29**	**19**	**3.0**
6600	Stew, chicken or turkey, with potatoes and vegetables (as above), gravy [1 cup]	252	8.9	217	16%	28	16	2.5
6601	**Stew, chicken or turkey, with potatoes and vegetables (including carrots, broccoli, and/or dark-green leafy), tomato-based sauce [1 cup]**	**247**	**8.7**	**218**	**16%**	**27**	**18**	**2.7**
6602	Stew, chicken or turkey, with potatoes and [above] vegetables, gravy [1 cup]	252	8.9	291	44%	24	15	2.0
6603	Stewed chicken with tomato-based sauce, Mexican style (Include Pollo guisado con tomate) [½ chicken breast with sauce]	128	4.5	135	46%	15	3	0.5
6604	Stuffed chicken, drumstick or breast, Puerto Rican style (Include Muslo de pollo o pechuga rellena) [1 breast (4"x3"x¾")]	210	7.4	470	30%	62	16	0.7
6605	Turkey with gravy [1 cup]	244	8.6	266	29%	38	6	0.5
	Fish Dishes							
6700	Biscayne codfish, Puerto Rican style (Include Bacalao a la Vizcaina) [1 cup]	175	6.2	341	54%	16	24	2.7
6701	Chow mein or chop suey, no noodles [1 cup]	220	7.8	284	51%	23	12	2.7
6702	Clam cake or patty (Include deviled clam cake) [1 cake or patty]	120	4.2	423	40%	24	38	1.2
6703	Clams Casino [2 clams]	60	2.1	70	40%	5	6	0.7
6704	Clams, stuffed [1 large (6 in 11 oz package)]	52	1.8	101	52%	5	7	0.4
6705	Codfish ball or cake [1 ball]	63	2.2	125	48%	9	8	0.7
6706	Codfish salad, Puerto Rican style (Include Ensalada de bacalao) [1 cup]	150	5.3	220	63%	12	9	1.7
6707	Codfish salad, Puerto Rican style (Gazpacho de bacalao) [1 cup salad and 1 slice toast]	170	6.0	270	53%	14	18	2.0
6708	Codfish salad, Puerto Rican style (includes oil, vinegar, onion, olives, tomatoes) (Include Serenata) [1 cup]	145	5.1	257	79%	10	5	0.9
6709	Codfish with starchy vegetables, Puerto Rican style (Serenata de bacalao) [1 cup]	173	6.1	239	35%	6	34	4.7

Food #	fat gm	sat fat gm	choles mg	sodium mg	potass mg	vit A	vit E	vit C	thia-min	ribo-flavin	nia-cin	vit B-6	fol-ate	vit B-12	cal-cium	phos-phorus	magne-sium	iron	zinc
														% of Daily Value					
6576	3	1	39	35	234	2	1	9	13	8	21	14	14	2	3	14	8	9	11
6577	10	3	41	919	195	2	2	0	9	7	23	8	8	1	2	14	7	10	11
6578	14	4	68	241	491	11	5	15	18	11	41	18	19	3	4	22	11	17	13
6579	16	4	63	374	391	16	6	57	14	12	36	16	23	3	7	21	10	15	13
6580	9	3	63	461	448	19	5	62	13	17	27	17	21	6	17	26	12	12	15
6581	15	4	68	421	365	16	5	43	15	11	37	17	22	3	6	21	10	14	13
6582	4	1	44	57	213	54	2	17	10	7	22	14	12	2	3	13	7	9	10
6583	10	3	41	707	252	125	2	2	7	8	20	13	8	1	4	12	7	9	9
6584	15	4	70	147	542	95	5	14	17	10	43	19	16	3	4	21	11	16	12
6585	14	3	58	582	482	66	6	11	18	16	40	24	14	4	6	23	14	16	14
6586	9	2	29	388	351	54	4	8	13	10	17	15	10	3	5	15	10	12	12
6587	16	4	51	836	360	16	5	6	14	14	34	18	11	4	6	18	8	12	14
6588	4	1	59	420	340	2	2	7	13	13	40	15	11	3	4	19	9	10	11
6589	10	3	39	38	88	3	1	0	1	4	15	10	0	2	1	7	2	3	6
6590	3	1	20	148	77	3	0	0	1	3	10	5	0	2	1	5	1	2	4
6591	28	6	305	537	911	36	19	38	10	30	55	16	26	63	7	37	15	52	49
6592	17	4	65	906	250	5	7	21	7	11	31	14	6	4	3	15	6	8	9
6593	31	5	64	907	428	6	13	13	10	9	66	29	11	4	5	26	16	11	10
6594	37	9	168	1527	443	6	9	14	16	23	71	31	10	9	5	33	13	18	22
6595	19	4	35	304	488	14	12	57	11	20	22	16	11	5	13	20	8	9	11
6596	6	1	45	974	355	4	4	39	8	9	30	18	3	3	3	14	10	9	9
6597	15	4	59	326	319	6	3	27	17	9	34	15	18	3	3	19	9	14	12
6598	14	3	46	881	1078	25	18	63	13	14	26	29	7	2	6	18	16	18	14
6599	4	1	83	246	780	8	2	42	15	15	55	28	9	5	5	27	14	14	16
6600	4	1	83	142	621	4	2	27	14	14	53	25	9	5	4	26	13	12	15
6601	4	1	82	226	822	72	3	38	12	14	54	28	6	5	5	26	14	12	15
6602	14	4	87	113	632	73	2	20	10	12	45	22	5	4	3	22	11	10	13
6603	7	1	46	174	244	3	4	11	4	7	27	11	2	3	1	12	5	5	7
6604	15	6	323	713	687	14	5	12	21	35	117	44	11	21	24	64	19	19	22
6605	9	3	93	805	491	0	2	0	7	19	41	28	3	9	3	29	8	17	31
6700	21	3	33	509	867	4	11	36	9	6	14	23	5	10	4	19	12	9	5
6701	16	4	60	941	524	12	7	39	19	16	27	22	12	18	4	22	10	14	21
6702	19	4	121	380	505	17	10	20	24	33	23	5	16	974	22	37	6	122	16
6703	3	1	10	118	163	5	2	21	5	5	5	4	3	192	3	5	2	20	3
6704	6	1	12	117	169	8	4	7	5	8	6	2	3	258	3	7	2	30	4
6705	7	1	35	175	275	1	3	4	5	4	7	8	2	6	2	11	5	2	2
6706	15	2	71	319	419	5	7	26	8	7	8	13	6	9	3	15	8	5	4
6707	16	2	72	427	468	6	8	33	12	11	12	14	9	9	4	18	10	8	5
6708	23	3	22	175	360	3	10	18	5	3	7	9	4	7	2	12	7	4	2
6709	9	1	10	87	716	63	7	30	7	6	6	19	6	3	4	11	9	5	3

Mixed Dishes & Fast Food

Food #	Food Description & Amount	wt gm	wt oz	calories	%cal fat	prot gm	carbo gm	fiber gm
6710	Crab cake [1 cake]	120	4.2	203	43%	27	1	0.1
6711	Crab imperial (Include stuffed crab) [1 stuffed crab]	194	6.8	292	48%	30	6	0.3
6712	Crab salad made with imitation crab [1 cup]	208	7.3	299	37%	18	28	0.8
6713	Crab salad [1 cup]	208	7.3	282	44%	27	11	0.7
6714	Crab, deviled [1 cup]	175	6.2	346	46%	23	23	1.0
6715	Crabs in tomato-based sauce, Puerto Rican style (Include Salmorejo de jueyes) [1 cup]	170	6.0	289	57%	27	4	0.5
6716	Fish a la creole, Puerto Rican style (Include Pescado frito con mojo) [1 slice (4"x3½"x½") with sauce]	213	7.5	324	59%	26	8	1.7
6717	Fish and noodles with cream of mushroom soup-based sauce [1 cup]	224	7.9	260	33%	18	25	1.0
6718	Fish and rice with cream of mushroom soup-based sauce [1 cup]	248	8.7	318	31%	19	34	0.7
6719	Fish and rice with cream sauce [1 cup]	248	8.7	366	35%	21	36	0.6
6720	Fish and rice with tomato-based sauce [1 cup]	248	8.7	283	16%	19	40	0.8
6721	**Fish and vegetables (no carrots, broccoli, dark-green leafy, or potatoes), tomato-based sauce [1 cup]**	**224**	**7.9**	**187**	**26%**	**28**	**7**	**1.7**
6722	Fish and vegetables (as above), soy-based sauce [1 cup]	162	5.7	146	26%	21	5	1.1
6723	**Fish and vegetables (including carrots, broccoli, and/or dark-green leafy, no potatoes), tomato-based sauce [1 cup]**	**224**	**7.9**	**195**	**25%**	**28**	**8**	**2.0**
6724	Fish and [above] vegetables, soy-based sauce [1 cup]	162	5.7	159	26%	23	5	1.0
6725	Fish, noodles, and [above] vegetables, cheese sauce [1 cup]	224	7.9	245	23%	24	22	2.0
6726	Fish, noodles, and vegetables (no carrots, broccoli, or dark-green leafy), cheese sauce [1 cup]	244	8.6	291	22%	27	29	3.0
6727	Fish cake tempura (Include kamaboko tempura) [2 oz, cooked]	56	2.0	94	33%	7	8	0.1
6728	Fish cake or patty [1 cake or patty]	120	4.2	237	48%	16	15	1.4
6729	Fish moochim (Korean style), dried fish with soy sauce [½ cup]	20	0.7	68	41%	7	2	0.2
6730	Fish timbale or mousse [1 cup]	175	6.2	331	69%	22	3	0.0
6731	Fish with cream or white sauce, not tuna or lobster [1 cup]	249	8.8	332	49%	28	13	0.3
6732	Fish with tomato-based sauce (Include fish with tomatoes) [1 cup]	222	7.8	223	28%	35	4	0.9
6733	Fish, tofu, and vegetables, tempura, Hawaiian style [1 cup]	63	2.2	146	68%	6	7	1.0
6734	Flounder, stuffed [1 piece]	210	7.4	334	29%	43	13	0.7
6735	**Gefilte fish balls [5 balls]**	**41**	**1.4**	**47**	**30%**	**7**	**0**	**0.0**
6736	Haddock cake or patty [1 cake or patty]	120	4.2	237	48%	16	15	1.4
6737	Kamaboko (Japanese fish cake) [2 slices]	32	1.1	37	5%	4	4	0.0
6738	Lau lau (pork and fish wrapped in taro or spinach leaves) [1 lau lau]	214	7.5	318	59%	30	2	1.4
6739	Lobster creole, Puerto Rican style (Include Langosta a la criolla) [1 cup]	242	8.5	395	57%	30	12	2.3
6740	Lobster newburg (Include lobster thermidor, lobster with cream or white sauce) [1 cup]	244	8.6	611	73%	30	11	0.1
6741	Lobster salad [1 cup]	182	6.4	150	46%	11	10	1.3
6742	**Lobster with butter sauce (Include Lobster Norfolk) [1 cup]**	**188**	**6.6**	**448**	**71%**	**30**	**2**	**0.0**
6743	Lobster, stuffed, baked [1 lobster]	400	14.1	730	40%	63	43	2.0
6744	Lomi salmon [1 cup]	234	8.3	151	32%	18	8	2.1
6745	Mackerel cake or patty [1 cake or patty]	120	4.2	297	54%	19	15	1.5
6746	Marinated fish, Puerto Rican style (Include Ceviche) [1 cup]	250	8.8	172	10%	29	10	1.3
6747	Mussels with tomato-based sauce [1 cup]	240	8.5	269	19%	30	24	3.5
6748	Octopus salad, Puerto Rican style (Include Ensalada de pulpo) [1 cup]	180	6.3	297	63%	17	10	1.7
6749	**Oyster fritter [2 fritters]**	**80**	**2.8**	**243**	**47%**	**8**	**24**	**0.8**
6750	Oyster pie (Include pot pie) [1/6 of pie]	109	3.8	274	58%	6	22	0.9
6751	Oysters Rockefeller [4 oysters]	96	3.4	129	51%	7	9	1.4
6752	Paella, with meat, Valenciana style (Include Paella Valenciana) [1 cup, boneless]	183	6.5	530	50%	35	28	0.9
6753	Paella, seafood Puerto Rican style (Include Paella a la marinera) [1 cup]	230	8.1	333	28%	37	22	1.7
6754	Salmon cake or patty (Include salmon croquette) [1 cake or patty]	120	4.2	261	54%	16	14	1.3
6755	Salmon loaf [1 slice]	105	3.7	208	49%	17	9	0.4

Food #	fat gm	sat fat gm	choles mg	sodium mg	potass mg	vit A	vit E	vit C	thia-min	ribo-flavin	nia-cin	vit B-6	fol-ate	vit B-12	cal-cium	phos-phorus	magne-sium	iron	zinc
						\multicolumn{14}{c}{% of Daily Value}												
6710	10	2	181	434	428	9	8	6	8	8	19	11	13	130	14	28	11	7	36
6711	16	4	244	504	517	15	10	17	12	17	21	14	20	157	19	34	13	9	38
6712	12	2	74	748	430	4	6	4	4	12	16	14	4	47	7	22	17	4	4
6713	14	2	142	700	536	4	9	12	10	5	23	14	20	163	16	29	12	8	38
6714	18	4	168	946	515	20	12	19	17	15	22	12	19	110	15	26	12	13	28
6715	18	2	132	375	539	3	13	21	10	5	24	15	18	161	15	28	13	9	38
6716	21	4	83	479	698	8	14	22	9	9	31	25	7	51	4	32	17	7	5
6717	9	3	38	769	240	4	5	1	10	12	40	10	9	27	8	18	8	13	9
6718	11	3	20	945	293	5	6	2	14	12	46	14	14	30	10	20	9	14	10
6719	14	4	26	411	364	18	7	1	16	17	46	15	15	31	17	25	11	14	9
6720	5	1	19	809	434	10	9	88	16	10	49	18	15	28	8	19	9	19	8
6721	5	1	67	443	712	11	14	40	11	9	23	20	6	34	4	24	12	6	5
6722	4	1	49	539	605	2	4	30	7	6	14	17	5	13	3	26	11	5	4
6723	5	1	68	432	721	76	14	40	12	9	24	21	5	34	4	24	13	6	5
6724	5	1	54	572	616	21	4	31	8	6	15	18	4	14	3	28	12	5	4
6725	6	3	52	684	393	12	3	23	12	17	47	16	12	37	20	29	12	12	8
6726	7	3	58	750	458	8	2	9	18	20	53	19	16	40	21	34	15	15	11
6727	3	1	29	33	132	0	2	0	2	4	6	5	1	17	2	8	6	2	1
6728	13	3	67	334	523	3	5	8	9	8	12	16	4	11	3	21	9	4	4
6729	3	0	17	1001	177	0	1	1	3	2	5	6	1	19	3	12	5	3	2
6730	25	15	212	163	423	29	8	3	7	15	14	11	5	27	8	25	9	4	5
6731	18	5	172	701	705	13	8	3	12	27	14	17	7	26	19	41	14	7	9
6732	7	1	87	334	857	12	15	26	13	10	30	22	5	37	6	35	17	6	6
6733	11	2	101	40	116	25	9	4	2	8	2	3	3	4	4	8	6	8	3
6734	11	2	160	470	803	10	16	10	18	16	34	21	14	90	12	44	19	11	19
6735	2	0	28	21	97	1	0	1	2	2	4	3	1	8	2	9	3	1	2
6736	13	3	67	334	523	3	5	8	9	8	12	16	4	11	3	21	9	4	4
6737	0	0	16	20	79	0	0	0	1	2	4	3	0	11	1	5	4	1	1
6738	21	6	90	212	762	40	12	19	29	19	29	22	21	25	8	29	19	13	15
6739	25	3	140	916	859	12	21	44	6	8	16	15	6	21	10	24	16	9	32
6740	50	30	369	647	607	52	7	1	7	24	8	8	9	67	24	40	14	6	27
6741	8	1	112	314	403	11	5	32	5	10	5	7	8	23	4	13	7	5	9
6742	35	22	198	905	523	36	7	0	1	7	8	6	4	76	10	28	13	4	28
6743	32	18	275	1751	1091	33	12	1	21	26	28	13	21	144	26	59	29	20	57
6744	5	1	45	467	603	9	5	44	7	13	31	18	12	60	20	31	12	9	6
6745	18	4	91	479	350	10	9	8	8	14	27	15	4	63	19	27	10	11	7
6746	2	0	50	90	734	20	3	121	7	1	3	34	6	68	6	29	14	3	4
6747	6	1	67	1489	913	14	13	42	28	31	22	10	26	432	7	39	22	50	26
6748	21	3	52	234	534	8	13	32	6	5	11	21	8	292	7	20	11	34	13
6749	13	3	73	294	117	5	6	2	14	13	11	3	9	128	12	15	7	26	279
6750	18	5	30	132	178	8	7	3	13	13	9	3	8	95	8	11	7	19	197
6751	7	3	37	303	250	34	3	19	11	9	8	5	14	150	8	11	12	25	280
6752	30	7	138	207	561	10	9	26	26	19	50	21	16	309	5	33	11	50	23
6753	10	2	168	423	554	18	10	62	12	8	17	22	12	147	12	29	15	33	20
6754	16	4	57	506	387	3	8	7	6	11	27	19	6	37	18	28	8	5	6
6755	11	3	122	506	292	11	6	4	6	17	23	11	7	39	19	28	8	7	7

Mixed Dishes & Fast Food

Food #	Food Description & Amount	wt gm	wt oz	calo-ries	%cal fat	prot gm	carbo gm	fiber gm
6756	Salmon salad [1 cup]	208	7.3	405	66%	27	6	1.3
6757	Sardines with mustard sauce [4 sardines (3"x1"x½") with sauce]	48	1.7	85	61%	8	0	0.0
6758	Sardines with tomato-based sauce [4 sardines (3"x1"x½") with sauce]	48	1.7	85	61%	8	0	0.0
6759	Scallops and noodles with cheese sauce [1 cup]	224	7.9	361	37%	31	27	0.8
6760	Scallops with cheese sauce [1 cup]	244	8.6	271	31%	35	14	0.4
6761	Seafood garden salad with seafood, eggs, tomato and/or carrots, other vegetables, no dressing (Include Hardee's Seafood Salad) [1 cup]	95	3.4	52	25%	7	2	0.9
6762	Seafood garden salad with seafood, tomato and/or carrots, other vegetables, no dressing [1 cup]	95	3.4	43	13%	7	3	1.0
6763	**Seafood garden salad with seafood, eggs, vegetables (no tomato or carrots), no dressing [1 cup]**	**95**	**3.4**	**54**	**26%**	**8**	**2**	**0.8**
6764	Seafood garden salad with seafood, vegetables (as above), no dressing [1 cup]	95	3.4	41	13%	7	2	1.0
6765	Seafood newburg (Include shrimp newburg, crabmeat thermidor) [1 cup]	244	8.6	613	74%	30	10	0.1
6766	Seafood restructured (Include Delicaseas, Sea Tails, Sea Stix, imitation crabmeat) [1 cup, chunks or flakes]	126	4.4	146	5%	17	16	0.2
6767	Seafood salad [1 cup]	208	7.3	328	63%	26	5	0.7
6768	Seafood souffle [1 cup]	159	5.6	252	57%	17	9	0.2
6769	Seafood stew with potatoes and vegetables (including carrots, broccoli, and/or dark-green leafy), tomato-base sauce [1 cup]	252	8.9	177	19%	21	15	2.1
6770	**Seafood stew with potatoes and vegetables (no carrots, broccoli, or dark-green leafy), tomato-base sauce [1 cup]**	**252**	**8.9**	**174**	**19%**	**20**	**15**	**2.0**
6771	Shellfish mixture and vegetables (as above), cream of mushroom soup-based sauce [1 cup]	244	8.6	244	41%	21	15	2.2
6772	Shellfish mixture and vegetables (as above), soy-base sauce [1 cup]	162	5.7	163	49%	10	12	2.7
6773	Shellfish mixture and noodles, tomato-based sauce [1 cup]	224	7.9	251	21%	15	34	1.9
6774	**Shellfish mixture and vegetables (including carrots, broccoli, and/or dark-green leafy, no potatoes), cream of mushroom soup-based sauce [1 cup]**	**224**	**7.9**	**216**	**48%**	**14**	**15**	**2.5**
6775	Shellfish mixture and [above] vegetables, soy-base sauce [1 cup]	162	5.7	164	50%	10	11	2.7
6776	Shrimp and [above] vegetables, soy-based sauce [1 cup]	162	5.7	175	54%	8	13	3.3
6777	Shrimp and vegetables (no carrots, broccoli, dark-green leafy, or potatoes), soy-based sauce [1 cup]	162	5.7	174	56%	8	12	3.0
6778	Shrimp and noodles with cheese sauce [1 cup]	224	7.9	348	38%	29	24	0.8
6779	Shrimp and pasta garden salad (shrimp, pasta salad, tomato &/or carrots, other vegetables), no dressing (Include Burger King Shrimp and Pasta Salad) [1 fast food order]	261	9.2	165	34%	13	15	2.8
6780	Shrimp cake or patty (Include shrimp burger, battered shrimp stick) [1 cake or patty]	120	4.2	247	48%	17	15	1.3
6781	Shrimp chow mein or chop suey with noodles [1 cup]	220	7.8	272	42%	17	24	2.8
6782	Shrimp chow mein or chop suey, no noodles [1 cup]	220	7.8	154	32%	16	11	2.0
6783	**Shrimp cocktail (shrimp with cocktail sauce) [1 cup]**	**230**	**8.1**	**218**	**11%**	**28**	**21**	**4.9**
6784	Shrimp creole, no rice [1 cup]	246	8.7	309	38%	36	11	1.5
6785	Shrimp creole, with rice (Include shrimp jambalaya) [1 cup]	243	8.6	310	27%	27	28	1.4
6786	Shrimp garden salad (shrimp, eggs, tomato and/or carrots, other vegetables), no dressing (Include McDonald's Shrimp Salad) [1 cup]	95	3.4	60	24%	9	2	0.7
6787	Shrimp garden salad (shrimp, eggs, vegetables but not tomato or carrots), no dressing [1 cup]	95	3.4	70	25%	11	2	0.6
6788	Shrimp in garlic sauce, Puerto Rican style (Include Camarones al ajillo) [1 cup]	212	7.5	653	74%	37	6	0.5
6789	Shrimp salad [1 cup]	182	6.4	282	54%	27	6	0.8
6790	**Shrimp scampi (Include shrimp in butter sauce) [1 cup]**	**136**	**4.8**	**311**	**64%**	**26**	**1**	**0.0**
6791	Shrimp teriyaki (shrimp with soy-based sauce) [1 cup]	201	7.1	248	11%	39	12	0.7
6792	Shrimp with lobster sauce [1 cup]	185	6.5	292	38%	35	7	0.6
6793	Shrimp, curried [1 cup]	236	8.3	297	43%	28	14	0.4
6794	Shrimp, stuffed [4 stuffed shrimp]	64	2.3	127	44%	13	4	0.1

Food #	fat gm	sat fat gm	choles mg	sodium mg	potass mg	vit A	vit E	vit C	thia-min	ribo-flavin	nia-cin	vit B-6	fol-ate	vit B-12	cal-cium	phos-phorus	magne-sium	iron	zinc
6756	30	6	216	837	501	11	16	6	7	24	38	29	12	87	27	45	12	10	11
6757	6	1	29	199	164	3	6	1	1	7	10	3	3	72	12	18	4	6	4
6758	6	1	29	199	164	3	6	1	1	7	10	3	3	72	12	18	4	6	4
6759	15	5	84	537	613	17	9	1	17	18	13	7	11	24	32	50	20	24	26
6760	9	4	88	1010	820	9	7	2	12	19	9	9	5	34	39	60	22	21	27
6761	1	0	71	82	199	16	2	13	3	5	4	4	8	5	4	9	4	5	6
6762	1	0	37	79	207	16	2	14	3	2	4	4	8	4	4	9	5	5	6
6763	2	0	78	88	194	5	2	18	3	5	4	5	10	6	4	10	4	5	6
6764	1	0	37	77	210	6	2	21	4	3	4	4	12	4	4	9	4	5	6
6765	50	30	426	551	533	53	6	5	9	23	15	11	12	83	25	39	14	13	27
6766	1	0	62	77	310	1	1	0	3	9	14	12	1	44	5	19	15	3	3
6767	23	3	132	352	503	5	13	21	5	6	12	9	8	31	9	28	14	11	22
6768	16	4	223	302	271	22	8	2	7	22	14	8	8	18	13	23	7	9	10
6769	4	1	97	521	817	43	6	50	13	13	18	17	9	404	8	23	11	52	13
6770	4	1	96	509	795	12	6	70	13	12	17	18	9	399	8	22	11	51	12
6771	11	3	77	754	565	13	7	25	11	19	17	8	8	620	10	28	9	77	15
6772	9	2	41	174	339	4	6	55	7	7	8	10	7	160	6	13	7	29	6
6773	6	1	81	348	284	8	4	15	18	10	15	7	22	150	5	20	12	28	10
6774	11	3	64	756	458	77	9	106	7	11	12	10	8	244	8	20	8	36	10
6775	9	2	43	185	388	61	6	59	9	7	9	9	8	165	6	14	8	29	6
6776	10	2	36	182	331	69	6	63	9	5	8	11	8	4	5	11	8	13	4
6777	11	2	37	197	313	2	7	65	8	5	7	10	8	4	6	11	8	13	4
6778	15	5	216	499	340	20	6	4	15	17	20	9	12	27	24	31	15	25	17
6779	6	1	73	384	411	20	6	36	10	6	11	8	22	8	6	15	10	13	7
6780	13	3	144	300	329	3	7	9	6	6	13	11	3	13	6	20	10	12	7
6781	13	2	82	710	391	2	4	16	15	14	22	9	16	10	6	22	13	19	9
6782	5	1	93	674	407	1	5	18	6	9	17	9	11	11	6	20	11	14	7
6783	3	0	196	1129	576	7	12	43	7	6	22	13	12	21	9	31	15	21	11
6784	13	2	256	521	580	19	11	40	9	7	26	14	5	28	13	38	19	27	14
6785	9	2	181	370	439	13	8	28	20	6	24	11	13	20	10	30	16	24	12
6786	2	0	88	72	184	8	2	11	3	4	5	4	6	7	3	10	5	7	4
6787	2	0	111	87	175	3	2	7	2	5	6	4	6	9	4	12	5	8	5
6788	54	9	269	536	417	39	28	60	5	4	22	14	3	33	12	38	18	26	14
6789	17	3	206	392	367	4	11	10	3	4	16	14	4	22	9	28	13	19	10
6790	22	13	247	392	240	21	5	4	2	3	15	6	1	21	7	27	12	17	9
6791	3	1	269	3104	486	9	5	8	6	8	30	14	4	31	11	39	22	31	15
6792	12	2	261	474	422	4	8	5	13	12	25	14	6	26	8	37	15	21	16
6793	14	4	177	342	443	18	8	6	8	17	16	8	5	23	23	37	15	17	12
6794	6	1	102	168	165	4	4	3	5	5	10	5	6	42	5	14	6	7	11

Mixed Dishes & Fast Food

Food #	Food Description & Amount	wt gm	wt oz	calories	%cal fat	prot gm	carbo gm	fiber gm
6795	Stewed codfish, Puerto Rican style (Include Bacalao guisado) [1 cup]	200	7.1	240	35%	18	21	3.1
6796	Stewed codfish, Puerto Rican style [1 cup]	227	8.0	322	27%	44	14	3.6
6797	Stewed salmon, Puerto Rican style (Include Salmon guisado) [1 cup]	212	7.5	318	45%	26	18	2.2
6798	Sushi rice (rice, vinegar, sugar, rice wine, salt) [1 cup]	145	5.1	256	1%	5	57	0.8
6799	Sushi (sushi rice w. seaweed, vegetables, raw fish) [2 pieces]	52	1.8	75	3%	2	16	0.4
6800	Sushi, with egg, no vegetables, no fish, rolled in seaweed [2 pieces, about 1/3 cup]	52	1.8	63	36%	3	7	0.1
6801	Sushi, with vegetables and fish [2 pieces, about 1/3 cup]	52	1.8	73	3%	3	15	0.6
6802	Sushi, with vegetables, no fish [2 pieces, about 1/3 cup]	52	1.8	75	2%	2	17	0.7
6803	Sushi, with vegetables, rolled in seaweed [2 pieces, about 1/3 cup]	52	1.8	61	2%	1	14	0.3
6804	Sweet and sour shrimp [1 cup]	176	6.2	481	56%	12	46	1.1
6805	Tuna and rice with cream of mushroom soup-based sauce [1 cup]	248	8.7	352	37%	20	34	0.8
6806	Tuna cake or patty [1 cake or patty]	120	4.2	300	52%	22	14	1.3
6807	Tuna casserole with vegetables, cream of mushroom soup-based sauce, no noodles [1 cup]	224	7.9	398	47%	29	23	2.0
6808	Tuna loaf [1 slice]	105	3.7	245	46%	22	10	0.5
6809	**Tuna noodle casserole with cream of mushroom soup-based sauce [1 cup]**	**224**	**7.9**	**401**	**40%**	**27**	**32**	**1.2**
6810	Tuna noodle casserole with cream or white sauce [1 cup]	224	7.9	425	40%	28	34	1.2
6811	Tuna noodle casserole with vegetables, cream of mushroom soup-based sauce [1 cup]	224	7.9	380	38%	25	33	2.2
6812	Tuna noodle casserole with vegetables, cream or white sauce [1 cup]	224	7.9	349	35%	21	35	2.7
6813	Tuna pot pie [1 cup]	252	8.9	563	53%	23	42	3.4
6814	Tuna salad with cheese [1 cup]	208	7.3	358	44%	30	20	0.8
6815	Tuna salad with egg [1 cup]	208	7.3	314	40%	28	19	0.8
6816	Tuna salad [1 cup]	208	7.3	296	33%	29	20	1.0
6817	Tuna with cream or white sauce [1 cup]	237	8.4	392	53%	32	12	0.3
	Other Mixed Dishes							
6900	Antipasto with ham, fish, cheese, vegetables [1 cup]	115	4.1	151	58%	11	4	1.1
6901	Bacon strips, meatless (Include Morning Star Breakfast Strips, Stripple) [4 strips]	20	0.7	62	86%	2	1	0.5
6902	Baked beans, homemade, with salt pork [1 cup]	253	8.9	390	30%	16	55	10.1
6903	Baked beans, canned, low sodium, low fat [1 cup]	253	8.9	235	4%	12	52	13.9
6904	Baked beans, canned, with pork and sweet sauce [1 cup]	253	8.9	281	12%	13	53	13.2
6905	Baked beans, canned, with tomato sauce (Include vegetarian baked beans) [1 cup]	255	9.0	237	4%	12	52	12.8
6906	**Beans and franks [1 cup]**	**259**	**9.1**	**368**	**42%**	**17**	**40**	**17.9**
6907	Beans, cooked with ground beef [1 cup]	266	9.4	416	25%	28	52	8.9
6908	Beans, cooked with pork [1 cup]	178	6.3	252	15%	12	43	6.8
6909	Bierock (turnover filled with ground beef and cabbage mixture) [1 bierock]	215	7.6	517	33%	21	64	3.7
6910	Biscuit with gravy (Include Hardee's biscuit with gravy) [1 biscuit with gravy]	221	7.8	429	49%	13	44	1.1
6911	Black beans, Cuban style (Include Habichuelas negras guisadas a la Cubana) [1 cup]	270	9.5	302	14%	16	50	11.8
6912	Boston baked beans [1 cup]	253	8.9	390	30%	16	55	10.1
6913	**Bread stuffing made with egg [1 cup]**	**170**	**6.0**	**300**	**44%**	**6**	**35**	**4.6**
6914	Breaded brains, Puerto Rican style (Include Sesos rebosados) [2 fritters (3½"x2½"x½")]	120	4.2	307	56%	13	20	0.6
6915	Breakfast links, patties, or slices, meatless (Include Prosage, Morningstar) [2 links]	50	1.8	128	64%	9	5	1.4
6916	Calzone, with cheese, meatless (Include stromboli, Pizza Hut Calizza) [1 calzone or stromboli]	424	15.0	1641	51%	81	117	5.0
6917	Calzone, with meat and cheese (Include stromboli, Pizza Hut Calizza) [1 calzone or stromboli]	424	15.0	1474	46%	64	131	5.7
6918	Cannelloni, cheese and spinach-filled, no sauce [1 cannelloni]	74	2.6	119	39%	5	13	0.9
6919	Cassava pie stuffed with crabmeat, Puerto Rican style (Include Empanada de jueyes) [1 empanada (5"x2½"x½")]	126	4.4	344	42%	12	39	2.1
6920	Chalupas with beans and cheese [1 chalupa]	164	5.8	285	48%	10	28	7.0
6921	Chalupas with chicken and cheese [1 chalupa]	150	5.3	296	47%	17	23	5.4

Food #	fat gm	sat fat gm	choles mg	sodium mg	potass mg	% of Daily Value													
						vit A	vit E	vit C	thia-min	ribo-flavin	nia-cin	vit B-6	fol-ate	vit B-12	cal-cium	phos-phorus	magne-sium	iron	zinc
6795	9	1	39	209	737	6	7	101	12	6	16	26	6	12	4	20	13	8	5
6796	10	1	102	4186	1063	9	9	122	16	12	28	39	11	106	11	55	22	12	7
6797	16	3	65	918	925	4	13	25	7	15	44	28	8	83	27	44	16	11	10
6798	0	0	0	6	78	0	0	0	20	2	13	5	26	0	2	7	5	15	5
6799	0	0	1	42	70	6	0	2	5	2	5	3	7	1	1	3	3	4	2
6800	3	1	70	176	43	5	1	1	3	6	2	2	5	2	1	4	2	3	2
6801	0	0	4	29	68	4	1	2	6	1	5	3	6	2	1	3	2	4	2
6802	0	0	0	28	53	5	0	2	6	1	4	2	7	0	1	3	2	4	2
6803	0	0	0	2	33	2	0	1	4	1	3	2	6	0	1	2	2	3	2
6804	30	4	71	2019	362	5	23	15	4	7	14	11	2	8	5	15	11	14	6
6805	15	4	13	928	278	7	7	11	12	13	42	8	10	22	10	27	9	13	10
6806	17	4	43	422	326	3	8	6	7	9	46	11	4	23	3	25	8	8	6
6807	21	5	18	1054	320	11	10	8	16	18	57	7	9	31	11	31	10	15	10
6808	13	3	99	346	193	11	6	4	7	15	38	5	6	24	7	22	6	8	6
6809	18	4	38	830	248	8	8	1	15	16	51	6	12	27	9	29	11	16	10
6810	19	4	42	461	296	16	8	1	17	20	51	6	13	28	14	32	12	16	10
6811	16	4	35	784	255	9	7	6	18	16	47	6	14	24	9	27	11	16	10
6812	14	3	33	663	318	10	7	16	18	19	36	7	14	17	14	27	11	16	10
6813	33	9	31	536	378	89	13	10	26	22	51	8	17	21	6	29	10	19	8
6814	18	6	54	1070	364	10	7	4	4	12	65	20	4	53	17	30	10	11	11
6815	14	3	130	810	332	9	7	4	4	12	65	20	6	54	4	22	8	12	7
6816	11	2	41	853	352	5	6	4	4	7	75	22	4	57	3	21	9	12	7
6817	23	6	134	779	403	13	10	2	9	28	53	9	7	41	18	42	11	10	10
6900	10	4	112	724	241	59	3	7	8	15	12	9	5	13	14	17	5	7	9
6901	6	1	0	293	34	0	5	0	59	6	8	5	2	0	0	1	1	3	1
6902	13	5	13	236	1082	0	2	4	14	5	3	13	31	1	18	20	33	35	16
6903	1	0	0	3	749	4	4	13	25	9	5	16	15	0	13	26	20	4	24
6904	4	1	18	850	673	3	5	13	8	9	4	11	24	0	15	27	22	23	25
6905	1	0	0	1012	755	4	5	13	25	9	5	16	14	0	13	27	20	4	24
6906	17	6	16	1114	609	4	4	10	10	9	12	6	19	0	12	27	18	25	32
6907	12	4	51	1146	987	4	4	11	12	14	20	16	19	23	13	26	23	32	32
6908	4	2	7	312	725	1	2	4	12	5	4	8	21	1	11	15	19	24	12
6909	19	6	44	48	319	1	4	15	38	32	38	12	31	23	4	20	8	29	22
6910	23	7	40	1373	405	5	7	3	24	27	16	5	11	15	24	44	36	15	7
6911	5	1	2	31	891	2	2	26	30	7	6	11	41	0	11	25	27	23	17
6912	13	5	13	236	1082	0	2	4	14	5	3	13	31	1	18	20	33	35	16
6913	15	3	43	881	131	15	8	0	15	13	12	4	41	2	6	9	5	10	4
6914	19	4	1499	102	340	1	10	20	17	24	23	8	7	132	7	28	5	16	10
6915	9	1	0	444	116	3	4	0	78	12	28	21	3	0	3	11	5	10	5
6916	93	44	253	2051	558	71	25	0	70	106	49	14	70	21	190	152	28	51	54
6917	76	26	190	1073	678	46	26	0	88	98	74	18	88	32	77	91	22	59	51
6918	5	2	34	60	129	16	2	3	7	10	4	4	11	2	9	8	5	8	4
6919	16	4	49	378	569	5	7	40	11	13	11	11	11	43	16	19	12	5	15
6920	15	6	23	165	476	9	6	12	12	8	4	11	33	2	18	23	15	13	10
6921	15	6	45	181	417	8	5	10	10	10	13	13	24	3	17	24	14	12	12

Mixed Dishes & Fast Food

Food #	Food Description & Amount	wt gm	wt oz	calories	%cal fat	prot gm	carbo gm	fiber gm
6922	Chayote relleno (stuffed christophine, Puerto Rican style) [¼ chayote (4½"x2"x1")]	123	4.3	252	66%	16	5	1.6
6923	Cheese fondue [1 cup]	215	7.6	446	59%	31	8	0.1
6924	Cheese souffle [1 cup]	95	3.4	196	69%	9	6	0.1
6925	Cheese turnovers, Puerto Rican style (Pastelillos de queso; Empandillas) [2 turnovers]	42	1.5	172	52%	4	16	0.5
6926	Chickpeas stewed with pig's feet, Puerto Rican style (Garbanzos guisados con patitos de cerdo) [1 cup, with bones]	202	7.1	268	51%	17	16	3.8
6927	**Chiles rellenos** [1 chili]	**143**	**5.0**	**365**	**74%**	**17**	**8**	**1.3**
6928	Chiles rellenos, filled with meat and cheese [1 chili]	143	5.0	222	65%	10	10	1.8
6929	Chili beans, barbecue beans, ranch style beans or Mexican-style beans (Include beans in chili sauce) [1 cup]	253	8.9	223	10%	13	43	10.6
6930	Chili con carne with beans and macaroni [1 cup]	253	8.9	336	31%	21	38	6.7
6931	Chili con carne with beans and rice [1 cup]	250	8.8	297	27%	11	45	7.2
6932	Chili con carne with chicken or turkey and beans [1 cup]	254	9.0	217	22%	17	27	7.4
6933	Chili con carne with venison and beans [1 cup]	254	9.0	251	17%	26	27	7.5
6934	Chilaquiles, with egg [1 cup]	232	8.2	441	64%	14	28	4.3
6935	Chilaquiles, without egg [1 cup]	232	8.2	445	65%	10	32	5.1
6936	Chimichanga with beans and cheese, meatless [1 chimichanga]	118	4.2	256	56%	8	21	3.2
6937	**Chimichanga with beef** [1 chimichanga]	**118**	**4.2**	**388**	**60%**	**13**	**25**	**1.7**
6938	Chimichanga with beef and beans [1 chimichanga]	118	4.2	241	52%	8	21	3.2
6939	Chimichanga with beef and cheese [1 chimichanga]	118	4.2	341	63%	13	19	1.5
6940	Chimichanga with beef and rice [1 chimichanga]	288	10.2	643	52%	19	59	4.4
6941	Chimichanga with chicken and cheese [1 chimichanga]	183	6.5	560	61%	24	31	2.3
6942	Chimichanga with chicken and sour cream, no cheese [1 chimichanga]	118	4.2	278	64%	9	17	1.2
6943	Chow fun noodles with meat and vegetables [1 cup]	152	5.4	192	34%	10	22	1.7
6944	Chow fun noodles with vegetables, meatless [1 cup]	152	5.4	160	12%	4	32	1.2
6945	**Chow mein** or chop suey, various types of meat, with noodles [1 cup]	**220**	**7.8**	**420**	**52%**	**21**	**31**	**3.7**
6946	Chop suey, meatless [1 cup]	220	7.8	248	26%	5	40	2.1
6947	Codfish fritters, Puerto Rican style (Bacalaitos) [2 fritters (3½"x3½")]	68	2.4	372	69%	12	17	0.6
6948	Corned beef patty [1 patty]	100	3.5	181	56%	9	11	0.5
6949	Cornmeal dressing with chicken or turkey and vegetables [1 cup]	161	5.7	383	55%	12	31	2.5
6950	Cornmeal fritters, Puerto Rican style (Arepa; arepitas) [2 fritters (2½"x2½"x4")]	80	2.8	219	60%	6	16	1.5
6951	Cornmeal sticks, Puerto Rican style (Surullos) [4 sticks (3"x¾")]	80	2.8	327	45%	6	38	3.6
6952	Cowpeas, cooked with pork (Include black-eyed peas or field peas with pork) [1 cup]	179	6.3	239	18%	24	25	7.9
6953	Creamed dried beef on toast [1 slice toast with sauce]	145	5.1	229	43%	11	21	0.7
6954	Crepe, with creamy chicken-mushroom filling, no sauce on top [1 crepe]	123	4.3	239	48%	18	13	0.6
6955	Crepe, with creamy beef-mushroom filling, creamy mushroom sauce on top [1 crepe]	154	5.4	292	52%	22	12	0.8
6956	Croissant, filled with broccoli and cheese [1 croissant]	113	4.0	303	51%	8	29	1.4
6957	**Dim sum**, egg roll type, meat filled (Include shrimp, pork, ham) [1 dim sum]	**28**	**1.0**	**31**	**20%**	**3**	**3**	**0.2**
6958	Dirty rice [1 cup]	198	7.0	281	31%	11	36	0.6
6959	Dressing with chicken and vegetables [1 cup]	161	5.7	351	47%	12	34	2.3
6960	Dressing with meat and vegetables (Include with sausage, ground beef, pepperoni, ham, bacon, salami) [1 cup]	161	5.7	421	58%	11	33	2.1
6961	Dressing with oysters [1 cup]	161	5.7	309	54%	8	28	2.0
6962	Dumplings, fried, pork [1 dumpling]	100	3.5	341	55%	13	25	0.8
6963	Dumplings, fried, Puerto Rican style [2 dumplings]	64	2.3	236	57%	4	22	0.7
6964	Dumplings, meat-filled (Include pierogi, piroshki, kreplach) [1 dumpling]	97	3.4	362	59%	11	25	0.9
6965	Dumplings, plain [2 dumplings]	64	2.3	80	23%	2	13	0.4
6966	Dumplings, potato or cheese-filled (Include pierogi) [1 dumpling]	57	2.0	104	21%	4	17	0.8
6967	Dumplings, steamed, filled with meat, poultry, or seafood (Include shui-mai, steamed dim sum) [2 dumplings]	74	2.6	81	20%	8	7	0.4

Food #	fat gm	sat fat gm	choles mg	sodium mg	potass mg	vit A	vit E	vit C	thia-min	ribo-flavin	nia-cin	vit B-6	fol-ate	vit B-12	cal-cium	phos-phorus	magne-sium	iron	zinc
6922	19	6	133	269	369	5	2	15	22	17	15	13	15	9	3	19	6	7	18
6923	29	19	97	286	225	27	2	0	3	25	2	5	3	17	103	66	13	5	28
6924	15	6	136	225	125	18	4	0	4	17	1	3	5	6	18	18	4	4	7
6925	10	4	15	137	31	3	2	0	8	7	5	1	5	1	11	9	2	6	3
6926	15	4	68	255	418	7	5	14	6	7	5	8	11	2	6	13	7	10	11
6927	30	12	168	522	386	25	16	188	6	23	5	13	7	8	40	31	9	9	14
6928	16	5	110	130	342	16	11	58	6	13	10	12	6	10	11	14	6	9	10
6929	3	0	0	1834	1139	0	2	7	7	22	5	34	16	0	8	39	28	26	34
6930	12	4	47	722	623	9	5	28	17	16	25	12	18	19	5	22	13	21	24
6931	9	4	26	1171	598	5	4	4	15	10	10	15	23	0	6	28	20	36	24
6932	5	1	33	874	682	12	6	36	15	13	26	18	14	2	6	20	13	15	10
6933	5	1	72	893	785	12	6	35	16	31	26	13	10	46	6	26	15	28	16
6934	32	9	198	217	416	26	12	24	9	23	6	13	14	8	20	25	13	12	11
6935	32	9	23	193	429	21	13	28	8	12	6	12	11	1	21	21	14	10	9
6936	16	5	17	305	291	8	9	18	9	9	7	6	9	2	15	14	7	10	7
6937	26	6	35	233	216	1	12	5	13	11	18	7	10	19	6	13	5	13	16
6938	14	3	17	230	323	4	8	18	9	8	11	8	8	8	5	10	7	11	10
6939	24	8	39	282	199	7	9	10	10	12	12	6	10	13	18	18	5	10	13
6940	37	8	39	573	668	12	23	41	30	20	33	18	28	21	11	22	14	26	22
6941	38	12	67	487	248	10	16	9	16	20	21	9	16	6	31	30	9	14	15
6942	20	6	30	155	179	8	8	9	9	9	11	4	8	2	7	9	4	7	5
6943	7	2	20	206	269	3	3	11	20	8	14	16	5	3	3	11	5	4	7
6944	2	0	0	80	94	1	1	8	5	1	6	9	4	0	2	6	6	3	3
6945	24	5	42	1150	477	11	6	33	36	23	32	19	17	11	4	25	13	20	17
6946	7	1	0	466	272	1	5	32	17	9	15	12	23	0	3	11	8	12	6
6947	29	4	24	51	253	1	17	1	11	8	11	7	6	8	2	14	6	7	3
6948	11	4	33	540	200	0	1	0	1	5	11	4	2	11	1	7	4	11	15
6949	23	5	140	357	228	77	11	7	13	27	13	9	34	47	16	18	7	21	12
6950	15	5	16	106	54	5	6	0	7	8	5	3	7	1	12	9	3	5	5
6951	17	4	8	57	90	4	10	0	17	12	11	6	15	1	6	8	6	12	4
6952	5	2	28	719	506	0	2	1	44	12	17	17	63	11	4	33	18	20	22
6953	11	3	16	865	278	12	4	1	12	18	11	6	8	13	16	16	7	10	10
6954	13	6	119	168	247	11	2	2	9	16	36	15	6	6	6	18	6	8	6
6955	17	6	109	515	282	12	5	2	8	20	26	11	5	20	17	26	9	11	19
6956	17	11	48	539	131	20	2	12	14	15	9	3	12	2	16	15	4	9	6
6957	1	0	15	123	50	0	0	1	3	2	4	2	1	1	1	3	1	2	2
6958	10	5	104	461	221	75	2	7	15	22	27	8	38	48	2	15	5	22	11
6959	18	4	104	494	200	68	8	7	19	27	17	8	35	41	10	13	7	22	11
6960	27	8	31	1105	215	8	5	3	27	16	19	5	15	3	9	11	6	18	8
6961	18	4	23	560	232	17	10	8	16	13	13	5	12	121	10	12	10	26	254
6962	21	5	27	86	198	1	8	1	35	16	18	10	9	5	3	13	5	10	7
6963	15	3	0	119	70	2	6	0	11	9	7	1	7	1	9	7	2	8	2
6964	24	6	28	119	115	0	7	0	15	12	13	5	9	14	1	10	3	13	15
6965	2	1	1	131	41	1	1	0	7	6	4	1	4	1	9	6	2	5	1
6966	2	1	33	101	84	3	1	2	9	8	6	3	6	2	3	6	2	6	2
6967	2	0	39	325	132	1	1	2	8	6	11	5	3	4	2	8	3	5	4

% of Daily Value

Mixed Dishes & Fast Food

Food #	Food Description & Amount	wt gm	wt oz	calo-ries	%cal fat	prot gm	carbo gm	fiber gm
6968	Egg foo yung, beef [1 patty]	86	3.0	119	60%	8	3	0.5
6969	Egg foo yung, chicken [1 patty]	86	3.0	121	59%	8	4	0.5
6970	Egg foo yung, pork [1 patty]	86	3.0	124	60%	8	4	0.5
6971	Egg foo yung, shrimp (Include Tortas de Carmaron) [1 cup]	175	6.2	317	70%	17	7	1.5
6972	Egg roll, meatless [1 egg roll]	64	2.3	101	52%	3	10	0.8
6973	Egg roll, with chicken or turkey [1 egg roll]	64	2.3	103	48%	4	9	0.6
6974	**Egg roll, with meat (Include Chinese rolls, spring rolls, lumpia) [1 egg roll]**	**64**	**2.3**	**113**	**49%**	**5**	**9**	**0.7**
6975	Egg roll, with shrimp [1 egg roll]	64	2.3	104	49%	4	10	0.7
6976	Eggplant parmesan casserole, low-calorie [1 cup]	198	7.0	181	44%	14	13	3.6
6977	Eggplant parmesan casserole, regular [1 cup]	198	7.0	319	62%	14	17	3.2
6978	Enchilada with beans, meatless [1 enchilada]	118	4.2	207	36%	6	29	6.4
6979	Enchilada with beans and cheese, meatless [1 enchilada]	131	4.6	252	46%	9	26	5.4
6980	Enchilada with beef, no beans [1 enchilada]	114	4.0	207	40%	11	21	3.0
6981	Enchilada with beef and beans [1 enchilada]	116	4.1	207	37%	8	25	4.9
6982	Enchilada with beef and cheese, no beans [1 enchilada]	105	3.7	209	50%	10	17	2.6
6983	Enchilada with beef, beans, and cheese (Include Taco Bell enchirito) [1 enchilada or enchirito]	129	4.6	242	45%	10	24	4.7
6984	Enchilada with cheese, meatless, no beans [1 enchilada]	102	3.6	225	55%	10	17	2.5
6985	**Enchilada with chicken [1 enchilada]**	**126**	**4.4**	**202**	**30%**	**14**	**22**	**3.2**
6986	Enchilada with chicken and beans [1 enchilada]	113	4.0	185	35%	9	22	4.6
6987	Enchilada with chicken and cheese, no beans [1 enchilada]	126	4.4	235	45%	14	20	3.0
6988	Enchilada with chicken, beans, and cheese [1 enchilada]	126	4.4	227	43%	11	23	4.5
6989	Enchilada with ham and cheese, no beans [1 enchilada]	105	3.7	201	45%	9	20	2.7
6990	Enchilada with seafood [1 enchilada]	126	4.4	179	24%	12	23	3.3
6991	Fajita with beef [fajita with 1 tortilla]	223	7.9	399	41%	23	36	3.2
6992	**Fajita with chicken [fajita with 1 tortilla]**	**223**	**7.9**	**363**	**30%**	**20**	**44**	**5.1**
6993	Falafel [4 patties (2¼"dia)]	68	2.4	227	48%	9	22	8.9
6994	Flauta with beef [1 flauta]	113	4.0	354	70%	14	13	1.9
6995	Flauta with chicken [1 flauta]	113	4.0	330	70%	13	12	1.7
6996	Flavored pasta (Include Lipton Beef Flavor, Lipton Chicken Flavor) [1 cup]	185	6.5	210	36%	7	27	1.0
6997	Flavored rice mixture (Include Ricearoni, all flavors; Liptons rice and sauce; Uncle Ben's Rice Oriental) [1 cup]	218	7.7	277	29%	4	44	0.9
6998	Flavored rice mixture with cheese (Include rice au gratin) [1 cup]	230	8.1	198	34%	5	29	1.8
6999	Flavored rice, brown and wild [1 cup]	217	7.7	236	24%	6	40	2.8
7000	Flavored rice, white and wild [1 cup]	182	6.4	172	17%	5	31	1.3
7001	Flavored rice and pasta mixture, beef flavor [1 cup]	184	6.5	207	27%	5	33	1.2
7002	**Flavored rice and pasta mixture, chicken flavor [1 cup]**	**208**	**7.3**	**234**	**27%**	**5**	**37**	**1.3**
7003	Fried chickpeas, Puerto Rican style (Garbanzos fritos) [1 cup]	120	4.2	377	58%	13	28	8.0
7004	Fried rice, Puerto Rican style (arroz frito) [1 cup]	173	6.1	222	25%	25	15	1.0
7005	Gnocchi, cheese [1 cup]	70	2.5	128	60%	7	6	0.2
7006	Gnocchi, potato [1 cup]	188	6.6	268	44%	5	33	1.8
7007	Grape leaves stuffed with rice [1 roll]	56	2.0	91	64%	1	8	1.7
7008	Gumbo with rice (New Orleans type with shellfish, pork, and/or poultry, tomatoes, okra, rice) [1 cup]	244	8.6	193	35%	14	17	1.9
7009	Gumbo, no rice (New Orleans type with shellfish, pork, and/or poultry, tomatoes, okra) [1 cup]	244	8.6	179	43%	15	11	2.0
7010	Hallacas, Puerto Rican style (hominy, pork or ham, vegetables) [1 hallaca (5¾"x2½"x½")]	95	3.4	148	62%	6	9	1.0
7011	Hash [1 cup]	190	6.7	344	56%	17	20	1.0

Food #	fat gm	sat fat gm	choles mg	sodium mg	potass mg	vit A	vit E	vit C	thia-min	ribo-flavin	nia-cin	vit B-6	fol-ate	vit B-12	cal-cium	phos-phorus	magne-sium	iron	zinc
																% of Daily Value			
6968	8	2	166	131	139	9	4	5	3	13	3	6	6	11	3	10	3	6	7
6969	8	2	167	132	136	9	4	5	3	14	4	6	6	6	3	10	3	5	5
6970	8	2	167	131	157	9	4	5	9	15	4	7	6	7	3	11	3	5	6
6971	25	5	379	522	329	49	11	6	6	28	8	12	10	16	7	24	7	13	10
6972	6	1	30	274	97	2	3	5	5	6	4	2	5	1	1	4	2	4	2
6973	6	1	38	164	73	2	2	4	5	6	5	2	5	1	2	4	2	5	2
6974	6	1	37	274	124	2	3	4	11	7	6	5	4	2	2	6	3	5	3
6975	6	1	40	293	100	2	3	4	5	6	5	3	5	2	2	5	2	5	2
6976	9	5	25	671	513	13	3	14	9	12	7	11	6	7	38	29	9	5	11
6977	22	9	55	684	447	17	9	13	9	15	8	10	8	7	37	28	9	7	10
6978	8	2	5	128	456	13	4	21	8	5	5	10	26	0	8	18	13	10	6
6979	13	6	21	262	464	23	5	26	7	8	5	11	22	2	20	25	13	9	9
6980	9	3	28	183	395	17	3	23	5	9	13	12	12	11	8	19	10	9	15
6981	9	3	15	152	428	15	4	22	7	7	8	11	20	5	8	18	11	10	10
6982	12	5	31	256	343	21	3	23	4	9	8	10	10	8	17	21	9	7	12
6983	12	5	25	242	459	22	4	27	7	9	8	12	19	6	16	23	12	10	11
6984	14	7	33	335	300	25	3	22	4	10	4	8	10	4	28	26	9	5	9
6985	7	1	35	197	381	18	4	24	5	8	18	14	12	1	8	20	11	8	9
6986	7	2	17	143	407	15	4	22	6	6	10	11	18	1	7	16	10	8	7
6987	12	5	39	301	382	25	4	27	5	10	12	12	11	3	21	25	10	7	10
6988	11	4	26	234	429	21	4	26	6	8	9	11	18	2	16	22	11	9	8
6989	10	4	25	471	336	19	3	21	10	9	9	10	11	4	17	24	9	6	8
6990	5	1	68	238	396	19	5	26	5	4	10	11	12	7	10	23	13	11	7
6991	18	6	45	316	479	4	6	45	26	18	27	19	21	34	8	24	9	21	23
6992	12	3	39	343	534	6	6	61	28	19	31	19	26	2	10	19	12	18	11
6993	12	2	0	103	275	0	8	2	6	6	3	4	13	0	4	13	13	11	7
6994	28	5	37	68	313	2	16	32	4	8	9	12	6	20	5	18	7	10	23
6995	26	4	35	71	269	3	15	30	3	6	15	11	5	1	5	14	7	5	8
6996	8	2	35	541	166	7	3	0	21	11	19	3	16	4	2	10	6	11	4
6997	9	2	2	653	99	7	5	2	16	2	12	6	21	0	3	7	4	14	5
6998	7	2	1	511	141	4	3	0	9	7	8	3	15	0	8	15	4	5	4
6999	6	1	0	789	304	5	4	2	8	6	18	12	3	0	2	20	17	7	9
7000	3	1	0	672	135	3	2	1	8	3	9	3	15	0	5	10	7	8	6
7001	6	2	3	546	119	8	3	3	17	7	11	6	15	0	5	7	5	13	4
7002	7	2	3	617	135	9	3	3	19	8	12	6	18	0	5	8	6	15	4
7003	24	8	25	217	463	0	2	3	20	8	8	14	64	4	5	21	14	17	13
7004	6	2	162	897	401	7	3	37	30	15	20	20	8	15	5	25	10	12	14
7005	8	3	49	206	51	9	3	0	3	8	2	1	3	4	15	11	2	3	4
7006	13	8	35	141	245	13	1	6	15	10	11	8	9	2	4	8	5	8	3
7007	6	1	0	4	90	26	3	6	2	3	3	4	5	0	5	2	4	4	1
7008	8	2	40	542	446	6	5	23	13	9	23	11	16	40	7	15	10	15	101
7009	8	2	45	607	489	7	5	25	11	10	23	11	13	45	8	16	10	14	112
7010	10	2	38	158	170	3	7	17	9	6	6	6	4	3	2	7	3	5	4
7011	21	7	63	1026	380	0	1	0	1	10	20	8	4	20	2	13	7	21	29

Mixed Dishes & Fast Food

Food #	Food Description & Amount	wt gm	wt oz	calories	%cal fat	prot gm	carbo gm	fiber gm
7012	Italian pie with meat (Include Priazzo; Pizza Hut Priazzo Roma, Priazzo Milano, Priazzo Portofino, Priazzo Verona) [1/8 of 12"dia]	191	6.7	569	36%	21	69	3.5
7013	Italian pie, meatless (Include Pizza Hut Priazzo Florentine) [1/8 of 12"dia]	163	5.7	444	30%	18	59	3.0
7014	Jambalaya with meat and rice [1 cup]	244	8.6	398	49%	26	23	1.2
7015	Julienne salad (meat, cheese, eggs, vegetables), no dressing (Include Burger King Chef's Salad; Hardee's Chef's Salad; McDonald's Chef's Salad) [1 cup]	76	2.7	72	52%	7	2	0.6
7016	Kibby, Puerto Rican style (beef and bulgur) (Plato Arabe) [2 fritters (3"x3"x½")]	110	3.9	190	39%	10	20	4.8
7017	Kidney bean salad [1 cup]	231	8.1	349	37%	13	45	11.2
7018	Kishke, stuffed derma [4 kishke (1 cubic inch, cooked)]	72	2.5	334	65%	3	25	1.2
7019	Knish, cheese [1 knish]	60	2.1	208	51%	6	19	0.6
7020	Knish, meat [1 knish]	50	1.8	175	55%	7	13	0.6
7021	Knish, potato [1 knish]	61	2.2	215	52%	5	21	0.9
7022	Kung Pao pork [1 cup]	162	5.7	451	68%	26	11	2.1
7023	**Lasagna** with meat (Include baked ziti) [1 piece (3½"x4")]	232	8.2	371	36%	22	38	2.6
7024	Lasagna with meat, canned [1 cup]	250	8.8	218	16%	8	39	1.7
7025	Lasagna with meat and spinach [1 piece (3½"x4")]	232	8.2	346	35%	21	35	3.0
7026	Lasagna with meat, spinach noodles [1 piece (3½"x4")]	232	8.2	351	37%	21	34	4.7
7027	Lasagna with meat, whole wheat noodles [1 piece (3½"x4")]	232	8.2	354	37%	22	36	4.1
7028	Lasagna, meatless [1 piece (3½"x4")]	256	9.0	360	28%	19	46	3.2
7029	Lasagna, meatless, spinach noodles [1 piece (3½"x4")]	256	9.0	335	29%	18	41	5.8
7030	Lasagna, meatless, whole wheat noodles [1 piece (3½"x4")]	256	9.0	339	29%	19	44	5.1
7031	Lasagna, meatless, with spinach [1 piece (3½"x4")]	256	9.0	334	28%	18	43	3.6
7032	Lasagna, with chicken or turkey, and spinach [1 piece (3½"x4")]	232	8.2	327	30%	22	35	3.0
7033	Liver dumpling [1 cup]	250	8.8	783	51%	57	37	1.7
7034	Liver hash (Include liver mush) [1 cup]	225	7.9	286	21%	32	23	1.9
7035	Lo mein with meat [1 cup]	200	7.1	283	43%	20	21	2.7
7036	Lo mein, meatless [1 cup]	200	7.1	135	5%	6	27	3.8
7037	Lo mein with shrimp [1 cup]	200	7.1	218	38%	13	22	4.2
7038	Macaroni, creamed, with cheese [1 cup]	200	7.1	396	39%	15	44	2.6
7039	Macaroni and cheese with egg [1 cup]	243	8.6	475	43%	19	48	1.7
7040	Macaroni or noodles with beans or lentils and tomato sauce [1 cup]	227	8.0	210	5%	9	41	9.0
7041	Macaroni or noodles with cheese (Include macaroni casserole) [1 cup]	243	8.6	477	43%	19	49	1.8
7042	Macaroni or noodles with cheese, canned [1 cup]	239	8.4	210	30%	7	29	1.1
7043	**Macaroni or noodles with cheese, made from dry mix** [1 cup]	191	6.7	397	43%	11	45	2.0
7044	Macaroni or noodles with cheese, from boxed mix with already prepared cheese sauce [1 cup]	217	7.7	358	28%	14	50	2.2
7045	Macaroni or noodles with cheese and beef (Include Hamburger Helper Cheeseburger Macaroni) [1 cup]	243	8.6	340	40%	28	22	1.1
7046	Macaroni or noodles with cheese and chicken or turkey [1 cup]	243	8.6	465	41%	31	37	1.3
7047	Macaroni or noodles with cheese and frankfurters [1 cup]	243	8.6	551	54%	21	41	1.5
7048	Macaroni or noodles with cheese and pork or ham [1 cup]	243	8.6	444	44%	25	36	1.3
7049	Macaroni or noodles with cheese and tomato [1 cup]	243	8.6	287	10%	12	54	4.0
7050	Macaroni or noodles with cheese and tuna (Include Tuna Helper Cheesy Noodles 'n' Tuna, Tuna Helper Tuna Au gratin) [1 cup]	243	8.6	417	44%	27	30	1.2
7051	Macaroni, creamed (Include fettuccine alfredo, macaroni cooked in milk, Noodles Romanoff) [1 cup]	200	7.1	274	34%	8	36	1.4
7052	Macaroni, creamed, with vegetables [1 cup]	200	7.1	232	34%	7	31	2.2
7053	Macaroni with tuna, Puerto Rican style (Macarrones con atun) [1 cup]	225	7.9	362	33%	21	38	1.5
7054	Macaroni salad with cheese [1 cup]	177	6.2	348	51%	10	35	3.6

Food #	fat gm	sat fat gm	choles mg	sodium mg	potass mg	vit A	vit E	vit C	thia-min	ribo-flavin	nia-cin	vit B-6	fol-ate	vit B-12	cal-cium	phos-phorus	magne-sium	iron	zinc
																% of Daily Value			
7012	23	8	39	1440	506	10	7	15	48	35	36	13	28	12	14	27	11	28	16
7013	15	6	29	638	358	13	6	13	33	29	23	7	24	3	31	30	10	22	11
7014	22	6	97	341	443	7	2	17	19	12	47	20	12	7	5	23	10	15	15
7015	4	2	74	138	143	13	1	5	6	8	5	6	7	5	6	9	3	3	5
7016	8	3	29	33	228	0	0	2	4	6	13	7	2	11	2	13	12	8	13
7017	14	3	0	614	680	5	10	8	16	6	5	11	48	1	6	22	17	25	11
7018	24	12	26	1	62	0	2	1	14	8	8	2	9	0	1	4	2	8	2
7019	12	3	56	204	62	13	5	0	11	12	6	2	8	3	2	8	2	7	2
7020	11	3	52	107	88	9	4	1	8	9	7	2	6	5	1	6	2	7	7
7021	12	3	59	140	96	13	6	2	11	10	7	3	8	2	2	6	3	7	2
7022	34	7	59	862	541	5	13	13	55	18	35	26	10	9	5	27	15	11	17
7023	15	8	55	370	435	15	4	23	15	19	20	12	16	15	26	28	12	16	21
7024	4	2	13	1404	311	8	1	36	17	10	13	7	14	5	5	10	7	9	7
7025	14	7	51	358	518	27	5	28	15	19	18	11	22	12	26	27	15	18	20
7026	15	8	55	377	440	16	4	23	8	16	16	12	5	13	27	32	20	11	24
7027	15	8	55	372	448	15	4	23	10	16	15	12	4	13	26	32	15	14	23
7028	11	7	38	428	438	18	4	28	18	19	15	10	19	3	31	29	13	15	14
7029	11	7	38	436	445	20	4	28	10	16	11	13	6	3	33	34	22	9	17
7030	11	7	38	431	454	18	5	28	12	16	9	13	5	3	32	33	17	13	17
7031	10	6	34	411	542	33	5	34	17	20	14	12	26	3	31	28	17	18	14
7032	11	6	52	361	509	27	5	28	15	19	21	15	22	4	26	28	15	17	16
7033	44	11	1040	609	527	896	18	78	36	171	77	49	284	1217	11	64	13	58	69
7034	7	2	767	93	463	597	6	70	31	127	35	46	237	393	3	42	11	59	37
7035	14	3	42	142	332	1	7	19	27	16	25	18	19	4	3	19	11	12	12
7036	1	0	0	564	386	13	1	20	16	14	14	10	23	0	5	11	8	11	6
7037	9	2	66	228	400	8	5	14	11	9	14	6	14	7	7	16	13	17	8
7038	17	8	30	416	99	14	4	0	22	15	13	4	27	5	28	25	10	13	10
7039	23	10	74	742	321	24	6	1	20	30	13	6	18	8	38	39	12	16	16
7040	1	0	5	642	538	4	7	11	20	12	15	7	12	0	8	13	12	23	11
7041	23	10	37	756	320	23	6	1	20	29	13	6	18	7	39	38	13	15	16
7042	7	3	14	1058	137	6	1	0	15	13	8	3	15	3	15	14	6	8	6
7043	19	5	9	749	153	16	8	1	21	14	12	4	25	3	15	18	9	11	8
7044	11	6	28	785	109	9	1	0	24	15	14	4	30	3	12	21	9	14	9
7045	15	8	92	736	348	7	1	0	14	18	20	13	13	33	19	34	9	19	31
7046	21	9	78	610	350	18	5	1	16	27	29	12	14	8	30	38	13	15	20
7047	33	14	55	1366	345	18	5	1	23	27	18	8	15	17	32	35	11	16	19
7048	22	9	55	1267	426	20	5	1	30	28	20	13	14	11	32	42	12	12	19
7049	3	2	6	514	526	12	7	30	21	14	18	13	20	2	13	18	14	17	9
7050	21	9	71	874	245	11	5	1	14	20	38	6	17	25	27	40	12	15	15
7051	10	3	7	138	174	12	4	1	18	15	10	4	20	4	11	14	8	9	6
7052	9	3	7	254	275	13	4	70	16	16	11	8	19	3	10	14	8	10	6
7053	13	3	14	309	280	12	6	2	16	18	36	5	16	18	12	28	11	14	9
7054	20	5	24	445	135	11	8	8	18	10	9	9	20	3	13	16	8	11	9

Mixed Dishes & Fast Food

Food #	Food Description & Amount	wt gm	wt oz	calo-ries	%cal fat	prot gm	carbo gm	fiber gm
7055	**Macaroni salad (Include made with celery, cucumber, lettuce, mushroom, olives, onion, peas, green or red pepper, pickles, radish, or relish) [1 cup]**	**177**	**6.2**	**271**	**30%**	**6**	**43**	**2.1**
7056	Macaroni salad with chicken (Include above vegetables) [1 cup]	177	6.2	304	38%	17	30	1.4
7057	Macaroni salad with crabmeat (Include above vegetables) [1 cup]	177	6.2	259	28%	10	37	1.8
7058	Macaroni salad with egg (Include above vegetables) [1 cup]	177	6.2	287	39%	8	36	1.6
7059	Macaroni salad with shrimp (Include above vegetables) [1 cup]	177	6.2	264	28%	10	38	1.8
7060	Macaroni salad with tuna (Include above vegetables) [1 cup]	177	6.2	261	27%	12	36	1.8
7061	Macaroni salad with tuna and egg (Include above vegetables) [1 cup]	177	6.2	273	35%	15	30	1.4
7062	Manapua, filled with bean paste, meatless [1 manapua]	103	3.6	233	15%	6	43	3.7
7063	Manapua, filled with meat [1 manapua]	93	3.3	214	37%	11	22	0.8
7064	Manicotti, cheese-filled, no sauce [1 manicotti]	127	4.5	275	42%	16	23	0.7
7065	Manicotti, cheese-filled, with meat sauce [1 manicotti]	143	5.0	242	42%	15	20	1.1
7066	**Manicotti, cheese-filled, with tomato sauce, meatless [1 manicotti]**	**143**	**5.0**	**231**	**40%**	**13**	**22**	**1.2**
7067	Manicotti, vegetable and cheese-filled, with tomato sauce, meatless [1 manicotti]	143	5.0	202	36%	11	22	1.6
7068	Matzo balls [2 matzo balls]	70	2.5	96	32%	4	12	0.4
7069	Meat loaf (Include meatball, with breading, no sauce) [1 slice]	108	3.8	231	54%	18	7	0.4
7070	Meat loaf made with beef, with tomato-based sauce [1 medium slice]	137	4.8	249	53%	19	9	0.9
7071	Meatloaf made with beef and pork (Include meatball or meat patty, made with beef and pork, with breading, no sauce) [1 slice]	108	3.8	214	50%	19	7	0.4
7072	Meatloaf made with beef and pork, with tomato-based sauce (Include meatball or meat patty, made with beef and pork, with breading, tomato-based sauce) [1 slice]	137	4.8	222	46%	20	9	0.9
7073	Meatloaf made with beef, veal and pork (Include meatball or meat patty, made with beef, veal, and pork, with breading, no sauce) [1 slice]	108	3.8	165	32%	20	7	0.4
7074	Meat pie, Puerto Rican style (Pastelon de carne) [1/8 of pie]	139	4.9	680	65%	22	36	1.5
7075	Meat turnovers, Puerto Rican style (Pastelillos de carne; Empanadillas) [2 turnovers]	56	2.0	191	48%	5	19	0.7
7076	Meat with barbecue sauce (Include with Sloppy Joe mix) [1 cup]	263	9.3	427	34%	59	8	0.7
7077	Meat with tomato-based sauce [1 cup]	249	8.8	349	47%	33	12	2.3
7078	Meatballs, Puerto Rican style (Albondigas) [2 meatballs with sauce]	100	3.5	253	65%	14	7	0.8
7079	Meatballs, with breading, with gravy (Include sweet and sour meatballs; Danish frikadeller) [2 meatballs with sauce]	86	3.0	131	51%	10	5	0.4
7080	Meatballs, with sauce [2 meatballs with sauce]	86	3.0	175	61%	16	0	0.0
7081	Meatless "chicken" (made with meat substitute) [1 cup]	168	5.9	370	57%	29	12	7.6
7082	Meatless "chicken," breaded, fried (Include Loma Linda brand) [1 cup]	168	5.9	286	64%	18	8	7.4
7083	Meatless luncheon slices, "beef, chicken, salami, or turkey" (Include vegetarian ham, Wham, Loma Linda, Worthington) [4 thin slices]	56	2.0	157	51%	14	5	2.9
7084	Meatless, "fish" stick [2 sticks]	56	2.0	162	56%	13	5	3.4
7085	Meatless, "frankfurter" [2 "frankfurters"]	70	2.5	140	45%	14	6	3.2
7086	Meatless, "meatball" [2 "meatballs"]	72	2.5	144	41%	15	6	3.3
7087	Meatless, "scallops," breaded, fried [1 cup]	168	5.9	507	56%	40	16	10.7
7088	Mexican casserole made with ground beef, beans, tomato sauce, cheese, taco seasonings, and corn chips [1 cup]	144	5.1	316	55%	16	20	3.7
7089	Mexican casserole made with ground beef, tomato sauce, cheese, taco seasonings, and corn chips (Include Frito pie) [1 cup]	144	5.1	358	64%	18	14	1.7
7090	Moo Shi Pork [1 cup]	151	5.3	517	81%	19	5	0.6
7091	Moussaka (eggplant and meat casserole) [1 cup]	203	7.2	300	58%	16	15	2.9
7092	**Nachos with beans and cheese [2 cups]**	**180**	**6.3**	**476**	**51%**	**17**	**42**	**10.5**
7093	Nachos with beans, no cheese [2 cups]	176	6.2	419	44%	12	49	12.2
7094	Nachos with beef and cheese [2 cups]	174	6.1	631	61%	39	23	2.3
7095	Nachos with beef, beans, and cheese [2 cups]	264	9.3	796	55%	38	52	10.8
7096	Nachos with beef, beans, cheese, and sour cream [2 cups]	362	12.8	1121	56%	38	91	13.7

Food #	fat gm	sat fat gm	choles mg	sodium mg	potass mg	% of Daily Value														
						vit A	vit E	vit C	thia-min	ribo-flavin	nia-cin	vit B-6	fol-ate	vit B-12	cal-cium	phos-phorus	magne-sium	iron	zinc
7055	9	1	6	331	119	3	4	4	15	7	9	4	21	1	2	7	6	10	4
7056	13	2	49	870	200	4	4	15	12	10	27	14	14	3	2	14	7	10	9
7057	8	1	29	353	180	2	4	5	15	7	12	5	21	30	4	11	7	10	11
7058	13	2	143	344	134	8	5	3	14	16	8	5	20	7	3	11	5	10	6
7059	8	1	45	327	152	3	4	4	14	7	11	4	18	5	3	12	7	12	6
7060	8	1	13	372	164	3	4	3	14	7	26	8	18	14	2	11	7	11	5
7061	11	2	128	387	182	7	5	2	12	14	26	9	17	21	3	14	7	11	6
7062	4	0	0	174	130	0	2	0	18	12	11	1	15	0	4	9	5	13	3
7063	9	3	28	140	163	0	2	1	25	15	16	4	9	5	2	10	3	10	10
7064	13	7	104	303	121	13	2	0	13	21	8	3	10	8	29	24	5	10	9
7065	11	6	86	447	259	13	3	8	11	18	11	7	9	11	22	21	6	10	11
7066	10	6	82	468	245	14	3	8	12	18	8	6	9	6	24	21	6	10	8
7067	8	4	74	416	273	20	3	12	12	17	8	6	11	5	19	17	7	11	7
7068	3	1	73	22	37	3	1	0	4	7	3	2	4	2	1	4	1	4	2
7069	14	5	90	133	295	2	0	1	5	16	20	7	4	28	4	16	6	11	24
7070	15	5	92	320	414	5	3	8	7	18	22	10	4	28	5	17	7	13	25
7071	12	4	87	129	317	2	1	1	12	17	20	9	4	23	4	18	6	10	21
7072	11	4	89	317	442	5	2	8	14	18	23	12	5	23	5	19	7	12	23
7073	6	2	86	125	305	2	1	1	17	17	25	14	5	17	5	18	6	8	17
7074	49	19	97	798	355	1	2	10	24	23	31	9	14	25	16	25	8	22	26
7075	10	2	34	58	83	2	4	2	13	10	8	2	7	2	2	6	2	7	3
7076	16	5	165	620	888	5	3	7	15	33	41	43	4	98	2	50	16	36	97
7077	18	6	100	661	798	5	7	18	40	21	38	28	5	34	5	28	13	17	32
7078	18	6	70	561	330	4	6	7	7	12	16	8	4	17	2	14	5	9	17
7079	7	3	46	244	177	1	0	1	3	9	11	4	2	15	2	9	3	7	15
7080	12	5	88	172	188	2	1	0	2	10	17	8	2	28	1	12	3	9	21
7081	24	4	0	1327	554	0	15	0	123	40	45	59	32	59	6	56	7	12	8
7082	20	3	0	672	504	0	11	0	78	47	39	42	24	59	4	41	5	16	7
7083	9	1	0	482	157	0	6	0	35	18	31	31	14	24	2	25	3	7	6
7084	10	2	0	274	336	0	7	0	41	30	34	42	14	39	5	25	3	6	5
7085	7	1	0	301	105	0	4	0	51	49	56	34	14	28	2	24	3	7	6
7086	6	1	0	396	130	0	4	0	43	25	36	43	14	29	2	25	3	8	9
7087	32	5	0	858	1050	0	23	0	128	93	105	131	45	123	17	79	10	19	16
7088	19	7	47	304	396	6	2	6	6	12	14	10	13	16	11	20	11	14	19
7089	26	9	67	364	345	7	3	6	3	14	18	10	3	23	11	20	9	11	24
7090	47	7	173	385	333	6	29	13	34	22	15	16	5	13	3	21	7	8	12
7091	19	5	45	220	512	9	8	19	11	14	20	11	9	20	10	17	10	12	21
7092	27	12	41	298	582	8	5	6	14	14	4	14	43	4	30	36	21	18	16
7093	20	7	12	139	644	1	5	7	16	9	4	15	49	0	10	25	22	20	12
7094	42	19	142	554	419	13	3	0	5	25	33	21	5	57	39	48	16	19	49
7095	49	21	119	590	771	15	6	5	16	27	22	25	43	37	50	61	29	27	43
7096	69	27	112	955	877	25	9	18	18	36	22	31	37	27	63	72	41	28	42

Mixed Dishes & Fast Food

Food #	Food Description & Amount	wt gm	wt oz	calo-ries	%cal fat	prot gm	carbo gm	fiber gm
7097	Nachos with beef, beans, cheese, tomatoes and onions (Include Taco Bell Nachos Supreme) [2 cups]	176	6.2	478	59%	13	38	6.2
7098	Nachos with cheese and sour cream [2 cups]	116	4.1	330	75%	9	13	1.0
7099	Nachos with cheese, meatless, no beans (Include Taco Bell Nachos) [2 cups]	116	4.1	516	61%	20	32	3.3
7100	Nachos with chicken and cheese [2 cups]	174	6.1	502	51%	40	20	2.0
7101	Nachos with chili [2 cups]	264	9.3	444	45%	16	51	12.4
7102	Noodle pudding (Include kugel) [1 cup]	144	5.1	298	30%	9	44	2.1
7103	Noodle pudding, with milk [1 cup]	144	5.1	392	36%	8	55	1.1
7104	**Paella** with chicken, salami, shrimp, clams [1 cup]	**240**	**8.5**	**348**	**28%**	**21**	**40**	**1.8**
7105	Pakora (vegetables, dipped in chick-pea flour batter, fried [3 pakoras]	36	1.3	44	35%	2	6	1.6
7106	Panzerotti, with meat, vegetables, and cheese [1 panzerotti]	396	14.0	1071	58%	40	71	4.3
7107	Panzerotti, with vegetables and cheese [1 panzerotti]	402	14.2	992	59%	28	73	5.3
7108	Pasta meat-filled with gravy (Include Chef Boy-ar-dee Mini Chicken Ravioli) [1 cup]	250	8.8	327	21%	12	51	1.9
7109	Pasta salad (macaroni or noodles, vegetables, dressing) [1 cup]	177	6.2	287	49%	5	32	2.2
7110	Pasta salad with meat (macaroni or noodles, vegetables, meat, dressing) [1 cup]	177	6.2	340	51%	12	30	1.9
7111	Pasta with carbonara sauce [1 cup]	201	7.1	356	28%	14	48	2.3
7112	Pasta with meat sauce and cheese (Include Cannelloni) [1 cup]	242	8.5	371	44%	19	32	1.9
7113	Pasta with tomato sauce and cheese, meatless [1 cup]	242	8.5	207	14%	8	37	3.0
7114	**Pasta with tomato sauce and cheese, canned** [1 cup]	**249**	**8.8**	**187**	**15%**	**5**	**36**	**1.9**
7115	Pasta with tomato sauce and meat or meatballs, canned [1 cup]	249	8.8	256	28%	10	36	1.5
7116	Pasta with tomato sauce and frankfurters or hot dogs, canned [1 cup]	253	8.9	259	40%	8	33	1.3
7117	Pasta with meat sauce (Include American chop suey) [1 cup]	255	9.0	303	30%	21	33	3.5
7118	Pasta with pesto sauce [1 cup]	122	4.3	358	58%	12	27	2.5
7119	Pasta with tomato sauce, meatless [1 cup]	248	8.7	189	4%	7	39	3.2
7120	Pasta, whole wheat, with meat sauce [1 cup]	255	9.0	302	20%	15	49	8.5
7121	Pasta, whole wheat, with tomato sauce, meatless [1 cup]	248	8.7	258	11%	10	53	9.0
7122	Pasta tetrazzini, dry mix prepared with water [1 cup]	202	7.1	187	6%	15	30	3.2
7123	Pastry, cheese-filled [2 pastries]	56	2.0	155	66%	5	8	0.2
7124	Pastry, filled with potatoes and peas, fried [1 samosa]	100	3.5	309	52%	5	33	1.9
7125	Peas cooked with pork [1 cup]	197	6.9	332	36%	16	38	15.0
7126	Pigeon pea asopao (Include Asopaode grandules) [1 cup]	178	6.3	242	22%	5	41	1.9
7127	Porcupine balls with cream of mushroom soup-based sauce [2 balls with sauce]	70	2.5	124	48%	8	8	0.3
7128	Porcupine balls with tomato-based sauce [2 balls with sauce]	70	2.5	115	41%	8	9	0.3
7129	**Pork and beans, canned** [1 cup]	**253**	**8.9**	**248**	**9%**	**13**	**49**	**12.1**
7130	Potato and ham fritters, Puerto Rican style (Include Frituras de papa y jamon) [1 fritter (2¾"x2½"x1")]	70	2.5	139	63%	4	9	0.8
7131	Potato chicken pie, Puerto Rican style (Include Pastelon de pollo) [¼ of 9" pie]	230	8.1	915	56%	42	58	3.0
7132	**Potato salad with egg** [1 cup]	**193**	**6.8**	**280**	**51%**	**6**	**30**	**2.8**
7133	Potato salad, German style [1 cup]	175	6.2	155	17%	4	29	2.6
7134	Puffs, fried, crabmeat and cream cheese filled [1 cup]	77	2.7	273	50%	9	25	0.8
7135	Puerto Rican stew (Include Sancocho) [1 cup, with bone (yield after bones removed)]	214	7.5	326	41%	17	32	3.8
7136	Puerto Rican style meat loaf (Include Albondigon) [1 serving (3"x1"x2")]	95	3.4	317	61%	19	10	0.6
7137	Puerto Rican style stuffed pot roast (larded meat) (Include Carne mechada con papas boliche) [1 slice (¾"x3") with ¼ cup potatoes]	190	6.7	675	62%	46	15	1.5
7138	Puerto-Rican style beef stew (Include Carne guisada con papas) [1 cup]	212	7.5	457	59%	31	14	1.6
7139	**Quesadilla** [1 quesadilla]	**54**	**1.9**	**183**	**47%**	**6**	**18**	**1.1**
7140	Quesadilla with meat and cheese [1 quesadilla]	60	2.1	196	44%	7	20	1.3
7141	Quiche with meat, poultry or fish (Include Quiche Lorraine) [1/8 of 9"dia]	192	6.8	574	70%	16	27	0.8
7142	Quiche, cheese, meatless [1/8 of 9"dia]	192	6.8	569	70%	17	27	0.8
7143	Quiche, spinach, meatless (Include broccoli quiche) [1/8 of 9"dia]	143	5.0	343	69%	11	17	1.2

Food #	fat gm	sat fat gm	choles mg	sodium mg	potass mg	vit A	vit E	vit C	thia- min	ribo- flavin	nia- cin	vit B-6	fol- ate	vit B-12	cal- cium	phos- phorus	magne- sium	iron	zinc
																% of Daily Value			
7097	32	7	26	515	341	5	15	7	7	9	9	14	19	6	22	38	16	12	16
7098	28	16	57	247	166	22	2	1	3	13	1	4	3	7	26	20	7	2	7
7099	35	16	69	673	164	19	3	0	4	20	3	10	4	9	55	44	16	7	19
7100	29	12	127	491	285	14	3	0	6	22	33	19	4	9	36	43	15	11	25
7101	22	7	38	1380	900	8	7	6	9	18	6	20	14	0	16	43	34	46	34
7102	10	2	144	111	193	11	4	4	13	13	8	6	14	5	4	14	7	14	7
7103	16	9	40	173	260	16	2	2	22	19	12	4	15	7	14	17	9	9	6
7104	11	2	47	454	371	13	5	60	20	12	33	13	20	207	4	20	8	35	13
7105	2	0	0	3	93	0	1	2	3	1	1	3	12	0	1	3	3	3	2
7106	69	23	82	2007	647	16	24	13	56	57	48	21	46	32	48	58	15	34	33
7107	66	18	33	2262	496	16	32	45	45	50	34	15	48	9	47	50	14	29	20
7108	8	3	17	1089	197	6	3	0	27	21	25	5	17	2	4	13	6	17	9
7109	16	2	0	951	159	41	12	19	15	7	9	5	19	1	3	7	6	9	4
7110	19	4	24	588	207	30	9	14	17	10	18	9	18	8	2	10	7	10	8
7111	11	4	92	217	154	4	1	1	27	17	17	7	31	6	7	18	9	15	10
7112	18	8	162	502	425	20	6	13	18	24	21	12	14	19	15	23	8	18	19
7113	3	2	7	262	345	9	3	27	18	10	13	8	20	1	9	12	9	12	7
7114	3	1	3	997	274	11	2	30	14	9	10	6	16	1	3	8	7	10	4
7115	8	3	28	907	340	6	2	32	14	12	17	8	11	13	2	11	6	12	12
7116	11	4	32	1152	328	7	1	30	11	9	11	11	7	7	6	11	6	8	7
7117	10	4	49	1056	903	16	9	47	23	21	31	20	16	16	4	19	15	21	26
7118	23	5	9	216	188	4	7	3	19	9	10	5	18	3	21	22	15	19	10
7119	1	0	0	231	356	8	3	28	19	9	14	9	21	0	4	9	9	12	6
7120	7	2	20	394	598	11	8	29	16	12	18	18	5	8	4	21	18	17	19
7121	3	0	0	403	560	12	8	31	16	9	13	16	5	0	5	18	18	15	11
7122	1	0	16	740	506	86	1	5	18	19	11	9	15	10	21	26	10	13	9
7123	11	4	48	327	58	11	4	0	6	14	3	4	4	4	11	10	2	4	5
7124	18	4	9	142	174	5	9	5	16	11	11	6	10	1	3	7	4	10	3
7125	13	5	14	228	666	0	3	1	24	6	9	5	29	1	3	19	17	13	13
7126	6	1	2	492	243	2	3	16	19	4	12	8	25	0	2	9	9	11	6
7127	7	2	26	180	114	0	1	1	3	4	10	5	4	14	1	6	2	6	11
7128	5	2	25	319	145	1	2	19	4	4	11	6	4	14	1	6	2	7	11
7129	3	1	18	1113	759	3	5	13	9	7	6	9	14	0	14	30	22	46	99
7130	10	2	36	171	294	1	6	10	9	5	6	9	2	3	1	6	3	3	3
7131	57	15	128	660	651	5	13	15	35	31	74	35	20	6	14	36	15	29	21
7132	16	3	106	214	557	6	8	35	11	9	10	26	7	5	3	11	8	5	5
7133	3	1	5	96	552	1	0	31	12	3	11	20	5	2	1	8	9	4	4
7134	15	8	71	122	125	14	2	0	12	14	10	3	9	8	4	11	5	11	3
7135	15	5	49	249	882	73	6	34	17	15	22	26	6	18	4	23	13	12	19
7136	22	7	155	61	219	4	6	2	14	19	15	8	7	18	2	14	4	11	20
7137	47	16	146	828	1181	0	7	21	16	24	42	36	6	70	2	48	17	26	47
7138	30	9	94	423	933	2	8	27	11	17	30	28	5	49	2	33	13	20	33
7139	10	4	13	230	77	4	3	25	9	8	5	2	7	1	13	11	3	7	4
7140	10	3	15	218	102	3	4	27	10	8	8	3	8	4	10	10	4	8	6
7141	45	21	241	241	261	30	7	1	19	31	11	6	12	11	25	29	7	11	11
7142	44	21	242	199	232	33	7	1	15	32	8	5	12	10	34	32	7	11	12
7143	26	12	158	112	278	42	6	9	12	24	6	7	19	7	25	21	10	12	9

Mixed Dishes & Fast Food

Food #	Food Description & Amount	wt gm	wt oz	calories	%cal fat	prot gm	carbo gm	fiber gm
7144	Ravioli, cheese and spinach-filled, with cream sauce [1 cup]	250	8.8	369	42%	15	38	1.9
7145	Ravioli, cheese-filled, no sauce [1 cup]	240	8.5	439	34%	21	49	1.7
7146	Ravioli, cheese-filled, with meat sauce [1 cup]	250	8.8	364	42%	17	35	2.1
7147	Ravioli, cheese-filled, with tomato sauce [1 cup]	250	8.8	341	38%	15	38	2.3
7148	**Ravioli, cheese-filled, with tomato sauce, canned** [1 cup]	246	8.7	234	21%	6	40	1.4
7149	Ravioli, meat-filled, no sauce [1 cup]	240	8.5	489	38%	30	43	1.6
7150	Ravioli, meat-filled, with tomato sauce or meat sauce [1 cup]	250	8.8	393	40%	22	37	2.6
7151	Ravioli, meat-filled, with tomato sauce or meat sauce, canned [1 cup]	251	8.9	220	17%	9	38	1.6
7152	Red beans and rice [1 cup]	224	7.9	251	22%	8	41	7.8
7153	**Refried beans** [1 cup]	253	8.9	488	43%	17	55	17.7
7154	Refried beans with cheese [1 cup]	253	8.9	502	44%	18	54	17.2
7155	Refried beans with meat (Include Old El Paso Refried Beans with Sausage) [1 cup]	253	8.9	385	46%	18	34	11.5
7156	Rice casserole with cheese (Include risotto) [1 cup]	204	7.2	368	31%	16	47	0.6
7157	Rice dressing (Include rice dressing combined with bread) [1 cup]	167	5.9	185	27%	3	30	0.9
7158	Rice meal fritters, Puerto Rican style (Include almojabanas) [2 crullers (3"x2"x½")]	60	2.1	379	78%	6	15	0.4
7159	Rice patty or croquette [1 patty (3¼"dia x ½")]	85	3.0	132	38%	3	17	0.8
7160	**Rice pilaf** [1 cup]	206	7.3	261	24%	4	45	1.3
7161	Rice pudding made with coconut milk, Puerto Rican style [1 cup]	256	9.0	694	60%	7	73	5.6
7162	Rice with beans and chicken [1 cup]	239	8.4	431	38%	26	39	4.6
7163	Rice with beans and pork [1 cup]	239	8.4	445	41%	25	41	4.9
7164	Rice with beans and tomatoes [1 cup]	239	8.4	308	24%	12	48	6.6
7165	**Rice with beans** [1 cup]	239	8.4	396	25%	15	60	8.0
7166	Rice with gravy [1 cup]	237	8.4	259	7%	7	52	0.9
7167	Rice with onions, Puerto Rican style (Include arroz con cebollas) [1 cup]	165	5.8	285	51%	6	31	2.1
7168	Rice with raisins [1 cup]	185	6.5	273	2%	5	62	1.4
7169	Rice with spanish sausage, Puerto Rican style [1 cup]	180	6.3	567	45%	17	59	1.3
7170	Rice with squid, Puerto Rican style (Include arroz con calamares) [1 cup]	160	5.6	405	37%	14	48	1.5
7171	Rice with stewed beans, Puerto Rican style [1 cup]	188	6.6	251	22%	5	42	1.4
7172	Rice with vienna sausage, Puerto Rican style (Include arroz con salchichas) [1 cup]	180	6.3	507	41%	12	61	1.3
7173	Rice, brown, with tomato sauce [1 cup]	243	8.6	229	15%	5	44	4.0
7174	Rice, cooked with coconut milk (Include Arroz con coco) [1 cup]	200	7.1	532	64%	7	46	3.9
7175	Rice, creamed [1 cup]	204	7.2	251	15%	6	45	0.6
7176	Rice, fried, meatless [1 cup]	166	5.9	271	41%	5	34	1.3
7177	**Rice, fried, with meat (Include Chinese pork or chicken fried rice)** [1 cup]	198	7.0	329	34%	12	41	1.3
7178	Rice, fried, with shrimp [1 cup]	198	7.0	319	33%	11	42	1.3
7179	Rice-vegetable medley (Include Italian-style rice) [1 cup]	206	7.3	281	33%	5	42	1.9
7180	Ripe plantain meat pie, Puerto Rican style (Include Pinon) [1 piece (4"x2"x2")]	190	6.7	629	61%	24	42	4.8
7181	Roll with meat and/or shrimp, vegetables and rice paper (not fried) [1 roll (4¼"x1½" dia)]	71	2.5	82	21%	6	10	1.8
7182	Sandwich spread, meat substitute type [2Tbs]	32	1.1	48	54%	3	3	1.1
7183	Sausage balls (pork sausage mixed with biscuit mix and cheese) [4 small balls]	56	2.0	228	58%	10	13	0.4
7184	Shad creole, with rice [1 cup]	249	8.8	413	50%	25	25	1.1
7185	**Shepherd's pie with beef** [1 cup]	243	8.6	278	30%	17	32	3.2
7186	Shepherd's pie [1 cup]	243	8.6	298	37%	17	31	3.3
7187	Somen salad [1 cup]	160	5.6	273	27%	20	28	1.6
7188	Soupy rice from Puerto Rican style (chicken parts reported separately) (Include Asopao de Pollo) [1 cup]	240	8.5	199	39%	8	22	2.1
7189	Soupy rice mixture with chicken and potatoes, Puerto Rican style [1 cup]	240	8.5	276	34%	18	27	1.5
7190	Soyburger (Include vegetarian burger) [1 patty]	70	2.5	140	41%	15	6	3.2
7191	Soyburger with cheese [1 sandwich]	140	4.9	319	34%	21	31	4.5

Food #	fat gm	sat fat gm	choles mg	sodium mg	potass mg	vit A	vit E	vit C	thia-min	ribo-flavin	nia-cin	vit B-6	fol-ate	vit B-12	cal-cium	phos-phorus	magne-sium	iron	zinc
						% of Daily Value													
7144	17	6	165	236	372	46	7	6	23	33	12	9	27	10	25	26	13	20	11
7145	17	9	251	159	191	21	3	0	28	36	17	6	23	12	24	30	7	21	13
7146	17	7	165	544	423	22	7	14	20	25	18	11	15	14	16	23	8	18	15
7147	15	6	162	574	405	24	7	16	21	25	15	10	16	6	17	22	8	17	10
7148	5	2	8	1112	133	10	3	6	16	12	11	4	10	1	7	9	4	11	4
7149	21	8	251	173	334	9	2	0	26	35	36	14	20	40	8	28	8	28	32
7150	18	6	170	180	528	17	9	12	21	26	30	15	15	28	7	22	10	24	23
7151	4	2	17	1354	337	7	1	36	15	12	14	7	10	8	3	9	6	11	8
7152	6	2	6	477	384	0	1	5	18	7	9	7	26	0	5	15	11	13	7
7153	23	9	21	6	999	0	7	11	24	11	4	19	81	0	11	33	28	29	15
7154	25	10	27	48	979	2	7	11	24	12	4	19	79	1	16	36	28	29	16
7155	20	7	50	1001	672	5	0	22	15	7	12	18	7	3	9	23	19	24	22
7156	13	8	42	254	365	16	1	2	18	24	11	7	22	8	42	36	11	12	14
7157	6	1	0	386	108	5	3	2	13	3	9	4	15	0	4	5	4	10	3
7158	33	7	78	233	50	10	17	0	4	9	3	4	3	4	14	12	3	4	4
7159	6	1	38	32	115	2	3	4	7	4	5	4	11	1	2	5	3	6	3
7160	7	1	0	151	111	6	4	2	18	2	12	6	22	0	3	8	5	13	5
7161	46	41	0	33	665	0	5	8	12	2	13	7	16	0	5	24	21	27	11
7162	18	4	63	277	567	23	5	1	18	14	26	15	31	11	8	24	16	26	17
7163	20	6	59	251	639	7	5	0	34	13	21	17	27	6	9	23	16	25	24
7164	8	2	0	185	669	11	5	14	18	4	9	11	31	0	11	15	18	26	12
7165	11	2	0	128	717	10	6	0	21	4	9	11	40	0	12	18	22	32	15
7166	2	1	2	359	112	0	0	0	20	3	15	8	25	1	2	9	6	14	10
7167	16	3	0	1111	160	14	8	3	10	3	10	7	12	0	4	7	5	9	7
7168	1	0	0	4	201	0	1	1	20	2	13	10	24	0	3	9	7	13	6
7169	28	9	46	913	338	2	6	8	41	11	28	19	29	15	3	17	8	22	17
7170	17	2	152	88	325	12	10	73	18	17	19	10	21	13	4	21	10	16	11
7171	6	1	2	43	157	0	4	4	17	2	11	8	22	0	2	8	6	12	6
7172	23	7	30	787	217	1	6	7	27	6	21	11	30	7	3	13	7	20	12
7173	4	1	0	463	337	9	8	15	14	5	17	17	3	0	3	16	22	7	8
7174	38	33	4	40	453	1	4	7	21	1	16	6	33	0	4	21	17	25	10
7175	4	1	5	191	145	2	2	1	18	7	12	8	22	3	9	12	7	10	6
7176	12	2	43	261	128	2	8	7	14	6	11	7	20	2	3	9	6	11	6
7177	12	2	102	821	182	5	7	6	20	11	18	12	23	4	4	15	8	15	9
7178	12	2	115	840	169	5	8	6	17	10	16	11	24	6	4	16	8	16	8
7179	10	2	0	906	147	16	6	32	17	4	12	6	22	0	4	7	6	13	4
7180	42	11	248	563	998	24	18	45	13	29	23	28	13	27	6	28	20	19	25
7181	2	1	15	43	183	47	1	14	11	4	6	7	2	2	5	5	3	3	4
7182	3	0	0	202	109	0	2	0	13	13	21	18	8	17	1	7	10	3	3
7183	15	7	35	580	96	7	2	0	12	12	7	3	5	6	24	27	4	5	8
7184	23	5	97	482	686	13	8	20	24	21	63	31	17	3	9	40	14	15	6
7185	9	3	37	312	764	8	4	27	13	11	19	29	5	21	4	19	12	12	26
7186	12	3	41	649	725	10	6	30	13	12	25	24	7	20	4	18	11	10	20
7187	8	2	218	499	330	10	3	6	19	20	14	14	12	19	5	24	11	10	12
7188	9	4	15	437	254	7	2	36	14	6	8	10	12	3	13	14	6	8	7
7189	10	3	49	188	450	4	1	31	12	7	25	17	12	2	2	14	8	11	11
7190	6	1	0	385	126	0	4	0	42	25	35	42	14	28	2	24	3	8	8
7191	12	4	9	956	251	4	7	1	56	36	43	44	27	30	16	35	7	17	13

Mixed Dishes & Fast Food

Food #	Food Description & Amount	wt gm	wt oz	calo-ries	%cal fat	prot gm	carbo gm	fiber gm
7192	Spaghetti sauce with beef, homemade-style (Include canned sauce, extra beef added) [1 cup]	249	8.8	288	52%	16	21	4.2
7193	Spaghetti sauce with combination of meats, homemade-style (Include canned sauce, extra meats added) [1 cup]	249	8.8	287	53%	17	19	3.8
7194	Spaghetti sauce with lamb or mutton, homemade-style [1 cup]	249	8.8	284	53%	15	21	4.2
7195	Spaghetti with corned beef, Puerto Rican style [1 cup]	215	7.6	408	39%	26	36	2.3
7196	**Spaghetti with tomato sauce and meat sauce and/or meatballs** [1 cup]	**248**	**8.7**	**325**	**27%**	**20**	**38**	**3.7**
7197	Spaghetti (spinach noodles) with tomato sauce and meat sauce and/or meatballs [1 cup]	248	8.7	311	27%	19	36	5.0
7198	Spaghetti (whole wheat noodles) with tomato sauce and meat sauce and/or meatballs [1 cup]	248	8.7	313	28%	20	37	5.5
7199	Spaghetti with tomato sauce and chicken or turkey [1 cup]	248	8.7	267	20%	18	34	3.3
7200	Spaghetti with tomato sauce and frankfurters [1 cup]	248	8.7	336	44%	11	35	3.3
7201	Spaghetti with red clam sauce [1 cup]	248	8.7	288	24%	13	41	3.1
7202	Spaghetti with white clam sauce [1 cup]	248	8.7	458	39%	25	43	2.5
7203	**Spaghetti with meatless tomato sauce** (Include marinara sauce; meatless tomato sauce with cheese, canned) [1 cup]	**248**	**8.7**	**229**	**14%**	**7**	**41**	**4.1**
7204	Spaghetti (spinach noodles) with meatless tomato sauce [1 cup]	248	8.7	213	14%	7	38	6.0
7205	Spaghetti (whole wheat noodles) with meatless tomato sauce [1 cup]	248	8.7	212	15%	8	40	7.0
7206	Spanakopitta (Include Greek spinach-cheese pie) [1 piece (3"x3"x1")]	108	3.8	223	67%	8	11	1.6
7207	Spanish rice (Include Mexican rice) [1 cup]	243	8.6	216	15%	5	42	3.0
7208	**Spanish rice with ground beef** [1 cup]	**230**	**8.1**	**306**	**37%**	**22**	**26**	**2.6**
7209	Spanish stew, Puerto Rican style (Cocido Espanol) [1 cup]	242	8.5	204	33%	15	20	4.7
7210	Spicy rice pudding, Puerto Rican style (arroz con dulce, arroz con especia) [1 cup]	240	8.5	330	7%	3	74	0.7
7211	Stewed chickpeas with Spanish sausages, Puerto Rican style (Garbanzos guisados con chorizos) [1 cup]	250	8.8	498	65%	15	31	8.7
7212	Stewed chickpeas, Puerto Rican style [1 cup]	260	9.2	233	41%	10	25	7.0
7213	Stewed chickpeas, with potatoes, Puerto Rican style [1 cup]	260	9.2	403	28%	19	57	15.3
7214	Stewed corned beef, Puerto Rican style ("Corned beef" guisado) (Include carne bif guisada) [1 cup]	280	9.9	617	55%	45	22	2.4
7215	Stewed cowpeas, Puerto Rican style (Include frijoles) [1 cup]	260	9.2	281	7%	19	49	8.6
7216	Stewed lima beans, Puerto Rican style [1 cup]	255	9.0	133	55%	6	10	2.2
7217	Stewed dry red beans, Puerto Rican style (Habichuelas coloradas guisadas) [1 cup]	250	8.8	414	34%	21	50	11.2
7218	Stewed green peas with pig's feet and potatoes, Puerto Rican style [1 cup (yield after bones removed)]	230	8.1	321	45%	21	23	6.5
7219	Stewed green peas, Puerto Rican style (Habichuelas del pais) [1 cup]	260	9.2	389	18%	25	57	23.7
7220	Stewed pigeon peas, Puerto Rican style (Gandules guisados, Gandur, Gandules) [1 cup]	260	9.2	254	26%	10	40	6.5
7221	Stewed pink beans with pig's feet, Puerto Rican style [1 cup, with bone (yield after bone removed)]	202	7.1	263	48%	18	16	5.1
7222	Stewed pink beans with viandas, ham, Puerto Rican style (Include pinto beans) [1 cup]	255	9.0	221	33%	11	27	9.2
7223	Stewed red beans with pig's feet and potatoes, Puerto Rican style [1 cup, with bone (yield after bone removed)]	220	7.8	306	45%	20	22	4.2
7224	Stewed red beans with pig's feet, Puerto Rican style [1 cup, with bone (yield after bone removed)]	202	7.1	262	49%	18	16	3.4
7225	Stewed rice, Puerto Rican style (arroz quisado) (Include red rice) [1 cup]	170	6.0	370	31%	7	55	1.2
7226	Stewed seasoned ground beef and pork, Mexican style (Picadillo de carne de rez y puerco) [1 cup]	222	7.8	360	57%	33	3	0.5
7227	Stewed seasoned ground beef and pork, with potatoes, Mexican style (Picadillo de carne de rez y puerco con papas) [1 cup]	222	7.8	334	52%	29	10	1.1
7228	Stewed white beans with pig's feet, Puerto Rican style [1 cup, with bone (yield after bone removed)]	202	7.1	261	49%	18	16	3.4
7229	Stewed white beans, Puerto Rican style [1 cup]	255	9.0	224	26%	8	33	3.6

Food #	fat gm	sat fat gm	choles mg	sodium mg	potass mg	% of Daily Value													
						vit A	vit E	vit C	thia-min	ribo-flavin	nia-cin	vit B-6	fol-ate	vit B-12	cal-cium	phos-phorus	magne-sium	iron	zinc
7192	17	5	47	872	1103	24	18	63	12	16	30	27	7	24	6	17	16	20	23
7193	17	4	47	889	1038	22	16	55	28	17	29	29	7	16	6	19	15	17	18
7194	17	5	45	866	1108	24	18	63	14	17	31	23	8	19	6	18	16	17	20
7195	18	6	59	1042	266	5	6	30	18	15	19	9	21	17	14	21	10	19	21
7196	10	3	69	711	653	10	7	26	24	19	24	17	19	17	13	24	14	21	18
7197	9	3	66	690	636	11	7	25	18	17	21	19	9	16	13	26	19	17	19
7198	10	3	69	712	661	10	7	26	19	17	21	19	8	17	14	26	16	19	19
7199	6	1	37	515	468	5	5	16	15	12	26	15	14	2	4	16	11	15	11
7200	16	5	23	1004	451	4	5	16	19	11	19	11	14	10	4	12	10	14	10
7201	8	1	17	170	411	10	5	30	22	15	18	8	25	420	6	17	10	53	10
7202	20	3	49	85	514	13	10	27	26	26	24	7	29	1213	8	32	10	126	18
7203	4	1	0	591	455	5	6	19	19	9	16	10	22	0	4	10	11	14	5
7204	3	0	0	565	440	7	6	18	11	6	13	12	6	0	5	15	19	9	8
7205	4	1	0	593	468	5	6	19	13	6	11	12	5	0	5	14	14	12	7
7206	16	8	91	374	322	41	6	16	8	21	5	8	22	5	18	14	11	12	8
7207	4	1	0	295	537	11	5	62	16	5	15	16	15	0	8	9	10	13	6
7208	13	5	63	385	719	11	5	38	12	17	28	17	9	20	5	19	12	19	31
7209	7	3	30	369	627	30	2	40	13	10	16	17	12	16	4	18	11	13	16
7210	3	1	0	130	194	2	1	0	13	3	9	3	16	0	6	5	6	15	4
7211	36	7	20	440	513	6	13	33	17	10	10	16	23	7	5	19	13	18	15
7212	11	2	9	189	356	2	4	9	11	6	5	10	33	1	5	16	11	14	10
7213	12	2	7	227	776	3	5	20	21	10	9	22	71	1	9	31	22	27	19
7214	38	12	135	1916	882	3	8	32	8	17	28	25	6	39	3	24	13	24	40
7215	2	0	0	18	798	4	3	19	32	10	7	12	81	0	9	32	32	34	17
7216	8	2	9	172	270	5	4	18	6	4	6	6	3	1	3	8	7	8	5
7217	15	3	16	479	1045	3	5	26	26	11	13	19	35	2	7	32	24	26	16
7218	16	5	77	221	543	2	4	21	11	6	9	11	11	2	5	14	9	10	11
7219	8	2	7	158	761	3	3	8	31	10	12	8	38	1	5	33	23	21	18
7220	7	2	8	235	889	9	3	70	28	13	14	12	37	1	6	18	23	12	10
7221	14	4	68	191	448	7	5	14	8	7	5	8	12	2	6	12	9	9	9
7222	8	2	9	203	551	2	3	15	13	6	6	11	23	1	5	17	14	13	8
7223	15	5	74	211	563	2	4	20	9	6	8	12	11	2	5	13	9	11	11
7224	14	4	68	192	464	7	5	14	8	7	6	8	11	2	5	13	8	10	10
7225	13	3	8	363	168	2	6	8	23	3	16	8	28	1	3	10	6	17	7
7226	23	9	115	111	616	2	2	16	33	24	38	22	3	32	3	31	10	15	34
7227	19	7	97	95	731	1	2	24	30	21	34	24	4	27	3	28	11	14	30
7228	14	4	68	193	524	7	5	13	7	6	5	7	11	2	8	11	10	14	11
7229	7	2	8	175	440	1	1	16	114	3	9	9	19	1	5	10	10	15	8

Mixed Dishes & Fast Food

Food #	Food Description & Amount	wt gm	wt oz	calo- ries	%cal fat	prot gm	carbo gm	fiber gm
7230	Stuffed cabbage, Puerto Rican style (Include Repollo relleno) [1 cup]	234	8.3	531	68%	27	17	4.6
7231	Stuffed cabbage, Syrian dish, Puerto Rican style (Include Repollo relleno Arabe Mihsy Melful) [1 cabbage roll]	110	3.9	94	37%	4	12	1.8
7232	Stuffed grape leaves with lamb and rice [2 rolls]	42	1.5	111	71%	4	5	1.4
7233	Stuffed green pepper, with meat [½ pepper with filling]	149	5.3	286	70%	14	8	1.8
7234	**Stuffed green pepper, with rice and meat [½ pepper with filling]**	**149**	**5.3**	**220**	**51%**	**12**	**14**	**1.7**
7235	Stuffed green pepper, with rice, meatless [½ pepper with filling]	149	5.3	230	57%	6	19	1.8
7236	Stuffed rice with chicken, Dominican (Include Arroz relleno Dominicano) [1 cup]	200	7.1	573	37%	43	43	1.7
7237	Stuffed pasta shell, cheese and spinach-filled, no sauce [1 jumbo shell]	60	2.1	115	33%	6	13	0.7
7238	Stuffed pasta shell, cheese-filled, no sauce [1 jumbo shell]	60	2.1	128	39%	7	12	0.4
7239	Stuffed pasta shell, cheese-filled, with meat sauce [1 jumbo shell]	85	3.0	140	39%	8	13	0.9
7240	Stuffed pasta shell, cheese-filled, with tomato sauce, meatless [1 jumbo shell]	85	3.0	130	37%	7	14	0.8
7241	Stuffed pasta shell, with chicken [1 jumbo shell]	83	2.9	117	22%	9	13	0.9
7242	Stuffed pasta shell, with fish and/or shellfish [1 jumbo shell]	83	2.9	103	14%	8	14	0.9
7243	**Stuffed tomato, with rice and ground beef [1 tomato with filling]**	**149**	**5.3**	**151**	**43%**	**7**	**16**	**1.4**
7244	Stuffed tomato, with rice, meatless [1 tomato with filling]	149	5.3	112	22%	2	20	1.5
7245	Sukiyaki [1 cup]	162	5.7	172	40%	19	7	1.3
7246	Tabbouleh/Tabbuli [1 cup]	160	5.6	199	68%	3	16	3.7
7247	Tamal in a leaf, Puerto Rican style (Include Tamales en hoja) [2 tamal (6"x2"x3½")]	82	2.9	131	50%	8	10	1.3
7248	Tamale casserole with meat [1 cup]	244	8.6	226	42%	14	18	2.4
7249	Tamale casserole, Puerto Rican style (Include Tamales en cazuela) [1 cup]	237	8.4	392	55%	17	28	3.9
7250	**Tamale with meat [1 small tamale]**	**70**	**2.5**	**134**	**48%**	**6**	**11**	**1.5**
7251	Tamale, meatless, Puerto Rican or Caribbean style [1 small tamale]	72	2.5	199	85%	1	8	1.3
7252	Tamale, plain, meatless, no sauce, Mexican style [1 small tamale]	72	2.5	150	47%	3	17	2.2
7253	Taquito [1 taquito]	72	2.5	185	49%	10	14	1.9
7254	Tortellini, cheese-filled, meatless, no sauce [1 cup]	150	5.3	354	21%	16	54	2.2
7255	Tortellini, cheese-filled, meatless, with tomato sauce [1 cup]	250	8.8	338	38%	14	38	2.3
7256	Tortellini, cheese-filled, meatless, with tomato sauce, canned [1 cup]	247	8.7	222	14%	9	39	1.6
7257	Tortellini, cheese-filled, meatless, with vinaigrette dressing [1 cup]	169	6.0	341	50%	12	30	1.1
7258	Tortellini, cheese-filled, meatless, with vegetables and vinaigrette dressing (Include Stouffer's Cheese Tortellini Vinaigrette) [1 cup]	169	6.0	364	63%	12	23	2.4
7259	**Tortellini, cheese-filled, with cream sauce [1 cup]**	**250**	**8.8**	**398**	**43%**	**16**	**39**	**1.3**
7260	Tortellini, meat-filled, no sauce [1 cup]	190	6.7	373	36%	25	33	1.1
7261	Tortellini, meat-filled, with tomato sauce [1 cup]	210	7.4	285	32%	15	34	2.0
7262	Tortellini, meat-filled, with tomato sauce, canned [1 cup]	233	8.2	218	17%	9	37	2.5
7263	Tortellini, spinach-filled, no sauce [1 cup]	122	4.3	232	35%	12	25	1.1
7264	Tortellini, spinach-filled, with tomato sauce [1 cup]	200	7.1	241	30%	10	33	2.3
7265	**Tostada salad with beef [1 salad]**	**232**	**8.2**	**435**	**59%**	**21**	**24**	**3.9**
7266	Tostada salad, meatless [1 salad]	232	8.2	350	56%	15	25	4.5
7267	Turnover, chicken, with gravy [1 turnover]	112	4.0	316	57%	11	23	0.7
7268	Turnover, chicken or turkey, and cheese-filled, no gravy (Include Hot Pockets Chicken and Cheddar with Bacon) [1 turnover]	128	4.5	453	57%	17	31	1.1
7269	Turnover, chicken- or turkey-, and vegetable-filled [1 turnover]	128	4.5	241	26%	10	34	1.8
7270	Turnover, meat and bean-filled, no gravy [1 turnover]	88	3.1	316	57%	10	23	1.5
7271	Turnover, meat and cheese-filled, no gravy (Include Hot Pockets Ham 'n Cheese, Hot Pockets Beef & Cheddar) [1 turnover]	96	3.4	356	59%	11	25	0.9
7272	Turnover, meat and cheese-filled, tomato-based sauce (Include Hot Pockets Pepperoni Pizza, Hot Pockets Sausage Pizza) [1 turnover]	73	2.6	265	62%	8	17	0.8
7273	Turnover, meat, potato, and vegetable-filled, no gravy [1 turnover]	88	3.1	267	57%	8	20	1.1
7274	Turnover, meat and vegetable- filled (no potatoes or gravy) [1 turnover]	88	3.1	279	58%	9	20	1.2

Food #	fat gm	sat fat gm	choles mg	sodium mg	potass mg	vit A	vit E	vit C	thia-min	ribo-flavin	nia-cin	vit B-6	fol-ate	vit B-12	cal-cium	phos-phorus	magne-sium	iron	zinc
7230	40	11	84	1405	1061	21	16	77	31	21	31	28	14	20	10	28	16	17	26
7231	4	1	8	87	228	2	1	32	5	3	6	5	9	3	4	4	4	6	5
7232	9	2	11	28	82	29	3	5	2	4	6	4	4	4	4	4	4	4	4
7233	22	8	51	276	312	20	7	110	6	10	14	16	7	19	14	17	6	9	17
7234	13	5	68	167	302	6	3	77	7	10	15	12	8	17	3	12	5	10	16
7235	15	5	16	228	203	18	7	102	9	6	6	12	11	1	13	12	5	6	5
7236	24	7	156	487	490	8	6	18	23	21	69	32	23	9	10	36	14	23	23
7237	4	2	49	111	95	13	1	2	8	11	4	3	9	3	11	10	4	7	4
7238	6	3	52	118	57	6	1	0	7	10	4	2	5	3	11	10	2	5	4
7239	6	3	51	117	172	8	3	4	7	10	7	4	5	6	11	11	4	7	6
7240	5	3	49	259	151	8	2	5	7	10	6	3	6	3	11	11	3	6	4
7241	3	1	53	47	180	5	3	5	8	9	13	6	6	2	2	8	4	8	5
7242	2	0	55	95	201	5	3	5	8	8	13	5	6	7	3	9	5	8	5
7243	7	2	17	379	305	8	3	35	8	5	11	9	8	8	1	8	5	8	8
7244	3	1	0	399	258	8	3	39	9	3	7	8	10	0	2	5	5	6	2
7245	8	3	148	675	463	26	2	8	9	24	16	18	15	25	6	20	12	18	24
7246	15	2	0	799	246	7	7	48	5	3	6	6	8	0	3	6	9	7	3
7247	7	2	49	110	262	4	3	10	14	9	9	6	4	5	2	10	6	5	8
7248	10	3	40	146	308	8	3	20	10	11	20	10	8	9	3	11	7	12	13
7249	24	8	57	283	506	9	5	68	12	17	24	14	13	22	4	17	11	19	23
7250	7	3	19	84	140	1	1	2	11	8	12	4	5	3	2	7	5	8	6
7251	19	7	17	252	180	5	3	40	2	2	3	4	3	0	1	3	3	4	2
7252	8	3	6	115	99	0	0	0	17	10	13	4	8	1	3	6	6	10	3
7253	10	3	27	76	170	3	3	1	3	7	10	8	6	11	6	15	7	7	14
7254	8	4	48	198	31	2	1	0	16	16	10	2	8	3	17	21	5	7	8
7255	14	6	162	553	406	24	7	16	21	25	15	10	16	6	15	21	8	17	10
7256	4	1	51	737	89	3	1	4	23	12	14	4	20	4	7	13	8	10	7
7257	19	7	148	94	121	12	7	0	16	21	10	4	14	6	14	18	4	12	8
7258	25	6	19	457	210	36	16	66	12	12	8	7	16	4	27	22	8	9	8
7259	19	8	167	378	252	18	5	2	22	31	12	6	16	10	25	27	7	15	11
7260	15	5	240	437	231	13	4	0	31	33	22	11	17	15	18	29	7	17	14
7261	10	3	91	506	277	11	5	9	23	14	17	10	21	7	11	20	10	15	11
7262	4	1	42	745	375	9	2	42	19	10	13	10	20	4	6	15	10	14	7
7263	9	3	158	252	138	18	3	2	16	22	9	5	16	8	14	17	6	13	7
7264	8	2	73	438	297	25	5	12	17	13	11	8	26	5	13	16	12	16	8
7265	29	10	63	455	518	12	8	21	15	20	23	13	21	24	24	26	11	20	24
7266	22	10	40	565	477	18	6	23	18	20	11	10	27	6	38	28	11	15	12
7267	20	4	23	217	146	4	8	1	13	14	15	5	8	3	7	11	4	9	6
7268	29	7	41	197	173	4	10	0	19	18	26	9	12	4	10	18	6	13	9
7269	7	1	31	601	205	15	8	2	19	18	21	8	10	2	11	15	6	14	6
7270	20	5	23	84	133	0	6	0	13	11	11	4	11	12	1	10	4	13	13
7271	24	6	26	125	134	3	8	0	14	15	14	4	9	9	8	12	4	11	11
7272	18	5	24	264	145	2	5	3	16	10	12	5	6	8	4	9	3	8	7
7273	17	4	20	75	133	17	5	2	11	9	10	6	7	10	1	8	3	10	11
7274	18	5	21	78	123	12	6	8	12	10	11	5	8	10	1	8	3	11	12

Mixed Dishes & Fast Food

Food #	Food Description & Amount	wt gm	wt oz	calo-ries	%cal fat	prot gm	carbo gm	fiber gm
7275	Turnover, meat-filled, no gravy [1 turnover]	88	3.1	339	60%	11	23	0.9
7276	Turnover, meat-filled, with gravy [1 turnover]	152	5.4	392	58%	13	27	1.1
7277	Vegetables and cheese in pastry [1 pastry]	103	3.6	327	68%	8	20	2.7
7278	Vegetables in pastry (Include Pepperidge Farm, all varieties) [1 pastry]	103	3.6	320	67%	7	22	3.0
7279	**Vegetarian chili** (made with soy meat-substitute) [1 cup]	**254**	**9.0**	**336**	**13%**	**45**	**36**	**11.8**
7280	Vegetarian fillets [1 fillet]	85	3.0	247	56%	20	8	5.2
7281	Vegetarian meat loaf or patties (meat loaf made with soy meat-substitute) [1 slice]	56	2.0	112	41%	12	4	2.6
7282	Vegetarian pot pie (Include beef-like pot pie, chicken-like pot pie) [1 pie]	227	8.0	510	57%	14	41	5.2
7283	Vegetarian stew [1 cup]	239	8.4	287	23%	41	17	2.6
7284	Vegetarian stroganoff (made with meat substitute) [1 cup]	125	4.4	231	59%	12	11	2.9
7285	Vienna sausages stewed with potatoes, Puerto Rican style (Include Salchichas guisadas) [1 cup]	175	6.2	393	68%	9	23	2.3
7286	Welsh rarebit [1 cup]	232	8.2	378	66%	18	14	0.1
7287	White rice with tomato sauce [1 cup]	243	8.6	253	11%	5	50	1.8
7288	Wonton, fried, meat filled [4 wonton]	76	2.7	219	42%	12	19	0.9
	Sandwiches (white bread, unless noted otherwise)							
7400	Bacon and cheese sandwich with mayonnaise [1 sandwich]	121	4.3	401	52%	18	30	1.2
7401	Bacon on biscuit (Include Arby's bacon on biscuit) [1 breakfast sandwich]	93	3.3	360	47%	8	40	1.1
7402	Bacon and egg sandwich [1 sandwich]	177	6.2	393	50%	21	27	1.1
7403	Bacon sandwich with mayonnaise [1 sandwich]	91	3.2	351	51%	13	29	1.3
7404	Bacon, chicken, and tomato club sandwich with lettuce, mayonnaise (Include Arby's Roast Chicken Club, Wendy's Chicken Club) [1 sandwich]	246	8.7	555	42%	31	48	2.8
7405	**Bacon, lettuce, and tomato sandwich** with mayonnaise [1 sandwich]	**164**	**5.8**	**350**	**49%**	**11**	**35**	**2.3**
7406	Beef barbecue submarine sandwich, on bun [1 submarine]	192	6.8	421	28%	31	43	2.4
7407	Bologna sandwich with margarine [1 sandwich]	83	2.9	256	47%	7	26	1.2
7408	Bologna and cheese sandwich with margarine [1 sandwich]	111	3.9	350	53%	13	28	1.2
7409	Bologna and cheese submarine sandwich, on bun with lettuce, mayonnaise (Include grinder, poor-boy) [1 submarine]	198	7.0	541	62%	21	29	1.6
7410	Cheese sandwich with margarine [1 sandwich]	83	2.9	262	44%	10	27	1.2
7411	**Cheese sandwich with margarine, grilled** [1 grilled cheese sandwich]	**83**	**2.9**	**292**	**49%**	**10**	**27**	**1.2**
7412	Cheese sandwich with lettuce, hoagie [1 hoagie]	156	5.5	464	49%	25	33	1.7
7413	Cheese spread sandwich [1 sandwich]	78	2.8	215	32%	9	27	1.2
7414	Chicken barbecue sandwich [1 sandwich]	119	4.2	251	22%	21	27	1.3
7415	Chicken fillet (breaded, fried) sandwich with lettuce, tomato, mayonnaise [1 sandwich]	174	6.1	466	51%	22	35	2.1
7416	Chicken fillet (breaded, fried) sandwich [1 sandwich]	126	4.4	327	34%	29	23	1.2
7417	Chicken fillet (broiled) sandwich, on whole wheat roll with lettuce, tomato, mayonnaise (Include Hardee's Grilled Chicken Sandwich) [1 sandwich]	173	6.1	331	23%	27	39	5.7
7418	Chicken fillet (broiled), sandwich, with lettuce, tomato, non-mayonnaise type spread (Include Wendy's Grilled Chicken Sandwich) [1 sandwich]	175	6.2	343	30%	27	32	1.9
7419	Chicken fillet (broiled), sandwich, on oat bran bun, with lettuce, tomato, mayonnaise (Include Burger King) [1 sandwich]	155	5.5	315	32%	30	23	2.4
7420	Chicken fillet (broiled), sandwich with cheese, on whole wheat roll, with lettuce, tomato and non-mayonnaise type spread (Include Wendy's) [1 sandwich]	193	6.8	380	27%	34	37	5.3
7421	Chicken fillet (broiled), sandwich with cheese, on bun, with lettuce, tomato and mayonnaise (Include Burger King, McDonald's) [1 sandwich]	229	8.1	530	38%	40	41	2.4
7422	Chicken patty (battered, fried) sandwich with lettuce, pickles, mayonnaise (Include McDonald's Crispy Chicken Deluxe) [1 sandwich]	208	7.3	595	45%	30	51	2.7
7423	Chicken patty (battered, fried) biscuit sandwich (Include Jimmy Dean Chicken Biscuit, Hardee's Chicken Biscuit) [1 biscuit sandwich]	146	5.1	434	42%	15	46	1.4
7424	Chicken patty (battered, fried) sandwich with cheese, on wheat bun with lettuce, tomato, mayonnaise (Include with onions; Jack-in-the-Box Chicken Supreme) [1 sandwich]	227	8.0	620	47%	35	46	3.9

Food #	fat gm	sat fat gm	choles mg	sodium mg	potass mg	% of Daily Value													
						vit A	vit E	vit C	thia-min	ribo-flavin	nia-cin	vit B-6	fol-ate	vit B-12	cal-cium	phos-phorus	magne-sium	iron	zinc
7275	22	6	26	93	106	0	7	0	14	12	12	4	9	13	1	9	3	13	14
7276	25	7	30	427	160	0	7	0	16	14	15	5	9	15	1	12	3	16	19
7277	25	7	14	180	244	6	17	10	11	18	11	4	9	2	14	18	13	10	7
7278	24	6	6	140	257	4	19	11	12	17	12	4	10	1	8	15	14	10	6
7279	5	1	0	843	868	18	10	22	19	9	14	18	49	0	13	52	21	58	20
7280	15	2	0	417	510	0	10	0	62	45	51	64	22	60	8	38	5	9	8
7281	5	1	0	308	101	0	3	0	34	20	28	34	11	22	2	19	3	7	7
7282	32	9	20	486	378	79	14	17	55	26	26	20	23	17	7	26	8	16	7
7283	7	1	0	956	287	0	4	0	112	84	143	131	62	88	7	53	76	17	18
7284	15	5	11	572	182	5	6	1	33	22	28	31	12	21	6	22	4	8	8
7285	30	8	34	801	765	3	10	44	11	7	15	20	5	9	2	10	8	9	10
7286	28	14	63	480	360	31	6	2	7	30	2	5	5	10	56	42	10	4	14
7287	3	1	0	526	360	11	5	18	21	4	16	14	25	0	3	9	9	14	7
7288	10	3	80	39	204	2	2	1	23	14	13	8	7	4	2	12	4	9	9
7400	23	11	48	1109	244	14	4	0	20	26	13	8	14	12	39	36	8	12	15
7401	19	4	9	1033	235	0	8	0	28	16	18	3	12	5	4	39	4	16	5
7402	22	7	418	781	277	23	6	0	25	42	15	10	21	19	14	28	7	17	12
7403	20	6	27	784	205	0	3	0	31	16	22	7	14	8	7	15	5	12	8
7404	26	6	72	855	463	5	9	16	40	26	60	30	26	9	12	30	12	23	11
7405	19	4	20	650	329	6	6	24	26	16	19	10	15	5	8	13	7	14	7
7406	13	4	70	711	506	2	5	3	30	24	33	15	27	50	12	27	11	29	40
7407	13	4	16	598	112	4	3	0	19	12	14	4	12	6	6	7	4	11	6
7408	20	8	35	940	185	10	3	0	20	20	14	6	13	11	22	21	6	12	11
7409	37	15	72	1585	349	8	5	2	27	24	21	12	20	26	25	28	8	18	20
7410	13	5	19	655	135	10	3	0	16	17	10	3	13	5	22	19	5	10	8
7411	16	6	19	696	137	13	5	0	12	16	9	3	8	3	22	19	5	10	8
7412	25	15	68	945	261	21	5	1	20	30	12	6	21	20	73	52	10	13	22
7413	8	4	16	642	127	5	1	0	17	17	10	3	12	2	21	24	5	9	7
7414	6	1	50	422	217	2	1	1	19	16	36	15	13	3	7	16	7	13	10
7415	26	5	67	593	283	5	13	7	24	16	46	22	23	5	10	18	8	16	7
7416	12	3	73	301	260	2	4	0	18	14	59	24	15	5	7	22	8	13	9
7417	9	2	53	699	400	2	5	5	22	14	57	26	13	4	7	32	22	19	14
7418	11	2	63	445	320	2	10	7	22	16	59	23	21	4	9	21	9	15	7
7419	11	2	72	578	290	2	5	2	20	15	68	27	15	5	6	24	10	18	9
7420	11	4	81	591	471	5	6	5	16	15	68	33	8	7	17	41	22	15	17
7421	22	7	100	889	461	9	10	6	30	27	76	34	28	11	29	42	13	21	15
7422	29	7	93	1042	327	4	12	1	34	26	51	20	32	6	14	23	10	23	15
7423	20	4	39	1484	163	1	9	0	23	18	28	8	14	3	14	17	6	16	8
7424	33	10	108	1151	413	10	9	5	30	28	50	22	22	9	29	41	16	23	21

Mixed Dishes & Fast Food

Food #	Food Description & Amount	wt gm	wt oz	calo-ries	%cal fat	prot gm	carbo gm	fiber gm
7425	Chicken patty (battered, fried) sandwich with mayonnaise, miniature (Include Kentucky Fried Chicken Chicken Little) [1 miniature sandwich]	52	1.8	164	47%	6	15	0.7
7426	Chicken salad (chicken, celery, mayonnaise) sandwich [1 sandwich]	141	5.0	335	44%	19	27	1.6
7427	**Chicken (roasted, sliced) sandwich with mayonnaise** [1 sandwich]	112	4.0	267	27%	22	26	1.2
7428	Corned beef sandwich with pickle relish [1 sandwich]	130	4.6	268	33%	19	25	1.7
7429	Crab cake sandwich, on bun [1 sandwich]	140	4.9	312	25%	20	37	1.9
7430	Croissant, filled with creamed chicken and broccoli [1 croissant]	128	4.5	347	49%	16	28	1.2
7431	Croissant, filled with creamed ham and cheese [1 croissant]	113	4.0	338	52%	15	25	0.8
7432	Croissant with mushrooms and cheese (Include Arby's) [1 croissant]	148	5.2	528	65%	14	33	2.3
7433	Croissant with sausage and egg (Include Arby's) [1 croissant]	142	5.0	497	62%	16	31	1.6
7434	Croissant with bacon and egg (Include Arby's, Hardee's) [1 croissant]	113	4.0	402	56%	14	30	1.6
7435	Croissant with ham, egg, and cheese (Include Burger King) [1 croissant]	144	5.1	402	53%	22	25	1.3
7436	Croissant with sausage, egg, and cheese (Include Burger King) [1 croissant]	159	5.6	538	65%	20	26	1.3
7437	Croissant with bacon, egg, and cheese (Include Burger King) [1 croissant]	118	4.2	386	58%	15	25	1.3
7438	Cuban sandwich, Puerto Rican style (roasted pork, cheese, ham, margarine on roll) (Include Sandwich Cubano) [1 sandwich (6" long)]	255	9.0	704	40%	44	58	3.1
7439	**Egg salad (chopped hard-boiled egg and mayonnaise) sandwich** [1 sandwich]	159	5.6	485	66%	14	27	1.2
7440	Egg (scrambled egg) sandwich [1 sandwich]	112	4.0	238	35%	11	27	1.2
7441	Egg and bacon on biscuit (Include Hardee's) [1 biscuit sandwich]	124	4.4	378	61%	14	24	0.6
7442	Egg and cheese on biscuit [1 biscuit sandwich]	140	4.9	425	55%	13	35	0.9
7443	Egg, cheese, bacon on biscuit (Include Swanson Great Starts Egg, Cheese & Bacon on a Biscuit breakfast sandwich) [1 biscuit sandwich]	119	4.2	340	50%	13	30	0.8
7444	Egg, cheese, ham on biscuit (Include Hardee's) [1 biscuit sandwich]	151	5.3	459	48%	19	43	0.7
7445	Egg, cheese, sausage on biscuit (Include Swanson Great Starts Sausage, Egg and Cheese on a Biscuit breakfast sandwich) [1 biscuit sandwich]	176	6.2	573	61%	21	34	0.8
7446	Egg and ham on biscuit (Include Hardee's) [1 biscuit sandwich]	138	4.9	317	55%	15	22	0.6
7447	Egg and sausage on biscuit (Include Hardee's, McDonald's) [1 biscuit sandwich]	162	5.7	523	60%	17	37	0.8
7448	Egg and steak on biscuit (Include Hardee's) [1 biscuit sandwich]	179	6.3	547	48%	20	50	1.3
7449	**Egg, cheese, and bacon on English muffin** (Include Burger King) [1 sandwich]	135	4.8	377	48%	19	29	1.5
7450	Egg, cheese, beef on English muffin (Include Swanson Great Starts Beefsteak, Egg & Cheese on a Muffin) [1 sandwich]	147	5.2	416	49%	22	30	1.6
7451	Egg, cheese, ham on English muffin (Include McDonald's Egg McMuffin, Swanson Great Starts Egg, Canadian Style Bacon & Cheese on a Muffin breakfast sandwich) [1 sandwich]	125	4.4	288	40%	19	24	1.3
7452	Egg, cheese, sausage on English muffin (Include McDonald's Sausage McMuffin with Egg) [1 sandwich]	165	5.8	476	58%	20	29	1.5
7453	Fajita-style beef sandwich with cheese, lettuce, onions, tomato, peppers in pita bread [1 pita sandwich]	207	7.3	292	35%	19	28	2.5
7454	Fajita-style chicken sandwich with cheese, lettuce, onions, tomato, peppers in pita bread (Include Jack-in-the-Box Chicken Fajita Pita) [1 pita sandwich]	207	7.3	311	35%	22	28	2.5
7455	Finger sandwich (tuna-egg-mayonnaise filling) [2 finger sandwiches]	46	1.6	104	24%	6	13	0.6
7456	Fish (breaded, fried) sandwich, on bun, with mayonnaise (Include Burger King) [1 sandwich]	185	6.5	497	36%	23	54	2.5
7457	Fish (breaded, fried) sandwich, on bun, with cheese and tartar sauce (Include Hardee's, McDonald's) [1 sandwich]	207	7.3	537	35%	30	56	2.8
7458	Fried egg sandwich [1 sandwich]	96	3.4	226	34%	10	26	1.2
7459	**Gyro sandwich** (pita bread, beef, lamb, tomato, and condiments) [1 gyro]	105	3.7	170	21%	12	21	1.0
7460	Ham on biscuit (Include Hardee's) [1 sandwich]	106	3.7	363	43%	13	41	0.7
7461	Ham and cheese on English muffin [1 ham and cheese muffin]	96	3.4	251	42%	17	18	1.0
7462	Ham and cheese sandwich with lettuce, margarine [1 sandwich]	155	5.5	380	46%	20	30	1.4
7463	Ham and cheese sandwich, grilled [1 sandwich]	141	5.0	381	46%	21	30	1.2

Food #	fat gm	sat fat gm	choles mg	sodium mg	potass mg	vit A	vit E	vit C	thia-min	ribo-flavin	nia-cin	vit B-6	fol-ate	vit B-12	cal-cium	phos-phorus	magne-sium	iron	zinc
									% of Daily Value										
7425	9	2	18	284	97	1	4	0	9	6	13	6	9	2	4	7	2	6	3
7426	16	3	52	415	226	2	7	3	19	16	27	13	15	3	8	14	7	13	9
7427	8	2	51	346	201	1	3	0	19	14	45	20	13	4	6	17	7	12	7
7428	10	4	46	1177	187	0	1	3	16	15	16	5	13	15	7	11	5	15	15
7429	9	2	97	637	341	6	7	7	27	17	25	8	28	70	18	22	10	18	22
7430	19	10	72	627	219	17	2	6	16	17	24	10	12	4	12	20	6	11	10
7431	20	11	65	877	234	17	2	0	27	19	17	6	10	6	16	26	5	10	11
7432	38	16	73	945	293	17	11	2	19	25	14	6	12	11	25	28	6	12	13
7433	34	15	242	878	207	19	3	2	28	24	14	7	15	13	5	20	5	15	12
7434	25	12	223	732	185	19	3	2	23	23	11	7	15	13	5	20	5	14	10
7435	24	12	265	1080	271	23	4	3	30	30	14	14	15	17	13	31	7	15	16
7436	39	17	281	1034	259	23	4	3	27	29	14	8	15	17	14	29	6	16	17
7437	25	12	252	751	199	23	4	3	18	26	8	8	15	15	13	26	5	14	12
7438	31	10	93	1466	591	17	13	1	99	44	52	31	38	20	37	48	14	26	28
7439	35	7	337	555	167	15	16	0	20	33	11	16	21	15	10	19	5	15	8
7440	9	2	213	447	145	12	3	0	18	26	10	5	17	8	10	15	5	13	6
7441	26	7	291	826	207	4	6	4	7	11	10	6	12	14	16	20	5	17	9
7442	26	7	174	1153	270	19	15	0	21	29	12	6	5	11	18	47	6	16	9
7443	19	6	135	1204	255	11	8	0	22	24	13	6	11	9	15	42	5	14	8
7444	25	14	145	1593	263	12	9	0	33	29	17	9	12	7	25	64	7	17	15
7445	39	12	201	1649	413	18	11	2	42	34	21	12	13	23	19	53	7	19	16
7446	19	4	215	994	229	17	5	0	32	25	7	10	12	14	16	23	6	18	11
7447	35	13	272	1027	288	15	8	0	30	24	16	9	15	21	14	44	6	20	13
7448	29	6	161	1544	410	13	15	0	33	33	24	12	19	22	8	58	8	27	19
7449	20	8	242	908	258	17	4	0	22	31	15	8	15	15	25	32	7	14	14
7450	22	8	183	900	289	18	6	0	17	28	20	9	13	22	25	30	7	16	22
7451	13	5	204	898	237	14	3	0	24	27	15	11	12	12	21	28	6	12	13
7452	31	12	207	1060	279	19	5	0	24	30	16	7	13	14	29	33	7	14	16
7453	11	4	39	778	464	9	5	56	22	18	21	21	16	28	18	25	10	14	18
7454	12	5	51	784	372	10	5	56	20	17	26	15	15	6	19	22	9	12	13
7455	3	0	21	213	66	1	1	0	8	7	14	3	6	8	3	5	2	6	2
7456	20	4	60	762	423	3	16	2	35	23	31	10	31	20	16	24	11	20	7
7457	21	5	75	1032	446	4	12	0	36	27	36	16	34	19	32	43	15	25	12
7458	9	2	207	433	120	11	3	0	18	24	10	5	16	7	8	14	4	12	6
7459	4	2	34	272	209	1	1	6	16	13	16	7	10	15	5	12	5	10	15
7460	17	11	23	1344	184	3	7	0	32	17	16	6	9	1	15	52	5	14	10
7461	12	7	46	739	170	8	1	0	25	17	15	9	9	8	28	26	6	8	13
7462	19	8	53	1449	350	11	4	1	51	27	26	14	15	14	23	34	8	14	16
7463	20	8	54	1465	337	11	4	0	48	26	25	13	11	14	23	34	8	13	16

Mixed Dishes & Fast Food

Food #	Food Description & Amount	wt gm	wt oz	calo-ries	%cal fat	prot gm	carbo gm	fiber gm
7464	Ham and cheese sandwich, on bun with lettuce, margarine (Include ham and cheese hero sandwich) [1 sandwich]	154	5.4	352	48%	19	25	1.5
7465	Ham and cheese submarine sandwich, on multigrain roll with lettuce, tomato, mayonnaise (Include Hardee's) [1 submarine]	219	7.7	476	60%	24	25	2.3
7466	Hot ham and cheese sandwich, on bun, with tomato, lettuce, mayonnaise (Include Arby's) [1 sandwich]	230	8.1	519	50%	30	34	2.2
7467	Ham and fried egg sandwich [1 sandwich]	124	4.4	277	38%	15	27	1.2
7468	Ham and tomato club sandwich with cheese, lettuce, french dressing [1 sandwich]	254	9.0	594	48%	30	47	2.2
7469	Ham salad (ham, celery, mayonnaise) sandwich [1 sandwich]	107	3.8	246	44%	13	20	1.2
7470	**Ham sandwich, with mayonnaise** [1 sandwich]	**112**	**4.0**	**282**	**41%**	**14**	**27**	**1.2**
7471	Ham sandwich with lettuce, margarine [1 sandwich]	127	4.5	285	38%	15	29	1.4
7472	Meat spread or potted meat sandwich [1 sandwich]	107	3.8	268	39%	8	32	1.3
7473	Meatball and spaghetti sauce on roll [1 submarine sandwich]	189	6.7	438	42%	29	32	2.3
7474	Midnight sandwich, Puerto Rican style (Media noche) (Includes roast pork, ham, cheese, pickle, margarine, mustard) [1 sandwich]	201	7.1	483	35%	34	42	2.2
7475	**Pastrami sandwich** [1 sandwich]	**134**	**4.7**	**331**	**49%**	**14**	**27**	**1.7**
7476	Pork barbecue or Sloppy Joe, on bun [1 sandwich]	186	6.6	322	27%	23	34	2.2
7477	Pork sandwich, plain [1 sandwich]	136	4.8	324	26%	26	32	1.5
7478	Pork sandwich, with gravy [1 sandwich]	218	7.7	326	25%	25	34	1.7
7479	Pork, barbeque sauce, onions, dill pickles on white roll [1 sandwich]	189	6.7	421	32%	28	40	2.5
7480	Puerto Rican sandwich (Sandwich criollo) (Includes cheese, mortadella, margarine) [1 sandwich]	160	5.6	550	50%	17	50	2.6
7481	Reuben sandwich (corned beef sandwich with sauerkraut and cheese) [1 sandwich]	181	6.4	464	56%	21	30	3.4
7482	**Roast beef sandwich** (Include Arby's, Hardee's, RAX) [1 sandwich]	**136**	**4.8**	**343**	**36%**	**27**	**26**	**1.2**
7483	Roast beef sandwich dipped in egg, fried in margarine, with gravy [1 sandwich]	258	9.1	521	51%	33	30	1.5
7484	Roast beef sandwich with bacon and cheese sauce (Include RAX) [1 sandwich]	189	6.7	588	47%	38	37	1.9
7485	Roast beef sandwich with cheese (Include Arby's) [1 sandwich]	175	6.2	460	41%	36	29	1.3
7486	Roast beef sandwich, with gravy [1 sandwich]	222	7.8	388	36%	30	30	1.5
7487	Roast beef submarine sandwich, on roll with lettuce, tomato, mayonnaise (Include Hardee's, Arby's) [1 sandwich]	202	7.1	440	46%	24	35	2.5
7488	Roast beef submarine sandwich, on roll, au jus (Include French Dip sandwich) [1 sandwich]	193	6.8	363	32%	25	34	1.8
7489	**Salami sandwich** with margarine [1 sandwich]	**82**	**2.9**	**234**	**43%**	**8**	**25**	**1.1**
7490	Sardine sandwich (filling of sardine in tomato sauce, celery, egg, mayonnaise, pickle, onion) with lettuce [1 sandwich]	214	7.5	492	52%	27	31	1.9
7491	Sausage and spaghetti sauce sandwich [1 sandwich]	189	6.7	469	49%	23	35	2.3
7492	Sausage on biscuit (Include McDonald's, Hardee's) [1 biscuit sandwich]	124	4.4	485	59%	12	40	1.4
7493	Sausage on biscuit, diet (Include Weight Watchers) [1 biscuit sandwich]	85	3.0	220	46%	10	19	0.6
7494	Sausage and cheese on English muffin (Include McDonald's Sausage McMuffin) [1 sandwich]	114	4.0	390	56%	15	29	1.5
7495	Sausage sandwich, plain [1 sandwich]	107	3.8	343	51%	15	26	1.2
7496	Steak and cheese sandwich [1 sandwich]	170	6.0	448	41%	34	30	1.5
7497	Steak and cheese submarine sandwich, on roll [1 submarine]	197	6.9	538	48%	41	27	1.2
7498	Steak and cheese submarine sandwich, with fried peppers. onions, on roll (Include Philadelphia-style cheese steak submarine sandwich; Arby's Philly Beef N' Swiss) [1 submarine]	311	11.0	749	39%	57	54	3.5
7499	Steak and cheese submarine sandwich, with tomato, lettuce on roll [1 submarine]	214	7.5	474	41%	35	33	2.0
7500	Steak on biscuit (Include Jimmy Dean Steak Biscuit) [1 sandwich]	57	2.0	170	37%	8	18	0.6
7501	Steak sandwich, plain, on roll [1 sandwich]	142	5.0	349	36%	30	24	1.3
7502	Steak submarine sandwich, with tomato and tomato, on roll [1 sandwich]	186	6.6	378	33%	30	31	2.1
7503	Tomato sandwich with lettuce, mayonnaise [1 sandwich]	134	4.7	237	39%	5	31	2.1

Food #	fat gm	sat fat gm	choles mg	sodium mg	potass mg	vit A	vit E	vit C	thia-min	ribo-flavin	nia-cin	vit B-6	fol-ate	vit B-12	cal-cium	phos-phorus	magne-sium	iron	zinc
7464	19	8	51	1357	357	11	5	2	47	24	23	13	18	13	23	32	7	12	16
7465	31	12	73	1587	496	16	8	13	46	30	24	20	16	17	35	46	13	16	21
7466	29	9	77	2016	592	10	10	9	63	35	39	22	24	16	25	44	11	20	22
7467	12	3	224	800	213	11	3	0	34	28	18	10	17	11	8	20	6	14	10
7468	32	12	76	2099	480	14	11	10	72	33	37	21	19	16	30	43	11	20	21
7469	12	2	29	817	226	1	5	2	31	14	18	14	11	5	5	13	5	9	9
7470	13	3	36	1033	245	1	4	0	47	18	24	13	13	8	6	18	6	12	10
7471	12	3	34	1103	276	4	3	1	51	20	26	12	15	8	7	20	6	13	11
7472	12	4	22	841	122	1	4	0	23	15	15	5	12	11	6	8	4	11	6
7473	20	7	86	591	497	2	6	6	22	22	41	17	21	47	10	23	10	25	36
7474	19	7	76	1379	458	8	7	1	74	32	39	25	25	14	22	36	10	19	22
7475	18	6	51	1335	243	0	1	3	19	16	24	7	13	16	7	14	6	15	18
7476	10	3	51	948	426	7	6	10	50	22	28	17	17	8	9	20	10	16	15
7477	9	3	62	392	343	0	1	0	60	27	31	17	17	9	9	23	9	15	17
7478	9	3	58	805	337	0	1	1	57	27	30	17	15	9	9	23	9	15	16
7479	15	5	81	891	460	3	6	6	57	30	30	13	23	12	13	20	9	22	29
7480	31	10	31	1285	251	21	12	0	33	27	21	5	31	11	32	26	8	19	13
7481	29	10	82	1348	261	9	3	7	16	21	17	11	13	22	30	29	10	16	27
7482	14	5	68	338	377	0	1	0	21	21	28	13	14	41	6	23	8	22	41
7483	29	9	173	973	478	15	7	0	23	30	30	15	17	47	8	30	9	27	48
7484	31	12	93	1047	549	4	5	0	39	31	39	16	25	48	20	39	11	28	47
7485	21	9	96	696	471	5	2	0	23	27	31	15	16	51	25	43	11	25	52
7486	16	6	70	821	446	0	1	0	22	23	31	13	14	42	7	25	9	25	47
7487	22	6	59	482	455	4	9	13	26	21	27	16	27	32	10	21	9	23	33
7488	13	5	54	616	380	0	4	0	26	22	30	11	23	34	10	21	8	23	34
7489	11	3	19	612	117	4	2	0	20	16	15	5	12	18	6	8	4	13	6
7490	29	5	228	895	480	12	10	4	23	30	31	16	21	117	37	47	12	24	11
7491	26	8	65	1295	472	2	6	9	56	24	32	18	21	19	11	21	9	19	16
7492	32	14	35	1071	198	1	10	0	26	17	16	6	11	8	13	45	5	14	10
7493	11	4	30	534	179	1	0	1	26	13	14	6	6	10	4	11	3	8	7
7494	24	10	58	1027	213	9	2	2	46	15	21	7	17	11	17	18	6	12	11
7495	19	6	47	998	262	0	1	2	44	19	23	11	12	16	7	15	5	12	11
7496	20	9	89	718	462	6	4	0	24	30	26	19	20	45	25	38	10	24	45
7497	29	14	116	1054	552	14	4	0	21	37	25	22	17	53	42	55	12	25	54
7498	32	12	142	939	642	11	10	31	40	44	45	29	37	60	43	61	16	43	57
7499	21	10	93	752	553	9	5	8	26	32	28	21	24	47	26	41	12	26	48
7500	7	2	17	353	141	0	3	0	11	10	10	5	6	9	5	18	3	9	9
7501	14	5	77	326	409	0	3	0	21	23	26	19	17	44	7	26	8	23	43
7502	14	5	74	391	481	2	4	8	26	25	28	20	24	42	9	26	10	25	42
7503	10	2	6	368	217	5	5	20	20	13	13	7	17	1	7	7	5	12	3

Mixed Dishes & Fast Food

Food #	Food Description & Amount	wt gm	wt oz	calo-ries	%cal fat	prot gm	carbo gm	fiber gm
7504	Tuna salad (tuna, celery, pickles, onion, mayo) sandwich, without lettuce [1 sandwich]	157	5.5	288	23%	19	36	1.7
7505	Tuna salad sandwich, with lettuce [1 sandwich]	167	5.9	289	23%	19	36	1.8
7506	Tuna salad submarine sandwich, on roll with lettuce [1 sandwich]	190	6.7	373	22%	20	51	2.9
7507	Turkey salad (turkey, celery, mayonnaise) sandwich [1 sandwich]	92	3.2	216	42%	13	18	1.0
7508	Turkey sandwich, with mayonnaise [1 sandwich]	143	5.0	331	31%	29	26	1.2
7509	Turkey sandwich, with gravy [1 sandwich]	284	10.0	392	23%	41	32	1.7
7510	Turkey submarine sandwich, on roll, with cheese, lettuce, tomato and mayonnaise (Include Arby's) [1 submarine]	277	9.8	583	38%	37	51	3.1
	Hamburgers & Hot Dogs (burgers on white bun unless noted otherwise)							
7600	Hamburger, 1 oz meat, with tomato and/or catsup, on miniature bun (including with lettuce, pickles, onions, and/or mustard) [1 baby burger]	47	1.7	97	36%	6	10	0.7
7601	Hamburger, 1 oz meat, plain, on miniature bun (Include Jimmy Dean Mini Burger) [1 baby burger]	49	1.7	137	37%	8	13	0.7
7602	Hamburger, with catsup, pickles, mustard (Include McDonald's Hamburger) [1 burger]	113	4.0	261	35%	13	28	1.7
7603	Hamburger, plain (Include Wendy's Kid's Meal Hamburger) [1 burger]	93	3.3	267	36%	14	27	1.5
7604	Hamburger, with mayonnaise or salad dressing (including with lettuce, pickles, onions, and/or mustard) [1 burger]	115	4.1	298	43%	14	28	1.7
7605	Hamburger, with mayonnaise or salad dressing and tomatoes (including with lettuce, pickles, onions, and/or mustard (Include Burger King Whopper Jr.) [1 burger]	153	5.4	342	43%	16	32	2.2
7606	Hamburger, 2½ oz meat, with mayonnaise or salad dressing and tomatoes (including with lettuce, pickles, onions, and/or mustard) [1 burger]	178	6.3	395	46%	20	32	2.3
7607	**Hamburger, ¼ lb meat, with tomato and/or catsup** (including with lettuce, pickles, onions, and/or mustard (Include McDonald's ¼-Pounder) [1 burger]	**192**	**6.8**	**446**	**41%**	**26**	**38**	**2.3**
7608	Hamburger, ¼ lb meat, plain [1 burger]	156	5.5	449	45%	28	32	1.7
7609	Hamburger, ¼ lb meat, with mayonnaise or salad dressing (including with lettuce, pickles, onions, and/or mustard) [1 burger]	200	7.1	542	51%	28	36	2.3
7610	Hamburger, ¼ lb meat, with mayonnaise or salad dressing and tomatoes (including with lettuce, pickles, onions, and/or mustard) (Include Jack-in-the-Box Jumbo Jack, Burger King Whopper) [1 burger]	244	8.6	595	51%	30	41	2.8
7611	Double hamburger (2 patties), plain [1 burger]	130	4.6	374	45%	23	27	1.4
7612	Double hamburger (2 patties), with tomato and/or catsup (including with lettuce, pickles, onions, and/or mustard) [1 burger]	164	5.8	378	42%	22	31	1.9
7613	Double hamburger (2 patties), with mayonnaise or salad dressing (including with lettuce, pickles, onions, and/or mustard) [1 burger]	159	5.6	430	53%	22	27	1.7
7614	Double hamburger (2 patties), with mayonnaise or salad dressing and tomatoes (including with lettuce, pickles, onions, and/or mustard) [1 burger]	197	6.9	478	52%	25	31	2.1
7615	Double hamburger (2 patties), with mayonnaise or salad dressing and tomatoes, on double-decker bun (including with lettuce, pickles, onions, and/or mustard) [1 burger]	241	8.5	593	49%	30	45	2.9
7616	Double hamburger (2 patties, ¼ lb meat each), with mayonnaise or salad dressing and tomato, catsup, lettuce, pickle, onion, on double-decker bun [1 double hamburger]	319	11.3	715	50%	44	43	3.0
7617	**Double hamburger (2 patties, ¼ lb meat each),** with tomato and/or catsup (Include with lettuce, pickles, onions, and/or mustard) [1 burger]	**314**	**11.1**	**780**	**48%**	**51**	**48**	**2.9**
7618	Cheeseburger, small, with catsup, lettuce, pickles, onions (Include McDonald's, Burger King) [1 burger]	127	4.5	299	40%	16	29	1.8
7619	Cheeseburger, plain (Include Wendy's Kid's Meal Cheeseburger) [1 burger]	107	3.8	314	41%	17	28	1.5
7620	Cheeseburger, with lettuce, pickles, onions, mayonnaise and/or mustard (Include Jack-in-the-Box Hamburger with Cheese) [1 burger]	129	4.6	345	46%	17	29	1.7
7621	Cheeseburger, with tomato and/or catsup, lettuce, pickles, onions, mayonnaise (Include Burger King Whopper Jr. with Cheese, Wendy's Jr. Cheeseburger Deluxe) [1 burger]	167	5.9	379	45%	18	34	2.2
7622	Cheeseburger (hamburger with cheese sauce), ¼ lb meat, with grilled onions, on rye bun, with lettuce, pickles, onions [1 burger]	183	6.5	411	47%	23	30	3.8

Food #	fat gm	sat fat gm	choles mg	sodium mg	potass mg	% of Daily Value												
						vit A	vit E	vit C	thia-min	ribo-flavin	nia-cin	vit B-6	fol-ate	vit B-12	cal-cium	phos-phorus	magne-sium	iron	zinc
7504	7	1	22	709	241	3	4	2	18	14	49	13	14	29	7	15	8	15	6
7505	7	1	22	710	257	3	4	3	18	14	49	13	16	29	7	16	8	15	6
7506	9	2	18	851	296	3	7	3	29	19	50	12	30	26	13	17	9	20	7
7507	10	2	32	271	188	1	4	2	13	11	16	12	10	3	5	11	5	10	9
7508	11	2	69	376	316	1	4	0	20	19	33	23	14	6	8	23	9	17	20
7509	10	3	89	1045	529	0	2	0	23	28	49	28	15	9	9	32	11	25	32
7510	25	7	70	2408	552	8	12	9	35	29	62	27	36	41	32	51	13	22	18
7600	4	1	14	160	101	1	1	1	7	5	8	3	7	6	3	4	2	5	7
7601	6	2	20	161	107	0	1	0	9	8	11	4	9	9	4	6	3	7	9
7602	10	4	33	478	240	1	3	3	18	14	21	7	19	18	8	11	5	15	15
7603	11	4	35	336	190	0	3	0	18	14	22	6	18	19	8	11	5	15	16
7604	14	4	37	435	215	1	5	1	18	14	21	8	19	19	8	12	5	15	16
7605	16	5	42	494	294	2	6	9	22	17	25	10	23	22	9	14	6	18	18
7606	20	6	58	596	355	3	6	9	22	19	30	13	23	31	10	17	7	20	24
7607	21	8	74	802	452	3	5	6	24	22	38	15	25	41	11	21	9	24	32
7608	22	8	82	437	358	0	4	0	23	22	39	14	23	45	10	21	8	24	34
7609	31	9	87	713	404	2	9	2	25	23	40	17	26	45	11	22	9	25	34
7610	34	10	94	779	498	4	10	10	28	26	44	20	30	49	12	25	10	28	37
7611	19	7	69	364	299	0	3	0	19	18	33	12	19	38	8	18	7	20	29
7612	18	7	66	677	391	2	4	5	19	19	32	13	20	36	9	18	8	20	28
7613	25	8	71	555	325	1	7	1	19	18	31	14	20	37	9	18	7	20	28
7614	28	8	79	614	406	3	8	9	21	21	35	16	23	41	9	20	8	23	31
7615	32	10	88	800	484	3	10	10	30	27	44	19	32	46	13	24	10	29	35
7616	40	14	142	1132	755	5	8	16	29	32	61	27	31	76	13	35	14	36	57
7617	41	16	161	1014	775	3	7	7	32	37	69	28	33	88	14	39	15	40	66
7618	13	5	40	676	272	4	4	3	18	17	21	8	19	20	15	18	6	15	17
7619	14	6	44	505	226	3	3	0	19	18	22	7	18	22	16	18	6	15	18
7620	18	6	46	601	251	4	5	1	19	18	22	9	20	22	16	18	6	16	18
7621	19	7	49	737	355	6	6	10	21	20	24	11	22	23	17	20	7	18	20
7622	21	7	68	727	387	5	4	2	19	22	31	13	16	36	9	23	11	19	30

Mixed Dishes & Fast Food

Food #	Food Description & Amount	wt gm	wt oz	calo-ries	%cal fat	prot gm	carbo gm	fiber gm
7623	**Cheeseburger, ¼ lb meat**, plain [1 burger]	184	6.5	543	48%	33	36	1.8
7624	Cheeseburger, ¼ lb meat, with mushrooms, lettuce, pickles, onions [1 burger]	205	7.2	464	50%	27	30	2.6
7625	Cheeseburger, ¼ lb meat, with lettuce, pickles, onions, catsup (Include McDonald's ¼-Pounder with Cheese) [1 burger]	220	7.8	526	46%	31	39	2.5
7626	Cheeseburger, ¼ lb meat, with ham [1 burger]	219	7.7	600	48%	41	35	1.8
7627	Cheeseburger, ¼ lb meat, with lettuce, pickles, onions, mayonnaise, and/or mustard [1 burger]	228	8.0	636	54%	33	38	2.3
7628	Cheeseburger, ¼ lb meat, with tomatoes, lettuce, pickles, onions, mayonnaise, and/or mustard (Include Jack-in-the-Box Jumbo-Jack with Cheese, Burger King Whopper with Cheese) [1 burger]	274	9.7	698	54%	37	43	2.8
7629	Double cheeseburger (2 patties), with tomato and/or catsup, with lettuce, pickles, onions, and/or mustard (Include McDonald's Double Cheeseburger) [1 burger]	192	6.8	463	46%	27	34	2.1
7630	Double cheeseburger (2 patties), plain [1 burger]	158	5.6	466	46%	27	34	1.7
7631	Double cheeseburger (2 patties), plain, on double-decker bun [1 burger]	186	6.6	548	46%	32	40	2.0
7632	Double cheeseburger (2 patties), with mayonnaise or salad dressing (including with lettuce, pickles, onions, and/or mustard) [1 burger]	187	6.6	523	52%	27	34	2.0
7633	Double cheeseburger (2 patties), with mayonnaise or salad dressing and tomatoes (including with lettuce, pickles, onions, and/or mustard) [1 burger]	225	7.9	575	52%	30	39	2.4
7634	Double cheeseburger (2 patties), with mayonnaise or salad dressing, on double-decker bun (including with lettuce, pickles, onions, and/or mustard) (Include **McDonald's Big Mac**) [1 burger]	224	7.9	615	52%	32	41	2.4
7635	**Double cheeseburger (2 patties, ¼ lb meat each)**, with mayonnaise or salad dressing (including with lettuce, pickles, onions, and/or mustard) (Include Jack-in-the-Box Ultimate Cheeseburger) [1 burger]	272	9.6	790	58%	46	35	2.0
7636	Triple cheeseburger (3 patties, ¼ lb meat each), with tomatoes, lettuce, pickles, onions, mayonnaise [1 burger]	400	14.1	1055	60%	66	38	2.5
7637	Bacon cheeseburger, ¼ lb meat, with tomato and/or catsup, lettuce, pickles, onions, and/or mustard (Include Wendy's Big Bacon Classic, Jack-in-the-Box Junior Bacon Cheeseburger) [1 burger]	208	7.3	557	52%	32	34	2.1
7638	Bacon cheeseburger, 1/4 lb meat, with mayonnaise or salad dressing and tomatoes (Include McDonald's Arch Deluxe with Bacon) [1 McDonald's Arch Deluxe]	255	9.0	609	51%	33	43	4.1
7639	Bacon cheeseburger with tomato, lettuce, pickle, onion, mayonnaise [1 burger]	288	10.2	751	51%	37	52	3.4
7640	Double bacon cheeseburger (2 patties) (including with lettuce, pickles, onions, and/or mustard) (Include Burger King Bacon Double Cheeseburger) [1 burger]	200	7.1	578	56%	37	25	1.4
7641	**Double bacon cheeseburger (2 patties, ¼ lb meat each)**, with mayonnaise or salad dressing and tomatoes (including with lettuce, pickles, onions, and/or mustard) (Include Jack-in-the-Box Bacon Ultimate Cheeseburger) [1 burger]	335	11.8	973	60%	56	39	2.4
7642	Chiliburger (Include hamburger with chili) [1 burger]	159	5.6	401	45%	24	30	2.8
7643	Pizzaburger (hamburger, cheese, pizza sauce) on ½ bun [1 burger]	137	4.8	327	47%	22	20	1.3
7644	Pizzaburger (hamburger, cheese, pizza sauce) on whole bun [1 burger]	165	5.8	409	40%	24	36	2.2
7645	Steak patty (breaded, fried) sandwich, with mayonnaise or salad dressing, lettuce, and tomato (Include Country Fried Steak Sandwich) [1 sandwich]	153	5.4	440	51%	15	39	2.3
7646	Taco burger, on bun (Include chiliburger with cheese) [1 burger]	127	4.5	286	33%	13	34	2.9
7647	Frankfurter, beef [1 frankfurter, thick (8 per lb)]	57	2.0	186	81%	7	1	0.0
7648	Frankfurter, beef, lowfat (Include Oscar Mayer Beef Franks - Light) [1 frankfurter]	57	2.0	136	74%	7	1	0.0
7649	Frankfurter, beef and pork (Include Smokie Links) [1 frankfurter (8 per lb)]	57	2.0	189	81%	7	2	0.0
7650	Frankfurter, beef and pork, lowfat [1 frankfurter]	57	2.0	92	58%	7	3	0.0
7651	Frankfurter, chicken [1 frankfurter (8 per lb)]	57	2.0	150	67%	8	4	0.0
7652	Frankfurter, low salt [1 frankfurter (8 per lb)]	57	2.0	186	81%	7	1	0.0
7653	Frankfurter, meat and poultry [1 frankfurter (8 per lb]	57	2.0	175	77%	7	2	0.0
7654	Frankfurter, meat and poultry, lowfat [1 frankfurter (8 per lb)]	57	2.0	72	20%	9	5	0.1
7655	Frankfurter, meat and poultry, fat free [1 frankfurter (8 per lb)]	57	2.0	72	20%	9	5	0.1

Food #	fat gm	sat fat gm	choles mg	sodium mg	potass mg	vit A	vit E	vit C	thia-min	ribo-flavin	nia-cin	vit B-6	fol-ate	vit B-12	cal-cium	phos-phorus	magne-sium	iron	zinc
7623	29	13	98	811	426	7	5	0	24	30	39	15	24	48	27	35	10	25	39
7624	26	10	80	993	398	9	6	1	21	22	33	12	21	38	26	36	10	21	33
7625	27	12	90	1204	516	9	6	6	24	28	37	16	25	44	27	34	11	25	37
7626	32	13	119	1388	578	7	5	0	43	36	50	21	24	52	27	46	12	27	44
7627	38	14	106	1072	478	9	9	2	25	31	39	19	27	50	29	37	11	27	40
7628	42	15	116	1169	578	11	11	10	28	34	44	22	30	54	31	41	13	30	43
7629	24	10	80	1034	453	8	5	5	21	25	33	14	22	39	23	30	10	22	32
7630	24	10	79	708	357	5	4	0	23	26	33	12	22	39	23	29	8	22	32
7631	28	12	93	833	420	6	5	0	27	30	39	15	26	46	28	35	10	26	37
7632	30	11	83	888	386	7	8	1	23	26	33	15	24	39	24	30	9	22	31
7633	33	12	90	1168	466	9	9	8	26	28	36	17	27	42	26	33	10	25	34
7634	36	13	97	1044	460	8	9	2	27	30	38	18	28	45	28	35	11	26	37
7635	51	20	155	1192	621	12	10	2	23	37	50	26	25	73	36	51	13	31	57
7636	70	29	227	1577	952	19	11	13	26	51	70	38	28	108	49	73	19	42	84
7637	32	13	93	1323	533	7	5	5	29	28	38	16	21	43	23	36	11	23	36
7638	34	12	99	1247	571	2	2	12	31	24	39	17	26	48	7	34	12	26	38
7639	43	15	101	1436	638	9	10	14	45	36	48	20	37	45	29	41	13	31	38
7640	36	15	117	1006	505	8	4	1	23	29	41	18	18	56	26	40	10	23	44
7641	65	25	185	1598	811	14	12	8	35	44	62	32	28	85	40	62	16	36	66
7642	20	7	72	523	409	1	4	1	19	20	32	13	20	37	10	22	10	25	32
7643	17	7	69	629	387	7	4	7	14	18	27	13	13	34	16	23	7	17	27
7644	18	8	66	790	420	7	6	6	24	24	32	13	23	33	20	25	9	22	28
7645	25	6	38	910	262	3	11	7	25	17	24	11	26	18	11	13	6	18	15
7646	11	4	30	638	266	4	6	9	21	16	20	7	23	13	14	14	6	15	13
7647	17	7	36	591	96	0	0	0	2	3	7	3	1	13	1	5	0	5	9
7648	11	5	24	600	74	0	0	1	2	3	6	2	1	12	0	11	2	4	8
7649	17	6	30	645	96	0	0	0	7	4	7	3	1	11	1	5	1	4	7
7650	6	2	26	716	86	0	0	0	6	4	6	2	1	11	1	8	1	4	8
7651	11	3	61	789	48	2	0	0	2	4	8	8	1	2	6	6	1	7	4
7652	17	7	36	179	96	0	0	0	2	3	7	3	1	13	1	5	0	5	9
7653	15	5	42	675	80	1	0	0	4	4	7	5	1	9	3	5	1	5	7
7654	2	1	25	532	141	0	0	0	10	5	8	6	0	4	1	8	2	3	7
7655	2	1	25	532	141	0	0	0	10	5	8	6	0	4	1	8	2	3	7

% of Daily Value

Mixed Dishes & Fast Food

Food #	Food Description & Amount	wt gm	wt oz	calo-ries	%cal fat	prot gm	carbo gm	fiber gm
7656	Frankfurter, turkey [1 frankfurter (8 per lb)]	57	2.0	132	69%	9	1	0.0
7657	Frankfurter, bacon and cheese-filled [1 frankfurter (8 per lb)]	57	2.0	186	80%	8	1	0.0
7658	Frankfurter, breaded, baked [1 frankfurter]	51	1.8	176	75%	6	4	0.1
7659	Frankfurter, cheese-filled [1 frankfurter (8 per lb)]	57	2.0	194	79%	8	1	0.0
7660	Frankfurter, chili-filled [1 frankfurter (8 per lb)]	57	2.0	155	77%	6	3	0.8
7661	Frankfurter and sauerkraut [1 frankfurter with sauerkraut]	120	4.2	140	74%	5	4	2.0
7662	Frankfurter with tomato-based sauce (Include barbecue or chili sauce) [1 frankfurter in sauce]	68	2.4	130	77%	5	3	0.4
7663	Chili dog, without bun (frankfurter with chili con carne, no bun) [1 frankfurter with sauce]	125	4.4	248	70%	10	10	3.2
7664	**Hot dog** (beef and/or pork frankfurter, plain, on bun) [1 hot dog]	**85**	**3.0**	**260**	**55%**	**9**	**20**	**1.0**
7665	Hot dog (frankfurter with catsup and mustard on bun) [1 hot dog]	105	3.7	295	54%	10	24	1.3
7666	Hot dog with cheese (frankfurter, with cheese, plain, on bun) [1 hot dog]	118	4.2	368	59%	14	23	1.1
7667	Hot dog (chicken frankfurter, plain, on bun) [1 hot dog]	85	3.0	229	44%	9	22	1.0
7668	Chili dog (frankfurter, with chili, on bun) [1 hot dog]	152	5.4	349	53%	13	28	3.7
7669	Chili cheese dog (frankfurter with chili and cheese on bun) [1 hot dog]	147	5.2	400	57%	16	26	2.4
7670	**Corn dog** (frankfurter with cornbread coating) [1 corn dog]	**88**	**3.1**	**274**	**58%**	**9**	**20**	**1.1**
7671	Corny dog, with chili, on bun [1 corny dog]	162	5.7	431	44%	13	47	4.1
7672	Pig in a blanket (frankfurter wrapped in dough) [1 pig in blanket]	85	3.0	283	69%	7	15	0.4
7673	Pochito (frankfurter and beef chili wrapped in tortilla) [1 pochito]	122	4.3	280	62%	10	18	3.1
	Pizza & Other Fast Foods							
7700	Pizza rolls (Include Pizza Bites) [6 miniature rolls]	84	3.0	252	41%	11	26	1.4
7701	Pizza, no cheese, thin crust (Include tomato pie) [1/8 of 12"dia]	194	6.8	430	25%	10	71	4.0
7702	Pizza, no cheese, thick crust (Include tomato pie, French bread pizza) [8"round]	248	8.7	661	23%	15	110	5.2
7703	White pizza, cheese, no sauce, thin crust [8"round]	194	6.8	721	31%	30	92	3.3
7704	White pizza, cheese, no sauce, thick crust [8"round]	184	6.5	675	29%	27	90	3.3
7705	**Pizza, cheese**, thin crust [8"round]	**184**	**6.5**	**477**	**34%**	**22**	**56**	**3.1**
7706	Pizza, cheese, thick crust (Include crust as English muffin or French bread) [8"round]	248	8.7	712	30%	26	97	4.5
7707	Pizza, cheese, with pineapple, thick crust [8"round]	276	9.7	732	29%	26	103	5.0
7708	Pizza, cheese, with vegetables, thin crust [[8"round]	212	7.5	452	35%	20	54	4.0
7709	Pizza, cheese, with vegetables, thick crust [8"round]	279	9.8	691	30%	25	95	5.5
7710	Pizza with beans and vegetables, thin crust (Include Pizza Hut taco pizza) [8"round]	234	8.3	567	34%	23	71	6.7
7711	Pizza with beans and vegetables, thick crust (Include Pizza Hut taco pizza) [8"round]	298	10.5	811	30%	28	114	7.9
7712	Pizza with ham (or Canadian bacon) and pineapple, thin crust [8"round]	234	8.3	501	34%	25	58	3.5
7713	Pizza with ham (or Canadian bacon) and pineapple, thick crust [8"round]	298	10.5	732	30%	30	98	5.0
7714	**Pizza with meat, thin crust (Include sausage, ground beef, pepperoni, ham, bacon, salami) [8"round]**	**191**	**6.7**	**564**	**44%**	**26**	**52**	**2.8**
7715	Pizza with [above] meat, thick crust [8"round]	255	9.0	792	37%	30	92	4.3
7716	Pizza with [above] meat and vegetables, thin crust [8"round]	234	8.3	575	44%	26	55	4.0
7717	Pizza with [above] meat and vegetables, thick crust [8"round]	298	10.5	805	37%	30	95	5.4
7718	Pizza with [above] meat and vegetables, lowfat, thin crust (Include Tombstone Light Supreme) [9"round]	261	9.2	530	38%	25	56	2.9
7719	Pizza with seafood, thin crust [8"round]	191	6.7	624	33%	33	68	2.4
7720	Pizza with seafood, thick crust [8"round]	255	9.0	854	29%	35	113	4.0
7721	Pizza, deep dish, with ground beef and tomato sauce on a crust (Include Pizzabake) [1/3 of 13"x9"x2" pan]	292	10.3	925	37%	53	88	3.8
7722	Burrito with beans, meatless [1 medium burrito]	142	5.0	341	31%	10	48	8.1
7723	**Burrito with beans and cheese**, meatless [1 medium burrito]	**142**	**5.0**	**409**	**45%**	**17**	**39**	**6.5**
7724	Burrito with beans and rice, meatless [1 medium burrito]	120	4.2	245	16%	8	43	4.2
7725	Burrito with rice, beans, cheese, sour cream, lettuce, tomato and guacamole, meatless (Include Taco Bell 7 Layer Burrito) [1 burrito]	270	9.5	527	42%	21	57	8.7

Food #	fat gm	sat fat gm	choles mg	sodium mg	potass mg	vit A	vit E	vit C	thia- min	ribo- flavin	nia- cin	vit B-6	fol- ate	vit B-12	cal- cium	phos- phorus	magne- sium	iron	zinc

Header spanning: "% of Daily Value" over the vitamin/mineral columns.

Food #	fat gm	sat fat gm	choles mg	sodium mg	potass mg	vit A	vit E	vit C	thia-min	ribo-flavin	nia-cin	vit B-6	fol-ate	vit B-12	cal-cium	phos-phorus	magne-sium	iron	zinc
7656	10	3	64	821	103	0	1	0	1	6	11	6	1	2	6	8	2	6	13
7657	17	6	39	617	117	2	1	0	9	5	8	4	0	16	3	10	2	3	9
7658	15	5	36	583	94	1	1	0	8	5	8	3	2	10	2	5	2	5	6
7659	17	6	41	623	117	2	1	0	8	5	8	3	0	15	3	10	2	4	9
7660	13	5	24	542	132	1	1	0	5	4	5	3	1	8	1	6	3	6	8
7661	12	4	20	973	203	0	1	20	6	4	6	8	5	8	3	5	4	9	6
7662	11	4	19	605	175	3	2	6	6	4	7	4	1	8	1	4	2	4	5
7663	19	7	38	964	353	2	2	2	9	8	8	8	5	11	4	16	10	17	16
7664	16	6	24	747	132	0	2	0	18	10	14	4	12	11	6	7	3	10	7
7665	18	6	27	963	185	1	3	2	21	11	15	5	14	12	7	9	4	11	9
7666	24	10	44	1127	212	6	3	0	20	18	15	6	14	16	21	21	5	11	13
7667	11	3	49	868	92	2	2	0	14	10	15	8	12	2	10	8	3	12	5
7668	21	8	36	1125	361	2	4	2	22	15	16	8	17	12	9	17	10	22	16
7669	25	11	49	1277	318	7	4	1	21	19	15	8	15	16	23	25	8	17	17
7670	18	7	47	609	140	2	2	0	10	11	11	5	7	13	10	11	3	10	9
7671	21	8	49	1284	320	4	8	9	25	19	21	9	23	15	15	16	6	18	11
7672	22	7	22	672	128	1	4	0	12	9	10	3	5	10	13	11	3	8	7
7673	19	7	35	851	278	2	2	1	9	7	9	8	10	10	7	19	10	13	14
7700	12	5	19	637	188	6	3	6	17	15	13	4	12	5	16	16	5	11	8
7701	12	3	0	98	453	10	11	22	40	25	29	9	27	0	4	13	10	26	6
7702	17	4	0	84	452	8	13	18	62	39	42	9	43	0	4	18	12	39	9
7703	25	13	57	470	200	14	5	1	52	46	32	6	37	5	55	49	12	32	20
7704	22	11	47	389	188	11	4	1	51	43	32	5	36	5	46	43	11	32	17
7705	18	8	28	447	393	16	9	16	31	29	22	8	21	4	43	37	11	21	15
7706	24	9	26	419	435	15	12	15	55	42	37	9	38	4	41	41	14	35	17
7707	24	9	26	419	481	15	12	21	57	43	37	10	38	4	42	41	15	35	17
7708	17	7	24	483	462	16	10	44	30	29	22	12	21	4	40	35	11	22	14
7709	23	8	24	476	517	16	13	44	53	43	37	13	37	4	40	40	14	36	17
7710	21	8	26	302	619	17	11	22	39	31	25	12	39	3	35	38	16	29	17
7711	27	9	24	281	643	16	14	21	64	46	41	13	56	3	34	42	19	43	19
7712	19	8	40	764	500	14	9	28	47	31	28	15	20	8	39	40	13	22	17
7713	24	9	39	746	550	14	11	27	69	44	42	16	36	7	39	45	16	35	20
7714	28	11	49	773	442	15	9	15	34	30	27	10	20	12	40	37	11	22	19
7715	33	12	47	744	488	14	11	14	56	43	41	11	36	12	39	42	14	35	21
7716	28	11	47	836	542	16	10	45	35	32	29	14	22	12	40	39	12	25	19
7717	33	12	46	815	590	15	13	43	57	46	43	15	37	11	40	44	15	38	22
7718	22	8	36	980	433	12	6	41	40	32	29	12	23	12	26	37	10	23	17
7719	23	9	81	565	218	14	8	1	38	36	26	6	27	17	48	51	13	27	21
7720	28	10	68	483	268	12	10	1	63	50	42	7	44	14	42	52	15	41	22
7721	38	14	161	164	803	3	6	10	54	50	82	31	49	87	4	45	16	49	74
7722	12	4	8	244	427	0	5	4	25	12	10	8	42	0	10	18	13	20	8
7723	21	10	41	403	378	9	4	3	21	17	9	7	35	4	32	32	13	17	13
7724	4	1	4	488	198	0	2	4	21	9	12	6	19	0	8	11	8	15	7
7725	24	12	52	846	586	16	5	19	27	24	16	14	29	6	40	37	18	25	19

Mixed Dishes & Fast Food

Food #	Food Description & Amount	wt gm	wt oz	calories	%cal fat	prot gm	carbo gm	fiber gm
7726	Burrito with beef and beans [1 medium burrito]	142	5.0	372	39%	18	39	6.5
7727	**Burrito with beef, beans, and cheese** [1 medium burrito]	142	5.0	413	48%	21	32	5.3
7728	Burrito with beef, beans, cheese, and sour cream (Include Taco Bell Burrito Supreme) [1 burrito]	234	8.3	578	48%	31	43	6.5
7729	Burrito with beef, no beans [1medium burrito]	142	5.0	454	41%	28	37	2.2
7730	Burrito with beef and cheese, no beans [1 medium burrito]	132	4.7	468	55%	29	23	1.3
7731	Burrito with beef and potato, no beans [1 medium burrito]	123	4.3	293	37%	14	32	2.2
7732	Burrito with chicken and beans [1 medium burrito]	142	5.0	330	32%	19	37	6.2
7733	Burrito with chicken and cheese [1 medium burrito]	142	5.0	388	48%	29	21	1.3
7734	**Burrito with chicken, beans, and cheese** [1 medium burrito]	134	4.7	329	43%	19	27	4.6
7735	Burrito with chicken, no beans [1 medium burrito]	142	5.0	340	27%	30	29	1.7
7736	Burrito with chicken and salsa, no beans [1 medium burrito]	142	5.0	275	26%	24	25	1.8
7737	Burrito with eggs, sausage, cheese and vegetables (Include McDonald's Breakfast Burrito) [1 burrito]	105	3.7	262	52%	10	21	1.3
7738	Burrito with eggs, cheese, no beans (Include Breakfast Burrito; Huevos Rancheros) [1 burrito]	188	6.6	386	53%	20	24	1.6
7739	Burrito with pork and beans [1 medium burrito]	142	5.0	355	37%	18	37	6.3
7740	Taco filling: beef, cheese, tomato, taco sauce [1 cup]	204	7.2	382	58%	26	15	3.7
7741	Taco or tostada with beans, meatless [1 small taco or tostada]	80	2.8	146	38%	4	20	4.6
7742	**Taco or tostada with beans and cheese, meatless** [1 small taco or tostada]	88	3.1	174	43%	6	20	4.7
7743	Taco or tostada with beans, cheese, and meat [1 small taco or tostada]	83	2.9	167	44%	8	16	3.2
7744	Taco or tostada with beef [1 small taco or tostada]	76	2.7	138	48%	8	11	1.7
7745	Taco or tostada with beef and cheese [1 small taco or tostada]	83	2.9	180	48%	9	14	2.4
7746	**Taco or tostada with beef, cheese and lettuce** (Include Taco Bell taco) [1 taco]	78	2.8	225	52%	11	16	2.1
7747	Taco or tostada with chicken or turkey [1 small taco or tostada]	72	2.5	125	34%	8	13	2.1
7748	Taco or tostada with chicken and cheese [1 taco or tostada]	79	2.8	153	41%	10	13	2.1
7749	Taco or tostada with fish, lettuce, tomato, salsa [1 taco or tostada]	76	2.7	100	32%	8	10	1.5
7750	Taco with crab meat, Puerto Rican style (Include Tacos de jueyes) [1 taco (4½" dia)]	121	4.3	270	49%	16	19	2.3
7751	Taco or tostada salad with beef, cheese, corn chips [1 cup]	122	4.3	198	57%	11	11	1.7
7752	**Taco or tostada salad with beef, cheese, fried flour tortilla** [2 cups]	244	8.6	458	59%	22	25	4.1
7753	Taco or tostada salad, meatless, with cheese, fried flour tortilla [2 cups]	244	8.6	368	56%	16	27	4.7
7754	Soft taco with beef, cheese, and lettuce (IncludeTaco Bell Soft Taco) [1 taco]	92	3.2	256	38%	13	25	1.6
7755	Soft taco with beef, cheese, lettuce, tomato and sour cream (Include Taco Bell Soft Taco Supreme) [1 taco]	124	4.4	304	46%	15	26	1.7
7756	Soft taco with chicken, cheese, and lettuce (IncludeTaco Bell Taco) [1 taco]	128	4.5	252	31%	22	20	1.5
	Your Additions							

Food #	fat gm	sat fat gm	choles mg	sodium mg	potass mg	vit A	vit E	vit C	thiamin	riboflavin	niacin	vit B-6	folate	vit B-12	calcium	phosphorus	magnesium	iron	zinc
						% of Daily Value													
7726	16	6	40	228	454	0	4	3	21	14	19	11	35	18	9	21	13	21	19
7727	22	10	61	353	398	7	4	3	18	18	16	10	29	18	27	31	12	18	21
7728	31	16	101	813	513	15	3	9	21	25	24	15	20	28	42	45	16	26	34
7729	21	7	83	391	354	0	3	0	24	21	38	13	20	43	9	24	9	25	35
7730	28	15	101	536	261	13	3	0	15	24	23	10	14	32	40	39	9	17	31
7731	12	4	34	227	338	0	4	10	18	12	21	13	13	17	6	13	7	13	16
7732	12	4	38	215	398	1	4	3	21	13	20	11	33	1	8	20	12	18	11
7733	21	11	91	569	244	15	3	3	15	21	24	10	12	8	37	35	9	12	18
7734	16	7	50	364	350	8	4	5	16	15	15	9	25	4	22	26	11	14	13
7735	10	3	80	327	286	1	3	0	22	18	50	22	16	5	8	24	9	16	15
7736	8	2	61	376	298	9	4	8	18	15	31	13	14	3	7	17	8	14	12
7737	15	5	130	565	165	10	6	10	15	18	8	5	13	7	13	17	5	10	7
7738	23	10	333	644	294	32	6	10	17	36	8	9	18	14	33	35	8	15	14
7739	14	5	36	208	473	0	4	3	35	15	16	13	33	3	9	21	12	18	12
7740	25	12	93	948	522	15	7	26	7	18	24	16	13	36	25	31	8	14	30
7741	6	2	3	233	259	2	4	9	7	3	3	7	18	0	4	9	8	7	4
7742	8	3	10	277	271	4	4	9	7	4	3	7	19	1	8	12	9	8	5
7743	8	3	21	317	219	4	4	9	6	5	7	8	12	4	8	12	7	6	7
7744	7	2	20	117	173	3	2	10	4	5	8	8	7	9	4	8	6	6	11
7745	10	4	28	363	212	5	4	9	5	7	9	8	8	9	8	13	7	7	12
7746	13	4	35	462	174	3	3	1	5	6	11	10	10	17	8	15	9	9	15
7747	5	1	21	286	164	3	4	8	4	4	10	8	7	1	3	8	6	5	5
7748	7	2	28	329	171	5	4	8	5	5	10	8	7	2	8	12	6	5	6
7749	4	1	39	164	174	3	3	10	4	2	5	6	7	4	5	11	7	6	7
7750	15	5	79	416	317	8	6	21	11	11	13	10	12	51	16	23	9	9	18
7751	13	4	35	166	310	21	2	17	3	8	11	9	6	16	8	13	7	7	14
7752	30	11	66	478	545	13	8	22	15	21	24	14	22	25	26	27	11	21	25
7753	23	10	42	594	501	19	6	24	19	21	11	10	28	6	40	29	11	16	13
7754	11	5	33	593	170	3	2	1	18	14	15	5	16	11	13	15	5	13	14
7755	16	8	44	605	223	8	3	5	18	17	15	6	17	12	17	18	6	13	15
7756	9	3	59	556	203	3	2	1	15	14	26	10	15	3	9	17	7	11	12

You only have a microwave and don't like to cook? This is about as homemade as it gets, considering your circumstance. The tomatoes and beans (garbanzo beans, kidney beans—whatever you like) make the chili more nutritious. Don't you dare look at the 3 cans and only eat the can of chili! If you feel ambitious, add some minced garlic, chopped onions, and chili powder to the recipe.

Dump Chili

1 can chili
1 can diced tomatoes
1 can beans, drained

The cans should be about equal size.
Dump everything into a bowl.
Stir. Microwave. Eat.

*   *   *   *   *   *   *   *   *   *   *   *

You only have a toaster oven and don't like to cook? These tacos are good in taste and nutrition.

Toaster Oven Tacos

Corn tortillas
Reduced-fat sharp cheddar cheese
Tomato wedges
Lettuce
Salsa

Put sliced cheese on half of the tortilla. Put two of these tortillas at a time on the rack in your toaster oven. If you have to overlap them a bit, overlap a part that doesn't have cheese. Toast until the cheese melts and the tortilla get crispy. Immediately fold each tortilla in half (if you wait, the tortilla will crack when you fold it). Put in the tomato wedges, lettuce, salsa, and enjoy.

Index

A

A1 sauce, see 5336
Abalone 4907-4908
Aburage, see 3870
Acerola, raw 2000
Acidophilus milk, see 554-555
Acorn squash, see 2759
Adobo fresco or criollo 5600
Ahi, see 4896
Air Heads candy, see 1966
Aku, see 4896
Akule, see 4833
Albondigas, see 7078
Albondigon, see 7136
Alcapurrias, see 2815
Alcohol, grain 404
Alcoholic beverages 380-446
Ale, see 383
Ale-type soft drink 200
Alewife, see 4793
Alexander cocktail 380
Alfalfa sprouts, raw 2350
Alfredo sauce 5300
Algae, dried 2351
All-Bran 3550-3552
Allspice, ground 5700
Almojabanas, see 7158
Almonds 3902-3906
    candy-coated, 1852-1853, see 1935
Almond
    butter 3900
    chicken 6500
    cookie 1200
    Joy candy, see 1884
    oil 5400
    paste 3901
    Roca candy, see 1969
    Smash soft drink, see 209
    toast, see 3000
Aloe vera juice 2
Alpha-Bits cereal 3553-3554
Alphabet vegetable soup, see 5236
Amaretto, see 408
Ambrosia 2001
Ambrosia juice 3
American Cheese Slices, see 861
American chop suey, see 7117
Anadama bread, see 3044
Anchovy 4750
Andes Mint Wafers 1855
Angel
    cup, see 1249
    food cake 1002-1004
    wings, see 1707
Angelfish, see 4771
Angelica, see 438
Animal cookie, see 1202
Animal cracker 3256

Anise seed 5701
Anisette
    sponge cookie/cake, see 1242
    toast 3000
    liqueur, see 408
Annona squamosa, see 2251
Antelope, see 4574
Antipasto 6900
Apples 2002-2014
Apple juices and drinks 4-21
Apple
    banana, see 2041
    -berry pie, see 1352
    betty, see 1660
    butter 1750
    -cabbage-mayonnaise salad 2007
    candied or caramel 2006
    chips 2008
    cobbler 1350, see1722
    crunch cake, see 1007
    dumpling, see 1722
    fried-pie or fritter 1354, see 1694
    Jacks cereal 3556
    Newton, see 1162
    nut loaf, see 1099
    pastry cake, see 1119
    -peach pie, see 1352
    pie 1351-1356
    pie filling, see 2018
    rings, fried 2015
    rolls, see 3196
    salad with dressing 2016
    snacks, see 1201
    turnover, see 1722
Applejack, see 389
Applesauce 2017-2019
Applesauce
    cake 1005-1007
    cookie 1201
Apricots 2020-2028
Apricot
    cake, see 1007
    cobbler 1357
    fried-pie 1360
    nectar 22
    oil, see 5400
    -orange juice 23
    pie 1358-1360
    -pineapple juice drink 24
    sour, see 431
Arepa, Arepitas, see 6950
Arepa Dominicana, see 3119
Armadillo 4550
Armenian cracker bread, see 3302
Arroz
    blanco, see 3826
    con calamares, see 7170
    con cebollas, see 7167
    con coco, see 7174
    con dulce or especia, see 7210
    con Pollo, see 6515
    con salchichas, see 7172

    frito, see 7004
    quisado, see 7225
    relleno Dominicano, see 7236
Artichokes 2353-2357
Artichoke salad 2352
Arugula 2358
Asiago cheese, see 856, 858, 888
Asopao de pollo, see 6597, 7188
Asopaode grandules, see 7126
Asparagus 2359-2365
Asparagus soup, cream of 5000-5001
Aspartame sweetener 1751-1752
Au gratin potatoes, see 2651
Avena con leche, see 3484
Avocado 2029-2030
Avocado dip, see 2129

B

Baba Ghanoush, see 5365
Babka, see 1666
Baby cookie 1202
Baby Ruth 1856
Bacalaitos, see 6947
Bacalao a la Vizcaina, see 6700
Bacalao guisado, see 6795
Bacardi cocktail 381
Bacon, pork 4150-4154, beef 4018-4020
Bacon
    cheeseburger 7637-7641
    chips, see 3257
    dressing 5500-5502
    -flavored cheese spread, see 801
    grease or meat drippings 5401
    on biscuit 7401
    sandwich 7400-7405
    soup, cream of 5002
    strips, meatless 6901
Bagels 3001-3013
Bagel chips 3014, see 3136
Bagoong, see 5311
Bailey's Irish Cream 382
Baked Alaska 1500
Baked beans 6902-6905, 6912
Baklava 1652
Ball cheese, see 840
Balsam pear, see 2380
Bamboo shoots 2366-2367
Bananas 2031-2047
Banana
    bread 3032-3033
    cake 1008-1009
    chips 2037
    chocolate-covered 2038
    cream pie 1361-1362
    flakes, dehydrated 2039
    fritter, see 1695
    Frost, see 531
    green, pickled 5628
    nectar 25
    Nut Crunch cereal 3557
    -orange drink 26
    whip 2040

Coconut (continued)
　custard pie　see 1387
　meat 3918-3919
　milk 3920
　mochiko, see 1075
　-pecan pie, see 1414
　pudding 1554
　water 3921
Cod 4763-4770
Codfish
　ball or cake 6705
　fritters, Puerto Rican style 6947
　salad 6706-6708
　soup 5095-5096
　with starchy vegetables 6709
Coffee 293-312
Coffee
　and chicory 285-287
　and cocoa (mocha) 288-292
　bread with icing, see 1121-1122,
　　3107-3108
　cake 1115-1123, 3107-3109
　cream, see 515- 516
　Royale, see 407
　whiteners, see 507-510
Cognac, see 389
Cointreau, see 408
Cola-type soft drink 205-206
Colby or Colby Jack cheese 814-818
Coleslaw 2415-1417
Coleslaw dressing 5510-5511
Collards 2466-2469
Combos crackers, see 3265, 3342
Complete Bran Flakes 3574-3575
Conch [fish] 4916-4917
Concord grapes, see 2124
Condiments 5600-5649
Cone shell for ice cream 1227-1228
Congo bar, see 1210
Cookies 1200-1288
Cookie Crisp cereal 3576
Cookie dough 1229
Cool Whip, see 589
Coon cheese, see Cheddar 812-813
Coquito, Puerto Rican 391
Coriander 5713-5714, see 2463
Corn 2471-2487
Corn
　and canola oil 5434
　beverage 313
　cake, puffed 3252
　Chex cereal 3577
　chips 3253-3254
　crackers 3262
　chowder, see 5170
　custard 1555
　dog 7670
　flakes 3578
　flour patties or tarts 3110
　fritter 2470
　meal beverage 207-208
　nuts 3255

oil 5433-5434
pone 3111-3112
Pops cereal 3579
relish 5614
rye, see 3084
souffle, see 2478
soup, cream of 5097-5098
syrup 1759
with cream sauce 2471
with peppers 2472
Cornbread 3114-3119
Cornbread
　boiled 3453
　chicken 6501
　fried, see 3132
　stuffing 3120
Corned beef 4042-4044, 4606
Corned beef
　mixed dishes 6095-6097
　hash 6094
　patty 6948
　sandwich 7428
　spread 4605
Cornish game hen 4450-4451
Cornmeal 3457-3458
Cornmeal
　bread, Dominican style 3119
　coconut dessert 1556
　dressing with chicken or
　　turkey and vegetables 6949
　dumplings 3453
　fritters 6950
　mush 3454-3456
　sticks 3459, 6951
Cornstarch, dry 3113
Cornstarch
　coconut dessert 1557
　pudding 1558
Corny dog, with chili 7671
Cottage
　cheese 819-832
　ham, see 4175-4176
　-style potatoes, see 2660
Cotto salami, see 4635
Cotton Candy, see 1910
Cottonseed
　bread 3045
　oil 5435
Cough drops, see 1910
Count Chocula cereal 3580
Country
　Corn Flakes 3581
　Fried Steak Sandwich, see 7645
　ham, see 4175-4176
Couscous 3460-3461
Cow head 4002
Cowpeas 2618-2620, 3853, 6952
Cowpeas with snap beans 2488
Crab 4918-4920
Crab
　bisque, see 5099
　cake 6710

cake sandwich 7429
deviled 6714
imperial 6711
salad 6712-6713
soup 5099-5100
stuffed, see 6711
in tomato-based sauce 6715
Crabmeat thermidor, see 6765
Cracked wheat bread 3046-3049
Crackers 3256-3304
Cracker Jacks, see 3322
Cracklin' Oat Bran cereal 3582
Cranapple-citrus juice drink 41
Cranberries 2077-2079
Cranberry
　juice, drink, or cocktail 41-47
　nut muffin, see 3163
　-orange relish 2081
　pie 1389-1391
　-raspberry sauce 5306
　salad 2080
　sauce, see 2077
Crappie, see Perch 4824-4828
Crayfish 4922-4923
Crazy bread, see 3026
Cream 511-517
Cream
　cake 1034
　cheese 833-835
　cheese dressing 5512
　cheese pie, see 1108
　horn, see 1708
　of rice 3462-3463
　of wheat 3464-3468
　puff, no filling or icing 1655
　soda 209-210
　substitute 507-510
Creamed
　beef soup, see 5032
　chipped or dried beef 6098
　dried beef on toast 6953
　potatoes, see 2671
Creamy salad dressing 5513-5516
Crème Brulèe 1559
Creme de menthe, see 408
Creme filling, see 1768
Cremora, see 509
Crenshaw melon, see 2065
Creole seasoning, see 5600
Crepe 1657-1659, 3401, 6954-6955
Crepe suzette 1656
Crescent biscuit or roll, see 3021, 3207
Cress 2464, 2489-2490
Crisco, see 5447, 5449
Crispbread 3300-3304
Crispix cereal 3583
Crisp, apple, blueberry, cherry, peach,
　or rhubarb 1660-1664
Croaker 4771-4774
Croissant 3121-3125
Croissant, filled, entrée-type
　6956, 7430-7437

Menudo, see 5158
Meringue 1699
Meringue cookie 1249
Mero en escabeche, see 4866
Mettwurst 4629
Mexican
    bread pudding 1592-1593
    casserole 7088-7089
    chocolate 1925
    crueller, see 1654
    eggnog, see 393
    rice, see 7207
    -style beef stew 6106
    -style corn, see 2472
    sweet bread, see 3196, 3200
Midnight sandwich, Puerto Rican 7474
Milk and milk beverages 521-577
Milk
    dessert, frozen 760-776
    candy, Puerto Rican style 1594
    ducts, see Udder 4573
    Duds, see 1863
    fruit drink 537-538
    shake 539-545
    -vinegar salad dressing 5544-5545
Milkfish, see Herring 4793-4799
Milky Way Bar 1926-1928
Millet 3473; puffed 3634
Millionaire's pie, see 1422
Mince pie 1402-1403
Minestrone soup 5135- 5136, see 5218
Mini-Wheats 3635-3637
Mint
    Jots, see 1929
    julep 414
Mints and buttercreams 1929-1930
Minute Rice, see 3818
Miracle Whip, see 5539, 5542-5543
Miso 5316
Miso sauce 5317
Mixed
    nuts 3928-3932
    salad greens, raw 2557
    vegetables 2558-2562
Mocha mix, see 507
Mock chicken leg , cooked 4563
Mofongo, see 2516
Molasses 1777
Molasses cookie 1250
Mole
    poblano 5318
    verde 5319
Mollejitas guisadas, see 6591
Mondongo, see 6119
Mondongo soup, see 5158
Mongo beans without salt 3859
Monkfish, see 4787
Monterey cheese 848-849
Moo Goo Gai Pan 6595
Moo Shi Pork 7090
Moon Cake 1700-1701
Moon pies, see 1246

Moose 4564
Mortadella 4630
Mostaccioli pasta, see 3800
Mother's Oat Bran, see 3477
Mounds, see 1884
Mountain Dew, see 211
Moussaka 7091
Mousse 1595-1597
Mozzarella cheese 850-852
Mrs. Butterworth, see 1796
Mr. Goodbar, see 1880
Mr. Phillips Tater Crisps, see 3333
Muenster cheese 853-855
Mueslix cereal 3638
Muesli cereal 3475
Muffins 3138-3175, 3220
Mulberries, raw 2156
Mullet 4809-4812
Multi-Bran Chex cereal 3639
Multi-grain
    bread 3063-3065
    cereal 3474
    cookie, high fiber 1251
    snack mix or chips 3305-3307
Mundo Nuevo, see 1555
Mung beans 3860, see 2370
Muscatel, see 438
Mushrooms 2563-2570; pickled 5618
Mushroom
    barley soup, see 5003
    soup 5138-5141
Muskellunge, see 4829
Muskmelon, see 2062
Muslo de pollo o pechuga rellena,
    see 6604
Mussels 4929-4930, 6747
Mustard 5619
Mustard
    cabbage 2571
    greens 2572-2575
    sauce 5620
    seed, yellow 5727
Mutton, see Lamb 4250-4262
M&M's 1916-1919

N

Nachos 7092-7101
Namasu, see 2491
Napa cabbage, see 2406
Napoleon, see 1708
Nara zuke, see 5642
Natilla Espanol, see 1629
Native lettuce, see 2534
Natto 5320
Navy
    bean soup, see 5005
    peas, see 3871
Necta Sweet, see 1780
Nectarine 2157-2158
Needlefish, see 4801
Nestle chocolate bar, see 1875-1877
Nestum, Puerto Rican cereal 3476

New York cheese, see 812
Newton bar, see 1162-1165
Nine-layer Chinese steamed rice and
    syrup pudding, see 1702
Nonpareils, see 1872
Noodles 3800-3812
Noodle(s)
    pudding 7102-7103
    Romanoff, see 7051
    soups 5142-5145
Nopal, see 2418
Norwegian flatbread, see 3300
Nougat 1931-1933
Now and Later, see 1966
Nut
    bread, 3068, 3082, 3096
    cake 1053-1054
    roll, fudge, nougat, or caramel 1934
Nutella, see 1758
Nutmeg, ground 5728
Nuts 3900-3948, 3961-3963
    coated 1935-1936
Nutty Buddy, see 713

O

Oat bran, plain, uncooked 3642
Oat bran
    bread 3069-3070
    cereal, cooked 3477-3478
    cookie 1252
    cracker 3278
Oatmeal
    beverage 217-218
    bread 3071
    cake 1055-1056
    cereal 3479-3485
    cookie 1253-1260
    cracker 3279
    Crisp cereal 3643-3645
    pie 1404
Oaxacan-style string cheese, see 883
Ocean Perch 4813-4818
October beans, see 3862
Octopus 4819-4823
Octopus salad, Puerto Rican style 6748
Oh Henry! bar, see 1894
Oh!s, Honey Graham cereal 3646
Oka cheese, see 808
Okinawan donut, see 1682
Okra 2576-2579; pickled 5621
Old fashioned
    cocktail 415
    loaf, see 4636
Olive oil 5442
Olives 5622-5624
Omelets or scrambled eggs 944-971
Onions 2583-2595
Onion
    bread 3072
    broth, see 5228
    cheese bread, see 3042
    dip, see 5367